Poorly Differentiated Neoplasms and Tumors of Unknown Origin

CLINICAL ONCOLOGY MONOGRAPHS

Series Editors

John W. Yarbro, M.D., Ph.D.
Richard S. Bornstein, M.D.
Michael J. Mastrangelo, M.D.

HUMAN MALIGNANT MELANOMA
edited by Wallace H. Clark, Jr., M.D., Leonard I. Goldman, M.D., and Michael J. Mastrangelo, M.D.

ONCOLOGIC EMERGENCIES
edited by John W. Yarbro, M.D., Ph.D., and Richard S. Bornstein, M.D.

SMALL CELL LUNG CANCER
edited by F. Anthony Greco, M.D., Robert K. Oldham, M.D., and Paul A. Bunn, Jr., M.D.

TOXICITY OF CHEMOTHERAPY
edited by Michael C. Perry, M.D., M.S., and John W. Yarbro, M.D., Ph.D.

Poorly Differentiated Neoplasms and Tumors of Unknown Origin

Edited by Mehmet F. Fer, M.D.

Assistant Professor
Department of Medicine
Division of Hematology/Oncology
University of Kentucky Medical Center
Lexington, Kentucky

F. Anthony Greco, M.D.

Professor of Medicine
Director, Division of Oncology
Department of Medicine
Vanderbilt University Medical Center
Nashville, Tennessee

Robert K. Oldham, M.D.

Director, Biological Therapy Institute
Franklin, Tennessee

GRUNE & STRATTON, INC.
Harcourt Brace Jovanovich, Publishers
Orlando   New York   San Diego   Boston   London
San Francisco   Tokyo   Sydney   Toronto

Library of Congress Cataloging-in-Publication Data
Main entry under title:

Poorly differentiated neoplasms and tumors of unknown
    origin.

   (Clinical oncology monographs)
   Bibliography: p.
   1. Cancer—Diagnosis.   2. Tumors—Diagnosis.
3. Carcinogenesis.   I. Fer, Mehmet F.   II. Greco,
F. Anthony (Frank Anthony), 1947–   . III. Oldham,
Robert K. IV. Series
RC270.P66   1986   616.99′2′075   85-24816
ISBN 0-8089-1755-2

Grune & Stratton, Inc.
Orlando, FL 32887

Distributed in the United Kingdom by
Grune & Stratton, Ltd.
24/28 Oval Road, London NW 1

Library of Congress Catalog Number 85-24816
International Standard Book Number 0-8089-1755-2
Printed in the United States of America

85   86   87   88   10   9   8   7   6   5   4   3   2   1

To our patients.

Contents

Contents

Contributors

PAUL G. ABRAMS, M.D., *Vice-President and Medical Director, NeoRx Corporation, Seattle, Washington*

ANDREW ARNOLD, M.D., *Medical Staff Fellow, Metabolism Branch, National Cancer Institute, National Institutes of Health, Bethesda, Maryland*

NORIO AZUMI, M.D., *Instructor, Department of Pathology, Stanford University, Stanford, California*

MARIA R. BAER, M.D., *Fellow in Hematology, Division of Internal Medicine, Vanderbilt University School of Medicine, Nashville, Tennessee*

AJAY BAKHSHI, M.D., *Senior Staff Fellow, Metabolism Branch, National Cancer Institute, National Institutes of Health, Bethesda, Maryland*

STEPHEN B. BAYLIN, M.D., *Associate Professor of Medicine and Oncology, The Johns Hopkins University Medical Institutions, Baltimore, Maryland*

ALISTAIR J. COCHRAN, M.D., *Professor of Surgery and Pathology, Division of Surgical Oncology, University of California at Los Angeles School of Medicine, Los Angeles, California*

ROBERT D. COLLINS, M.D., *Professor of Pathology, Department of Pathology Vanderbilt University School of Medicine, Nashville, Tennessee*

MICHAEL A. CORNBLEET, M.D., M.R.C.P., *Senior Registrar, Department of Medical Oncology, Western General Hospital and Royal Infirmary, Lothian Health Board, Edinburgh, Scotland*

JOHN B. COUSAR, M.D., *Associate Professor of Pathology, Director of Clinical Hematology Laboratory, Department of Pathology, Vanderbilt University School of Medicine, Nashville, Tennessee*

GEORGE FARROW, M.D., *Professor, Department of Surgical Pathology, Mayo Clinic, Rochester, Minnesota*

MEHMET F. FER, M.D., *Assistant Professor, Department of Medicine, Division of Hematology/Oncology, University of Kentucky Medical Center, Lexington, Kentucky*

EMIL FREI, III, M.D., *Professor of Medicine, Harvard Medical School, Physician-in-Chief, Division of Medical Oncology, Dana-Farber Cancer Institute, Boston, Massachusetts*

MARC B. GARNICK, M.D., *Associate Professor of Medicine, Harvard Medical School, Associate Physician, Brigham and Women's Hospital, Division of Medical Oncology, Dana-Farber Cancer Institute, Boston, Massachusetts*

KEVIN C. GATTER, M.D., *Nuffield Department of Pathology, John Radcliffe Hospital, The University of Oxford, Headington, Oxford, England*

GERALD S. GILCHRIST, M.D., *Consultant in Pediatric Hematology and Oncology, Mayo Clinic and Foundation, Professor and Chairman, Department of Pediatrics, Mayo Medical School, Rochester, Minnesota*

ARMANDO E. GIULIANO, M.D., *Associate Professor of Surgery, Division of Surgical Oncology, University of California at Los Angeles School of Medicine, Los Angeles, California*

ALAN D. GLICK, M.D., *Associate Professor of Pathology, Vanderbilt University School of Medicine, Nashville, Tennessee*

HARVEY M. GOLOMB, M.D., *Professor and Chairman, Division of Hematology/ Oncology, University of Chicago, Chicago, Illinois*

F. ANTHONY GRECO, M.D., *Professor of Medicine, Director, Division of Oncology, Department of Medicine, Vanderbilt University Medical Center, Nashville, Tennessee*

WILLIAM W. GROSH, M.D., *Assistant Professor of Medicine, Division of Oncology, Department of Medicine, Vanderbilt University Medical Center, Nashville, Tennessee*

JOHN D. HAINSWORTH, M.D., *Assistant Professor, Division of Oncology, Department of Medicine, Vanderbilt University Medical Center, Nashville, Tennessee*

MICHAEL R. HENDRICKSON, M.D., *Associate Professor, Department of Pathology, Stanford University Medical Center, Stanford, California*

ALLAN JONES, M.D., F.R.C.P. (C.), *Department of Hematology-Oncology, Foothills Hospital, Calgary, Alberta, Canada*

RICHARD P. KADOTA, M.D., *Senior Clinical Fellow in Pediatric Hematology and Oncology, Mayo Clinic and Foundation, Instructor in Pediatrics, Mayo Medical School, Rochester, Minnesota; Division of Hematology/Oncology, Children's Hospital, San Diego, California*

RICHARD L. KEMPSON, M.D., *Department of Pathology, Stanford University, Stanford, California*

STANLEY J. KORSMEYER, M.D., *Senior Investigator, Metabolism Branch, National Cancer Institute, National Institutes of Health, Bethesda, Maryland*

BRUCE MACKAY, M.D., Ph.D., *Professor of Pathology, Department of Anatomic Pathology, University of Texas System Cancer Center, M.D. Anderson Hospital and Tumor Institute, Texas Medical Center, Houston, Texas*

JAMES E. MARKS, M.D., *Professor and Chairman, Department of Radiotherapy, Mallinckrodt Institute, Washington University School of Medicine, St. Louis; Loyola Hines Department of Radiotherapy, Edward Hines Junior Hospital, Loyola University, Stritch School of Medicine, Maywood, Illinois*

DAVID Y. MASON, M.D., *Nuffield Department of Pathology, John Radcliffe Hospital, The University of Oxford, Headington, Oxford, England*

MARY J. MATTHEWS, M.D., *Navy Medical Oncology Branch, National Cancer Institute, Bethesda, Maryland*

GEOFFREY MENDELSOHN, M.D., *Associate Professor of Pathology, Director, Surgical Pathology, Case Western Reserve University, University Hospitals of Cleveland, Cleveland, Ohio*

JOHN S. MEYER, M.D., *Department of Pathology, Jewish Hospital of St. Louis, Professor of Pathology, Washington University Medical Center, St. Louis; Chief Pathologist and Director of Laboratories, Department of Pathology, St. Luke's Hospital, Chesterfield, Missouri*

DONALD L. MORTON, M.D., *Professor and Chief, Division of Surgical Oncology, University of California at Los Angeles School of Medicine, Los Angeles, California*

JAMES MULSHINE, M.D., *Navy Medical Oncology Branch, National Cancer Institute, Bethesda, Maryland*

ROBERT K. OLDHAM, M.D., *Director, Biological Therapy Institute, Franklin, Tennessee*

NELSON G. ORDÓÑEZ, M.D., *Associate Professor of Pathology, Department of Anatomic Pathology, Director, Immunocytochemistry Laboratory, University of Texas System Cancer Center, M.D. Anderson Hospital and Tumor Institute, Texas Medical Center, Houston, Texas*

RONALD L. RICHARDSON, M.D., *Associate Professor of Oncology, Mayo Clinic, Rochester, Minnesota*

Q. SCOTT RINGENBERG, M.D., *Assistant Professor of Medicine, Division of Hematology/Medical Oncology, Department of Medicine, School of Medicine, University of Missouri-Columbia, Columbia, Missouri*

NICHOLAS J. ROBERT, M.D., *Assistant Professor, Department of Medicine and Pathology; Clinical Director, Medical Oncology, Division of Hematology-Oncology, New England Medical Center, Boston, Massachusetts*

JON C. ROSS, M.D., *Assistant Professor Pathology, Laboratory of Surgical Pathology, Stanford University Medical Center, Stanford, California*

RAYMOND W. RUDDON, M.D., Ph.D., *Professor and Chairman, Department of Pharmacology, University of Michigan Medical School, Ann Arbor, Michigan*

MATTHEW L. SHERMAN, M.D., *Clinical Fellow in Medicine, Harvard Medical School, Brigham and Women's Hospital, Dana-Farber Cancer Institute, Boston, Massachusetts*

STEPHEN A. SHERWIN, M.D., *Genentech Corporation, South San Francisco, California*

CRAIG L. SILVERMAN, M.D., *Assistant Professor, Department of Radiotherapy, Division of Radiation Medicine, Evanston Hospital, McGaw Medical Center, Northwestern University Medical School, Chicago, Illinois; Loyola Hines Department of Radiotherapy, Stritch School of Medicine, Edward Hines Junior Hospital, Loyola University, Maywood, Illinois*

KATHERINE A. SIMINOVITCH, M.D., *Medical Staff Fellow, Metabolism Branch, National Cancer Institute, National Institutes of Health, Bethesda, Maryland*

DANIEL D. VON HOFF, M.D., *Associate Professor of Medicine, Division of Oncology, The University of Texas Health Science Center at San Antonio, San Antonio, Texas*

THOMAS A. WALDMANN, M.D., *Chief, Metabolism Branch, National Cancer Institute, National Institutes of Health, Bethesda, Maryland*

LESTER E. WOLD, M.D., *Consultant in Surgical Pathology, Mayo Clinic and Foundation, Assistant Professor of Pathology, Mayo Medical School, Rochester, Minnesota*

ELLEN P. WRIGHT, M.D., *Fellow in Surgical Pathology, Department of Pathology, Vanderbilt University School of Medicine, Nashville, Tennessee*

JOHN J. WRIGHT, M.D., *Medical Staff Fellow, Metabolism Branch, National Cancer Institute, National Institutes of Health, Bethesda, Maryland*

JOHN W. YARBRO, M.D., Ph.D., *Professor and Chief, Division of Hematology/ Medical Oncology, Department of Medicine, School of Medicine, University of Missouri-Columbia, Columbia, Missouri*

JOHN C. YORK, M.D., *Director, DeYor Laboratories, Youngstown, Ohio*

Poorly Differentiated Neoplasms and Tumors of Unknown Origin

1
INTRODUCTION

Mehmet F. Fer
F. Anthony Greco
Robert K. Oldham

In planning the therapeutic strategies in clinical oncology, the physician largely relies on the histologic type and anatomical origin of the tumor. Although it is widely recognized that tumors of a given "type" can vary greatly in their biologic behavior in different patients, these two guidelines have endured as the most useful and practical tools for predicting the natural history of a given neoplasm and for planning therapy. Undifferentiated neoplasms and cancers of unknown primary site, however, lack at least one of these distinguishing features. The common denominator for both of these heterogeneous groups is that the cell or site of origin is unclear, and it is difficult to classify these neoplasms into an established descriptive category.

The management of patients who present with such neoplasms pose a major challenge, since the oncologist is forced to plan therapy without the benefit of the most valued conventional guidelines. Early and accurate recognition of tumors has become especially important over the past decade, since several types of cancer have become potentially curable, including some that lack either histologic features of cellular differentiation or a detectable primary site. Certain lymphomas, germinal tumors, and small cell carcinomas may fall within this category. Several other cancers

POORLY DIFFERENTIATED NEOPLASMS AND TUMORS OF UNKNOWN ORIGIN   ISBN 0-8089-1755-2

can be effectively palliated. Many patients with these cancers are young, and the impact of recovery can be dramatic. In addition to advances in therapy, diagnostic methods have vastly improved with the advent of techniques such as electron microscopy, immunocytochemistry, computerized tomography, and nuclear magnetic resonance. Thus, the clinician is often faced with a wide selection of diagnostic tests, along with various possibilities for therapeutic action.

This monograph will summarize some of the methods that may assist in the evaluation and therapy of undifferentiated neoplasms, and cancers of unknown primary site. Some of the diagnostic methods, such as electron microscopy and immunocytochemistry, have become better established; thus the sections addressing them are more factual or didactic. Other newer approaches are in an earlier stage of development. Accordingly, discussions on these concepts will focus on potential directions rather than on reviewing data already acquired. In certain cases, rational therapeutic trials are indicated, and some will be addressed in this book.

While biologic considerations are discussed in the book, the emphasis has been placed on practical applications. We have also stressed the clear distinction between undifferentiated neoplasms and cancers of unknown primary site. Both categories of tumors share certain diagnostic uncertainties, but they clearly represent different clinical syndromes, which occasionally overlap. It is hoped that this book will assist physicians in developing organized clinical approaches to patients with these heterogeneous, perplexing neoplasms, while stimulating research where additional information is needed.

2

THE ROLE OF THE PATHOLOGIST IN THE EVALUATION OF POORLY DIFFERENTIATED TUMORS AND METASTATIC TUMORS OF UNKNOWN ORIGIN

Bruce Mackay
Nelson G. Ordóñez

The primary objective of a surgical pathologist examining a tumor specimen by light microscopy is to provide a specific diagnosis that will allow the clinician to treat the patient appropriately. The pathologist will seek to confirm that the lesion is neoplastic, to determine if it is benign or malignant and primary or metastatic, and to classify the tumor as precisely as possible. If the tumor is metastatic, the histology may indicate the site of origin. It may also be possible for the pathologist to give some indication of how the tumor is likely to behave—the process of histologic grading. The information provided by the pathologist aids the clinician in deciding what other investigations may be necessary before treatment can be instituted, and in planning the therapy and assessing prognosis.

For various reasons, the amount of data which the pathologist is able to provide on a particular specimen is sometimes limited. The specimen may not be representative, or the amount of tumor it contains can be too

POORLY DIFFERENTIATED NEOPLASMS AND TUMORS OF UNKNOWN ORIGIN   ISBN 0-8089-1755-2
© 1986 by Grune & Stratton.   All rights of reproduction in any form reserved.

small for adequate evaluation, or the tumor cells might be severely distorted from squashing or from delayed or inadequate fixation. Even with suitable material, there are frequent situations where the pathologist is not able to provide a confident histopathologic diagnosis: some tumors simply do not possess sufficiently distinctive features to allow a firm classification by routine light microscopy, irrespective of the skill and experience of the pathologist examining the microscopic sections.

In such cases, the pathologist must resort to using nomenclature that reflects his uncertainty, and terms like "poorly differentiated" and "undifferentiated" appear in the reports. In some instances, it may not be possible to decide if a particular tumor has arisen at the site where it has presented, resulting in additional dubiety in the pathology report. Some tumors are truly undifferentiated in that they do not possess any histological features that can be used in their classification. The term "undifferentiated" is also applied to certain tumors that are known to fit within a particular category yet lack identifiable "differentiating" features at the light microscopic level: large cell and small cell undifferentiated bronchogenic carcinomas provide an example, since each can be diagnosed from histopathologic features, even though the tumors lack the specific characteristics of a bronchogenic squamous carcinoma or adenocarcinoma.

It might be more appropriate to use the term "unclassified" as an umbrella designation for tumors that cannot be assigned to a particular category, such as carcinoma or sarcoma, but that term is also limiting, since a tumor that cannot be identified by conventional light microscopy may ultimately be classified by more sophisticated procedures, such as electron microscopy. The term "poorly differentiated" is therefore convenient to describe the tumors that are reviewed in this chapter: they range from neoplasms that remain completely unclassified after all pathologic studies have been completed, to those that can be recognized to fall within a particular broad tumor group, yet cannot be more accurately labelled. A metastatic adenocarcinoma of undetermined primary source would be an example of the latter category.

The implications of an imprecise diagnosis for clinician and patient vary, and they are, of course, more serious in the case of malignant tumors. If the pathologist can supply at least some information, his report is usually more useful than one that is totally noncommittal. Thus, the knowledge that a patient has a metastatic adenocarcinoma of unknown primary site, or a sarcoma of undetermined cell type, may be sufficient to enable the clinician to plan suitable therapy. Under these circumstances, provided the pathologic material has been of adequate quality and all the available or indicated procedures have been performed, it is unlikely that additional tissue would yield more information on the nature of the tumor. When a metastatic tumor is totally unclassified on the initial biopsy, further procedures are generally performed in an attempt to determine the nature of the tumor, and if metastatic, the primary location. These additional tests are often time-consuming and expensive. The surgical pathologist should therefore consider whether rebiopsy, assuming it is feasible, would significantly improve the chances of reaching a definite diagnosis.

Traditionally, tumors have been identified by light microscopy using histologic criteria developed over many decades by pathologists using paraffin sections stained with hematoxylin and eosin. The recognition of some cell types was facilitated by employing special staining procedures to demonstrate substances within the cells, such as glycogen, mucin or fat. Many tumors inevitably still remained unclassified or were only tentatively labelled. A fundamental problem was and still is the lack of specific cytologic or architectural features of some tumors in histologic preparations. In addition, there is a progressive disappearance of, or failure to manifest, distinguishing characteristics as a tumor dedifferentiates. A further limiting factor in the past was the limited resolution of the light microscope: since this is a function of the wavelength of light, it cannot be compensated for by improvements in the optical quality of the instrument.

In the past two decades, pathologists have dramatically improved their ability to derive clinically relevant information from tumor specimens. Although some credit for this must be given to the progressive accumulation of histopathologic and clinical pathologic data on human tumors in the medical literature, it must particularly be attributed to the introduction and development of new techniques.

The electron microscope has greatly enhanced the pathologist's ability to identify tumor cells and characterise the details of their structure. Although this instrument was developed and made commercially available almost 50 years ago, it has only been used extensively in surgical pathology in the last 15 years. Electron microscopy has, however, provided enormous contributions to our knowledge of the structure of normal cells and tissues since it was first introduced.

Throughout the past half-century, there have been conflicting views over the potential of the electron microscope as a practical tool in diagnostic medicine. Many skeptics doubted that the instrument would provide a significant advantage over conventional light microscopy, while others believed it might dramatically alter the field of surgical pathology. Experience has shown that the truth lies somewhere between the two extremes. The practical contributions of the instrument as a diagnostic tool have not been realized to the degree anticipated by some of the more optimistic pathologists, but electron microscopy has nevertheless proved invaluable in revealing the cellular changes responsible for particular light microscopic appearances. Used in conjunction with routine light microscopy, the electron microscope has proved to be a very useful diagnostic tool in a limited number of areas, including the interpretation of renal biopsies and the identification and classification of many human neoplasms. Its range of contributions in tumor diagnosis is now being redefined with the expansion of immunocytochemistry, as we discuss in detail later in this chapter.

The transmission electron microscope utilizes extremely thin sections of tissues and offers an enormous increase in resolution over the light microscope, enabling the study of intracytoplasmic components of cells and their nuclei and detailed analysis of the cell periphery and intercellular contacts. Two other forms of electron microscope, the scanning and the analytical electron microscopes, have proved useful in areas of research in the biological and physical sciences, but have not been significantly effective in clinical diagnostic work. The former visualizes the surface of cells and tissues and produces micrographs which convey a three-dimensional concept of these surfaces, but it has little application in surgical pathology and is of virtually no value in tumor diagnosis. The analytical electron microscope permits the identification of some of the molecular components of cells, but again does not have routine diagnostic applications. Subsequent references in this chapter to the electron microscope (EM) therefore refer to the transmission electron microscope.

Pure morphologic studies are limited in the extent to which they are able to reveal the functional activities of cells. It is possible, for example, to deduce from the presence of extensive ribosome-bearing endoplasmic reticulum that a cell is forming proteins which will be passed out of the cell for use elsewhere in the body—the products of exocrine and endocrine gland cells provide an illustration—and recognition of the presence of dense-core granules of a particular caliber could establish that the secretory product is a hormonal polypeptide. It might even be possible to determine the nature of the secretory product from the size and appearance of the granules, though this is generally not possible.

A new and fruitful method to identify a wide range of biochemical components of cells came with the introduction of immunocytochemistry. The first specific histologic demonstration of a fixed tissue antigen occurred in 1942 when Coons et al.[1] reported the use of fluorescein-labeled antibodies to localize antigens in tissues. The method was at first applied to research problems, but its potential in diagnostic pathology soon came to be recognized, and a rapidly expanding array of immunofluorescent, and more recently, immunoperoxidase techniques have been developed and applied to the solution of problems in surgical pathology. By being able to selectively apply immunohistochemical procedures and electron micros-copy as adjuncts to routine light microscopy, the surgical pathologist has greatly expanded and improved his ability to classify tumors.

In this chapter, we describe the role of the pathologist in evaluating poorly differentiated neoplasms, including metastatic tumors that can be classified, but for which the primary site is undetermined. We place particular emphasis on the contributions of immunocytochemistry and electron microscopy. Since the effectiveness of these procedures is in large part determined by the material provided for study, the discussion is preceded by a brief review of proper specimen procurement.

Tissue Procurement

If the material provided for pathologic study is less than optimal in quantity or quality, the information that the pathologist can provide may be compromised. Poorly selected or handled tissue may turn out to be as useless as a specimen that does not contain tumor. It is highly frustrating to have to wrestle with a problem case in which the tissue has been squashed or poorly fixed, and the prudent pathologist faced with this situation may reluctantly decline to offer an opinion, when a carefully procured, optimally processed specimen might have been diagnostic. Some clinicians are surprisingly ill-informed or unconcerned about the needs of the pathologist or the consequences of an inadequate tissue specimen. Good tissue is, in fact, the single most important factor in deciding the results of the pathologist's study. The amount of tissue is also important in that a needle biopsy, whether an aspirate or a cutting needle core, rarely gives as much information by light microscopy as an open biopsy of a tumor.

Clinicians should therefore be aware of the indications for the different types of biopsy procedures in particular clinical situations, and prior consultation with a pathologist often pays dividends and saves unneces-sary additional procedures. The indications for the most widely used and best known methods, such as cytology smears, brushings, and washings, are often appreciated, but the limitations of a needle biopsy when com-pared with open biopsy are not always as well-realized, and indications for electron microscopy or immunocytochemistry are certainly not familiar to many clinicians. Fortunately, some immunoperoxidase procedures can be carried out on formalin-fixed, paraffin sections, but for others, the results are better with frozen sections, and electron microscopy on formalin-fixed tissue produces distinctly inferior results compared with those obtained by using specimens that have been promptly fixed in glutaraldehyde.

Solid tissue for light microscopy should be brought to the pathologist as soon as it has been excised in order that thin (3 mm) slices can be promptly fixed in 10 percent buffered formalin and, where indicated, a portion frozen for rapid diagnosis or subsequent immunocytochemistry, or placed in glutaraldehyde for electron microscopy. Needle biopsies are particularly vulnerable to squashing, often by being held with forceps, or from drying out as a result of not being immediately immersed in fixative solution. A specimen can be kept moist for a short time if it is covered with a piece of gauze soaked in saline, but prolonged immersion of a small biopsy in saline will introduce a severe degree of cytologic distortion and may render it unsuitable for electron microscopy. Blood smears are usually air–dried, but cytology smears should be promptly fixed in 95 percent alcohol. Effusions and fine needle aspiration biopsies require special handling, and prior consultation with the pathologist is necessary: in some institutions, a cytologist or cytotechnologist is in attendance when the aspiration biopsies are performed, or the pathologist may even perform the biopsies if the lesions are superficially located. Rapid smears can then be made and stained immediately to confirm that the material that has been obtained is representative. It may be worthwhile to take some tissue from a fine needle aspiration biopsy for electron microscopy when there is an indication from examination of the smears that the diagnosis is likely to be a problem.

The main requirement for specimens for electron microscopy is small pieces of tissue totally free of drying artifact or squashing effect which have been rapidly fixed in a suitable medium. Buffered glutaraldehyde in a 2–4 percent solution is usually employed as the fixative for specimens for electron microscopy. When the specimen is a piece of solid tumor, a cut surface of the lesion should be exposed and a tapering wedge not more than 1 mm in thickness gently sliced from the surface with a sharp scalpel or razor blade, lifted carefully on the knife blade, and immersed immediately in the fixative solution. The glutaraldehyde is usually kept chilled in the laboratory, but as long as it is fresh (prepared within the past two weeks), it can be used at room temperature. The advantage of using chilled fixative is that autolytic changes are retarded as the fixative slowly penetrates. Where the need for electron microscopy is anticipated, a specimen bottle containing the proper fixative should be obtained before the biopsy procedure is begun.

Needle biopsies of soft tissue or bone can also be placed directly in glutaraldehyde, but bone marrow and fine needle aspirates should be taken in a heparinized syringe and carried directly to the electronmicroscopy (EM) laboratory where they will be centrifuged to separate the significant cells. Core biopsies of bone should not be decalcified as this procedure introduces extensive cytologic distortion. It is preferable to separate the soft tissues from the marrow spaces of the fixed specimen with fine needles or forceps under a dissecting microscope. If cells from an effusion are to be studied ultrastructurally, the specimen can be taken to the laboratory in the bottle in which it is collected: the cells will retain their morphology for many hours, particularly if the bottle is kept cool. In the pathology department, part of the specimen can be allocated for routine cytology studies, and the portion reserved for electron microscopy will be centrifuged before the cells are fixed. Prior hemolysis may be necessary if there are many contaminating blood cells, but the hemolysis should be as brief as possible.

Approach to the Study of a Problem in Tumor Diagnosis

The first indication that a tumor is likely to pose a problem in diagnosis comes with examination of the initial tissue specimen. It is commonly a routine paraffin section stained with hematoxylin and eosin for light microscopy, but it may be a cytology smear or a frozen section. In the case of a frozen section, the pathologist will give an interim verbal report indicating that the diagnosis presents difficulties, and will defer his final opinion until permanent (paraffin) sections of the tissue have been studied. These sections may be obtained either through processing the residual frozen material or, preferably, by using nonfrozen tissue which provides preparations that are devoid of freezing artifact and consequently of much better quality and easier to interpret. With cytology smears, there is also an opportunity for permanent sections if a cell block can be prepared, and these sections will show more of any architectural arrangement of the cells which may be present, than can usually be perceived in the smears.

If the diagnosis remains in doubt after cytology preparations have been studied, it is advisable to then obtain a tissue biopsy, since light microscopic sections of solid tissue will give more information. As fine needle aspiration biopsies continue to be favored, and this technique gains wider acceptance, it is likely that many more diagnoses in the future will hinge on examination of preparations of this type.[2] There is a valid argument for also processing tissue from fine needle aspirations for electron microscopy, since ultrastructural study in problem cases will often indicate the tumor cell type.

The importance of providing adequate tissue for examination by the pathologist has already been emphasized. If the sample is less than acceptable, the amount of information that the pathologist can provide is severely restricted. For the conscientious pathologist who on the one hand wishes to aid patient and clinician as much as possible, and on the other is concerned with rendering an honest evaluation of the biopsy material, there may be no alternative to giving a noncommittal opinion and recommending that another specimen be obtained. Again, the amount of tissue taken is important in that needle biopsies, including fine needle aspiration biopsies, rarely give as much information as an incisional or excisional biopsy: where feasible, the latter should be the procedure of choice whenever it is known that there is a diagnostic problem or if one is anticipated.

A pathologist examining sections or smears of a tumor by light microscopy has a number of questions in mind. Is the lesion truly neoplastic? Some non-neoplastic proliferations in soft tissues can simulate neoplasms. If it is tumor, is it benign or malignant? If it is tumor and a diagnostic problem, is it totally undifferentiated, or can the tumor be placed with reasonable confidence in one of the broad tumor groups such as carcinoma or sarcoma? It would be impossible in the available space to review all of the issues each of these questions can raise in practice, but some brief comments will be made.

To determine whether a particular tumor is benign or malignant, the pathologist uses established cytologic criteria that include the cellularity, the degree of pleomorphism, and amount of mitotic activity of the tumor cells. The importance of each of these criteria varies with the type of tumor. A reactive lesion of fibroblasts, such as nodular fasciitis, can look ominous histologically because of the alarming cytologic appearance of its cells and frequent mitotic figures, but the histologic features correlated with the clinical presentation should indicate the diagnosis. Similarly, mitoses are found without difficulty in an atypical fibrous histiocytoma of the skin, yet this lesion rarely metastasizes. In dealing with a poorly differentiated tumor of undetermined cell type, the pathologist may elect to lean on the side of caution and interpret a moderate amount of mitotic activity as an indication of at least a low grade of malignancy. Other histologic features, however, such as infiltration of surrounding tissues at the periphery of the lesion, or the presence of tumor cells in vessels, may be detected and provide reassuring support. The presence of pleomorphic tumor cells is not of itself a reliable indication of malignancy.

It may be obvious that a tumor is metastatic, as when a carcinoma is present within a lymph node. Even when the histology does not provide a clear indication of the cell type, the occurrence of tumor in regional nodes will prompt careful clinical and, if appropriate, radiologic examination of the territory drained by the nodes. If the cell type of an intranodal tumor cannot be identified, it may not be possible to decide whether the tumor is indeed metastatic or is primary within the node: a sinusoidal pattern has been observed in some large cell lymphomas, for example, and in these cases the common initial histologic diagnosis was metastatic melanoma.[3] A carcinoma may present as a solitary metastasis in a peripheral site where clinically a sarcoma would be the more probable diagnosis, and the histology of the tumor must then determine whether the tumor is primary or metastatic.

An extensive range of histologic appearances is seen among well–differentiated human tumors, and it becomes even broader when alterations occurring with loss in differentiation (or failure to differentiate) are taken into account. It would, of course, be impossible to list in one chapter all the combinations of histologic features that can be seen in particular types of tumors, and pathologists must mentally juggle a multitude of histopathologic permutations and combinations in assessing a problem tumor. Essentially pathologists will assemble all the information they can glean from the tissue sections and will try to match the histology with what they know to be the characteristics of particular neoplasms. Both the cytologic features and the patterns of the tumor cells must be taken into account, with the awareness that there are relatively few histologic features that can be considered completely specific as diagnostic criteria for any one type of tumor. Thus gland-like formations usually indicate that a tumor is an adenocarcinoma, but they are also seen in biphasic synovial sarcomas.[4] Squamous differentiation may be seen in a bronchogenic or endometrial adenocarcinoma. When a tumor lacks any architectural arrangement of the component cells, the diagnostic decision must be based on evaluation of the cytologic features of the individual cells, bearing in mind that absence of a pattern could indicate loss of differentiation, but is also seen in a variety of tumor types where it constitutes the regular histologic appearance.

In examining the cells of a tumor, the pathologist observes their size and shape and whether these features are regular or variable, and the relationship of the cells to one another and to the surrounding stroma. Uniform small round or ovoid cells in a pediatric patient will raise the likelihood that the tumor falls within the "small round cell" group,[5] whereas a similar appearance in an adult will bring to mind an alternative differential diagnosis. Large pleomorphic cells are more suggestive of a carcinoma or sarcoma, but occasionally a lymphoma can present with this appearance.[6] Although round cells are commonly associated with carcinomas, and spindle cells with sarcomas, there are many exceptions. Spindle cell transformation of a carcinoma is often, but by no means exclusively, seen in squamous carcinoma and the appearance can occasion considerable difficulty in distinguishing a carcinoma from a sarcoma.[7] Conversely, round cell sarcomas do occur. When Enzinger first described a series of epithelioid sarcomas,[8] he commented on the frequency with which the tumors had been misdiagnosed as squamous carcinomas or foci of granulomatous inflammation. A mixture of spindle cells, often in a radiating (storiform) pattern, with large cells containing bizarre or multiple nuclei, is seen in malignant fibrous histiocytomas which have emerged in the past decade as the most common soft tissue sarcoma in older patients.

Histochemistry

Many special staining procedures are available to the surgical pathologist, but in practice only a few are used regularly. They are methods of proven value for demonstrating substances that are frequently found in the cytoplasm of certain cells.[9] In the typical situation, a special stain will not be requested unless there is good reason to believe it may be contributory, but when the cells of a poorly differentiated tumor have moderate amounts of cytoplasm, and especially if it looks in any way unusual, a blind search for mucin and glycogen may be undertaken in the hope that something positive turns up. Usually, however, special stains are deliberately planned to support a diagnostic suspicion, while histochemical fishing expeditions are only occasionally rewarding.

Since melanoma is a tumor whose cells can mimic a broad range of other neoplasms, melanin stains are performed frequently. If a metastatic tumor is recognized or strongly suspected to be a carcinoma, mucin stains may be performed in an attempt to narrow the list of possible primary sites. The value of a positive result is often limited, since adenocarcinomas from many locations can produce mucin, and similarly, the presence of glycogen in tumor cells is of itself relatively nonspecific since this substance can occur in many different cell types. Demonstration of glycogen in tumor cells can be helpful when there is no indication of the nature of a tumor from its histology. As an example, in the differential diagnosis of small round cell tumors in children, plentiful glycogen will favor Ewing's tumor or rhabdomyosarcoma, and is much less common in neuroblastomas or lymphoma-leukemias.[10]

Certain other stains are used more selectively in diagnosis. If an endocrine tumor of polypeptide-forming cells is considered on clinical or histologic grounds to be a possibility, the silver impregnation techniques such as that of Fontana-Masson for enterochromaffin cells or the Grimelius or Sevier-Munger stains for argyrophilic cells may be useful. Their specificity is limited, however, and they are not invariably positive in endocrine tumors. If the nature of the functional product of the tumor cells can be suspected, as is often the case with adenomas of the anterior pituitary, an appropriate immunohistochemical procedure will give more information. The congo red stain, or thioflavine T fluorescence, can be useful to confirm an impression that amyloid is present in a patient with an endocrine or plasma cell tumor. Stains for stromal components are sometimes used to classify soft tissue sarcomas: examples are the use of a reticulin stain if a tumor of vasoformative cells is suspected, Masson's trichrome stain if a mixture of smooth muscle cells and fibroblasts is recognized, or stains such as oil red O or sudan black if liposarcoma is a reasonable possibility. Special stains are no substitute, however, for good quality hematoxylin and eosin stained sections in the microscopic evaluation of soft tissue tumors.

When light or electron microscopy suggests that a soft tissue lesion might be granulocytic leukemia (granulocytic sarcoma), the naphthol ASD chloroacetate (NASD) stain for the demonstration of esterase is indicated. If electron microscopy is not available, the profusion of ribosomes that characterizes the cells of a large cell lymphoma can be shown with the methyl green pyronin (MGP) stain.

Immunocytochemistry

Direct and Indirect Immunofluorescence

Immunofluorescence methods are being increasingly used in diagnostic pathology. Initially their major application was in the classification of renal disease,[11,12] but direct and indirect methods of immunofluorescence are now being used for the demonstration of a variety of cell products, including hormones, enzymes, oncofetal antigens, and other tumor markers.[13] Specimens selected for immunofluorescence should be in the form of fresh tissue that is oriented in a standard frozen section, embedding compound on a piece of cork and snapfrozen by immersion in a beaker of isopentane surrounded by liquid nitrogen or dry ice. Frozen sections are cut in a cryostat and stained either by the direct method of immunofluorescence, which is the more simple technique and satisfactory for routine purposes, or by the indirect method when extra sensitivity is needed. In the direct method, a fluorochrome (fluorescein or rhodamine) conjugated to a primary antibody is applied directly to the tissue. The indirect method is a two-step staining procedure: first a primary, unconjugated antibody is applied, and then a secondary fluorochrome-labeled antibody derived from a second species is directed against the globulin fraction of the first antibody. The site of the antigen-antibody reaction is visualized under ultraviolet light using a dark field microscope.

While immunofluorescent techniques have proven invaluable to diagnostic pathology, various limiting factors have prevented their expansion. Among these difficulties are the need for elaborate and expensive equipment, impermanence of the sections, problems of background interference, need for frozen sections of tissues to obtain optimal results, and the frequent inability to correlate the fluorescent images with conventional histology. Fortunately, the introduction of enzyme-labeled antibodies which could elicit reactions in sections fixed, processed, and embedded using conventional histologic methods provided a new impetus to diagnostic immunopathology. A number of enzymes were used successfully, but horseradish peroxidase conjugates became the most popular. By employing a direct and indirect immunofluorescence procedure, the enzyme-labeled methods appeared to have at least as much sensitivity as the fluorescent techniques.[14]

Unconjugated Techniques

Unconjugated techniques, another major development in the field of immunocytochemistry, circumvented some of the disadvantages inherent in conjugation procedures such as denaturation of antibody, inactivation of enzyme, residual free enzyme, and residual free unlabeled antibody. Free antibody, or antibody conjugated to inactivated enzyme, binds competitively with active conjugated antibody, reducing the sensitivity of the reaction, while the denatured antibody and free enzyme increase nonspecific staining. The most important unconjugated procedures have been the immunoglobulin-enzyme bridge method of Mason et al.[15] and the peroxidase-antiperoxidase (PAP) method of Sternberger et al.[16] The immunoglobulin-enzyme method involves the sequential application of a primary antibody, an antibody (bridge) with the specificity directed toward the globulin fraction of the primary antibody, and an antibody against horseradish peroxidase raised in the same species as the primary antibody. It is completed with the addition of free horseradish peroxidase and reaction with a chromogenic substance. The main problem with this method is that it is difficult to produce a purified antibody against horseradish peroxidase; consequently, there is considerable binding of the bridge antibody by nonperoxidase-specific immunoglobulins.

Like the Mason et al. method, the PAP method utilizes the same sequence of reactions, except that instead of using an antibody against peroxidase, it employs a soluble peroxidase-antiperoxidase complex. With this technique, the nonspecific binding by nonperoxidase-specific immunoglobulins is virtually eliminated. Advantages of the unlabeled antibody procedures over the enzyme conjugated method are increased sensitivity and a considerable reduction in background reaction. The latter can be almost totally eliminated with the PAP method.[14,17]

Avidin–Biotin Technique

A more recent development in immunoperoxidase methodology is the avidin–biotin technique. This procedure is based on the ability of the egg-white glycoprotein avidin (mol wt 68,000) to bind four molecules of biotin. A comprehensive review of the uses of the avidin–biotin system in enzyme immunoassay and immunoperoxidase techniques has recently been published.[18] The most common immunocytochemical method using avidin–biotin is the avidin–biotin peroxidase complex (ABC) process developed by Hsu et al.[19] As with the PAP method of Sternberger, there are three basic steps in the ABC technique. In the first, the primary antibody specific for the antigen to be localized reacts with the specimen. This is followed by a biotin-labeled secondary antibody capable of binding to the first. The third step involves the use of a complex of peroxidase-conjugated biotin and avidin: the free sites on the avidin molecule allow binding of the biotin on the secondary antibody. Then the peroxidase (and consequently the original antigen) is visualized with the use of an appropriate chromogen. The method allows greater dilution of the primary antibody and, as a result, there is lower background staining. By virtue of its ability to enhance staining reactions in either frozen or paraffin sections, the avidin–biotin technique is ideally suited for use with monoclonal antibodies. Five of the most common immunoperoxidase methods used in immunocytochemistry are illustrated in Fig. 2-1.

Staphylococcal Protein A

Another immunocytochemical method uses staphylococcal protein A, a cell wall constituent of *Staphylococcus aureus* that specifically binds to the Fc portion of IgG.[20] It can be conjugated to fluorescein,[21] alkaline phosphatase,[22] or horseradish peroxidase,[23] without altering its binding ability.

Diagram of Immunoperoxidase Methods

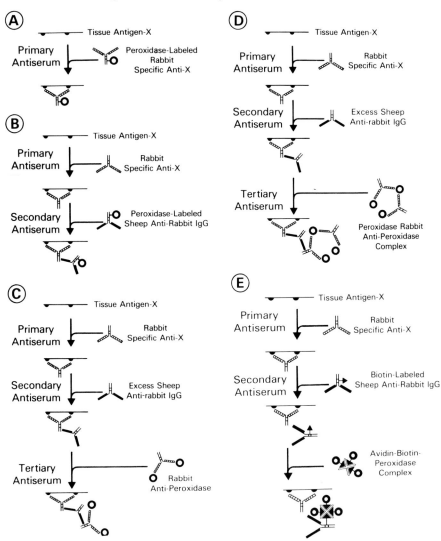

Figure 2-1. *(A) Diagrammatic representation of the direct peroxidase-conjugated method: (B) indirect peroxidase-conjugated method: (C) unlabeled antibody bridge method: (D) peroxidase-antiperoxidase (PAP) method: (E) and avidin-biotin peroxidase complex (ABC) method. The site of the immunoreaction is visualized by the use of chromogenic substances (diaminobenzidine, chloro-naphthol, or aminoethyl-carbazole), and the reaction product appears as a brown, blue, or red granular deposit.*

This has the advantages of being a relatively rapid technique, requiring little nonspecific background staining, and it can be used with any kind of primary antibody, regardless of the animal species in which it was produced, because of its binding affinity for the Fc portion of IgG.

The introduction of hybridoma-produced monoclonal antibodies has resulted in an exponential expansion in the application of immunohistochemical procedures in diagnostic pathology. A single antigen molecule contains several antigenic determinants or epitopes. When an animal is immunized, its B lymphocytes produce antibodies against the antigen. Each B cell (clone) produces antibody for a single epitope. Since there are many B cell clones producing antibodies to each epitope, the antibody is termed polyclonal. In contrast, a monoclonal antibody is the product of a clone of cells secreting chemically-homogeneous immunoglobulin of definable specificity.[24] Because of these characteristics, a monoclonal antibody is much easier to characterize and more reproducible in its behavior than conventional polyclonal antibodies.

At present, several methods using hybridization technology are available for the production of monoclonal antibodies.[25-27] As the first step in the production of a monoclonal antibody, a mouse is immunized with the antigen of interest. Once large amounts of antibodies are being produced, the mouse is sacrificed and the spleen removed. B lymphocytes from the mouse spleen are mixed with mouse myeloma cells that have previously been adapted to grow continuously in culture. Polyethylene glycol is added to the mixture to promote fusion of cell membranes, and the cells are suspended in tissue culture medium. The desired hybridomas will live and grow in the culture. Then the hybridoma is tested to determine which clone is producing antibody against the desired epitope. Once the appropriate cell clone is identified, it can be injected back into a mouse where it will produce a tumor. The ascitic fluid formed by the tumor will contain high concentrations of the desired antibody. Unfortunately, the presence of other mouse proteins in the ascitic fluid tends to increase nonspecific background staining in immunocytochemical techniques. Another method for producing monoclonal antibodies is to grow the hybridoma in tissue culture: the antibody accumulates in the supernatant fluid, and although it is present in lower concentrations than in the mouse ascitic fluid, it produces less nonspecific background staining since undesired proteins are eliminated.

The main advantage of monoclonal antibodies over conventional polyclonal antibodies is their enhanced ability to distinguish slightly different antigens.[23] The intensive work that is required to produce specific hetero-antisera has restricted their availability to a few sources. In contrast, the immortality of immunoglobulin-producing hybridomas permits the manufacture of purified antibodies in large quantities, and batch variations which are often encountered with conventional antisera can be avoided. On the other hand, monoclonal antibodies are associated with certain problems. Although cross-reactivity of the type encountered with poly-clonal antibodies does not occur, the monoclonal antibody may recognize as identical antigenic determinants parts of totally different molecules in cells that are unrelated to one another. OKT-6, for example, reacts with immature thymocytes, and also with Langerhans' cells in the skin.[29] Conversely, antibodies against an epitope that is subject to allotypic variability may fail to react with a target, even when the antigen of interest is present.[28]

Double–labeling immunofluorescent techniques using fluorescein and rhodamine labels have been widely used in the past for the localization of two different antigens in the same specimen. With this method, it is necessary to switch to the excitation wavelength of the incident light to sequentially study the distribution of fluorescein- or rhodamine-labeled compounds. With the newly developed immunoenzymatic techniques, however, both antigens can be visualized and examined simultaneously. These techniques also have the advantage over immunofluorescence of producing a permanent preparation with excellent morphologic detail. Double immunoenzymatic labeling may be achieved by two fundamentally different approaches which can be referred to as the single-enzyme and double-enzyme methods. In the single-enzyme procedure, both antigens are labeled using an immunoperoxidase technique; two different enzyme substrates yielding distinctively-colored reaction products are used to reveal each antigen.[30] In the two-enzyme approach, two different and unrelated enzymes (horseradish peroxidase, alkaline phosphatase, or glucose oxidase) are used to label the two antigens.[31–34] Double–labeling immunohistochemical methods are not usually applied in routine diagnos-tic pathology and are therefore beyond the scope of this chapter, but the interested reader can refer to publications in which the technical aspects and applications of the methods are discussed.[35–36]

Lectins

As new immunocytochemical techniques and monoclonal antibodies develop, there has been at the same time great interest in the potential applications of lectins in diagnostic pathology. Lectins are sugar-binding proteins primarily found in plants and some lower animals, which have the ability to recognize complex carbohydrate structures in glycoproteins and glycopeptides, particularly those of the cell membrane. Although the specificity of a particular lectin is generally established in terms of its binding to a free monosaccharide, lectins also have the ability to recognize differences in more complex structures. There is increasing evidence that the carbohydrate components of cell membrane molecules are important in defining cell types, and that changes in these components are associated with cellular maturation, differentiation, and neoplastic transformation.[37]

Lectins have potential for use as histochemical markers of cells of different types. Because lectins are non-immune proteins, they are used in standard histochemical procedures[37,38]: the lectin, conjugated with peroxidase or fluorescein, is reacted directly with the tissue. On occasion, however, lectins can be used in association with an immunohistochemical technique, such as the PAP method. The tissue is incubated with purified lectin, then reacted with an antibody against the lectin, such as rabbit anti-lectin serum. In the sequential reaction which follows, a secondary antibody with the specificity directed towards the globulin fraction of the primary antibody combines with an antibody against horseradish peroxidase raised in the same animal species as the primary antibody. The site of the reaction is visualized with a chromogen.

A great many lectins derived from plants and animals have been described, and a considerable number are well–characterized and commercially available. It is important to remember that the determinants characterized by lectins may be common to several different glycoproteins or glycolipids, and therefore can be present in a variety of cell types. For example, peanut agglutinin (PNA), a lectin isolated from the peanut (*Archis hypogaea*) which possesses a marked affinity for glycoproteins containing the terminal sequence beta-D-galactose (1-3)-N-acetyl-D-galactosamine, has been demonstrated on immature murine thymocytes,[39] bone marrow and splenic stem cells,[40] human thymocytes and leukemic blast cells,[41] mammary breast epithelium,[42] and histiocytes.[43] Ulex europaeus agglutinin I (UEAI), a lectin obtained from *Ulex europaeus* seeds, which has a specific affinity for alpha-L-fucose residues of sugar moieties and is used to evaluate antigen H in individuals with blood group O,[44] also binds to vascular endothelium and does so independently of the blood group of the tissue donors.[45] UEAI has proven to be a useful tissue marker for the diagnosis of tumors of endothelial cells.[46] Detailed information on the use of lectins in pathology is contained in the recent comprehensive review by Goldstein and Hayes.[47]

Several immunohistochemical techniques have been modified for use at the ultrastructural level,[48,49] but they are still experimental and are being applied in research rather than in diagnostic pathology. The commonest are methods which employ peroxidase or colloidal metals, especially colloidal gold.[49] Both have been shown to be excellent markers for transmission electron microscopy. In these procedures, antibodies of a particular protein are linked to the peroxidase or the colloidal gold particles, and the use of various monoclonal antibodies linked to gold particles of different sizes offers the potential for performing double or multiple labelling experiments. Colloidal gold particles are capable of strong emission of secondary electrons, making them a useful marker for scanning electron microscopy.[50] The reader who is interested in immuno-electron microscopy can refer to a number of publications which provide detailed discussion and practical guidelines on the techniques.[17,48,49]

These developments in immunocytochemistry have permitted its widespread use in diagnostic pathology, but a clear understanding of the techniques and a thorough awareness of a number of pitfalls are essential. While immunocytochemical methods can in general be applied to a wide range of specimens, including formalin-fixed, paraffin-embedded tissue,[17] frozen sections,[51] cytologic preparations (imprint, smear, or cytospin),[52–55] and plastic-embedded tissue,[56,57] it is critical to select a procedure that is appropriate to the type of specimen to be studied. For example, formalin-fixed, paraffin-embedded sections are adequate for the demonstration of most polypeptide hormones, but they are not suitable for the detection of surface antigens on cells in lymphoproliferative disorders, and cryostat sections are preferable for the demonstration of membrane immunoglob-ulins and other lymphocyte surface antigens.[58]

A great advantage of immunoperoxidase techniques is that many of them are applicable to formalin-fixed, paraffin-embedded tissue, which is of course a standard type of preparation in any pathology department. Although buffered formalin is the most convenient and practical fixative for routine light microscopy in most laboratories, it may not be the best fixative for immunoperoxidase staining. Sections of tissue fixed in Bouin's solution or B5 fixative provide superior preparations for immunoglobulins and polypeptides and are associated with the lowest amount of nonspecific background staining. Formalin fixation will reduce or even inactivate immunostaining for some intermediate filaments, notably the cytokeratins, but ethanol is suitable as a fixative for the detection of these antigens.[59] Some monoclonal antibodies can be used with formalin-fixed, paraffin-embedded tissue sections, but many others are suited only to frozen tissue sections. Decalcifying solutions do not interfere with immunostaining to a significant degree, provided the tissue has been adequately fixed prior to decalcification.[51]

For the recognition of false–positive and false–negative staining results in immunocytochemistry, appropriate controls[51,60] and considerable experience are necessary. Errors in interpretation can be caused by poorly fixed, necrotic, or hemorrhagic tissue.[51] Even when antisera are obtained from reliable sources, the pathologist must be aware of the possibility of cross-reactivity of antibodies producing false–positive results, and a good quality control program is imperative.

Applications in Diagnostic Pathology

Endocrine System

The immunoperoxidase method can be very helpful in the differential diagnosis of endocrine tumors, some of which look alike but differ in prognosis and response to treatment. Sera against hormones have been successfully used in the classification of many endocrine tumors. Most medullary thyroid carcinomas have a typical histologic appearance and an associated amyloid stroma, but amyloid is not a constant feature and this tumor can occur as a small cell carcinoma that resembles an anaplastic carcinoma or a lymphoma, or as a gaint cell, pleomorphic, follicular, or papillary carcinoma mimicking other types of primary thyroid carcinoma or intrathyroid metastasis from other sites.[61,62] A positive immunoperoxidase stain for calcitonin will identify the tumor as medullary carcinoma.[63,64] Some thyroid carcinomas of follicular origin are also difficult to identify by conventional light microscopy, and immunostaining for thyroglobulin has proved extremely helpful in the diagnosis of primary and metastatic follicular, papillary, clear cell, and spindle and giant cell carcinomas of the thyroid[65-68] (see Fig. 2-2).

Parathyroid tumors are occasionally a source of diagnostic difficulty. An intrathyroid adenoma can be confused with some primary thyroid neoplasms, or a "nonfunctioning" parathyroid carcinoma which is not associated with hypercalcemia may be confused with a metastasis from another site.[69] Immunostaining for parathormone can then establish the diagnosis.

A functional classification of endocrine tumors of the pancreas and gastrointestinal tract is possible with the use of immunoperoxidase methods. Islet cell tumors of the pancreas, both primary and metastatic, display a broad range of variation in their histology, and may closely resemble endocrine tumors of the gastrointestinal tract.[70] Three commonly recognized histologic patterns seen in islet cell tumors are trabecular, pseudoacinar, and solid,[71] but infrequently a tumor may be pleomorphic,

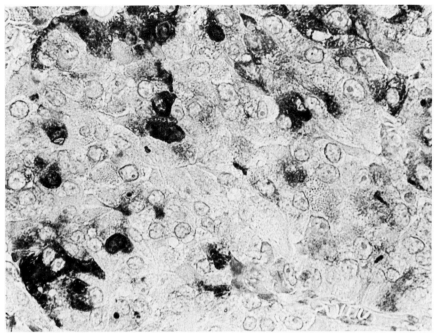

Figure 2-2. *Metastatic thyroid carcinoma to the neck showing immunoreactivity for thyroglobulin.* (× 250)

oncocytic, composed of clear cells (similar to a clear cell renal cell carcinoma), or consist of undifferentiated cells similar to those of small (oat) cell carcinoma of the lung.[72–74] It has been suggested that the histology of islet cell tumors can be correlated with their hormonal activity, but we do not agree with the suggestion that it is possible to predict the secretory products from the tumor architecture.[73,74] Histochemical staining methods, as well as the ultrastructural characteristics of the secretory granules, have been used to classify endocrine tumors of the pancreas and gastrointestinal tract, but these criteria are limited by a lack of specificity of the histochemical reactions and by variations in size and shape of the secretory granules from tumor to tumor, or within cells of the same tumor.[74,75]

A pathologic classification of islet cell and enterochromaffin cell tumors has been achieved using immunocytochemical procedures to identify their hormonal products.[72,73,76,77] While some of these tumors have been categorized on the basis of the predominant secretory product (gastrin, insulin, glucagon, etc.) which is generally responsible for the patient's clinical symptoms, it should be kept in mind that the great majority of these tumors are multihormonal, and that they sometimes produce hormones not normally present in the pancreas or gastrointestinal tract. A case in point is the demonstration of pituitary hormones in some pancreatic and foregut endocrine neoplasms.[74,78–80] The incidence of nonfunctioning pancreatic endocrine tumors is approximately 15-20%, if one considers all clinically silent tumors to be "nonfunctioning."[76,77,81,82]

If a tumor demonstrating hormone production (as by immunocyto-chemical methods) is viewed as evidence of function, however, the incidence of truly nonfunctioning tumors is undoubtedly much lower. In two recent large series of pancreatic endocrine tumors studied by immu-nocytochemistry,[76,77] the majority of clinically "nonfunctioning" tumors were shown to produce at least one hormone. The most common hor-mones demonstrated in clinically silent tumors in order of frequency were pancreatic polypeptide, insulin, glucagon, and somatostatin. The reason for the absence of symptoms in these patients is not well understood, but possibilities are that insufficient hormone is being secreted to elicit clinical manifestations, that the appropriate releasing factor is lacking, that the tumor cells are failing to respond to such a factor, or that the hormone is being inactivated before it can cause a biochemical disturbance. Immuno-cytochemical identification of secretory products does, nevertheless, per-mit a functional classification of these neoplasms, and in the case of a metastatic tumor, may lead to identification of the primary site when it is not already known (Fig. 2-3).

A major advance in diagnostic endocrine pathology has been the introduction of specific antisera directed against neuron-specific enolase (NSE), an isoenzyme of the glycolytic enzyme enolase, which is localized in neurons[83] and neuroendocrine cells.[84] NSE immunocytochemistry al-lows immediate recognition of neuroendocrine cells and their tumors independently of the hormones or neurotransmittors produced.[84–86] NSE has been demonstrated in a variety of endocrine neoplasms, including carcinoids and islet cell tumors, pituitary adenomas, medullary carcinoma of the thyroid, pheochromocytoma, oat cell carcinoma, ganglioneuroblas-toma, paraganglioma, and endocrine carcinoma of the skin (Merkel cell tumor).[85,86–88]

Genitourinary System

Immunocytochemical methods have contributed to the classification of germ cell tumors.[89–91] The occurrence of high levels of human chorionic gonadotrophin (HCG) and alpha fetoprotin (AFP) in the serum of patients

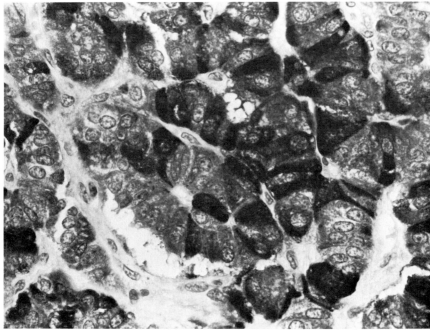

Figure 2-3. *Metastatic "silent" islet cell carcinoma to the liver stained with antiserum against pancreatic polypeptide. (× 250)*

with certain types of germ cell tumor has been used for some years to monitor response to chemotherapy and detect early evidence of recurrence. The first attempts to correlate tumor markers with the morphology of germ cell tumors produced confusing results for several reasons. One is that mixed germ cell tumors are common. While pure choriocarcinomas were always associated with HCG and pure endodermal sinus tumors with AFP, it was found that some patients with seminoma had high levels of HCG while others with embryonal carcinoma had elevated HCG, AFP, or both. It was only when immunocytochemical techniques were applied that the tumor cell types responsible for the serum marker elevations were precisely identified. The high serum levels of HCG were always associated with syncytiotrophoblastic giant cells which can be identified in some seminomas, embryonal carcinomas, and teratomas[89–93] (Fig. 2-4), whereas elevations of AFP were due to the presence of embryonal carcinoma or its derivative, endodermal sinus tumor.[89,90] Germ cell tumors metastatic to or originating in the retroperitoneum or mediastinum can be difficult to

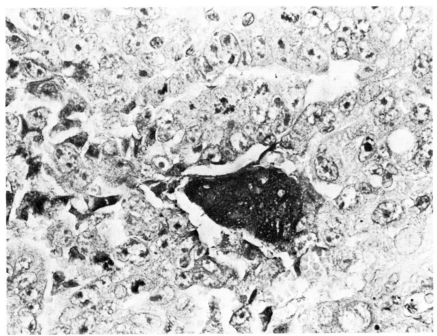

Figure 2-4. *Embryonal carcinoma with a syncytiotrophoblastic giant cell that is staining for HCG. (× 280)*

identify if the tissue available for study is scanty. Since roughly half of the patients have no measurable elevation in serum tumor marker levels, immunocytochemistry can be extremely helpful in establishing that the neoplasm is a malignant germ cell tumor.[94] The immunoperoxidase technique can be used to identify steroid hormones in paraffin-embedded tissues. Estrogen, progesterone, and testosterone have been demonstrated by Taylor and colleagues in ovarian and testicular tumors, and have been used to classify these neoplasms.[95]

Another application of immunoperoxidase methods to tumors of the genitourinary system is in the diagnosis of prostatic carcinoma, which can be a problem when the tumor presents in metastatic sites. The detection of prostate-specific acid phosphatase (PSAP) using the immunoperoxidase technique is a simple way of establishing the prostatic origin of a metastatic carcinoma.[96,97] The identification of PSAP in certain primary prostatic tumors has led to a clearer understanding of the pathogenesis of these neoplasms. For example, most so-called "carcinosarcomas" of the prostate are now recognized to represent adenocarcinomas with sarcomatoid change, as a result of the demonstration of positive staining for PSAP in cells of the sarcomatoid areas.[98] Immunostaining for PSAP may be used to distinguish rectal carcinomas infiltrating the prostate, or bladder tumors invading the rectum, from prostatic adenocarcinoma, since only the prostatic carcinomas will be producing PSAP. While only some prostatic tumors secrete CEA, all rectal adenocarcinomas do so, and negative staining for CEA can therefore be used to exclude the possibility of a rectal tumor.[99,100] Recently, Wang and colleagues isolated a prostate-specific antigen (PSA) from human prostate tissue,[101] and the diagnostic applications of antiserum against PSA are similar to those of PSAP.[102–104]

Hematopoietic System

Tumors of the lymphoid and hematopoietic systems, have been extensively investigated by immunocytochemical methods.[105–110] The major systems for the classification of non-Hodgkin's lymphomas depend primarily on histologic patterns and cytologic features, but some are partly based on immunologic considerations.[111,112] All have been shown to successfully separate lymphomas into groups with survival rates ranging from relatively good to poor, and none has been found to be significantly superior to the others.[113] Reasons for poor reproducibility of the histology-based classifications in different hands include observer error resulting from imprecision in the light microscopic criteria, morphologic variability of the tumors, and variations in the quality of fixation and staining of the specimens.[114] Furthermore, certain histologic types, such as the diffuse histiocytic and diffuse mixed lymphocytic and histiocytic lymphomas of the Rappaport classification, are recognized to be heterogenous in character.[113–115]

Additional parameters to supplement conventional histology have been needed for some time, and immunologic studies of lymphomas were performed with the anticipation that they would enhance the existing histologic classification systems. Conventional lymphocyte marker studies are performed on cell suspensions, but the introduction of a large number of commercially available monoclonal antibodies to T and B lymphocytes has permitted the immunotyping of lymphomas using immunoperoxidase techniques applied to frozen tissue sections.[107,109] Many of the cellular antigens can now be identified using immunocytochemical methods that work with sections of paraffin-embedded tissue.

The tissue antigens that are useful in the study of lymphoreticular tumors can be divided into two major groups. The first consists of cytoplasmic antigens which can be demonstrated in routinely-fixed and paraffin-embedded tissue, and the second comprises membrane antigens which, since they are inactivated by fixation, must be localized in frozen sections. The cytoplasmic antigens which have been utilized in the diagnosis of lymphoreticular tumors include the different heavy and light chains of immunoglobulins (Ig), J chain, alpha-1-antitrypsin (A AT), alpha-1-antichymotrypsin (A AChy), and muramidase (lysozyme).[116,117] A wide variety of cell membrane antigens can be demonstrated in frozen tissue sections, and since the emergence of monoclonal antibodies, their number has been progressively increasing. Antibodies commonly used in the diagnosis of lymphorecticular tumors include those to surface immunoglobulins (sIg),[107] thymocytes,[118] peripheral T lymphocytes and their helper and suppressor-cytotoxic subsets,[118–120] B cells and B cell-associated antigens such as HLA-DR (Ia),[121] common ALL (Calla) antigen,[122] and a common leukocyte antigen.[123]

One clearly useful application of a frozen section-immunoperoxidase study in hematopathology is the distinction between reactive and neoplastic B lymphocytic proliferations. On occasion, it may be difficult to distinguish, by histology alone, a reactive lymphoid proliferation from a lymphoma. While more than one heavy Ig chain is occasionally synthesized by malignant B cells, the finding of single light chain staining of lymphocytes is indicative of monoclonality and therefore neoplasia.[107,122,124] The demonstration of a monotypic staining pattern of immunoglobulin light chains on the surface or within the cytoplasm of cells of a lymphoid proliferation thus facilitates the distinction between B cell lymphoma and reactive proliferations of B cell lymphocytes. Immunohistochemical typing of B cell lymphomas using paraffin-embedded, formalin-fixed tissue has, at least in our hands, been of little value. Lymphomas have generally either shown negative immunostaining for Ig, or they have stained nonspecifically for both kappa and lambda light chains. Proliferations of plasma cells or plasmacytoid lymphocytes, on the other hand, can generally be typed for immunoglobulin light and heavy chains using sections of routinely-fixed and paraffin-embedded tissue. Neoplasms of these cells usually show a monotypic staining pattern[125] (Fig. 2-5). Immunocytochemical studies can be extremely helpful in the identification of the type of protein secreted by myeloma cells in cases of nonsecretory multiple myeloma.[126,127]

Commercially available monoclonal antibodies permit the recognition of lymphocytes in frozen sections as T cell or B cell. Antibodies purporting to distinguish helper and suppressor-cytotoxic T lymphocyte subsets[118–120] and natural killer cells[128] are also available. It is impossible, however, to

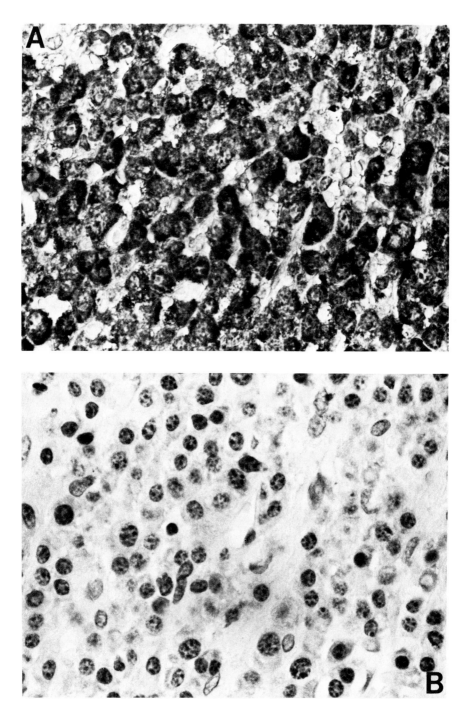

Figure 2-5. *Plasmacytoma of the larynx showing positive staining for (A) lambda light chains and (B) absence of staining for kappa light chains. (× 250)*

prove clonality of T lymphocyte proliferations with monoclonal antibodies at present. To show that a lymphoma is T cell (or B cell in the case of immature B cell-directed neoplasms without demonstrable sIg), it is necessary to demonstrate T cell (or B cell) marking of the malignant cells. Typing of lymphomas by immunologic methods has the inherent limitation of measuring phenotypic parameters. Techniques employing molecular genetics, such as analysis for Ig gene rearrangement, and cytogenetics, offer the advantage of detecting genotypic parameters and the potential of greater sensitivity. They may also serve to complement histologic and immunologic phenotyping in the classification of lymphomas.[129,130]

The pathologist is occasionally faced with the question of whether an apparently undifferentiated malignant neoplasm might be a lymphoma, and identification of the human homologue of murine T200 glycoprotein or leukocyte common antigen has proved useful in this situation.[123,131,132] These antigens have been shown to be expressed exclusively on the surface of hematopoietic cells. A monoclonal antibody—T29-33—against common leukocyte antigen is commercially available. Unfortunately, the value of this antibody (and most other monoclonal antibodies to surface antigens) is, in our experience, limited because it cannot be used with sections of formalin-fixed and paraffin-embedded tissue, and requires frozen tissue sections.

While it is well recognized that nearly all lymphomas classified in the Rappaport system as diffuse histiocytic lymphoma are in fact neoplasms of transformed lymphocytes, true histiocytic "lymphomas" (i.e., extramedullary neoplasms of monocyte-macrophage origin) do occur, albeit uncommonly, and they can be difficult to recognize on morphologic grounds. The initial enthusiasm for muramidase (lysozyme) as a marker for this tumor group[133] has ebbed somewhat.[134,135] In our experience, as well as that of others, A AT and A AChy are more sensitive markers for histiocytic tumors.[116,117,136] Muramidase can be helpful in the diagnosis of acute myelocytic leukemia when it presents in an extramedullary site, and particularly if staining for naphthol AS-D chloracetate (NASD) is negative.[137] OKM-5 is a monoclonal antibody which, it is claimed, will stain monocytic cells, but not those of granulocytic lineage.[138] Interpretation of immunoperoxidase marker studies for lymphomas on frozen sections requires some experience, and it is important to be aware that almost all B cell lymphomas contain a variable admixture of T lymphocytes,[120–121] and that the latter can occasionally be even more numerous than B lymphocytes in lymph nodes involved by follicular (B cell) lymphomas.

It must also be recognized that many, if not all, monoclonal antibodies, though pure, are not necessarily "specific" for a particular cell type. As an example, anti-Leu-1, which is regarded as a Pan T cell antibody, also stains most B cell lymphocytic lymphomas (chronic lymphocytic leukemia, well-differentiated lymphocytic lymphoma of Rappaport).[139,140] OKT-6, an antibody used to identify cortical thymocytes, also stains epidermal Langerhans' cells, paracortical (T zone) histiocytes, and the tumor cells of histiocytosis-X.[141,142] We have observed that OKM-5, which recognizes monocytes, will also stain endothelial cells. Anti-Leu-3, used to identify helper T cells, also stains histiocytes; and anti-Leu-2, which identifies suppressor-cytotoxic T lymphocytes, stains splenic sinusoidal cells.[119] Lymphocytes showing positive staining for anti-HLA-DR (OKIa) are usually B lymphocytes, but activated T lymphocytes reportedly can also show positive staining, and tumor cells derived from peripheral T lymphocytes, as in mycosis fungoides, can stain with anti-HLA-DR.[120,121]

Nonspecific background staining presents a particular problem in the frozen section-immunoperoxidase study of lymphomas. Our experience has been that immunoglobulin and particularly kappa and IgG are often present in large amounts in the fibrous stroma, while lymphoma cells can be nonspecifically bound to or even absorbed by associated histiocytes.

Normal Tissue Components

A number of normal cellular components are confined to one or a few tissues and can be detected using antibodies, and these tumor markers have been found useful in establishing the histogenesis of certain poorly differentiated tumors or in determining the source of metastatic neoplasms of unknown origin. Factor VIII-related antigen, one of the three components of coagulation factor VIII, is synthesized by endothelial cells, and it has been used as a marker for endothelial cell neoplasms (Fig. 2-6).[143–145] Antibodies to myoglobin, normally present in skeletal and cardiac muscle cells, are useful to distinguish rhabdomyosarcoma from other small round cell malignant neoplasms[146,147] (Fig. 2-7).

The milk proteins, casein and alpha lactalbumin, are synthesized in breast epithelial cells, and breast tumors derived from mammary epithelium may also express these substances; consequently they can be used in the diagnosis of metastatic breast carcinoma[148,149] and mammary Paget's disease.[148,150] It should be noted that while a positive staining for these tumor-specific markers is significant, a negative reaction does not carry the same diagnostic weight. Absence of staining for alpha-lactalbumin in a neoplasm clinically suspected to be breast carcinoma does not exclude the diagnosis.

Recently, immunocytochemical studies on components of the cyto-

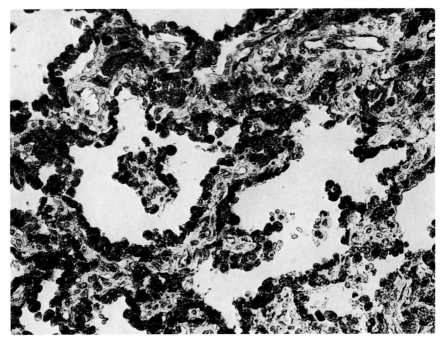

Figure 2-6. *Angiosarcoma of the breast showing positive staining for factor VIII-related antigen. (× 150)*

skeleton have been employed in the identification of unclassified neoplasms.[151–170] Different types of filaments are to some degree associated with different tissues. Three major systems are found in the cytoplasm of eukaryotic cells—microfilaments, microtubules, and intermediate filaments—and these structures account for most of the static cell cytoskeleton and may also have contractile functions. Microfilaments are the thinnest filaments with an average diameter of 6 nm, and they are mainly composed of actin. Microtubules are hollow, noncontractile structures with an external diameter of 25 nm and variable length; they are involved in various motile events, such as the beating of cilia, phagocytosis, and mitosis. Intermediate filaments (IFs) are structures with a diameter of 8–11 nm. They are insoluble under physiological conditions, and may be subclassified on the basis of chemical composition and immunologic properties. Five major intermediate subclasses have been defined: the keratins (mol wt 40,000-68,000) in epithelial cells; desmin (mol wt 53,000) in smooth, cardiac and skeletal muscle; vimentin (mol wt 57,000) in most mesenchymal cells;

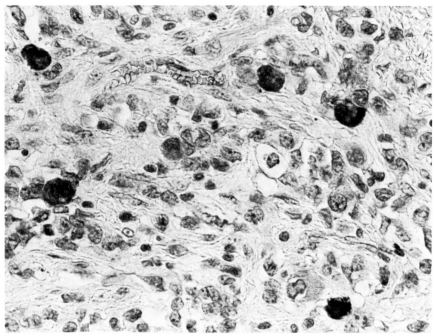

Figure 2-7. *Rhabdomyosarcoma showing immunoreactive cells for myoglobin. (× 200)*

Table 2-1
Localization of Intermediate Filament Protein in Human
Tumors

Type of Intermediate Filaments	Diagnostic Application
Keratin	Carcinoma,[151–156,172] mesothelioma,[157,158] adenomatoid tumor,[159] epithelioid sarcoma,[178] synovial sarcoma[178,179]
Vimentin	Sarcoma,[160,172] lymphoma,[161] melanoma[162,163]
Desmin	Rhabdomyosarcoma,[160,164,172] leiomyosarcoma[160,164]
GFAP	Gliomas[165,166]
Neurofilaments	Neuroblastoma,[167,168] ganglioneuroblastoma,[167–169] Pheochromocytoma,[167–169] Merkel cell carcinoma[170]

neurofilaments (mol wt 200,000, 150,000, and 68,000) in neurons; and glial fibrillary acidic protein (GFAP) (mol wt 55,000) in astrocytes.[171,172]

The tissue distribution of IFs is, in fact, more complex than this simplified scheme implies. Thus, epithelial cells in tissue culture will produce both keratin and vimentin.[173] Desmin is found in skeletal and cardiac muscle cells, in the smooth muscle cells of the uterus and gastrointestinal tract, and in some, but not all, vascular smooth muscle cells.[172,174] Some vascular smooth muscle cells are characterized by the simultaneous presence of desmin and vimentin, while others only possess a single type.[174–176] Keratins have been reported in some sarcomas, including epithelioid sarcoma[177] and synovial sarcoma.[178,179]

Several studies have indicated that neoplastic cells maintain the intermediate filaments characteristic of the original tissues.[172,180] Since the different classes of intermediate filaments may be characteristic of certain tissues, they can serve as cell markers for the identification of tumors of unknown origin. Specific polyclonal and monoclonal antibodies against the different types of IFs are now commercially available, but there is a drawback to their widespread application in surgical pathology. With the exception of glial fibrillary acidic protein, most of these antibodies unfortunately tend to work poorly in formalin-fixed tissue, and optimal staining requires cryostat sections. Recently, however, good results have been reported using ethanol-fixed, paraffin-embedded tissue.[59] Table 2-1 summarizes some of the applications of immunostaining for intermediate filaments in tumor diagnosis (Fig. 2-8,2-9).

Other Tumor Markers

It should be stressed that the occurrence of a tumor marker is not necessarily restricted to a particular tumor type. Markers such as AFP or A AT can be found not only in gonadal and extragonadal cell tumors, but also in hepatocellular carcinomas and certain other neoplasms.[181–184] Another example is S-100 protein, a soluble acidic protein first described in glial cells of the central nervous system. The name derives from the observation that this protein is soluble in 100% ammonium sulphate solution at neutral pH.[185] Its presence has been demonstrated in different cell types, including neurons,[186,187] Schwann cells,[186,188] Langerhans' cells of the epidermis,[186] chondrocytes,[186,190] and the interdigitating reticulum cells of lymph nodes.[186,189] Although it has been demonstrated in a variety of neoplasms (glioma,[191,192] granular cell tumor,[188,193] chordoma,[188,194] pleomorphic adenoma of salivary gland,[195] chondrosarcoma,[186,194] and histiocytosis-X,[186,188]) the most important applications of S-100 protein as a tumor

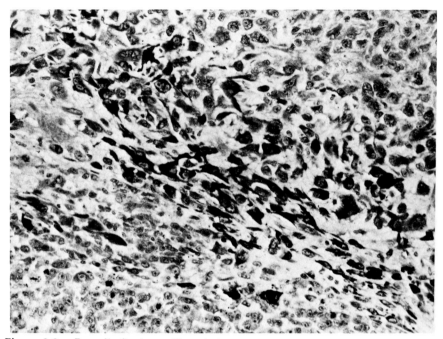

Figure 2-8. *Formalin-fixed, paraffin embedded astrocytoma showing positive staining for glial fibrillary acidic protein (GFAP). (× 120)*

marker in surgical pathology are in the diagnosis of amelanotic melanoma,[186,196-199] and neurogenic sarcoma[186,188,200] (Fig. 2-10). Other tumors which stain positively for S-100 protein can usually be separated from melanoma and neurogenic sarcoma by their histopathology.

Carcinoembryonic antigen (CEA) has been located in most carcinomas of the gastrointestinal tract, lung, pancreas, urothelium, breast, and biliary tract, and in medullary carcinoma of the thyroid.[201-204] In contrast, staining for it is usually negative in mesotheliomas, and in adenocarcinomas of prostate and kidney. Based on the observation that adenocarcinomas of the lung usually stain positively for CEA while mesotheliomas are generally negative or at best weakly positive, several authors have suggested that CEA could be helpful in the differential diagnosis of these two tumors.[167,205,206]

Other tumors in which antigens have been studied using immunocytochemistry include carcinoma of the breast (estrogen and progesterone

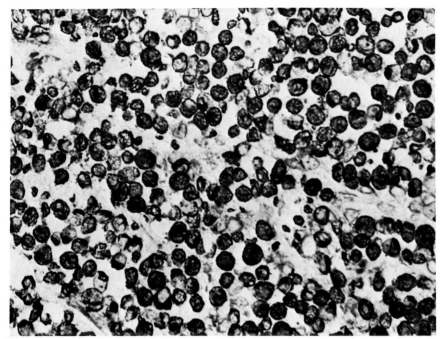

Figure 2-9. *Frozen section tissue from a poorly differentiated carcinoma involving the urinary bladder staining with polyclonal antiserum against keratin. (× 250)*

receptors,[207]) bladder,[208-210] cervix,[211-212] and prostate[213] (blood group antigens), but their use has not as yet contributed significantly in diagnosis.

Selection of the appropriate marker(s) to study a particular neoplasm requires experience and an awareness of current information. Choice of antisera should be made in conjunction with available data from the patient's clinical history, laboratory, and radiographic findings, and after assessing the histologic appearance of the tumor and its ultrastructural features. Indiscriminate use of batteries of antibodies escalate the cost of medical care and can produce confusing results.

The rapidly increasing availability of commercial antisera, some of them arranged in the form of diagnostic kits ready for use, has facilitated the incorporation of immunohistochemistry into routine diagnostic oncology. Table 2-2 lists the tumor markers most commonly used and some of their applications. The reliability of the results depends on rigorous quality control of the reagents and all the technical procedures, and on the inclusion of confirmed positive and negative controls each time the

Table 2-2
Tumor Markers Most Commonly Used for Classification of
Neoplasms of Unknown Origin

Tissue Marker	Diagnostic Application
Enzymes	
Prostatic acid phosphatase[96–98]	Identification of metastatic carcinomas of prostate
Muramidase (lysozyme)[117,137]	Myelogenous leukemia, Paneth cells
Alkaline phosphatase (Regan lysozyme)[216]	Ovarian carcinoma, other tumors
Amylase[217,218]	Some pancreatic and salivary tumors, and serous carcinoma of ovary
Histaminase[219,220]	Medullary thyroid carcinoma, undifferentiated small (oat) cell carcinoma of the lung
Neuron-specific enolase[85,86,221,222]	Endocrine and neuroendocrine carcinomas, other tumors
Creatine kinase[223]	Tumors derived from skeletal muscle
Hormones	
Anterior pituitary hormones (ACTH, prolactin, TSH LH, etc.)[224–227]	Functional classification of pituitary tumors. Differentiation of pituitary tumors from poorly differentiated neoplasms originating from the ethmoidal and sphenoidal sinuses
Calcitonin[63,64]	Medullary carcinoma of thyroid. C-cell hyperplasia
Thyroglobulin[66–68]	Metastatic thyroid carcinoma, poorly differentiated follicular carcinomas
Parathormone[69]	Parathyroid tumors
Pancreatic islet cell, lung and gastrointestinal hormones (insulin, glucagon, somatostatin, serotonin, etc.)[75–77,228,229]	Functional classification of pancreatic islet cell and carcinoid tumors
Human chorionic gonadotropin (HCG)[90–93,230]	Identification of trophoblastic elements in gonadal germ cell tumors, other neoplasms
Testosterone[95]	Sertoli-Leydig tumors
Estradiol[95]	Granulosa and theca cell tumors
Oncofetal antigens	
Alpha fetoprotein[89,90,95]	Differential diagnosis and classification of gonadal and extra-gonadal germ cell tumors. Hepatocellular carcinoma, other tumors
Carcinoembryonic antigen (CEA)[201–204]	Adenocarcinoma of colon, other tumors

36

Table 2-2 (*Continued*)

Tissue Marker	Diagnostic Application
Serum proteins	
Immunoglobulins[117,125]	Differentiation of large (B) cell lymphomas from carcinomas. Differentiation of atypical lymphocytic proliferations from lymphomas. Characterization of multiple myeloma
Alpha-l-antitrypsin[117,181–184,231–233]	Hepatocellular carcinoma, gonadal and extragonadal germ cell tumors, histiocytic lymphoma and other neoplasms
Alpha-l-antichymotrypsin[117,136,231]	Fibrous histiocytoma, malignant histiocytosis, histiocytic lymphoma, and other tumors
Intermediate filaments[152,160,162,170]	
keratin, vimentin, and GFAP, etc.	Differential diagnosis of carcinoma from sarcoma. Gliomas and other tumors
Other products	
myoglobin[146,147]	Tumors derived from skeletal muscle
actin, myosin[234–236]	Tumors derived from smooth and skeletal muscle, other neoplasms
Factor VIII-related antigen[143–145]	Tumors derived from endothelial cells
Alpha lactalbumin, casein[148–150]	Metastatic breast carcinoma. Differentiation of extramammary Paget's disease from other tumors
S-100 Protein[186,196–199]	Diagnosis of melanoma, neurogenic sarcoma and other tumors
Surfactant apoprotein[237]	Lung tumors derived from type II pneumocytes
Prostate specific antigen[102–104]	Metastatic carcinomas of prostate

staining is performed. False-negative and false-positive reactions have been reported in some commercial kits.[214,215] The pathologist should be aware that the pattern and intensity of immunostaining for a given cell marker depend on a number of variables including the nature of the tissue and the type of fixation. Staining patterns can vary considerably depending on whether frozen sections or paraffin sections are used. The accuracy of the findings from an immunocytochemical study hinge on the experience

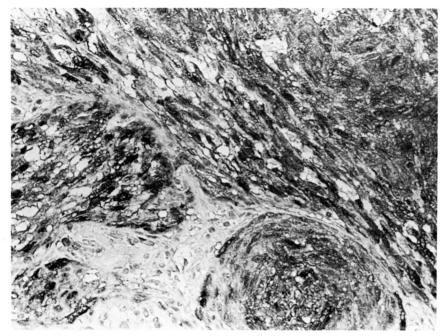

Figure 2-10. *Neurotropic melanoma showing strong immunoreactivity for S-100 protein.* (× 120)

of the pathologist and his awareness of the limitations of the technique and the pitfalls of misinterpretation of false-negative or false-positive findings.

Electron Microscopy

The great increase in resolution that the electron microscope provides compared with the light microscope enables the pathologist to study the detailed structure of diseased cells and tissues, but specimens must be very carefully prepared. The light microscopist accepts the distortion that is always present in formalin-fixed material, and the quality of light microscopic sections is often further impaired by the delay that almost inevitably occurs before excised specimens are placed in the fixative solution. In fact, the light microscopist is so accustomed to a minor degree of distortion that tissues lacking it appear strange, and consequently some mental adjustment must be made in order to evaluate the plastic-embedded tissues that are used in electron microscopy. A hematologist may find the transition less of an effort, since glycol methacrylate embedding is now used in many pathology departments for bone marrow biopsies.

The fixative commonly used in electron microscopy is glutaraldehyde, and it can be employed in concentrations ranging from less than 1 percent to over 6 percent. A 2 percent or 4 percent buffered solution is usual, and the buffer can be phosphate, cacodylate, or a more elaborate mixture. Since much of diagnostic electron microscopy is performed at relatively low magnifications, the minimal changes that result from using different buffers are not of practical importance. The quality of preservation achieved with glutaraldehyde is a marked improvement over that provided by formalin, but there are also disadvantages to its use. Glutaraldehyde penetrates tissues slowly, and therefore a tissue block should not be more than 1 mm thick if it is to fix within an hour. Beyond this time, the autolytic changes occurring within the cells may render the tissue unacceptable for ultrastructural study, though the degenerative changes are retarded if the solution is kept cool. Also, glutaraldehyde renders tissues brittle, and paraffin blocks of glutaraldehyde-fixed tissue are difficult to cut, with the result that the sections tend to split or fragment. Still another disadvantage of using these sections is that they stain differently from conventional light microscopic sections: the cytoplasm assumes a markedly eosinophilic hue in hematoxylin-eosin stained sections when contrasted with similar tissue that has been fixed in formalin, and special stains may not produce the same effects, or be difficult to interpret.

Attempts have been made to devise multipurpose fixatives that would be usable for both light and electron microscopy, the idea being that a piece of tissue could then be placed in one solution and subsequently used for light and, if it proved indicated, ultrastructural studies. Mixtures of glutaraldehyde and formaldehyde such as those devised by Karnovsky,[238] or McDowell and Trump,[239] can produce very good preservation, but the solutions should be carefully prepared and buffered, and specimens must still be kept small. Ten percent formalin is an acceptable alternative when nothing better is available, and it will often produce perfectly adequate preservation of fine structure—less immaculate than with glutaraldehyde, but good enough for most diagnostic purposes.[240] The quality of the preparations is greatly influenced by the speed with which the tissue is fixed after it has been excised, and it is therefore advisable to routinely cut small (not more than 3 mm thick) slices of tissue from surgical pathology specimens and immerse them promptly in a buffered formalin solution. Tissue can even be recovered from a paraffin block, or as an extreme measure, from a microscope slide, but the results do not compare with those obtainable by glutaraldehyde fixation.

The tissue used for electron microscopy is diced into small pieces each roughly 1 mm in size. An important preliminary to the ultrastructural study is the cutting of sections of the plastic-embedded blocks for examination by light microscopy. The sections are cut with an ultramicrotome using glass knives, and they are heat-sealed to microscope slides and stained, usually with methylene blue or toluidine blue, since use of these stains does not require that the embedding resin be removed.[241] To utilize more elaborate staining procedures, the surface of the section must first be etched to remove some of the plastic, but for routine purposes the monochromatic stains are perfectly acceptable. The sections are roughly one micrometer thick, and they are referred to as thick, semi-thin, or blue sections. As the pathologist studies these sections, a number of questions must be kept in mind. Clearly, the tissue block which is selected for study with the electron microscope must be representative, and it is highly desirable that preservation be at least good; a significant degree of squashing or fixation artefact cannot be tolerated. Since the tissue block must be trimmed to produce a smaller surface before the thin sections for electron microscopy are cut with a diamond knife, it is also important to assess whether the entire block is representative, and if not, to indicate to the technician which portions of it can be cut away during trimming.

The surgical pathologist receives a variety of types of specimens, including incisional and excisional biopsies, larger surgical resections, cutting needle biopsies of soft tissue or bone, aspirations of solid tumors or bone marrow, effusions, and cerebrospinal fluid.[242] It is possible to harvest tumor cells from any specimen and retain them through processing for electron microscopy, but special techniques must sometimes be used.

When specimens are studied with the electron microscope, the procedure is to sit down at the instrument and examine the thin sections of the selected blocks, taking photographs of areas of interest or importance. It follows that information will be obtained more readily if a pathologist performs the ultrastructural study, having first examined the light microscopic sections (paraffin and plastic), ascertained the clinical situation, and determined the nature of the particular specimen under study and the anatomic location from which it was obtained. We do not recommend having a technician view the sections and take photographs which are subsequently interpreted by the pathologist. When a pathologist performs the study, it is often possible to obtain the required diagnostic information while perusing the section, and an immediate verbal report can then be given. This policy is also considerably less expensive, since the pathologist will be able to document the significant ultrastructural features of the tissue with a small number of select micrographs.

When providing a written report of diagnostic electron microscopy, the pathologist should keep in mind that his clinical colleagues are often unfamiliar with the terminology used in ultrastructural studies, and they may not be able to assess the significance of the ultrastructural findings, particularly when the results differ from those found through routine light microscopy. It is therefore advisable to correlate the findings from light and electron microscopy in a single report, or an initial report of the light microscopy may be followed by a supplemental account of the ultrastructural findings if the latter is delayed. At the M.D. Anderson Hospital, the report of the electron microscopy is sent to the pathologist handling the light microscopy who is then responsible for integrating and reporting the findings. Specimens sent only for electron microscopy are reported directly by the pathologist who performs the ultrastructural study.

Applications of Diagnostic Electron Microscopy

Before the use of immunocytochemistry gained wide acceptance, it was common practice to submit tissue for electron microscopic study whenever difficulty was experienced identifying a tumor by light microscopy. Much of the information that used to be sought by ultrastructural study can now be obtained at the light microscopic level using immunoperoxidase methods. Meanwhile, the role of electron microscopy in tumor diagnosis has diminished noticeably in recent years, even while ultrastructural diagnostic criteria were still being established and before the full potential of electron microscopy had been realized.

The advent of immunocytochemistry has proved beneficial to patient, clinician, and pathologist, since the information obtained by immunocytochemical methods can usually be gathered more rapidly and with less expense than by electron microscopy. A further advantage of immunocytochemistry is the relative ease with which a surgical pathologist in a small laboratory can perform immunoperoxidase staining procedures using commercially available kits. The same pathologist can interpret the preparation with limited prior experience, provided he observes the cautionary advice offered in the section of this chapter on immunocytochemistry.

At present, there are strong arguments for pathologists to make use of both immunocytochemistry and electron microscopy as complementary diagnostic aids to routine light microscopy. Until the range of contributions and degree of specificity of immunocytochemical procedures has been established for the different types of human tumors, and while new antibodies are being produced and assessed, it is often useful to have data from both procedures so that one can monitor the other. There are also many situations in which one technique will be informative while the other is not. The economic factor must also be considered: electron microscopic study of a specimen is costlier than a single immunocytochemical staining procedure, but not necessarily more expensive than a battery of stains. The prices of some of the antibodies used in immunocytochemistry are currently quite high.

It follows that a pathologist must be aware of the relative contributions of these diagnostic methods, and must select, to the best of his ability, the test or tests most likely to provide the required information in a particular case. All the while, he should keep in mind the importance of expediting the report and minimizing expense to the patient. There are situations where it is possible to anticipate that electron microscopic examination of a tumor is more likely to contribute helpful data than any special light microscopic staining methods.

If, for example, the pathologist suspects clinically or by routine light microscopy that a patient has an endocrine tumor, there are several ways to seek confirmation of this impression. Silver impregnation methods on light microscopic sections are the most convenient and least expensive for the purpose, but they are not consistently reliable and may be negative. If the primary location of the tumor is known or suspected, one or more appropriate immunocytochemical procedures for hormonal polypeptides may be selected, again with the awareness that they are not consistently positive, and that an endocrine tumor often forms more than a single secretory product. It may suffice to demonstrate the presence of dense-core granules of the caliber seen in endocrine cells in order to establish the nature of the tumor, and electron microscopy is then the procedure of choice, even when the only tissue available has been fixed in formalin. The onus is on the pathologist to keep abreast of the contributions of, and indications for, the various specialized diagnostic procedures that are available—no simple task, with the unabated explosion of information and accumulation of data that have occurred in the past few years.

The percentage of problem diagnoses in which electron microscopy is contributory has decreased with the development of immunocytochemistry. Four years ago at the M.D. Anderson Hospital, 8 percent of the accessioned specimens were processed for electron microscopy, approximately half of them because the need for its aid was realized at the time of biopsy or surgery. This figure has to be viewed in the context of the fact that more than one third of the more than 25,000 specimens received annually in the department were from outside the hospital, and in many instances electron microscopy would have been helpful, but tissue was not available. A rough estimate would be that electron microscopy is currently useful in 5 percent of the tumors examined in this department.

Carcinomas

Immunostaining for keratins will usually indicate whether a tumor is or is not epithelial, but nonkeratinizing carcinomas may stain only for keratins of intermediate molecular weight. EM can reveal whether squamous or glandular features are present, and for this purpose the surface features of the tumor cells are particularly important. All but the most poorly differentiated carcinomas have cell junctions, but in squamous carcinomas they are typically frequent and prominent with the structure of mature desmosomes, and are associated with prominent bundles of prekeratin filaments that run through the adjacent cytoplasm, forming a cytoskeleton that helps maintain the structural integrity of the cells. In a nonkeratinizing carcinoma, such as may arise in the nasopharynx (lymphoepithelioma), the junctions are, in contrast, small or so inconspicuous as to be hard to detect, while the filament bundles are wispy or absent. Cells of adenocarcinomas tend to form acinar spaces bordered by cells that are united by tight junctions which seal off the intercellular spaces from the lumen. Microvilli varying in number and complexity protrude into the lumen from the apices of the cells.

In adenocarcinomas from the gastrointestinal tract, the microvilli contain cores of filaments that unite in the apical cytoplasm to form bundles which insert into the lateral cell membrane at the zonula adherens: the presence of these filament cores, often accompanied by small (glycocalyceal) vesicles between the microvilli, is a strong though not an absolute indication that a metastatic adenocarcinoma is from the gastrointestinal tract.[243] True microvilli must be distinguished from the irregular cytoplasmic projections (filopodia) that protrude from the surface of the cells of most squamous carcinomas, and can be seen in occasional sarcomas, including some malignant fibrous histiocytomas. Long, sinuous, branching microvilli are present on the cells of the better differentiated mesotheliomas, and electron microscopy can usually help in making the distinction between a mesothelioma and an adenocarcinoma[244]: in the minority of instances in which the ultrastructure does not allow a firm distinction between the two tumors, immunostaining for both keratin and CEA may serve the purpose.[167,168]

The features described in the preceding paragraph are, in fact, a considerable simplification of the degree of complexity that can be encountered among carcinomas, partly because there is a range of natural variation within individual tumor types at the ultrastructural level, just as differences are seen by conventional light microscopy, and also because poorly differentiated tumors tend to lose many of the specific morphological characteristics that would serve to identify their better differentiated counterparts. Surface microvilli may be lost, for example, though the nature of the tumor is sometimes still evident from the presence of intracytoplasmic acini containing microvilli: they are seen more frequently in breast carcinomas, but can occur in many different forms of adenocarcinoma.[245] Both squamous carcinomas and adenocarcinomas may undergo spindle cell transformation, and distinction from a sarcoma may then be difficult by EM, or the cells may become large and highly variable in size and shape—this pleomorphism can create a similar diagnostic problem.[246] Finally, mixture of squamous and adenocarcinomatous features can occur in a differentiated carcinoma: in more than 10 percent of bronchogenic adenocarcinomas, for example, foci of squamous differentiation can be detected at the ultrastructural level.[247]

Most squamous carcinomas that are well or moderately differentiated look similar regardless of the location, and it is not possible to determine the primary site of a metastatic squamous carcinoma by electron microscopy. Some adenocarcinomas have features that help locate the primary tumor when the tissue for examination is from a metastasis: the microvilli of gastrointestinal adenocarcinomas have already been mentioned. Other identifying characteristics are usually found within the cytoplasm. For example, an accumulation of mitochondria is seen in Hurthle cell carcinoma of the thyroid,[248] and less frequently in tumors originating in salivary,[249] endocrine,[250,251] and renal tissues.[252] The appearance of the mitochondria may also be informative: in some tumors of steroid–forming cells, they have tubular cristae, and the cells may also contain extensive zones of smooth endoplasmic reticulum.[253]

Secretory material within the cytoplasm of tumor cells can be helpful in diagnosis, and small quantities of mucin, glycogen, or lipid are readily identified by EM. Their significance may be limited, however, just as it is at the light microscopic level, because these substances are found in cells of many different tumors. An accumulation of dense-core granules can be very informative, since the caliber of the granules provides some indication of the cell type.[254] Exocrine cells of the salivary glands and pancreas contain large granules (over 500 nm in diameter) that are accompanied by abundant granular endoplasmic reticulum, and a similar appearance is seen in a salivary acinic cell carcinoma or an acinar cell carcinoma of the pancreas.

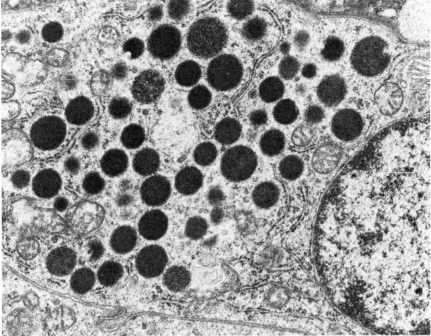

Figure 2-11. *Numerous secretory granules in the cytoplasm of a bronchial carcinoid cell. (original magnification × 24,960)*

The secretory granules of polypeptide-forming endocrine cells are smaller than those of exocrine cells, and they range from approximately 150 to 400 nm in caliber. In a particular endocrine tumor, the granules will fall within a relatively narrow range of diameters (Fig. 2-11). Many tumors, however, form more than a single secretory product, and there is little value in trying to predict the nature of the secretions from the fine structure of the cells. There are a few exceptions. The granules of insulinoma cells may have a crystalline center like those of the normal beta islet cell, and in norepinephrine-forming pheochromocytomas, granules are ovoid with an eccentrically–positioned dense core.[255] Care must be taken to avoid confusing primary lysosomes with secretory granules, since the two can appear identical. Lysosomes are rarely numerous in viable carcinoma cells, but dense bodies should only be accepted as authentic secretory granules when they are present in the majority of the cells of a tumor and fall within a narrow range of diameters. Again, an exception exists in the endocrine tumors of the midgut which often have large, pleomorphic secretory granules.

Small cell carcinomas of the lung have been known for many years from light microscopy, but it was only with the advent of electron microscopy that primary small cell undifferentiated carcinomas in other locations were convincingly demonstrated. Granules are present in these tumors, but they vary in frequency. In many small cell lung carcinomas, granules are sparse or absent, and when present they are smaller in caliber (120 nm) than those of most endocrine carcinomas, including bronchial carcinoids.[247] In some peripheral bronchial carcinoids, however, granules are only slightly larger than those in small cell carcinomas, and distinction between the tumors depends on other fine structural criteria.

Among extrapulmonary small cell carcinomas, attention has recently been focused on those arising in the skin, where the presumed cell of origin is a tactile receptor, the Merkel cell. In cutaneous neuroendocrine carcinomas, accumulations of small granules roughly 120 nm in size are found within dendritic processes of the tumor cells, and the ultrastructural features are therefore helpful in establishing the diagnosis[256] (Fig. 2-12). It is not possible to distinguish among small cell undifferentiated carcinomas arising in different location from their ultrastructure alone, and there is overlap in the hormonal polypeptides they produce. Consequently, the clinical evidence is important in determining whether a tumor in, for example, the skin is arising there or is metastatic from some internal organ, such as the lung.

Melanoma

A frequent and often difficult problem for the surgical pathologist is the diagnosis of metastatic melanoma when the tumor cells do not manifest or have lost their ability to form melanin identifiable by light microscopy. In the cytoplasm of melanocytes, melanin is deposited on a protein framework within specific organelles, and four stages in the formation of these melanosomes have been defined ultrastructurally. The first stage is merely a membrane-bound sac or vesicle, but in stage two and three melanosomes, a protein framework (premelanosome) with a distinctive periodicity is present.[257] In stage four melanosomes, the deposition of melanin totally obscures the banded body, and distinction from a lysosome is difficult or impossible. Thus, the identification of stage two or three melanosomes can serve to establish that a tumor is forming melanin, and in the proper clinical and light microscopic context will indicate the diagnosis of metastatic amelanotic melanoma.

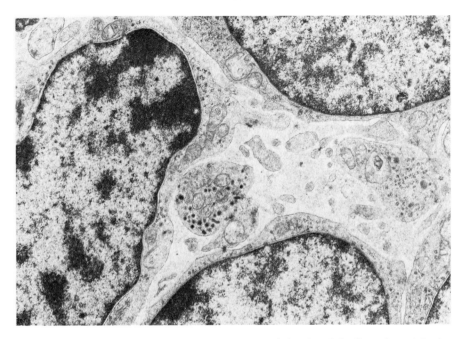

Figure 2-12. *Metastatic neuroendocrine carcinoma of skin (Merkel cell carcinoma) in the testicle of a 72-year-old male. Small dendritic processes containing dense core granules lie between the tumor cells. (original magnification × 24,000)*

It is well known that a primary cutaneous malignant melanoma can undergo spontaneous regression, and that absence of a demonstrable primary does not exclude the possibility that a metastatic tumor is melanoma. Rarely, a melanoma arises from a mucosal surface,[258,259] or develops within soft tissues. The so-called clear cell sarcoma, formerly attributed to tendons or aponeuroses, is now recognized to be a tumor of melanocytes, and the name has been revised to malignant melanoma of soft parts.[260] Presumably, the melanocytes from which these tumors arise became sequestered in the soft tissues in the course of their embryologic migration from neural crest or skin. Occasionally, melanosomes are found in cells of a squamous carcinoma or a Schwann cell tumor.[261]

If a diagnosis of metastatic melanoma is suspected, immunostaining for S-100 protein should be performed. It appears that all melanoma cells will stain positively,[197] but staining is also manifested by other cells of neural crest derivation and by some histiocytes and mesenchymal cells.[186,188]

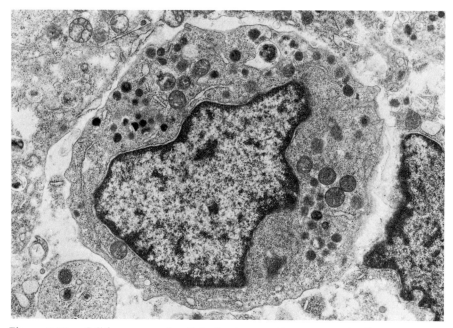

Figure 2-13.   *Cell from a granulocytic leukemia presenting as a mass in the paranasal soft tissues. (original magnification × 12,000)*

Lymphoma-Leukemia

Diagnostic electron microscopy on a tumor within the broad group of lymphomas and leukemias must be correlated with the results of immunocytochemical stains, conventional light microscopy, and the clinical data. The cell type can usually be determined by EM, but confirmation that the cells are neoplastic requires examination of the light microscopic sections. Areas where EM is helpful in this category of tumors include the recognition of an unsuspected granulocytic leukemia involving soft tissues (Fig. 2-13) (the naphthol AS-D chloroacetate (NASD) stain will then be performed to add light microscopic confirmation of the diagnosis), and the identification of cells of monocytic or of hairy cell leukemia from the presence of cytoplasmic complexes of endoplasmic reticulum and ribosomes.[262] In hairy cell leukemia, true ribosome-lamellar complexes can be found in about half the cases, which is a considerably higher frequency than for the other forms of leukemia in which they have been described. The complexes in monocytic leukemia are superficially similar to the ribosome-lamellar complexes but differ in details of the arrangement of the reticulum which does not have the usual spiral configuration (personal observations).

Probably the greatest contribution of EM in diagnosing lymphomas is confirmation of a suspected diagnosis of large cell lymphoma. The proliferating transformed lymphocytes can closely resemble cells of a poorly differentiated carcinoma by light microscopy, especially if the biopsy material is scanty or of poor quality, if the neoplastic cells are mainly within lymph node sinusoids, or when the clinical presentation is atypical and the diagnosis is not suspected. EM will usually serve to identify the cells as transformed lymphocytes from the paucity of organelles, abundant free ribosomes, cell and nuclear shape including the occasional presence of nuclear blebs, and prominent nucleoli.[262] The cells may also have irregular peripheral projections which by EM can simulate microvilli and lead the unwary to believe that the tumor is a poorly differentiated adenocarcinoma.

If plasmacytoid transformation of the lymphocytes is occurring, its presence and degree can be accurately determined by EM. Some true plasma cell neoplasms are not recognized as such by routine light microscopy, and again the ultrastructural findings will establish the diagnosis. Nuclear-cytoplasmic asynchrony is frequently observed in myeloma cells, and accumulations of immunoglobulin within the cytoplasm may be identified.[263] The latter can also be seen occasionally in other lymphoproliferative disorders: IgG inclusions appear as tiny vesicles within coalescing larger vacuoles in a signet–ring cell lymphoma, and IgM inclusions form dense aggregates within cisternae of the endoplasmic reticulum. Immunostaining is also helpful in the distinction of lymphoma from carcinoma through the use of monoclonal antibody T29-33 against common leukocyte antigen and the absence of staining for cytoplasmic keratins.[132]

Other contributions of EM in this broad tumor group are the confirmation of a suspected diagnosis of histiocytosis X by revealing the presence of Langerhans' granules in the cytoplasm of the cells,[264] and the identification of a mediastinal tumor as a thymoma.[265]

Small Round Cell Tumors

This is a convenient designation for a heterogeneous group of malignant tumors in pediatric patients that are composed of small round or ovoid cells. There may be some distinguishing features by light microscopy to indicate the diagnosis, such as rosettes in neuroblastoma or copious glycogen in Ewing's tumor, but in the absence of definite criteria, ultrastructural study should be undertaken. There is some overlap in the fine structure of the tumors, but specific ultrastructural features do aid in their identification. They include dendritic processes containing microtubules and small dense-core vesicles in neuroblastoma, and skeletal muscle myofilaments in some rhabdomyosarcomas. Immunostaining is also useful: neuron-specific enolase may serve to identify a neuroblastoma, and many rhabdomyosarcomas contain myoglobin. A small proportion of the tumors remain unclassified even after immunocytochemical and ultrastructural studies.

Central Nervous System Tumors

This is a difficult diagnostic area for the general surgical pathologist who does not see many examples of primary brain and spinal cord tumors, and even the experienced neuropathologist must resort to special techniques like EM in many cases. Immunostaining is useful, since the glial fibrillary acidic protein and vimentin stains are usually positive in gliomas.[152,175] Tumors in which EM is helpful include ependymomas and meningiomas, especially the latter when it presents in an extracranial site[266] (Fig. 2-14). Filament-filled processes encircling small vessels, and small lumens bordered by cells with long tight junctions, microvilli, and occasional cilia, are characteristics of ependymomas, while meningioma cells are distinguished by their undulating cytoplasmic extensions and plasma membranes, and by the masses of intermediate filaments that occupy the cytoplasm of some cells.

Soft Tissue Tumors

A wide range of histologic appearances can be seen within this extensive and complex group of neoplasms, and it is often difficult to append a designation to a soft tissue tumor, particularly one that is malignant. Probably as many as one in three sarcomas cannot be accurately classified by light microscopy. Some immunostaining methods are selectively helpful, notably factor VIII-related antigen and Ulex Europeaus I for endothelial cell neoplasms,[46,144] myoglobin for rhabdomyosarcomas,[146] and S-100 protein which stains many schwann cell tumors but is not highly specific.[188,199] By studying the ultrastructure of the component cells, an experienced pathologist will be able to identify most soft tissue tumors, but roughly 10 percent of the sarcomas do not have sufficiently characteristic features to allow their classification. Since it is not possible to be certain by light microscopy that these truly are primitive tumors lacking any specific

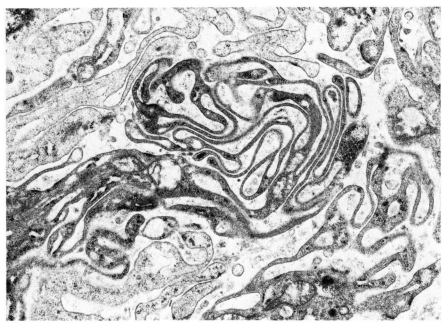

Figure 2-14. *A large mass in the neck of a 19-year-old male was composed of cells with long, slender, curving cytoplasmic extensions. This appearance is characteristic of meningioma cells. (original magnification × 5740)*

cellular differentiation, the ultrastructural findings are needed to confirm the impression.

It may be questioned whether precise subclassification of a soft tissue sarcoma is of value to the clinician treating the patient. Often, it suffices to state that a tumor is of soft tissue origin and is benign or malignant. Reproducible, prognostically significant histologic features have been defined for a few soft tissue tumors, but reliable grading criteria are not available for the majority. Nevertheless, with the emergence and development of elaborate forms of combination therapy, it is desirable that the pathologist provide as specific a designation as possible for each tumor in the hope that relationships between cell type and response to particular forms of treatment may ultimately emerge. With the gradual accumulation of data on the fine structure of the soft tissue sarcomas,[267] subclassification by electron microscopy is becoming more feasible, but the field is a complex one, and there is overlap among related types. More work on larger groups of cases than have so far been studied is required. Regretably, only the larger institutions have the opportunity to collect extensive series of cases with material for electron microscopy to pursue these clinico-pathologic investigations.

Discussion

It is evident that the surgical pathologist has in recent years acquired powerful tools to aid in the diagnosis of human tumors. The full impact of the burgeoning discipline of immunocytochemistry has not yet been realized, and some years must elapse before the extent of its contribution can be accurately defined. Clearly, it has enormous potential, and by using carefully selected immunohistochemical methods and, where appropriate, electron microscopy, the pathologist is much better able to diagnose problem cases than in the past. Also, the additional information that is being gathered about the structure and function of tumors is clarifying their histogenesis and refining, or even revising, classifications. Some new entities have been discovered, an example being the neuroendocrine carcinomas, and doubtless more will emerge. As these newer techniques are further investigated and applied, the pathologist must be mindful of the importance of clinical correlation, and relate the morphologic and functional data that accrue on specific tumors to their biologic behavior and response to different forms of therapy. The enhanced precision with which the pathologist can classify tumors will in turn improve the accuracy of reports of clinical studies which in the past have often suffered from erroneous light microscopic diagnoses.

In this chapter, we have briefly reviewed applications of immunocyto-chemistry and electron microscopy to the investigation of tumors that pose a problem in identification by routine light microscopy. The information is pertinent both for tumors that have arisen at the site where they are biopsied or resected, and for those known or suspected to be metastatic. In the latter situation, when the primary site is not known, the pathologist has the added responsibility of providing an indication of possible locations.

The identification of a poorly differentiated tumor, and determination of the primary location of a metastatic tumor, require integration of all the available information on the case. Both pathologist and clinician can help by sharing their respective views on the possibilities and the implications for the further investigation of the patient and institution of treatment. The clinician must weigh the diagnostic information available and decide if it is sufficient to select and begin therapy, or whether the delay and additional expense of obtaining more tissue is likely to be worth the effort.[268,269]

There is no convenient formula that will indicate the cost-effectiveness of additional diagnostic procedures, and studies have suggested that a low yield of positive findings and limited impact on management or patient survival do not justify an intensive search for the primary site of a metastatic tumor.[268] The pathologist will probably be intent on reaching as precise a diagnosis as possible, but academic enthusiasm must be subordinated to economic considerations and the other factors that are pertinent to patient care, particularly with the current emphasis on cost-containment. If it is concluded that more tissue is needed for pathologic study, a procedure should be undertaken only after the clinician has, in dialogue with the pathologist, ascertained what type of specimen would be most useful, how much tissue is necessary, and how the specimen should be optimally handled and subdivided for the appropriate studies. A surgeon performing a biopsy is often poorly informed on which tests are indicated, and how material for each should be submitted. It is frustrating and can be tragic when mishandling of a diagnostic specimen is the reason an accurate and clinically meaningful interpretation cannot be achieved.

There have been a number of studies of relative probabilities in the differential diagnosis of metastatic tumors in various sites.[270–275] The age and sex of the patient are sometimes helpful. A small round cell tumor in a child will raise a different group of possibilities in the minds of pathologist and clinician than a similar tumor in an adult. A carcinoma in axillary lymph nodes in a female patient will lead the physician to suspect a primary in breast. Among 60 patients with axillary metastases from unknown primary sites reviewed by Copeland and McBride,[274] 19 were found to have breast cancer. A primary tumor was found antemortem in only 3 of the other 42 patients. The location of a distant metastasis can be significant, as when a metastatic prostatic adenocarcinoma presents in a left supraclavicular lymph node.

Holmes and Founts[270] investigated 686 patients with metastatic cancer and found that the average age was 60, 58 percent were female, 10 percent of the patients were alive at 2 years, and 5 percent survived for 5 years. In the 254 patients reviewed by Didolkar et al.,[271] the primary site was determined in 30 percent, but usually at autopsy: adenocarcinoma was the most common histologic type, and the primary was in the lung in 40 percent, followed by stomach, pancreas, kidney, ovary, and colon. Lung, then stomach, were the most common primary locations when the tumor was in lower cervical nodes. The study of Krementz et al.[272] revealed that most nodal metastases with unknown primaries involve the head and neck region, and that a primary tumor is found in approximately one–third and is within the head and neck in 60 percent. If the tumor is a squamous carcinoma, origin in the head or neck is more likely than when it is an adenocarcinoma which is more often from a primary located below the level of the clavicles. One percent of the 2232 patients with inguinal node metastases reviewed by Zaren and Copeland[275] were from an unknown primary site, and the source of the tumor was only determined in one patient. The 22 patients had a 50 percent five-year survival.

Analyses of this type are undeniably helpful, but malignant tumors do not play according to rigid rules, and instances of variations in their behavior are legion. Pathologists must not allow their judgment to be biased by probabilities at the expense of ignoring relevant histologic clues, and they should not speculate beyond the limits warranted by their microscopic findings. They must be mindful of an obligation to communicate with clinicians as soon as possible on any problem case in which the results of the pathology studies are likely to influence the management of the patient. If a precise diagnosis has not been reached, a prompt interim verbal assessment may serve to narrow the differential diagnosis sufficiently to allow therapy to be commenced, and reduce or even eliminate the need for additional diagnostic procedures. The verbal report must be followed by an expedited report for the patient's medical record in which the findings and conclusions from all the pathology studies are clearly summarized.

References

1. Coons AH, Creech HJ, Jones RN, et al: The demonstration of pneumococcal antigen in tissue by the use of fluorescent antibody. J Immunol 45:159–170, 1942
2. Christopherson WM: Cytologic detection and diagnosis of cancer; its contributions and limitations. Cancer 51:1201–1208, 1983
3. Osborne BM, Butler JJ, Mackay B: Sinusoidal large cell ("histiocytic") lymphoma. Cancer 46:2484–2491, 1980
4. Mickelson MR, Brown GA, Maynard JA, et al: Synovial sarcoma—an electron microscopic study of monophasic and biphasic forms. Cancer 45:2109–2118, 1980
5. Mackay B, Osborne BM: The contribution of electron microscopy to the diagnosis of tumors. Pathobiol Annu 8:359–405, 1978
6. Weinbor DS, Pinkus GS: Non-Hodgkin's lymphoma of large multilobulated cell type. A clinicopathologic study of ten cases. Am J Clin Pathol 76:190–196, 1971
7. Battifora H: Spindle cell carcinoma—ultrastructural evidence of

squamous origin and collagen production by tumor cells. Cancer 37:2275–2282, 1976

8. Enzinger FM: Acidophilic fascial sarcoma: A sarcoma simulating a granuloma—An analysis of 62 cases. Cancer 26:1029–1041, 1970

9. Lillie RD: Conn's Biological Stains (ed 9). Baltimore, Williams and Wilkins, 1977

10. Triche TJ, Ross WE: Glycogen-containing neuroblastoma with clinical and histopathologic features of Ewing's sarcoma. Cancer 41:1425–1432, 1978

11. Thoenes GH: The immunohistology of glomerulonephritis—distinctive marks and variability. Curr Top Pathol 61:61–106, 1976

12. Spargo BH, Seymour AE, Ordonez NG: Renal Biopsy Pathology with Diagnostic and Therapeutic Implications. John Wiley and Sons, Inc., New York, 1980

13. DeLellis RA: Diagnostic Immunohistochemistry. Masson Publishing USA Inc., New York, 1981

14. DeLellis RA, Sternberger LA, Mann RB, et al: Immunoperoxidase techniques in diagnostic pathology. Am J Clin Pathol 71:483–484, 1979

15. Mason TE, Phifer RF, Spicer S, et al: An immunoglobulin enzyme bridge method for localizing tissue antigens. J Histochem Cytochem 17:565–569, 1969

16. Sternberger LA, Hardy PH Jr., Cuculis JJ, et al: The unlabeled antibody method of immunohistochemistry. Preparation and properties of soluble antigen-antibody complex (horseradish peroxidase-anti-horseradish peroxidase) and its use in the identification of spirochetes. J Histochem Cytochem 18:315–333, 1970

17. Sternberger LA: Immunocytochemistry (ed 2). John Wiley and Sons, New York, 1979

18. Guesdon J-L, Ternynck T, Avrameas S: The use of avidin-biotin interaction in immunoenzymatic techniques. J Histochem Cytochem 27:1131–1139, 1979

19. Hsu SM, Raine L, Fanger H: Use of avidin-biotin-peroxidase complex (ABC) in immunoperoxidase techniques: A comparison between ABC and the unlabeled antibody (PAP) procedures. J Histochem Cytochem 29:577–580, 1981

20. Goding JW: Use of staphylococcal protein A as an immunological reagent. J Immunol Methods 20:241–253, 1970

21. Biberfeld P, Ghetie V, Sjoquist J: Demonstration and assaying of IgG antibodies in tissues and in cells by labeled staphylococcal protein A. J Immunol Methods 6:249–259, 1975

22. Crowther JR, Elzein EM: Detection of antibodies against foot-and-mouth disease virus using purified staphylococcus A protein conjugated with alkaline phosphatase. J Immunol Methods 34:261–267, 1980

23. Dubois-Dalcq M, McFarland H, McFarlin D: Protein A-peroxidase: A valuable tool for the localization of antigens. J Histochem Cytochem 25:1201–1206, 1977

24. Kohler G, Millstein C: Continuous cultures of fused cells secreting antibodies to predefined specificity. Nature 256:495–497, 1975

25. Kohler G: The technique of hybridoma production, in Lefovits I, Pernis B (eds): Immunological Methods, vol. 4. New York, Academic Press Inc., 1981, pp 285–298

26. Diamond BA, Dale E, Yelton BA, et al: Monoclonal antibodies—A new technology for producing serologic reagents. N Engl J Med 304:1344–1349, 1981

27. Winger L, Winger C, Shastry P, et al: Efficient generation in vitro, from human peripheral blood cells, of monoclonal Epstein-Barr virus transformants producing specific antibody to a variety of antigens without prior deliberate immunization. Proc Natl Acad Sci USA 80:4484–4488, 1983

28. Borowitz MJ, Stein RB: Diagnostic applications of monoclonal antibodies to human cancer. Arch Pathol Lab Med 108:101–105, 1984

29. Murphy GF, Bhan AK, Sato S, et al: A new immunological marker for human Langerhan's cells. N Engl J Med 304:791–792, 1981

30. Nakane PK: Simultaneous localization of multiple tissue antigens using the peroxidase-labeled antibody method: A study on pituitary gland of the rat. J Histochem Cytochem 16:557–560, 1968

31. Campbell GT, Bhatnagar AS: Simultaneous visualization of light microscopy of two pituitary hormones in a single tissue section using a combination of indirect immunohistochemical methods. J Histochem Cytochem 24:448–452, 1976

32. Mason DY, Sammons R: Alkaline phosphatase and peroxidase for double immunoenzymatic labelling of cellular constituents. J Clin Pathol 31:454–460, 1978

33. Suffin SC, Muck Yuong JC, et al: Improvement of the glucose oxidase immunoenzyme technique: Use of a tetrazolium whose formagen is stable without heavy metal chelation. Am J Clin Pathol 71:492–496, 1979

34. Falini B, DeSolas I, Halverson C, et al: Double labeled-antigen method for the demonstration of intracellular antigens in paraffin-embedded tissues. J Histochem Cytochem 30:21–26, 1980

35. Falini B, Taylor CR: New developments in immunoperoxidase. Arch Pathol Lab Med 107:105–117, 1983

36. Mason DY, Abdulaziz Z, Falini B, et al: Double immunoenzymatic labeling, in Polak JN, Noorden SV (eds): Immunocytochemistry, Practical Applications in Pathology and Biology. Bristol, Wright PSG, 1983, pp 113–128

37. Ponder BAJ: Lectin histochemistry in immunocytochemistry, in Polak JN, Noorden SV (eds): Practical Applications in Pathology and Biology. Bristol, Wright PSG, 1983, pp 129–142

38. Kocourch J, Horejsi V: Defining a lectin. Nature 290:188–189, 1981

39. Reisner Y, Linker-Israeli M, Sharon S: Separation of mouse thymocytes into two subpopulations by the use of peanut agglutinin. Cell Immunol 25:129–134, 1976

40. Reisner Y, Itzinovitch L, Meshorer A, et al: Hematopoietic stem cell transplantation using mouse bone marrow and spleen cells fractioned by lectins. Proc Natl Acad Sci USA, 75:2933–2936, 1978

41. Reisner Y, Biniaminov M, Rosenthal E, et al: Interaction of peanut agglutinin with normal human lymphocytes and with leukemic cells. Proc Natl Acad Sci USA 76:447–451, 1979

42. Newman RA, Klein PJ, Rudland PS: Binding of peanut lectin to breast epithelium, human carcinomas and cultured rat mammary stem cell: Use of the lectin as a marker of mammary differentiation. J Natl Cancer Inst 63:1339–1346, 1979

43. Howard DR, Batsakis JG: Peanut agglutinin: A new marker for tissue histiocytes. Am J Clin Pathol 77:401–408, 1982

44. Pereira MEA, Kisalus EC, Grueso G, et al: Immunohistochemical studies on the combining site of the blood group H-specific lectin I from Ulex europaeus seeds. Arch Biochem Biophys 185:108–115, 1978

45. Holtofer H, Virtanen I, Kariniemi AL, et al: Ulex europaeus I lectin as a marker for vascular endothelium in human tissues. Lab Invest 47:60–66, 1982

46. Ordonez NG, Batsakis JG: Comparison of Ulex europaeus I lectin and factor VIII-related antigen in vascular lesions. Arch Pathol Lab Med 108:129–132, 1984

47. Goldstein IJ, Hayes CE: The lectins: Carbohydrate-binding proteins of plants and animals. Adv Carbohydr Chem Biochem 35:127–340, 1978

48. Nakane PK: Recent progress in the immunoperoxidase labeled antibody method. Ann NY Acad Sci 254:203–210, 1975

49. De Mey J: Colloidal gold probes in immunocytochemistry. Polak JM,

Van Noorden SV (eds): Practical Applications in Pathology and Biology. Bristol, Wright PSG, 1983, pp. 82–112

50. Horisberger M, Roset J, Bauer H: Colloidal gold granules as markers for cell surface receptors in the scanning electron microscope. Experientia 31:1147–1149, 1975

51. Fenoglio CM, Tlasma G: Application of immunoperoxidase techniques to diagnostic surgical pathology. NY State J Med 83:293–299, 1983

52. Nadji M: The potential value of immunoperoxidase techniques in diagnostic cytology. Acta Cytol 24:442–447, 1980

53. Walts AE, Said JW: Specific tumor markers in diagnostic cytology. Acta Cytol 27:408–416, 1983

54. Orell SR, Dowling KD: Oncofetal antigens as tumor markers in the cytologic diagnosis of effusions. Acta Cytol 27:625–629, 1983

55. Banks PM, Caron L, Morgan TW: Use of imprints for monoclonal antibody studies. Suitability of air-dried preparations for lymphoid tissues with an immunohistochemical method. Am J Clin Pathol 79:438–442, 1983

56. Carnegie JA, McCully ME, Robertson HA: Embedment in glycol methacrylate at low temperature allows immunofluorescent localization of a labile tissue protein. J Histochem Cytochem 28:308–310, 1980

57. Giddins J, Griffin RL, Maciner AG: Demonstration of immunoproteins in Araldite-embedded tissues. J Clin Pathol 35:111–114, 1982

58. Isaacson P, Wright DH: Immunohistochemistry of lymphoreticular tumors. In Polak JM, Van Noorden SV (eds): Immunocytochemistry. Practical Applications in Pathology and Biology. Bristol, Wright PSG, 1983, pp. 249–273

59. Altmannsberger M, Osborn M, Schauer A, et al: Antibodies to different intermediate filament proteins: Cell type-specific markers in paraffin-embedded human tissues. Lab Invest 45:427–434, 1981

60. Mukai K, Rosai J: Applications of immunoperoxidase technique in surgical pathology. In Fenoglio CM, Wolff M (eds): Progress in Surgical Pathology, Vol 1, New York, Masson Publishing USA Inc., 1980, pp 15–49

61. Bussolati G, Monga G: Medullary carcinoma of the thyroid with atypical patterns. Cancer 44:1769–1777, 1979

62. Norman T, Johannessen JV, Gautvik KM: Medullary carcinoma of the thyroid: Diagnostic problems. Cancer 38:366–377, 1977

63. Mendelsohn G, Bigner SH, Eggleston JC, et al: Anaplastic variants of medullary thyroid carcinoma. Am J Surg Pathol 4:333–341, 1980

64. Nieuwenhuijzen Kruseman ACN, Bosman FT, van Bergen Henegouw JC, et al: Medullary differentiation of anaplastic thyroid carcinoma. Am J Clin Pathol 77:541–547, 1982

65. Logerfo P, LiVolsi V, Collachio D, et al: Thyroglobulin production in thyroid cancers. J Surg Res 24:1–6, 1978

66. Bocker W, Donalle H, Husselman H, et al: Immunohistochemical analysis of thyroglobulin synthesis in thyroid carcinomas. Virchows Arch (Pathol Anat) 385:187–200, 1980

67. Albores-Saavedra J, Nadji M, Civantos F, et al: Thyroglobulin in carcinoma of the thyroid: An immunohistochemical study. Human Pathol 14:62–66, 1983

68. Civantos F, Albores-Saavedra J, Nadji M, et al: Clear cell variant of thyroid carcinoma. Am J Surg Pathol 8:187–192, 1984

69. Ordonez NG, Ibanez ML, Samaan NA, et al: Immunoperoxidase study of uncommon parathyroid tumors—Report of two cases of nonfunctioning parathyroid carcinomas and one intrathyroid parathyroid tumor producing amyloid. Am J Surg Pathol 7:535–541, 1983

70. Soga J, Tazawa K: Pathological analysis of carcinoids. Histologic evaluation of 62 cases. Cancer 28:990–998, 1971

71. Greider NH, Rosai J, McGuigan JE: The human pancreatic islet cells and their tumors. II. Ulcerogenic and diarrheogenic tumors. Cancer 33:1423–1443, 1974

72. Guarda LA, Silva EG, Ordonez NG, et al: Clear cell islet cell tumor. Am J Clin Pathol 79:512–517, 1983

73. Dayal Y, O'Brian DS: The pathology of the pancreatic endocrine cells. In DeLellis RA (ed): Diagnostic Immunocytochemistry. New York, Masson Publishing USA, Inc., 1981, pp 208–230

74. Creutzfeldt W: Endocrine tumors of the pancreas: Clinical, chemical and morphological findings, in Fitzgerald PJ, Morrison AB (eds): The Pancreas. Baltimore, Williams and Wilkins Co., 1980, pp 208–230

75. Woodtli W, Hendinger C: Histologic characteristics of insulinomas and gastrinomas. Value of argyrophilia, metachromasia, immunohistology, and electron microscopy for the identification of gastrointestinal and pancreatic endocrine cells and their tumors. Virchows Arch (Cell Pathol) 16:95–109, 1974

76. Mukai K, Greider MH, Grotting JC, et al: Retrospective study of 77 pancreatic endocrine tumors using an immunoperoxidase method. Am J Surg Pathol 6:387–399, 1982

77. Heitz PU, Kasper M, Polak JM, et al: Pancreatic endocrine tumors. Human Pathol 13:263–271, 1982

78. Sundler F, Alumets J, Hakason R: Growth hormone-like immuno-reactivity in gastrin cells and gastrinomas. Histochemistry 59:343–346, 1973

79. Pearse AGE, Polak JM, Heath CM: Polypeptide hormone production in "carcinoid" apudomas and their relative cytochemistry. Virchows Arch (Cell Pathol) 16:95–109, 1974

80. Dayal Y, O'Brian DS, DeLellis RA, et al: Carcinoid tumors of the gastro-intestinal tract and extra-intestinal sites. A comparative study of polypeptide hormonal profiles. Regulatory Polypeptides 1(Suppl):22–34, 1980

81. Broder LG, Carter SK: Pancreatic islet cell carcinoma. I. Clinical features of 52 patients. Ann Intern Med 79:101–107, 1973

82. Raleigh BK, Heerden JA, Weiland LH: Nonfunctioning islet cell tumors. Ann Surg 193:185–190, 1981

83. Schmechel DE, Marangos PJ, Zis AP, et al: Brain enolases as specific markers of neural and glial cells. Science 199:313–315, 1978

84. Schmechel DR, Marangos PJ, Brightman MW: Neuron-specific enolase is a marker for central and peripheral neuroendocrine cells. Nature 276:834–836, 1978

85. Tapia FJ, Polak JM, Barbosa AJA, et al: Neuron-specific enolase is produced by neuroendocrine tumors. Lancet 1:808–811, 1981

86. Carlei F, Polak JM: Antibodies to neuron-specific enolase for the delineation of the entire neuroendocrine system in health and disease. Semin Diagnostic Pathol 1:59–70, 1984

87. Gu J, Polak JM, van Noorden SV, et al: Immunostaining of neuron-specific enolase as a diagnostic tool for Merkel cell tumor. Cancer 52:1039–1043, 1983

88. Asa SL, Ryan N, Kovacs K, et al: Immunohistochemical localization of neuron-specific enolase in the human hypophysis and pituitary adenomas. Arch Pathol Lab Med 108:40–43, 1984

89. Kurman RJ, Scardino PT: Alpha fetoprotein and human chorionic gonadotropin in ovarian and testicular tumors, in DeLellis RA (ed): Diagnostic Immunocytochemistry. New York, Masson, 1981, pp 277–298

90. Jacobsen GK, Jacobsen M, Clausen PP: Distribution of tumor-associated antigens in the various histologic components of germ cell tumors of the testis. Am J Surg Pathol 5:257–277, 1981

91. Kurman RJ, Scardio PT, McIntire KR, et al: Cellular localization of alpha fetoprotein and human chorionic gonadotropin in germ cell

tumors of the testis using an indirect immunoperoxidase technique. A new approach to the classification utilizing tumor markers. Cancer 40:2136–2151, 1976

92. Ueda G, Hamanaka N, Hayakawa K, et al: Clinical, histological and biochemical studies of an ovarian dysgerminoma with trophoblasts and Leydig cells. Am J Obstet Gynecol 114:748–754, 1972

93. Nochovitz LE, Lange PH, Fraley EE, et al: Testicular seminoma with human chorionic gonadotropin (HCG) production. A study of 16 cases with special reference to anaplastic seminoma. Lab Invest 42:140, 1980

94. Skinner DG, Scardino PT: Relevance of biochemical tumor markers and lymphadenectomy in management of non-seminomatous testis tumor. Current Perspective. J Urol 123:278–283, 1980

95. Taylor CR, Kurman RJ, Warner NE: The potential value of immunocytochemical techniques in the classification of ovarian and testicular tumors. Human Pathol 9:417–427, 1978

96. Nadji M, Tabei SZ, Castro A, et al: Prostatic origin of tumors. An immunohistochemical study. Am J Clin Pathol 73:735–739, 1979

97. Li C-Y, Lan WKW: Immunohistochemical diagnosis of prostatic cancer with metastasis. Cancer 46:706–717, 1980

98. Ordonez NG, Ayala AG, von Eschenbach A, et al: Immunoperoxidase localization of prostatic acid phosphatase in carcinoma of the prostate with sarcomatoid changes. Urology 19:210–214, 1982

99. Heyderman E, Neville AMA: A shorter immunoperoxidase technique for the demonstration of carcinoembryonic antigen and other cell products. J Clin Pathol 30:138–140, 1977

100. Heyderman E: Tumor markers, in Polak JM, van Noorden SV (eds): Immunocytochemistry. Practical applications in pathology and biology. Bristol, Wright PSG, 1983, pp 274–294

101. Wang MC, Valenzuela LA, Murphy GP, et al: Purification of human prostatic specific antigen. Invest Urol 17:159–163, 1979

102. Kuriyama M, Loor R, Wang M, et al: Prostatic acid phosphatase and prostatic-specific antigen in prostate cancer. Int Adv Surg Oncol 5:29–49, 1982

103. Allhof EP, Proppe KH, Chapman CM: Evaluation of prostatic-specific acid phosphatase and prostatic-specific antigen. J Urol 129:316–319, 1983

104. Stein BS, Vangore S, Paterson RO, et al: Immunoperoxidase localization of prostatic-specific antigen. Am J Surg Pathol 6:553–557, 1982

105. Bloomfield CD, Gajl-Peczalska KJ, Frizzera G, et al: Clinical utility of

lymphocyte surface markers combined with the Lukes-Collins histologic classification in adult lymphoma. N Engl J Med 301:512–518, 1979

106. Pinkus GS, Said JW: Characterization of non-Hodgkin's lymphomas using multiple cell markers: Immunologic, morphologic, and cytochemical studies of 72 cases. Am J Pathol 94:349–380, 1979

107. Harris NL, Poppemas S, Data RE: Demonstration of immunoglobulin in malignant lymphomas: Use of an immunoperoxidase technique on frozen sections. Am J Clin Pathol 78:14–21, 1982

108. Stein H, Bonk A, Tolksdorf G, et al: Immunohistochemical analysis of the organization of normal lymphoid tissue and non-Hodgkin's lymphomas. J Histochem Cytochem 28:746–760, 1980

109. Tubbs RR, Fishleder A, Weiss RA, et al: Immunohistologic cellular phenotypes of lymphoproliferative disorders. Comprehensive evaluation of 546 cases including 257 non-Hodgkin's lymphomas classified by the International Working Formulation. Am J Pathol 113:207–221, 1983

110. Warnke R, Miller R, Grogan T, et al: Immunologic phenotype in 30 patients with diffuse large cell lymphoma. N Engl J Med 303:293–300, 1980

111. Lennert K, Mohri N, Stein H, et al: The histopathology of malignant lymphoma. Brit J Hematol 31:(Suppl):193–203, 1975

112. Lukes RJ, Collins RD: Immunologic characterization of human malignant lymphomas. Cancer 34:1488–1503, 1974

113. National Cancer Institute sponsored study of classification in non-Hodgkin's lymphomas. Summary and description of a working formulation for clinical usage. Cancer 49:2112–2135, 1982

114. Whitcomb CC, Cousar JB, Flint A, et al: Subcategories of histiocytic lymphoma: Associations with survival and reproducibility of classification. The Southwestern Cancer Study Group experience. Cancer 48:2464–2474, 1981

115. Strauchen JA, Young RC, DeVita VT, et al: Clinical relevance of the histopathological subclassification of diffuse "histiocytic" lymphoma. N Engl J Med 299:1382–1387, 1978

116. Isaacson P, Jones DB, Millward-Sadler GH, et al: Alpha-1-antitrypsin in human macrophages. J Clin Pathol 34:982–990, 1981

117. Isaacson P, Wright DH: Immunocytochemistry of lymphoreticular tumors, in Polak JM, van Noorden SV (eds): Immunocytochemistry. Practical applications in pathology and biology. Bristol, Wright PSG, 1983, pp 249–273

118. Hsu A-M, Cossman J, Jaffe ES: Lymphocyte subsets in normal human lymphoid tissue. Am J Clin Pathol 80:21–30, 1983

119. Harris NL, Bahn AK: Distribution of T-cell subsets in follicular and diffuse lymphomas of B-cell type. Am J Pathol 113:172–180, 1983

120. Dvoretsky P, Wood GS, Levy R, et al: T-lymphocyte subsets in follicular lymphomas compared with those in non-neoplastic lymph nodes and tonsils. Human Pathol 13:618–625, 1982

121. Kadin ME: Ia-like (HLA-DR) antigens in the diagnosis of lymphomas and undifferentiated tumors. Arch Pathol Lab Med 104:503–508, 1980

122. Anderson KC, Bates MP, Slaughenhoupt BL, et al: Expression of human B-cell differentiation. Blood 63:1424–1433, 1984

123. Dalchau R, Fabre JW: Identification with monoclonal antibody of a predominantly B-lymphocyte specific determinant of the human leukocyte common antigen. J Exp Med 153:753–765, 1981

124. Levy R, Warnke R, Dorfman RF, et al: Monoclonality of B-cell lymphomas. J Exp Med 145:1014–1028, 1977

125. Taylor CR: Immunocytochemical methods in the study of lymphoma and related conditions. J Histochem Cytochem 26:496–512, 1978

126. Turesson I, Grubb A: Non-secretory myeloma with intracellular kappa light chains. Acta Med Scand 204:445–451, 1978

127. Dreicer R, Alexanian R: Nonsecretory multiple myeloma. Am J Hematol 13:313–318, 1982

128. Lanier LL, Lee AM, Phillips JH, et al: Subpopulations of human natural killer cells defined by expression of the Leu-7 (NHK-1) and Leu-11 (NK-15) antigens. J Immunol 131:1789–1796, 1983

129. Arnold A, Cossman J, Bakhshi A, et al: Immunoglobulin-gene rearrangements as unique clonal markers in human lymphoid neoplasms. N Engl J Med 309:1593–1599, 1983

130. Yunis J: Chromosomal basis of human neoplasia. Science 221:227–235, 1983

131. Trowbridge IS: Interspecies spleen-myeloma hybrid producing monoclonal antibodies against mouse lymphocyte surface glycoprotein, T-200. J Exp Med 148:313–323, 1978

132. Battifora H, Trowbridge IS: A monoclonal antibody useful for the differential diagnosis between malignant lymphoma and nonhematopoietic neoplasms. Cancer 51:816–821, 1983

133. Taylor CR: Immunoperoxidase techniques: Theoretical and practical aspects. Arch Pathol Lab Med 102:113–121, 1978

134. Risdall RJ, Sibley RK, McKenna RW, et al: Malignant histiocytosis. A light- and electron-microscopic and histochemical study. Am J Surg Pathol 4:439–450, 1980

135.   Mendelsohn G, Eggleston JC, Mann RB: Relationship of lysozyme (muramidase) to histiocytic differentiation in malignant histiocytosis. Cancer 45:273–279, 1980

136.   Meister P, Huhn D, Natharath W: Immunohistochemical characterization in paraffin-embedded tissue. Virchows Arch (Pathol Anat) 385:233–246, 1980

137.   Neiman RS, Barcos M, Berard C, et al: Granulocytic sarcoma: A clinical pathologic study of 61 biopsied cases. Cancer 48:1426–1437, 1981

138.   Shey HH, Talle MA, Goldstein G, et al: Functional subsets of human monocytes defined by monoclonal antibodies: A distinct subset of monocytes contains the cells capable of inducing the autologous mixed lymphocyte culture. J Immunol 130:698–705, 1983

139.   Burns BF, Warnke RA, Doggett RS, et al: Expression of a T-cell antigen (Leu-1) by B-cell lymphoma. Am J Pathol 113:165–171, 1983

140.   Foon KA, Schroff RW, Gale RP: Surface markers in leukemia and lymphoma cells. Recent advances. Blood 60:1–29, 1982

141.   Fithian E, Kung P, Goldstein G, et al: Reaction of Langerhan's cells with hybridoma antibody. Proc Natl Acad Sci USA 78:2541–2544, 1981

142.   Fox JL, Berman B: T6-antigen-bearing cells in eosinophilic granuloma. JAMA 249:3071–3072, 1983

143.   Guarda LA, Silva EG, Ordonez NG, et al: Factor VIII in Kaposi's sarcoma. Am J Clin Pathol 76:197–200, 1981

144.   Guarda LA, Ordonez NG, Smith JL, et al: Immunoperoxidase localization of factor VIII in angiosarcomas. Arch Pathol Lab Med 106:515–516, 1982

145.   Ordonez NG, del Junco GW, Ayala AG, et al: Angiosarcoma of the small intestine: An immunoperoxidase study. Am J Gastroenterol 78:218–221, 1983

146.   Mukai K, Rosai J, Hallaway BE: Localization of myoglobin in normal and neoplastic skeletal muscle cells using an immunoperoxidase method. Am J Surg Pathol 3:373–376, 1979

147.   Corson JM, Pinkus GS: Intracellular myoglobin. A specific marker for skeletal muscle differentiation in soft tissue sarcomas. Am J Surg Pathol 103:384–389, 1981

148.   Clayton F, Ordonez NG, Hanssen GM, et al: Immunoperoxidase localization of lactalbumin in malignant breast neoplasms. Arch Pathol Lab Med 106:268–270, 1982

149.   Lee AK, DeLellis RA, Rosen PP, et al: Alpha lactalbumin as an

immunohistochemical marker for metastatic breast carcinoma. Am J Surg Pathol 8:93–100, 1984

150. Bussolati G, Pick A: Mammary and extramammary Paget's disease. An immunocytochemical study. Am J Pathol 80:117–128, 1975

151. Miettinen M, Lehto VP, Virtanen I: Nonpharyngeal lymphoepithelioma. Histological diagnosis as aided by immunohistochemical demonstration of keratin. Virchows Arch (Cell Pathol) 40:163–169, 1982

152. Nagle RB, McDaniel KM, Clark VA, et al: The use of antikeratin antibodies in the diagnosis of human neoplasms. Am J Clin Pathol 79:458–466, 1983

153. Battifora H, Sun T-T, Bahu R, et al: The use of antikeratin antiserum in tumor diagnosis. Lab Invest 42:100, 1980

154. Pinneys NS, Nadji M, Ziegels-Weissman J, et al: Prekeratins in spindle tumors of the skin. Arch Dermatol 119:476–479, 1983

155. Ramaekers F, Puts J, Moesker O, et al: Demonstration of keratin in human adenocarcinomas. Am J Pathol 111:213–223, 1983

156. Said JW: Immunohistochemical localization of keratin protein in tumor diagnosis. Human Pathol 14:1017–1019, 1983

157. Corson JM, Pinkus GS: Mesothelioma, profile of keratin proteins and carcinoembryonic antigens. Am J Pathol 108:80–87, 1982

158. Walts AR, Said JW, Shintaku PI, et al: Keratins of different molecular weight in exfoliated mesothelial and adenocarcinoma cells. An aid to cell identification. Am J Clin Pathol 81:442–446, 1984

159. Said JW, Nash G, Lee M: Immunoperoxidase localization of keratin proteins, carcinoembryonic antigen, and factor VIII in adenomatoid tumors. Evidence of a mesothelial derivation. Human Pathol 13:1106–1108, 1982

160. Denk H, Krepler R, Artlieb U, et al: Proteins of intermediate filaments. An immunohistochemical and biochemical approach to the classification of soft tissue tumors. Am J Pathol 110:193–208, 1983

161. Gabbiani G, Kapanci Y, Barazzone P, et al: Immunohistochemical identification of intermediate-sized filaments in human neoplastic cells. Am J Pathol 104:206–216, 1981

162. Caselitz J, Janner M, Breitbart E, et al: Malignant melanomas contain only the vimentin type intermediate filaments. Virchows Arch (Pathol Anat) 400:43–51, 1983

163. Ramaekers FS, Puts JG, Moesker O, et al: Intermediate filaments in melanoma. J Clin Invest 71:635–643, 1983

164. Miettinen M, Lehto VP, Badley RA, et al: Alveolar rhabdomyosar-

coma. Demonstration of the muscle type of intermediate filament protein, desmin, as a diagnostic aid. Am J Pathol 108:246–251, 1982

165. Velasco ME, Dahl D, Roessman U, et al: Immunohistochemical localization of glial fibrillary acidic protein in human glial neoplasms. Cancer 45:484–494, 1980

166. Marsden HB, Kumar S, Kahn J, et al: A study of glial fibrillary acidic protein (GFAP) in childhood brain tumors. Int J Cancer 31:439–445, 1983

167. Osborn M, Altmannsberger M, Shaw G, et al: Various sympathetic derived human tumors differ in neurofilament expression: Use in diagnosis of neuroblastoma, ganglioneuroblastoma and pheochromocytoma. Virchows Arch (Cell Pathol) 40:141–156, 1982

168. Trojanowsky JQ, Lee VMY, Schlaepfer WW: An immunohistochemical study of human central and peripheral nervous system tumors, using monoclonal antibodies against neurofilaments and glial filaments. Human Pathol 15:248–257, 1984

169. Osborn M, Altmannsberger M, Shaw G, et al: Various sympathetic derived human tumors differ in neurofilament expression. Virchows Arch (Cell Pathol) 40:141–156, 1982

170. Miettinen M, Lehto VP, Virtanen I, et al: Neuroendocrine carcinoma of the skin (Merkel cell carcinoma): Ultrastructural and immunohistochemical demonstration of neurofilaments. Ultrastruct Pathol 4:219–225, 1983

171. Rungger-Brandle E, Gabbiani G: The role of cytoskeletal and cytocontractile elements in pathologic processes. Am J Pathol 110:361–392, 1983

172. Osborn M, Weber K: Biology of disease. Tumor diagnosis by intermediate filament types: A novel tool for surgical pathology. Lab Invest 48:372–394, 1983

173. Osborn M, Franke WW, Weber K: Direct demonstration of the presence of two immunologically distinct intermediate-sized filament systems in the same cell by double immunofluorescence technique: Vimentin and cytokeratin fibers in culture of epithelial cells. Exp Cell Res 125:37–46, 1980

174. Gabbiani G, Schmid E, Winters S, et al: Vascular smooth muscle cells differ from other smooth muscle cells. Predominance of vimentin filaments and of specific alpha type actin. Proc Natl Acad Sci USA 78:298–302 1978

175. Frank ED, Warren L: Aortic smooth muscle cell contain vimentin instead of desmin. Proc Natl Acad Sci USA 78:3020–3024, 1981

176. Schmid E, Osborn M, Rungger-Brandle E, et al: Distribution of

vimentin and desmin filaments in smooth muscle tissues of mammalian and avian aorta. Exp Cell Res 137:329–240, 1982

177. Chase DR, Enzinger FM, Weiss SW, et al: Keratin in epithelioid sarcoma. An immunohistochemical study. Am J Surg Pathol 8:435–441, 1984

178. Miettinen M, Lehto VP, Virtanen I: Keratin in the epithelial-like cells of classic biphasic synovial sarcoma. Virchows Arch (Cell Pathol) 40:157–161, 1982

179. Corson JM, Weiss LM, Banks-Schlegel SP, et al: Keratin proteins in synovial sarcoma. Am J Surg Pathol 7:107–109, 1983

180. Altmannsberger M, Osborn M, Schauer A, et al: Antibodies to different intermediate filament proteins: Cell type specific markers on paraffin-embedded human tissues. Lab Invest 45:427–434, 1981

181. Palmer PE, Wolfe HJ: Immunocytochemical localization of oncodevelopmental proteins in human germ cell and hepatic tumors. J Histochem Cytochem 26:523–531, 1978

182. Kodama T, Kemeya T, Hirota T, et al: Production of alpha fetoprotein, normal serum proteins, and human chorionic gonadotropin in stomach cancer: Histologic and immunohistochemical analysis of 35 cases. Cancer 48:1647–1655, 1981

183. Ordonez NG, Manning JT, Hansson G: Alpha-1-antitrypsin in islet cell tumors of the pancreas. Am J Clin Pathol 80:277–282, 1983

184. Ordonez NG, Manning JT: Comparison of alpha-1-antitrypsin and alpha-1-antichymotrypsin in hepatocellular carcinoma. An immunoperoxidase study. Am J Gastroenterol 79:959–963, 1984

185. Moore BW: A soluble protein characteristic of the nervous system. Biochem Biophys Res Commu 19:739–744, 1965

186. Kahn HJ, Marks A, Thom H, et al: Role of antibody to S-100 protein in diagnostic pathology. Am J Clin Pathol 79:341–347, 1983

187. Haglid K, Hamberger A, Hansson HA, et al: S-100 protein in synapses of the central nervous system. Nature 251:532–534, 1974

188. Nakajima T, Shaw W, Sato Y, et al: An immunoperoxidase study of S-100 protein distribution in normal and neoplastic tissues. Am J Surg Pathol 6:715–727, 1982

189. Takahashi K, Yumaguchi H, Ishizeki J, et al: Immunohistochemical and immunoreaction microscopic localization of S-100 protein in the interdigitating reticulum cells of the human lymph node. Virchows Arch (Cell Pathol) 37:125–135, 1981

190. Stafansson K, Wollmann RL, Moore W, et al: S-100 protein in human chondrocytes. Nature 295:63–64, 1982

191. Haglid K, Hamberger A, Hansson HA, et al: An immunohistochemi-

cal study of human brain tumors concerning the brain specific proteins S-100 and 14-3-2. Acta Neuropathol (Berlin) 24:187–196, 1978

192. Jacque CM, Kujas M, Poreau A, et al: CGA and S-100 proteins levels and index of malignancy in human gliomas and neurinomas. J Natl Cancer Inst 62:479–483, 1979

193. Mukai M: Immunohistochemical localization of S-100 protein and peripheral nerve myelin proteins (P2 protein, PO protein) in granular cell tumors. Am J Pathol 112:139–146, 1983

194. Nakamura Y, Becker LE, Marks A: S-100 protein in human chordoma and human and rabbit notocord. Arch Pathol Lab Med 107:118–120, 1983

195. Nakazato Y, Ishizeki J, Takahashi K, et al: Localization of S-100 protein and glial fibrillary acidic protein-related antigen in pleomorphic adenoma of the salivary glands. Lab Invest 46:621–626, 1982

196. Gaynor R, Irie R, Morton D, et al: S-100 protein is present in cultured malignant melanomas. Nature 286:400–401, 1982

197. Nakajima T, Watanabe S, Sato Y, et al: Immunohistochemical demonstration of S-100 protein in malignant melanoma and pigmented nevus, and its diagnostic applications. Cancer 50:912–918, 1982

198. Springall DR, Gu J, Cocchia D, et al: The value of S-100 immunostaining as a diagnostic tool in human malignant melanomas. A comparative study using S-100 and neuron-specific enolase antibodies. Virchows Arch (Pathol Anat) 400:331–343, 1983

199. Steffansson K, Wollmann R, Jerkovic M: S-100 protein in soft tissue tumors derived from Schwann cells and melanocytes. Am J Pathol 106:261–268, 1982

200. Weiss SW, Langloss JM, Enzinger FM: Vale of S-100 protein in the diagnosis of soft tissue tumors with particular reference to benign and malignant Schwann cell tumors. Lab Invest 49:299–308, 1983

201. Goldenberg DM, Sharkey RM, Primus FJ: Immunocytochemical detection of carcinoembryonic antigen in conventional histopathology specimens. Cancer 42:1546–1553, 1978

202. Walker RA: Demonstration of carcinoembryonic antigen in human breast cancer by immunoperoxidase technique. J Clin Pathol 33:356–360, 1980

203. Hamada S, Hamada S: Localization of carcinoembryonic antigen in medullary thyroid carcinomas by immunofluorescence technique. Brit J Cancer 36:572–576, 1977

204. Prumus FJ, Clark CA, Goldenerg DM: Immunohistochemical detec-

tion of carcinoembryonic antigen, in DeLellis RA (ed): Diagnostic Immunocytochemistry. New York, Masson Publishing USA Inc., 1981, pp 263–276

205. Holden J, Churg A: Immunohistochemical staining for keratin and carcinoembryonic antigen in the diagnosis of malignant mesothelioma. Am J Surg Pathol 8:277–279, 1984

206. Whitaker D, Sterrett GF, Shilkin KB: Detection of tissue CEA-like substance as an aid in the differential diagnosis of malignant mesothelioma. Pathology 14:255–258, 1982

207. Hanna W, Ryder DE, Mobbs BG: Cellular localization of estrogen binding sites in human breast cancer. Am J Clin Pathol 77:391–395, 1982

208. Lange PH, Limas C, Fraley EE: Tissue blood-group antigens and prognosis in low stage transitional cell carcinoma of the bladder. J Urol 119:52–55, 1978

209. Weinstein RS, Alroy JM, Davidsohn I: Tissue-associated blood group antigens in human tumors, in DeLellis RA (ed): Diagnostic Immunocytochemistry. New York, Masson Publishing USA Inc., 1981, pp 239–267

210. Coons JS, Weinstein RS, Summers JL: Blood group precursor T-antigen expression in human bladder carcinoma. Am J Clin Pathol 77:679–699, 1982

211. Stafl A, Mattingley RF: Isoantigens ABO in cervical neoplasia. Gynecol Obstetr 1:26–35, 1972

212. Davidsohn I, Kovarik S, Li LY: Isoantigens A, B and H in benign and malignant lesions of the cervix. Arch Pathol 87:306–314, 1969

213. Gupta RK, Schuster R, Christian WD: Loss of isoantigens A, B and H in prostate. Am J Pathol 70:439–447, 1973

214. Bentz MS, Cohen C, Mudgeon LR, et al: Evaluation of commercial immunoperoxidase kits in diagnosis of prostate carcinoma. Urology 23:75–78, 1984

215. Wilson AJ: Factor VIII-related antigen staining by immunoperoxidase technique in smaller laboratories: A potential problem. Am J Clin Pathol 81:117–120, 1984

216. Lin C-W, Sasaki M, Orcutt ML, et al: Plasma membrane localization of alkaline phosphatase in HeLa cells. J Histochem Cytochem 24:659–667, 1976

217. Bruns DE, Mills SE, Savoroy J: Amylase in fallopian tube and serous ovarian neoplasms. Immunohistochemical localization. Arch Pathol Lab Med 106:17–20, 1982

218. Batsakis JG, Ordonez NG, Krueger JJ, et al: Acinic cell carcinoma of

investigations of tumors of supposed fibroblastic-histiocytic origin. Human Pathol 13:834–840, 1982

233. Brooks JJ: Immunohistochemistry of soft tissue tumors: Progress and prospects. Human Pathol 13:969–974. 1982

234. Miller F, Lazarides E, Elias J: Application of immunological probes for contractile proteins to tissue sections. Clin Immunol Immuno-pathol 5:416–428, 1976

235. Donner L, Lanerolle P, Costa J: Immunoreactivity of paraffin-embedded normal tissues and mesenchymal tumors for smooth muscle myosin. Am J Clin Pathol 80:677–681, 1983

236. Bures JC, Barnes L, Mercer D: A comparative study of smooth muscle tumors utilizing light and electron microscopy, immunocyto-chemical staining and enzymatic assay. Cancer 48:2420–2426, 1981

237. Singh G, Katyal SL, Ordonez NG, et al: Type II pneumocytes in pulmonary tumors. Implications for histogenesis. Arch Pathol Lab Med 108:44–48, 1984

238. Karnovsky MJ: A formaldehyde-glutaraldehyde fixative of high osmolarity for use in electron microscopy. J Cell Biol 27:137A, 1965

239. McDowell EM, Trump BF: Histologic fixatives suitable for diagnostic light and electron microscopy. Arch Pathol Lab Med 100:405–412, 1976

240. Carson F, Martin JH, Lynn JA: Formalin fixation for electron micros-copy: a re-evaluation. Am J Clin Pathol 59:365–373, 1978

241. Baur PS, Mackay B: Technical procedures, in Mackay B (ed): Intro-duction to Diagnostic Electron Microscopy. New York, Appleton-Century-Crofts, 1981, pp 29–45

242. Akhtar M, Ali MA, Owen EW: Application of electron microscopy in the interpretation of fine-needle aspiration biopsies. Cancer 48:2458–2463, 1981

243. Hickey WF, Seiler MW: Ultrastructural markers of colonic adenocar-cinoma. Cancer 47:140–145, 1981

244. Susuki Y, Churg J, Kannerstein M: Ultrastructure of human malig-nant diffuse mesothelioma. Am J Pathol 85:241–252, 1976

245. Battifora H: Intracytoplasmic lumina in breast carcinoma. Arch Pathol 99:614–617, 1975

246. Newland JR, Mackay B, Hill CS, et al: Anaplastic thyroid carcinoma: An ultrastructural study of 10 cases. Ultrastruct Pathol 2:121–129, 1981

247. Mackay B: Ultrastructure of lung neoplasms, in Straus MJ (ed): Diagnosis and Treatment of Lung Carcinoma (2nd ed). New York, Grune & Stratton, 1983, pp 85–96

248. Feldman PA, Horvath E, Kovacs K: Ultrastructure of three Hurthle cell tumors of the thyroid. Cancer 30:1279–1285, 1972

249. Johns ME, Regesi JA, Batsakis JG: Oncocytic neoplasms of salivary glands—ultrastructural study. Laryngoscope 87:862–871, 1977

250. Ordonez NG, Ibanez ML, Mackay B, et al: Functioning oxyphil cell adenomas of parathyroid gland. Immunoperoxidase evidence of hormonal activity in oxyphil cells. Am J Clin Pathol 78:681–689, 1982

251. Sajjad SM, Mackay B, Lukeman JM: Oncocytic carcinoid tumor of the lung. Ultrastruct Pathol 1:171–176, 1980

252. Klein JJ, Valensi QJ: Proximal tubular adenomas of kidney with so-called oncocytic features—clinicopathologic study of 13 cases of a rarely reported neoplasm. Cancer 38:906–914, 1976

253. Silva EG, Mackay B, Samaan NB, et al: Adrenocortical carcinomas—an ultrastructural study of 22 cases. Ultrastruct Pathol 3:8, 1982

254. Osborne BM, Culbert S, Cangir A, et al: Acinar cell carcinoma of the pancreas in a 9 year old child: Case report with electron microscopic observations. South Med Assoc J 70:370–372, 1977

255. Mackay B: Tumor diagnosis, in Mackay B (ed): Introduction to Diagnostic Electron Microscopy. New York, Appleton-Century-Crofts, 1981, pp 221–255

256. Silva EG, Mackay B: Neuroendocrine (Merkel cell) carcinomas of the skin: An ultrastructural study of nine cases. Ultrastruct Pathol 2:1–9, 1981

257. Mazur MT, Katzenstein A-LA: Metastatic melanoma: The spectrum of ultrastructural morphology. Ultrastruct Pathol 1:337–356, 1980

258. Carle G, Alastair M: Malignant melanoma in the gallbladder. A case report. Cancer 48:2318–2322, 1981

259. Robertson AJ: Primary melanocarcinoma of the lower respiratory tract. Thorax 35:158–159, 1980

260. Chung EB, Enzinger FM: Clear cell sarcoma of tendons and aponeuroses: Further observations. Lab Invest 38:8, 1978

261. Mennemeyer RP, Hammar SP, Tytus JS, et al: Melanotic schwannoma. Clinical and ultrastructural studies of three cases with evidence of intracellular melanin synthesis. Am J Surg Pathol 3:3–10, 1979

262. Osborne BM: Hematologic disorders, in Mackay B (ed): Introduction to Diagnostic Electron Microscopy. New York, Appleton-Century-Crofts, 1981, pp 171–196

263. Bernier GM, Graham RC Jr: Plasma cell asynchrony in myeloma: Correlation of light and electron microscopy. Semin Hematol 13:239–245, 1976

264. Cutler LS, Krutchkoff D: An ultrastructural study of eosinophilic granuloma: The Langerhans cell—its role in histogenesis and diagnosis. Oral Surg Med Pathol 44:246–252, 1977

265. Rosai J, Levine GD: Tumors of the Thymus. Atlas of Tumor Pathology. Washington, Armed Forces Institute of Pathology, Fasc 13, 1976

266. Schmidt D, Mackay B, Luna MA: Aggressive meningioma with jugular vein extension. Arch Otolaryngol 107:635–637, 1981

267. Mackay B: Electron microscopy of soft tissue tumors, in Management of Primary Bone and Soft Tissue Tumors—M.D. Anderson Hospital and Tumor Institute. Chicago, Year Book, 1977, pp 259–269

268. Moertel CG: Adenocarcinoma of unknown origin. Ann Intern Med 91:646–647, 1979

269. Steward JF, Tattersall MHN, Woods RL, et al: Unknown primary adenocarcinoma: Incidence of overinvestigation and natural history. Br Med J 1:1530–1533, 1979

270. Holmes FF, Fouts TI: Metastatic cancer of unknown primary site. Cancer 46:816–830, 1970

271. Didolkar S, Fanous N, Elias EG, et al: Metastatic carcinomas of occult primary tumors. A study of 254 cases. Ann Surg 186:625–630, 1977

272. Krementz ET, Cerise EJ, Ciaravella JM Jr, et al: Metastases of undetermined source. Cancer 27:289–300, 1977

273. Batsakis JG: The pathology of head and neck tumors. x. The occult primary and metastases to the head and neck. Head Neck Surg 3:409–423, 1981

274. Copeland EM, McBride CM: Axillary metastases from unknown primary sites. Ann Surg 178:25–27, 1973

275. Zaren HA, Copeland EM: Inguinal node metastases. Cancer 41:919–923, 1978

3

IMMUNOLOGIC AND BIOCHEMICAL MARKERS IN THE DIAGNOSIS AND MANAGEMENT OF POORLY DIFFERENTIATED NEOPLASMS AND CANCERS OF UNKNOWN PRIMARY

Raymond W. Ruddon

Tumor markers have been used clinically in a number of ways: to aid in differential diagnosis, to give an index of stage of disease and patient prognosis, and to provide an indicator of response to therapy and disease recurrence. In some instances, the pattern of marker production gives an idea of the differentiation state of the tumor and may suggest the tissue of its origin. By definition, malignant tumors are phenotypically abnormal compared to their normal counterparts, and the malignant phenotype often tends to reflect a more poorly differentiated state than that of the normal cells of the originating tissue. There is, however, a great deal of biochemical heterogeneity among the cells of a given tumor. Moreover, the more anaplastic a tumor becomes, the more it may resemble other undifferentiated cancers. For example, Knox[1] measured 30 biochemical indices in rat tumor cells and found that poorly differentiated mammary

POORLY DIFFERENTIATED NEOPLASMS AND TUMORS OF UNKNOWN ORIGIN   ISBN 0-8089-1755-2

carcinomas more closely resembled themselves and undifferentiated hepatomas than they did a well–differentiated mammary carcinoma or normal mammary tissue. Thus, the pattern of biochemical marker production by poorly differentiated tumors may be more indicative of an immature proliferating tumor cell population than of the tissue of origin of the tumor. With the development of monoclonal antibodies that recognize tissue and differentiation-stage specific cell surface antigens for a variety of cell types, however, there is hope that, with appropriate panels of monoclonal antibodies, a fingerprint for each tumor type will be possible.

It has been frequently stated as a generalization that malignant tumors tend to have a genetic program that is more characteristic of an earlier state of tissue differentiation. How this comes about is in some dispute. One school of thought maintains that it happens by means of a "dedifferentiation" of normal cells that have been damaged by a carcinogenic agent or a combination of carcinogenic agents to produce a population of cells with a more fetal-like phenotype. Another school holds that the committed but not yet fully differentiated "stem" cells of normal adult tissues are the targets for carcinogenic agents and that after carcinogenic insult the progeny of these cells are prevented from differentiating further and continue to multiply in an uncontrolled manner. There is some evidence to support both of these possibilities, although the clearest evidence supports the latter point of view. For example, data on the transformation of hematopoietic stem cells by the oncogenic Friend virus or the avian erythroblastosis virus indicate that the target cell in these virus-induced leukemias is the erythroid precursor cell of the CFU-E type.[2,3] At any rate, the observation that malignantly transformed cells have an altered phenotype reflecting an earlier state of differentiation of the organism is widely supported by both clinical and cell culture studies. The markers that reflect the immature phenotype of cancer cells are sometimes called "oncodevelopmental" markers and include oncofetal antigens, such as alpha fetoprotein (AFP), placental hormones, such as chorionic gonadotropin (hCG) and placental lactogen (hPL), and developmental isoenzymes, such as placental alkaline phosphatase. Each of these classes of markers will be discussed below.

It should be emphasized at the outset that no clear pattern of "ectopic" (i.e., gene product not normally made in tissue of origin) oncodevelopmental gene expression occurs in cancer cells. There is a significant amount of data from both clinical and cell culture studies that indicate a large degree of discordance in expression of such genes.[4–6] For instance, in a study of 67 malignant cell lines derived from a wide variety of human cancers, Neuwald et al.[6] found that 68 percent of these cell lines produced markedly elevated levels of at least one oncodevelopmental marker, but that there was no predictable coexpression of any two of these markers. Moreover, although the production of oncodevelopmental markers by human cancers is a common phenomenon, it is by no means restricted to cancer cells, but may also occur in nonmalignant diseases. As illustrations, about 8 percent of patients with regional enteritis or ulcerative colitis, 11 percent with cirrhosis of the liver, and 17 percent with duodenal ulcers have elevated levels of hCG in their blood.[7] Similarly, serum AFP levels have been reported to be elevated in 15–51 percent of patients with chronic hepatic disorders and in 33 percent of patients with acute hepatitis.[8] These data indicate that the increased production of so-called oncodevelopmental markers is not specific for neoplastic disease, but may also be triggered by tissue damage by any of a number of disease processes.

Another point to consider is that ectopic expression of certain normally repressed genes varies to some extent with the tissue of origin of the tumor. For example, ectopic ACTH secretion most commonly occurs with bronchogenic carcinomas, whereas ectopic hCG secretion is more commonly seen with gastrointestinal (GI) tract cancers. This may reflect the fact that the pathways of differentiation (or "dedifferentiation") are different in different tissues and that tissues have different populations of cell types, but this cannot be the complete explanation because lung cancers of various histologic types may produce hCG,[9] some GI cancers produce ACTH,[10] and a variety of other oncodevelopmental markers (e.g., AFP, placental alkaline phosphatase, CEA) are produced by both kinds of cancers.

Based on these observations, there is apparently no predictable pattern of ectopic gene re-expression in cancer cells. Advancing knowledge in oncology, and specifically in the field of oncogene expression by various human cancers, however, may reveal a more predictable pattern of gene expression that relates to the tissue of origin of the tumor. If the products of the onc genes circulate in body fluids in detectable levels, a whole new class of diagnostic tumor markers would become available.

The incidence of oncodevelopmental gene expression is high for certain markers in neoplasms in which their production is "eutopic" (i.e., expected gene product). For example, AFP is much more likely to be produced by germ cell tumors of the testis or ovary or by hepatocellular carcinoma than by other tumors. hCG is almost invariably produced by trophoblastic malignancies. Thus, production of AFP or hCG is more likely to indicate the presence of endodermal sinus (yolk sac) elements or trophoblastic cells, respectively, than it is to predict the degree of differentiation of the whole population of cancer cells in a given malignant neoplasm.

It would be helpful to know whether the production of a given tumor marker can be used to predict the sensitivity of various tumors to chemotherapeutic agents. In other words, is a bronchogenic carcinoma or a breast carcinoma that produces hCG or placental alkaline phosphatase or CEA, for example, more or less likely to respond to various anticancer agents? There is as yet very little clinical data to answer this question.

Tissue and Differentiation-Stage Specific Markers

There are now several tissue cell types for which panels of monoclonal antibodies have been developed. These antibodies can be used to type the stage of differentiation in a tissue–specific manner. A few examples will suffice to make this point.

Lymphoid Cells

Using monoclonal antibodies, it has been possible to define a series of specific cell surface glycoproteins that appear at discrete stages of human T lymphocyte differentiation. Despite the morphologic similarity of T lymphocytes, a great degree of functional heterogeneity exists. Tumors arising from such a functionally diverse cellular compartment would also be expected to show considerable heterogeneity, and they do. It is now possible to type the stage of differentiation of a lymphoid leukemia cell population utilizing the monoclonal antibodies to recognize antigens restricted in their pattern of expression to cells of T cell lineage.[11]

In the human thymus gland where T cell differentiation occurs, the earliest cells in the T lineage are rapidly proliferating and bear two distinct antigens, T_9 and T_{10} (Stage I). These antigens are shared by some other bone marrow cells, but are not present on mature T cells. During the next step in maturation, T lymphocytes lose T_9, maintain T_{10}, and acquire a T cell-specific antigen, T_6. These cells (called Stage II cells) also express additional markers defined by anti-T_4 and anti-$T_{5/8}$. With further differentiation, the T cells lose T_6, gain T_1, T_3, and T_{12} antigens, and separate into T_4 and $T_{5/8}$ subsets of T cells, which have inducer and cytotoxic/suppression functions, respectively (Stage III).

T cell malignancies reflect the same degree of heterogeneity and the differentiation profile seen in normal T cell ontogeny.[11-13] In these studies, 41 of 60 T cell acute leukemias (ALLs) possessed antigens found on prothymocytes or early T cells; 13 of 60 T cell ALLs expressed antigens found in Stage II of differentiation, and only 2 of 60 expressed Stage III differentiation antigens. The stage of differentiation as indicated by the expression of these stage-specific antigens appears to have both therapeutic and prognostic implications.

Myeloid Cells

Acute myelogenous leukemia (AML) is a heterogeneous disease that has traditionally been classified into subsets based primarily on cell morphology and cytochemistry. This approach, however, has yielded limited information regarding prognosis or response to therapy. As in the case of lymphoid cells, monoclonal antibodies have now been developed that demonstrate the presence of cell surface antigens restricted to myeloid cells.[14-16] These antigens, which also appear to be differentiation stage-specific, may identify subsets of myeloid leukemia that correlate with cell morphology, clinical course, and response to therapy.

Melanoma

Although the study of differentiation antigens on T and B lymphocytes of mouse and man is relatively advanced, the characterization of differentiation antigens displayed on normal and neoplastic cells of other cellular lineages is still in its beginning stages. One cell type which has been well-characterized is the melanocyte and its corresponding malignant cell type, the melanoma cell.[17] The availability of a large number of melanoma-derived cell lines has now made possible a detailed analysis of melanoma surface antigens.

There are at least three distinct stages in melanocyte differentiation, based on surface antigenic phenotype, morphology, and biochemical markers: precursor, intermediate, and mature. Similarly, on the basis of surface antigens, morphology, pigmentation, and tyrosinase activity, three classes of melanoma can be defined corresponding to the early, intermediate, or mature phases of melanocyte differentiation. In one study of 25 melanoma cell lines,[17] 5 melanomas expressed early markers, 10 intermediate markers, and 10 late melanocyte markers. One surface antigen, M-18, was found at all stages of melanocyte differentiation and was present on all melanoma cells, but almost no cross-reactivity with other fetal or adult normal tissues or other neoplastic cell types was seen. Thus, this marker is an example of an ideal candidate for typing of tumors of unknown primary source.

Melanomas expressing the early differentiation phenotype have M-2, M-3, M-18, and HLA-DR antigens on the surface, have an epithelioid morphology, lack pigmentation, and have low levels of tyrosinase. Melanomas with an intermediate differentiation stage phenotype express M-4, M-6, and M-18 antigens, and generally have spindle morphology, little pigmentation, and low levels of tyrosinase. Melanomas expressing late markers, M-9 and M-10, as well as the general tissue-specific marker M-18, are spindle-shaped or polydendritic, pigmented, and have high tyrosinase activity.

An interesting question raised by these data is whether melanomas arise at various stages of differentiation (i.e., is the target cell for the carcinogenic event potentially any cell in the differentiation pathway?), or is there one target cell type for malignant transformation? In the latter case, one would have to postulate that the early differentiation stage-transformed cell could progress to various stages of differentiation before being arrested in that stage. Data showing that different metastatic sites from an individual patient vary in their phenotype[18] support the hypothesis that transformation occurs at an early stage of differentiation and that the progeny of transformed cells have variable capacity to differentiate toward later stages (assuming that the clonal hypothesis of cancer development is correct for melanomas). It will be interesting to see whether normal melanocytes at different stages of differentiation can be transformed by viruses or chemical carcinogens.

Renal Cancer

Based on monoclonal antibody probes, a number of human kidney differentiation stage and kidney cell type-specific antigens have been identified.[19] Some of these determinants are also expressed by renal tumors. It is now literally possible to "immunodissect" the urinary tract based on cell type-specific monoclonal antibodies directed against renal cells of various types, e.g., glomerulus, proximal tubule, collecting duct, and urinary bladder epithelium,[20] and one would presume that renal tumors arising from these various cell types would be similarly distinguishable based on their cell surface antigenic phenotype.

Interestingly, although a number of tissue type-specific antigens have been identified by monoclonal antibody "mapping," antigens that are truly tumor-specific (in the sense that they appear only on cancer cells of a certain type and not also on normal cells from some stage of differentiation of the tissue of origin) have not been found. This does not mean that they don't exist, but it will be most difficult to find markers that are cancer-specific in addition to being tissue type-specific.

Oncofetal Antigens

Alpha Fetoprotein (AFP)

AFP is one of the most thoroughly studied oncofetal antigens from a clinical point of view. It is a serum protein similar to size and amino acid composition to serum albumin, is produced in high amounts by fetal liver and yolk sac, and can be detected in amniotic fluid and maternal serum. In the normal adult, AFP is present in small amounts (less than 20 ng/ml) in the serum. Elevated serum concentrations occur in the adult after exposure to hepatotoxic agents or in patients with hepatocellular carcinomas or tumors containing yolk sac-type cells. AFP was first detected in fetal cord blood in 1957 by Berstrand and Czar[21] and later found in mice and patients with hepatocellular carcinomas.[22,23] Abnormally high concentrations of AFP occur in amniotic fluid and maternal serum in certain fetal malformations, such as neural tube defects, anencephaly, esophageal atresia, and congenital nephrosis.[5] In the adult, serum concentrations greater than 1000 ng/ml are almost always indicative of malignant neoplasm. Lower, transitory elevations may be present with liver injury, whereas sustained or increasing elevations are more often seen with cancer.

AFP is elevated in about 80 percent of patients with primary hepatocellular carcinomas and in almost all teratocarcinomas that contain endodermal sinus (yolk sac) elements. Highly elevated levels of serum AFP also occur in patients with extragonadal tumors containing yolk sac elements. There is a good correlation between the levels of AFP and the amount of yolk sac elements in the tumor.[24] Patients with gonadal tumors of non-germ cell origin generally have normal AFP levels. Slightly elevated levels of AFP (60 ng/ml) have been observed in a few patients with "pure" embryonal carcinomas of the testes[24] or with pure seminoma,[25] but these tumors probably have minor populations of yolk sac-like cells. In some of these latter cases, modest elevations of AFP may be due to liver metastases when active liver regeneration is occurring.[25]

Concomitant use of AFP and hCG as markers detects about 90 percent of nonseminomatous testicular cancers.[26] Serial assays of hCG and AFP provide an accurate monitor of disease activity and response to therapy in those patients with marker-positive tumors. Discordance between the two markers, however, can occur,[27] showing that different cell types, presumably with different drug sensitivities, produce the two markers. Falling marker levels usually reflect response to treatment and rising levels indicate progression of disease, and they may predict disease recurrence by as much as six months before clinical evidence for recurrence.[28] Persistently high marker levels after orchiectomy or chemotherapy invariably indicate residual disease (after taking into account the metabolic clearance rates of the markers). Normal marker levels, however, may occur in about 9 percent of patients with nonseminomatous metastases.[28] A persistent mass in a treated patient with previously elevated marker levels that have returned to the normal range often indicates a residual mature teratoma. Surgical removal of the residual tumor may then lead to long-term survival.[28]

Elevated serum AFP levels have also been reported for 15 percent of 95 patients with gastric, 3 percent of 191 patients with colorectal, 24 percent of 45 patients with pancreatic, and 25 percent of 8 patients with biliary tract carcinomas.[29] Most of the patients in this study had advanced metastatic disease, and a number had liver metastases. The presence of AFP in a primary, moderately well-differentiated adenocarcinoma of the lung has also been reported.[30] Presumably, these latter tumors contained some yolk sac-like elements, but this was not demonstrated.

CEA

Carcinoembryonic antigen (CEA) was first described by Gold and Freedman,[31] who detected it in colon carcinomas and fetal gastrointestinal tract tissue. Although CEA is frequently described as an oncofetal tumor antigen, it really is not, at least in the sense that AFP is. CEA or CEA-like material is produced by a variety of mucin-producing normal epithelial tissues[32] and has been identified in colon lavages of healthy individuals.[33] Furthermore, its production is not limited to a particular cancer cell type, but is produced by a wide variety of cancers of epithelial origin. Also, it is more likely to be produced by well-differentiated gastric or colon carcino-mas than by anaplastic ones.[34] Less well-differentiated gastric tumors may also produce CEA, but at a lower level.[35] CEA does not appear to be produced by germ cell tumors and is a poor marker for testicular carcinomas.[26,36]

The use of CEA in the management of colorectal cancer is well-documented.[37] It also has some usefulness in determining tumor burden, prognosis, and response to therapy in other epithelial cancers, including breast carcinomas, bronchogenic carcinomas, and gynecological malignancies. Immunofluorescent staining for CEA of specimens obtained by biopsy or surgery has been used to determine whether a poorly differentiated gastric neoplasm is anaplastic carcinoma or histiocytic lymphoma, since the former shows membrane staining for CEA-like material, whereas histiocytic lymphomas do not contain this material.[35] A similar example is the use of CEA immunofluorescent staining to distinguish between lung tumors arising from bronchial epithelium and mesotheliomas or carcinoid tumors.[38] In this study, all 13 cases of bronchogenic carcinoma examined were positive for CEA-like material, whereas 12 out of 12 cases of mesothelioma and a carcinoid tumor were negative.

There is some evidence for the presence of different antigenic determinants on CEAs isolated from colon carcinoma and other cancerous tissues such as breast and ovarian carcinomas,[39] but these differences appear to be subtle and they have not been exploited clinically.

Other Tumor-Associated Antigens

A large number of tumor-associated antigenic substances have been identified in human cancer cells. Some of these have been biochemically characterized; others have not. Many of them also appear to be present in fetal tissues and so may be oncodevelopmental antigens like AFP. To date, however, none of these tumor-associated antigens have been widely used in the clinic. The human cancers for which tumor antigens have been found include melanoma,[40-43] neuroblastoma,[44] glioma,[45] colorectal carcinoma,[46] gastric carcinoma,[47,48] mammary carcinoma,[49-52] bronchogenic carcinoma,[53-58] pancreatic carcinoma,[59-62] ovarian carcinoma,[63-65] Wilms' tumor,[66] renal cell carcinoma,[67] transitional cell carcinoma of the bladder,[68] osteogenic sarcoma,[69] carcinoma of the uterine cervix,[70] and lymphoma.[71] Monoclonal antibody technology is providing a new way to detect tumor-associated antigens, and more and more of them are being reported. Monoclonal antibodies should provide greater specificity for tumor-associated antigenic substances, and these antibodies may provide more specific probes to determine if cancer cells are present in a biopsy or a body fluid sample and to establish the tumor cell type, although, as noted above, it has proven difficult to do both because tumor-*specific* antigens have not been identified for most tumor types.

Hormones

Hormone production by malignant neoplasms is basically of two types: that which is appropriate to the tissue in which the tumor arises (eutopic) and that which is inappropriate to the tissue of origin of the tumor (ectopic). These distinctions are not necessarily clearcut. For example, the cells that make up a small cell carcinoma of the lung, tumors which may produce a variety of ectopic polypeptide hormones, have some characteristics of cells of neuroectodermal origin, the so-called amine precursor uptake and decarboxylation (APUD) cell type.[72] Populations of cells derived from primitive neuroectoderm may reside in the lung and become clonally expanded during carcinogenesis. Thus, the production of hormones in this case may not be truly ectopic in the sense that the tumor may be derived from a more primitive cell type programmed to produce the hormone(s).

Although the APUDoma hypothesis cannot explain the inappropriate production of hormones of non-neuroectodermal origin by tumors, similar arguments could be made for their production. For instance, certain primitive stem cells that still produce small amounts of placental or fetal proteins could reside in tissues, and, after carcinogenic damage, this population could be expanded to make up a significant percentage of the tumor cells. Other explanations, of course, are also possible. A mutation in a regulatory gene leading to the "derepression" of oncodevelopmental genes, amplication of these genes in tumor cells, or alterations in rates of mRNA transcription, processing, or degradation could also explain the increased expression of certain more primitive gene products. Regardless of the mechanism, the fact is that many human cancers produce extra amounts of hormones. In the cases where the hormonal form produced has biological activity, a clinical syndrome reflecting hormone overproduction may result. This, however, is a small percentage of the total number of cancer patients whose tumors produce hormones[73] because in many cases the form of the hormone produced has minimal biological activity, e.g., "big" ACTH.

The placental hormones hCG and hPL are secreted by a variety of human cancers.[6,7,9,74] Of these, hCG has been the most thoroughly studied. HCG and its subunits have been shown to be produced by many cancer types both in cancer patients[7,9] and in cultured human malignant cell lines.[75,76] The use of serum hCG levels to track the course of malignant disease and to determine response to therapy is clearly established for gestational choriocarcinoma and nonseminomatous testicular cancer. The value of hCG as a marker to follow tumor response to therapy and disease recurrence is not well-established for cancers that produce it ectopically.

A recent study by Fer et al.[77] utilized immunoperoxidase staining of tissue specimens and serum radioimmunoassays (RIA) for hCG-β subunit and AFP in 28 patients with poorly differentiated carcinomas of suspected extragonadal germ cell type. Positive staining for hCG-β was observed in 9 cases and for AFP in 11; 5 tumors were positive for hCG only, 7 for AFP only, and 4 for both markers. In a number of instances, patients with positive-staining tumors had normal serum marker levels, suggesting that marker secretion by the tumor cells was low, that the form secreted into the blood was not detectable by the RIA used, or that the secreted form was rapidly cleared from the blood. Although this approach could help detect germ cell elements in such undifferentiated tumors, it did not, unfortunately, predict response to therapy or patient survival in the cases studied.[77]

Tumor-Derived Growth Factors

The recent findings that the products of a number of onc genes are closely related to a number of growth factors[78] and that certain types of animal and human cancer cells produce transforming growth factors called TGFs suggest a number of interesting possibilities about the mechanisms of malignant transformation and about the regulation of cancer cell proliferation. It will be important to determine if tumor-derived growth factors are shed into the circulation and thus be detectable as tumor markers, and, of course, if tumor growth depends on production of these TGFs, one could envisage strategies to block or inhibit this action in vivo. Sherwin et al.[79] have reported the presence of a high molecular weight TGF activity (M_r = 30,000–35,000) in the urine of patients with disseminated cancer. This factor was detected in the urine of 18 of 22 patients with cancer (carcinomas of lung, breast, colon, and ovary as well as melanomas and sarcomas), but only in 5 of 22 patients with nonmalignant diseases. Thus, the presence of such growth factors may have some general diagnostic significance for malignant neoplastic disease, but whether there may be tissue-specific or tumor-specific growth factors that might be of use in diagnosing tumors of unknown primary origin is still an open question.

Enzymes

The use of enzymes and isoenzymes as tumor markers offers another possibility for determining the tissue of origin of cancers of unknown primary. Several examples will be used to demonstrate this point.

Acid Phosphatase

The acid phosphatases are a family of isoenzymes that originate in various tissues. Measurement of prostatic acid phosphatase in the serum has been used for many years to indicate metastatic prostatic carcinoma.

The use of specific substrates can improve the discrimination between prostatic acid phosphatase and the nonprostatic forms.[80] The immunologic specificity of prostatic acid phosphatase has made possible the development of an RIA for the prostatic form. Utilizing such an RIA, Belville et al.[81] have shown that the presence of prostatic adenocarcinoma in the bone marrow can be detected by RIA of bone marrow aspirates. It has also been reported that an RIA for prostatic acid phosphatase can detect a significant percentage of patients with Stage I or Stage II prostatic cancer.[82]

Alkaline Phosphatase

Serum alkaline phosphatase (AP) activities are frequently elevated in patients with osteogenic sarcoma, parathyroid carcinoma, and cancers metastatic to bone or liver. The greatest elevations are seen in patients with osteoblastic bone involvement, the type usually seen with metastatic prostate carcinoma, whereas patients with the osteolytic metastases more often seen with breast carcinoma metastatic to bone may have normal levels.[80] Isoenzymes of alkaline phosphatase isolated from different human tissues can be distinguished by various techniques, including electrophoresis, heat stability, specific inhibitors, or immunochemistry.

At least three different structural genes appear to code for AP activity.[83] Additional differences between various isoenzymes of adult tissues may result from post-translational modifications to the three polypeptide chains. Isoenzymes from bone, kidney, intestine, and liver can be detected.[80] The distinction between bone and liver isoenzymes, however, is difficult. Thus, the pattern of AP isoenzymes extracted from tumor tissue may give some clues as to the origin of the tumor. In cases of metastatic carcinoma with elevated serum AP levels, distinction between bone and liver metastases can be made by measuring serum 5'-nucleotidase or gamma glutamyl transpeptidase levels. These will frequently be elevated in patients with liver involvement, but are usually in the normal range if only bone is involved.[80,84]

There are, in addition, at least three AP electrophoretic patterns characteristic of different phases in the developing human trophoblast.[85] The most well-studied of the placental isoenzymes is the Regan heat-stable, phenylalanine-sensitive form. Serum levels of the Regan isoenzyme have been reported to be elevated in choriocarcinoma, in 30–40 percent of patients with carcinomas of the ovary, testis, or pancreas, and in a smaller percentage of patients with certain other carcinomas or lymphomas.[86] The expression of the placental form of AP probably also reflects the presence of immature cells in the tumor cell population and/or the derepression of oncodevelopmental genes, as discussed above for hCG and AFP.

Adenosine Deaminase

Three distinguishable forms of adenosine deaminase exist in human tissues and can be resolved by electrophoretic migration: type A (M_r = 200,000), type B (M_r = 100,000), and type C (M_r = 35,000). In humans, erythrocytes contain exclusively the type C form, and other tissues contain a mixture of high and low molecular weight forms with the ratio varying from tissue to tissue.[87] Differences between normal and malignant tissues have also been observed. In normal human colon, most of the adenosine deaminase exists as type A; whereas colon carcinomas contain a high proportion of type C and type B, and the proportion of these forms varies from tumor to tumor.[88]

Aldolase

The proportion of the three isoenzymes of aldose (A, B, and C) differs in various human cancers. Primary hepatocellular carcinomas contain the A form whereas the predominant form in normal liver is B.[89] The serum of cancer patients contains a greater proportion of aldolase A (muscle-type) than does normal serum.[90] Gliomas and normal brain tissue contain aldolase C (nerve and brain variant). Aldolase A (liver and fetal form) is the predominant form in meningiomas and cancer metastatic to the brain.[91]

Amino Acid Naphthylamidase

Human tissues and body fluids contain a family of enzymes that hydrolyze L-amino acid naphthylamides. A number of isoenzymes have been identified by electrophoresis. Certain disease states are characterized by the appearance in the serum of various molecular forms of the enzyme. In patients with liver metastases, the isoenzyme forms present in serum are of greater molecular weight than that of the major component present in normal serum.[92] Two deviant isoenzymes (B and C) have been found in peripheral blood leukocytes of 25 of 25 patients with acute (AML) or chronic (CML) myelogenous leukemia.[93] In the AML group, the amount of the altered isoenzyme correlated with the number of blast cells in the blood, and after remission, the normal B isoenzyme pattern returned. The abnormal B isoenzyme was found in only 1/14 acute lymphoblastic leukemia (ALL) patients, suggesting a way to differentiate between AML and ALL.

Creatine Kinase

Creatine kinase (CK) reversibly catalyzes the transfer of a high energy phosphate bond from creatine phosphate to ADP. The enzyme is a dimer consisting of three possible combinations of two antigenically distinct subunit chains: the M (muscle) form and B (brain) form. The relative proportions of the three isoenzyme types varies from tissue to tissue, with the MM form predominant in skeletal muscle, MB in cardiac muscle, and BB in brain, gastrointestinal tract, genitourinary tract, lung, and thyroid gland. In normal serum, the MM form predominates, with the BB form being barely detectable. In patients with a variety of cancers, however, serum CK-BB levels rise dramatically, particularly in patients with small cell carcinoma of the lung[94,95] and in patients with prostate cancer.[96] Using sensitive radioimmunoassay techniques, CK-BB has also been found in abnormal amounts in the sera of patients with cancer of the breast, kidney, testes, stomach, ovary, and hematopoietic system.[96]

Although elevated serum CK-BB levels do not appear to be specific for a given type of cancer, the isoenzyme patterns derived from tissue extracts may provide an indication of the histological type. For example, the tissue CK isoenzyme patterns for normal lung, small cell carcinoma, adenocarcinoma, and squamous cell carcinoma of the lung are distinct from one another.[95]

Glycosyltransferases

This is a family of enzymes that catalyzes the addition of monosaccharides to glycoprotein or glycolipid acceptors. Most of the clinical studies have been done by measuring activities that transfer sugars to glycoprotein acceptors. Three enzymes in this class have been studied as tumor markers in patients: sialyltransferase, galactosyltransferase, and fucosyltransferase. These enzymes are ubiquitous in tissues, and elevated serum levels have been found in a wide variety of cancer patients. Certain isoenzymes of interest have also been discovered. Three fucosyltransferase activities have been identified in normal plasma by isoelectric focusing.[97] An activity that focused at pH = 4.7 was elevated during rapid proliferation of myeloid cells, such as in AML and in certain infectious diseases. Additional isoenzymes (pH = 6.0, 6.9, and 7.8) were detected in the plasma of patients with certain solid tumors and multiple myeloma. The level of an enzyme activity that focused at pH = 5.6 was elevated in untreated CML and rose markedly prior to onset of blast crisis.[98]

An isoenzyme of galactosyltransferase (isoenzyme II or gal II) has been identified by Weiser et al.[99] and is elevated in the serum of patients with metastatic carcinomas. Patients with localized primary disease had lower serum levels as a rule.

Histaminase

High histaminase (diamine oxidase) activity is found in the placenta and in certain human tumors. Histaminases from human placenta, kidney, medullary thyroid carcinoma (MTC), and small cell lung carcinoma (SCLC) are immunologically identical, whereas the activity isolated from gastrointestinal tract cross-reacted weakly with antisera made to the placental form.[100] Serum levels of histaminase are frequently high in patients with MTC and SCLC, both of which are classified as APUD-type tumors. A high percentage of elevated histaminase activities, however, has also been reported in malignant effusion fluids of patients with cancers of the ovary (87 percent), colon (73 percent), and stomach (88 percent).[101] Levels were not elevated in patients with lymphoma. Measurement of CEA, hCG-β, and the Regan isoenzyme of AP together with histaminase indicated different patterns of elevation of these markers among patients with different types of primary tumors. In patients with colon cancer, for example, high levels of histaminase in ascitic fluid correlated with elevated CEA in the majority of cases, whereas in patients with ovarian carcinoma, elevated histaminase tended to concur with the production of hCG-β.[101]

Lactic Dehydrogenase

Ratios of lactic dehydrogenase (LDH) isoenzymes have been used to differentiate normal from cancerous tissue. Five common forms of LDH are identified in homogenates of human tissue. The enzyme is a tetramer made up of two subunits specified by two genetic loci (LDH-A and LDH-B). The proportion of the muscle variant (LDH_5) is higher in some tumors than in the corresponding normal tissue. In normal uterine tissue, for example, LDH_5 was reported to be 4 percent of the total activity, whereas it was 13 percent in leiomyoma, 38 percent in leiomyosarcoma, and 42 percent in cervical carcinoma.[102] A predominance of the LDH_5 form has also been observed in cancers of the prostate, brain, lung, stomach, and kidney.[80]

Measurement of LDH isoenzymes in cerebrospinal fluid (CSF) is a diagnostic aid in patients suspected in harboring a central nervous system neoplasm. The proportion of LDH_5 is abnormally increased in leptomeningeal infiltration by metastatic carcinomas of the breast and lung and by malignant melanoma but not by other types of CNS metastases.[103] In the absence of infection (which may also produce abnormal LDH isoenzyme patterns), an elevated LDH_5/LDH_1 ratio suggests leptomeningeal tumor, and when used with other markers measured in the CSF such as β-glucuronidase and CEA, LDH isoenzyme patterns can aid in the early detection of CNS metastases.[103]

A unique electrophoretic form of LDH, called LDH-Z, has been identified in placenta and choriocarcinoma cells.[104] LDH-Z has also been found in hydatidiform mole and choriocarcinoma metastatic to the liver. It has not been observed in other human tissues nor in cell lines derived from a wide variety of human neoplasms. This had led Siciliano et al.[104] to conclude that LDH-Z is an isoenzyme associated with choriocarcinoma and indicative of the trophoblastic origin of the cells.

Other Isoenzymes of Carbohydrate Metabolism

Isoenzyme forms of several enzymes involved in carbohydrate metabolism have been reported, and, in some cases, altered patterns of these have been observed in human cancer. In hepatoma tissue, for instance, an increased level of hexokinase II (HK II) and a decreased level of HK III has been observed.[105] In cell lines derived from hepatoma and esophageal cancers, the proportion of HK II was also increased compared with the normal tissues of origin of the tumors. Type IV hexokinase has been found only in liver and kidney. Brain contains mainly type I. Type II HK is not normally found in human brain, but it reappears in certain malignant gliomas; it may account for a significant amount of total HK activity in grade IV astrocytomas, but appears to be absent or very low in less malignant gliomas.[106]

Alterations of pyruvate kinase (PK) isoenzyme patterns have also been observed in malignant tissues. Hepatomas have additional PK bands on electrophoresis that migrate between PK L and PK M_2 bands.[105] Other tumor tissues had PK M_2 only.

Neuron-specific Enolase

Enolase is a glycolytic enzyme, widely distributed in mammalian tissues, and has three dimeric forms: $alpha_2$, alpha-gamma, and $gamma_2$[107] The gamma subunit has been found to be identical with the nervous system-specific protein 14-3-2, and the $gamma_2$ isozyme has been termed neuronspecific enolase (NSE). The form of brain enolase containing one alpha and one gamma subunit is called hybrid enolase. NSE has been detected in a number of tissues that contain neuroendocrine cells including pituitary, thyroid, adrenal, and pancreatic tissues. It has also been found in tumors containing neuroendocrine cell types such as carcinoid tumors, insulinomas, glucagonomas, medullary thyroid carcinomas, neuroblastomas, and small cell lung carcinomas.

The non-neuronal enolase (NNE) is identical to liver enolase and contains two alpha subunits. NNE is also found in glial cells but not in neuronal cells, the opposite of NSE. Serum levels of NSE have proven to be a useful marker for following the course of certain tumors such as small cell lung carcinoma, and NSE levels in amniotic fluid can serve as a diagnostic index for fetal neural tube defects. NSE levels in biopsy specimens have been used to distinguish between neuroblastoma and Wilms' tumor in children.[108]

Terminal Deoxynucleotidyl Transferase

TdT is a specific intracellular marker for immature lymphocytes,[109] and is not found in measurable levels in other cell types. The enzyme catalyzes the polymerization of deoxynucleoside triphosphates, but does not require a DNA template for the polymerization step. It can be detected by catalytic assay or immunocytochemical staining. High levels of enzyme and an increased proportion of cells staining for TdT are found in lymphoblastic leukemias and lymphomas. TdT$^+$ cells represent the major population in acute lymphoblastic leukemia and frequently appear in the blast crisis phase of chronic myelogenous leukemia. They may also be a significant percentage of the leukocyte population in acute nonlymphocytic leukemia. Patients with non-Hodgkin's lymphoma may also have elevated TdT levels in extracts of lymph nodes and bone marrow.

Conclusion

A variety of tumor marker substances have been reviewed in this chapter. Much of this information has been derived from tumors with an established origin and histology. In some instances, the detection of these substances can provide clues regarding the biology or histogenesis of a neoplasm that cannot otherwise be defined. Although biomarkers alone are not considered diagnostic of specific tumor types, the presence of one or more of the markers reviewed above can suggest or support the diagnosis of a cancer with which they are associated. On occasion, treatment may be selected on this basis, particularly when other diagnostic criteria are inconclusive, as is the case in undifferentiated tumors, or in cancers of unknown primary site.

Since most of these markers lack specificity, their implications should be judged within the context of the overall clinical setting. As an example, an elevated alpha-fetoprotein in an elderly man with a liver tumor would support the diagnosis of a primary hepatocellular carcinoma, while in a younger patient with a mediastinal mass, a germinal neoplasm should be considered.

After therapy is instituted, markers may also be useful in follow-up and in assessing response. Moreover, as treatment modalities are developed that successfully exploit specific tumor-related substances, the presence or absence of the target substance within the neoplastic tissue or serum may correlate with response. Examples already exist. The correlation between hormone receptor proteins and response to hormonal manipulation in breast cancer, for example, is well-established. Through the recent advances in immunodiagnosis and the introduction of monoclonal antibodies to clinical oncology, similar correlations are likely to be made between the presence of certain tumor antigens and the response to therapy based on monoclonal antibodies directed against those antigens. Consequently, the diagnostic and predictive value of tumor markers should increase considerably in the future as such developments are made.

References

1. Knox WE: Convergent chemical grades of neoplasticity in two types of neoplasm, in Ruddon RW (ed): Biological Markers of Neoplasia: Basic and Applied Aspects. New York, Elsevier North Holland, 1978, p 547
2. Kost TA, Koury MJ, Hankins WD, et al: Target cells for Friend virus-induced erythroid burst in vitro. Cell 18:145–152, 1979
3. Graf T, Ade N, Beug H: Temperature-sensitive mutant of avian erythroblastosis virus suggests a block of differentiation as a mechanism of leukemogenesis. Nature 275:496–501, 1978
4. Rosen SW, Weintraub BD, Vaitukaitis JL, et al: Placental proteins and their subunits as tumor markers. Ann Intern Med 82:71–83, 1975
5. Sell S, Becker FF: Alpha-fetoprotein. J Nat Cancer Inst 60:19–26, 1978
6. Neuwald PD, Anderson C, Salivar WO, et al: Expression of oncodevelopmental gene products of human tumor cells in culture. J Nat Cancer Inst 64:447–459, 1980
7. Vaitukaitis JL, Ross GT, Braunstein GD, et al: Gonadotropins and their subunits: Basic and clinical studies. Recent Prog Horm Res 32:289–331, 1976

8. Chen DS, Sung JL: Relationship of hepatitis B surface antigen to serum alpha-fetoprotein in nonmalignant disease of the liver. Cancer 44:984–992, 1979

9. Blackman MR, Weintraub BD, Rosen SW, et al: Human placental and pituitary glycoprotein hormones and their subunits as tumor markers: A quantitative assessment. J Nat Cancer Inst 65:81–94, 1980

10. Rees LH, Ratcliffe JG: Ectopic hormone production by nonendocrine tumors. Clin Endocrinol 3:263–299, 1974

11. Reinherz EL, Kung PC, Goldstein G, et al: Discrete stages of human intrathymic differentiation: Analysis of normal thymocytes and leukemic lymphoblasts of T lineage. Proc Natl Acad Sci USA 77:1588, 1980

12. Nathwani BN, Kim H, Rappaport H: Malignant lymphoma. Lymphoblastic. Cancer 38:964, 1976

13. Jaffe ES, Berard CW: Lymphoblastic lymphoma, a term rekindled with new precision. Ann Int Med 89:415, 1978

14. Civin CI, Mivvo J, Banquerigo ML: MY1, a new myeloid specific antigen identified by a mouse monoclonal antibody. Blood 57:842, 1981

15. Griffin JD, Ritz J, Nadler LM, et al: Expression of myeloid differentiation antigens on normal and malignant myeloid cells. J Clin Invest 68:932, 1981

16. Roberts MM, Greaves MF: Maturation linked expression of a myeloid cell surface antigen. Br J Hematol 38:439, 1978

17. Houghton AN, Eisinger M, Albino AP, et al: Surface antigens on melanocytes and melanomas: Markers of melanocyte differentiation and melanoma subsets. J Exp Med 156:1755–1766, 1982

18. Albino AP, Lloyd KO, Houghton AN, et al: Heterogeneity in surface antigen expression and glycoprotein expression of cell lines derived from different metastases of the same patient: Implications for the study of tumor antigens. J Exp Med 154:1764, 1981

19. Ueda R, Ogata S-I, Morrissey DM, et al: Cell surface antigens of human renal cancer defined by mouse monoclonal antibodies: Identification of tissue-specific kidney glycoproteins. Proc Natl Acad Sci USA 78:5122–5126, 1981

20. Cordon-Cardo C, Bander NH, Fradet Y, et al: Immunoanatomic dissection of the human urinary tract by monoclonal antibodies. J Histochem Cytochem (in press)

21. Berstrand CG, Czar B: Demonstration of a new protein fraction in serum from the human fetus. Scand J Clin Lab Invest 8:174–179, 1956

22. Abelev GI, Perova SD, Khramkova NI, et al: Production of embry-

onal alpha-globulin by transplantable mouse hepatomas. Transplantation 1:174–180, 1963

23. Tatarinov YS: Detection of embryo-specific alpha-globulin in the blood sera of patients with primary liver tumors. Vopr Med Khim 10:90–91, 1964

24. Talerman A, Haije WG, Baggerman L: Serum alphafetoprotein (AFP) in patients with germ cell tumors of the gonads and extragonadal sites: Correlation between endodermal sinus (yolk sac) tumor and raised serum AFP. Cancer 46:380–385, 1980

25. Javadpour N: Significance of elevated serum alphafetoprotein (AFP) in seminoma. Cancer 45:2166–2168, 1980

26. Bosl GJ, Lange PH, Nochomovitz LE, et al: Tumor markers in advanced nonseminomatous testicular cancer. Cancer 47:572–576, 1981

27. Braunstein GD, McIntire KR, Waldmann TA: Discordance of human chorionic gonadotropin and alpha fetoprotein in testicular teratocarcinoma. Cancer 31:1065–1068, 1973

28. Fraley EE, Lange PH, Kennedy BJ: Germ-cell testicular cancer in adults. New England J Med 301:1370–1377, 1979

29. McIntire KR, Waldmann TA, Moertel CG, et al: Serum alpha-fetoprotein in patients with neoplasms of the gastrointestinal tract. Cancer Res 35:991–996, 1975

30. Yasunami R, Hashimoto Z, Ogura T, et al: Primary lung cancer producing alpha-fetoprotein: A case report. Cancer 47:926–929, 1981

31. Gold P, Freedman SO: Demonstration of tumor-specific antigens in human colonic carcinomata by immunological tolerance and absorption techniques. J Exp Med 121:439–462, 1965

32. Von Kleist S, Chavanel G, Burtin P: Identification of an antigen from normal human tissue that crossreacts with carcinoembryonic antigen. Proc Nat Acad Sci USA 69:2492–2494, 1972

33. Egan ML, Pritchard DG, Todd CW, et al: Isolation and immunochemical and chemical characterization of carcinoembryonic antigen-like substances in colon lavages of healthy individuals. Cancer Res 37:2638–2643, 1977

34. Denk H, Tappeiner G, Eckerstorfer R, et al: Carcinoembryonic antigen (CEA) in gastrointestinal and extragastrointestinal tumors and its relationship to tumor-cell differentiation. Int J Cancer 10:262–272, 1972

35. Ejeckam GC, Huang SN, McCaughey WTE, et al: Immunohistopathologic study on carcinoembryonic antigen (CEA)-like material and

immunoglobulin A in gastric malignancies. Cancer 44:1606–1614, 1979

36. Talerman A, Van Der Pompe WB, Haije WG, et al: Alpha-fetoprotein and carcinoembryonic antigen in germ cell neoplasms. Br J Cancer 35:288–291, 1977

37. Monograph: CEA as a cancer marker. National Institutes of Health Consensus Development Conference Summary, Vol. 3, No. 7. Office of Medical Applications of Research, National Institutes of Health, Bethesda, MD, 1980

38. Wang NS, Huang SN, Gold P: Absence of carcinoembryonic antigen-like material in mesothelioma: An immunohistochemical differentiation from other lung cancers. Cancer 44:937–943, 1979

39. Chism SE, Warner NL, Wells JV, et al: Evidence for common and distinct determinants of colon carcinoembryonic antigen, colon carcinoma antigen-III, and molecules with carcinoembryonic antigen activity isolated from breast and ovarian cancer. Cancer Res 37:3100–3108, 1977

40. Stuhlmiller GM, Seigler HF: Enzymatic susceptibility and spontaneous release of human melanoma tumor-associated antigens. J Nat Cancer Inst 58:215–221, 1977

41. McCabe RP, Ferrone S, Pellegrino MA, et al: Purification and immunologic evaluation of human melanoma-associated antigens. J Nat Cancer Inst 60:773–777, 1978

42. Carrel S, Accolla RS, Carmagnola AL, et al: Common human melanoma-associated antigen(s) detected by monoclonal antibodies. Cancer Res 40:2523–2528, 1980

43. Dippold WG, Lloyd KO, Li LTC, et al: Cell surface antigens of human malignant melanoma: Definition of six antigenic systems with mouse monoclonal antibodies. Proc Nat Acad Sci USA 77:6114–6118, 1980

44. Seeger RC, Zeltzer PM, Rayner SA: Onco-neural antigen: A new neural differentiation antigen expressed by neuroblastoma, oat cell carcinoma, Wilms' tumor, and sarcoma cells. J Immunol 122:1548–1555, 1979

45. Schnegg JF, Diserens AC, Carrel S, et al: Human glioma-associated antigens detected by monoclonal antibodies. Cancer Res 41:1209–1213, 1981

46. Herlyn M, Steplewski Z, Herlyn D, et al: Colorectal carcinoma-specific antigen: Detection by means of monoclonal antibodies. Proc Nat Acad Sci USA 76:1438–1442, 1979

47. Bara J, Paul-Gardais A, Loisillier F, et al: Isolation of a sulfated

glycopeptidic antigen from human gastric tumors: Its localization in normal and cancerous gastrointestinal tissues. Int J Cancer 21:133–139, 1978

48. Hakkinen IPT, Heinonen R, Inberg MV, et al: Clincopathological study of gastric cancers and precancerous states detected by fetal sulfoglycoprotein antigen screening. Cancer Res 40:4308–4312, 1980

49. Gorsky Y, Vanky F, Sulitzeanu D: Isolation from patients with breast cancer of antibodies specific for antigens associated with breast cancer and other malignant diseases. Proc Nat Acad Sci USA 73:2102–2105, 1976

50. Lopez MJ, Thomson DMP: Isolation of breast cancer tumor antigen from serum and urine. Int J Cancer 20:834–848, 1977

51. Mesa-Tejada R, Keydar I, Ramanarayanan M, et al: Detection in human breast carcinomas of an antigen immunologically related to a group-specific antigen of mouse mammary tumor virus. Proc Nat Acad Sci USA 75:1529–1533, 1978

52. Schlom J, Wunderlich D, Teramoto YA: Generation of human monoclonal antibodies reactive with human mammary carcinoma cells. Proc Nat Acad Sci USA 77:6841–6845, 1980

53. Frost MJ, Rogers GT, Bagshawe KD: Extraction and preliminary characterization of a human bronchogenic carcinoma antigen. Br J Cancer 31:379–386, 1975

54. Bell Jr CE, Seetharam S: A plasma membrane antigen highly associated with oat-cell carcinoma of the lung and undetectable in normal adult tissue. Int J Cancer 18:605–611, 1976

55. Veltri RW, Mengoli HF, Maxim PE, et al: Isolation and identification of human lung tumor-associated antigens. Cancer Res 37:1313–1322, 1977

56. Akeson R: Human lung organ-specific antigens on normal lung, lung tumors, and a lung tumor cell line. J Nat Cancer Inst 58:863–869, 1977

57. Kempner DH, Jay MR, Stevens RH: Human lung tumor-associated antigens of 32,000 daltons molecular weight. J Nat Cancer Inst 63:1121–1127, 1979

58. Gaffar SA, Princler GL, McIntire KR, et al: A human lung tumor-associated antigen cross-reactive with α_1–antichymotrypsin. J Biol Chem 255:8334–8339, 1980

59. Banwo O, Versey J, Hobbs JR: New oncofetal antigen for human pancreas. Lancet 1:643–645, 1974

60. Chu TM, Holyoke ED, Douglass HO: Isolation of a glycoprotein

antigen from ascites fluid of pancreatic carcinoma. Cancer Res 37:1525–1529, 1977

61. Gelder FB, Reese CJ, Moossa AR, et al: Purification, partial characterization, and clinical evaluation of a pancreatic oncofetal antigen. Cancer Res 38:313–324, 1978

62. Hobbs JR, Knapp ML, Branfoot AC: Pancreatic oncofetal antigen (POA): Its frequency and localization in humans. Oncodev Biol Med 1:37–48, 1980

63. Order SE, Thurston J, Knapp R: Ovarian tumor antigens: A new potential for therapy. Nat Cancer Inst Monogr 42:33–43, 1975

64. Imamura N, Takahashi T, Lloyd KO, et al: Analysis of human ovarian tumor antigens using heterologous antisera: Detection of new antigenic systems. Int J Cancer 21:570–577, 1978

65. Knauf S, Urbach GI: Identification, purification, and radioimmunoassay of NB-70K, a human ovarian tumor-associated antigen. Cancer Res 41:1351–1357, 1981

66. Beierle JW, Wise KS, Trump GN, et al: Isolation of Wilms' tumor antigens by chelation. Clin Chim Acta 61:411–414, 1975

67. Wright Jr GL, Schellhammer PF, Faulconer RL: Isolation of a soluble tumor-associated antigen from human renal cell carcinoma by gradient acrylamide gel electrophoresis. Cancer Res 37:4228–4232, 1977

68. Schneider MU, Troye M, Paulie S, et al: Membrane-associated antigens on tumor cells from transitional-cell carcinoma of the human urinary bladder. I. Immunological characterization by xenogeneic antisera. Int J Cancer 26:185–192, 1980

69. Byers VS, Johnston JO: Antigenic differences among osteogenic sarcoma tumor cells taken from different locations in human tumors. Cancer Res 37:3173–3183, 1977

70. Chiang W-T, Alexander ER, Kenny GE: Identification of a tumor-associated antigen in cervical carcinoma by two-dimensional (crossed) immunoelectrophoresis. J Nat Cancer Inst 58:43–48, 1977

71. Nadler LM, Stashenko P, Hardy R, et al: Serotherapy of a patient with a monoclonal antibody directed against a human lymphoma-associated antigen. Cancer Res 40:3147–3154, 1980

72. Pearse AG: Neurocristopathy, neuroendocrine pathology, and the APUD concept. Z Krebsforsch 84:1–18, 1975

73. Vaitukaitis JL: Peptide hormones as tumor markers. Cancer 37:567–572, 1976

74. Sheth NA, Adil MA, Schinde SR, et al: Paraendocrine behavior of tumors of the gastrointestinal tract with reference to human placental lactogen. Br J Cancer 42:610–612, 1980

75. Ruddon RW, Anderson C, Meade KS, et al: Content of gonadotro-
    pins in cultured human malignant cells and effects of sodium
    butyrate treatment on gonadotropin secretion by HeLa cells. Cancer
    Res 39:3885–3892, 1979

76. Rosen SW, Weintraub BD, Aaronson SA: Nonrandom ectopic pro-
    tein production by malignant cells: Direct evidence in vitro. J Clin
    Endocrinol Metab 50:834–841, 1980

77. Fer MF, Forbes JT, Oldham Rk, et al: The detection of intracellular
    β-human chorionic gonadotropin (β-hCG) and α-fetoprotein (α-FP)
    in suspected extragonadal germ cell tumors by immunoperoxidase
    staining. Proc Am Assoc Cancer Res 22:82, 1981

78. Heldin C-H, Westermark B: Growth factors: Mechanism of action
    and relation to oncogenes. Cell 37:9–10, 1984

79. Sherwin SA, Twardzik DR, Bohn WH, et al: High-molecular-weight
    transforming growth factor activity in the urine of patients with
    disseminated cancer. Cancer Res 43:403–407, 1983

80. Schwartz MK: Enzymes in cancer. Clin Chem 19:10–22, 1973

81. Belville WD, Cox HD, Mahan DE, et al: Bone marrow acid phospha-
    tase by radioimmunoassay. Cancer 41:2286–2291, 1978

82. Foti AG, Cooper JF, Herschman H, et al: Detection of prostatic
    cancer by solid-phase radioimmunoassay of serum prostatic acid
    phosphatase. New England J Med 297:1357–1361, 1977

83. McKenna MJ, Hamilton TA, Sussman HH: Comparison of human
    alkaline phosphatase isoenzymes. Structural evidence for three
    protein classes. Biochem J 181:67–73, 1979

84. Schwartz MK: Laboratory aids to diagnosis—enzymes. Cancer
    37:542–548, 1976

85. Fishman L, Mayayama H, Driscoll SG, et al: Developmental phase-
    specific alkaline phosphatase isoenzymes of human placenta and
    their occurrence in human cancer. Cancer Res 36:2268–2273, 1976

86. Fishman L, Inglis NR, Vaitukaitis J, et al: Regan isoenzymes and
    hCG in ovarian cancer. Nat Cancer Inst Monogr 42:63–73, 1975

87. Ma PF, Magers TA: Comparative studies of human adenosine
    deaminases. Int J Biochem 6:281–286, 1975

88. Trotta PP, Balis ME: Characterization of adenosine deaminase from
    normal colon and colon tumors. Evidence for tumor-specific vari-
    ants. Biochemistry 17:270–278, 1978

89. Schapira F, Dreyfus JC, Schapira G: Anomaly of aldolase in primary
    liver cancer. Nature 200:995–997, 1963

90. Tsonematsu K, Shiraish T: Aldolase isozymes in human tissue and
    serum. Cancer 24:637–642, 1969

91. Sato S, Sugimura T, Chien TC, et al: Aldolase isozyme patterns of human brain tumors. Cancer 27:223–227, 1971
92. Smith EE, Rutenberg AM: The heterogeneity of serum amino acid naphthylamidase in liver metastases. Biochem Med 4:418–424, 1970
93. Roos G, Sinna GA, Bjorksten B, et al: Discriminative value of isozymes of amino acid naphthylamidase in the diagnosis of myeloid leukemias. Cancer 46:325–329, 1980
94. Coolen BR, Pragay DA, Nosanchuk JS, et al: Elevation of brain-type creatine kinase in serum from patients with carcinoma. Cancer 44:1414–1481, 1979
95. Gazdar AF, Zweig MH, Carney DN, et al: Levels of creatine kinase and its BB isozyme in lung cancer specimens and cultures. Cancer Res 41:2773–2777, 1981
96. Zweig MH, Van Steirteghem AC: Assessment by radioimmunoassay of serum creatine kinase BB (CK-BB) as a tumor marker: Studies in patients with various cancers and a comparison of CK-BB concentrations to prostate acid phosphatase concentrations. J Nat Cancer Inst 66:859–862, 1981
97. Kessel D, Ratanatharathorn V, Chou T-H: Electrofocusing patterns of fucosyltransferases in plasma of patients with neoplastic disease. Cancer Res 39:3377–3380, 1979
98. Kessel D, Shah-Reddy I, Mirchandani I, et al: Electrofocusing patterns of fucosyltransferase activity in plasma of patients with chronic granulocytic leukemia. Cancer Res 40:3576–3578, 1980
99. Weiser MM, Podolsky DK, Isselbacher KJ: Cancer-associated isoenzyme of serum galactosyltransferase. Proc Nat Acad Sci USA 73:1319–1322, 1976
100. Baylin SB: Histaminase (diamine oxidase) activity in human tumors: An expression of a mature genome. Proc Nat Acad Sci USA 74:883–887, 1977
101. Lin C-W, Inglis NR, Rule AH, et al: Histaminase and other tumor markers in malignant effusion fluids. Cancer Res 39:4894–4899, 1979
102. Okabe K: Study of lactate dehydrogenase in the normal uterus and in uterine tumor tissues of humans. Seikagaku 39:291–300, 1965
103. Fleisher M, Wasserstrom WR, Schold SC, et al: Lactic dehydrogenase isoenzymes in the cerebrospinal fluid of patients with systemic cancer. Cancer 47:2654–2659, 1981
104. Siciliano MJ, Bordelon-Riser ME, Freedman RS, et al: A human trophoblastic isozyme (lactate dehydrogenase-Z) associated with choriocarcinoma. Cancer Res 40:283–287, 1980
105. Hammond KD, Balinsky D: Isozyme studies of several enzymes of

carbohydrate metabolism in human adult and fetal tissues, tumor tissues, and cell cultures. Cancer Res 38:1323–1328, 1978

106. Bennett MJ, Timperley WR, Taylor CB, et al: Isoenzymes of hexokinase in the developing, normal and neoplastic human brain. Europ J Cancer 14:189–193, 1978

107. Marangos PJ, Polak JM, Pearse AG: Neuron specific enolase in biological fluids: A probe for neuronal and neuroendocrine pathology. Protides Biol Fluid Proc Colloq 36:65–70, 1983

108. Odelstad L, Pahlman S, Lackgren G, et al: Neuron specific enolase: A marker for differential diagnosis of neuroblastoma and Wilms' tumor. J Pediatr Surg 17:381–385, 1982

109. Bollum FJ: Terminal deoxynucleotidyl transferase as a hematopoietic cell marker. Blood 54:1203–1215, 1979

4

PRESENTATIONS AND CLINICAL SYNDROMES OF TUMORS OF UNKNOWN ORIGIN

Q. Scott Ringenberg
John W. Yarbro

Few situations are more frustrating to the oncologist than being forced to make a therapeutic decision in a patient with cancer from an unknown site or unknown cell of origin. We can cure over a dozen malignancies with proper chemotherapy and palliate many others, but often the initial therapeutic regimen is decisive in determining the success of our treatment. Yet all too often we are forced to treat patients before a definitive diagnosis can be made.

A review of the literature of cancers of unknown primary reveals inconsistency of definition and reporting. Some authors define the entity as a metastatic cancer in which the primary site is unknown after routine physical examination, screening laboratory, and chest radiograph. Others demand an extensive list of examinations. We prefer to define tumors of unknown origin (TUOs) as those in which the origin is unknown at the time a therapeutic decision must be made.

Tumors of unknown origin account for 3 percent of cancers and are the eighth most common cancer diagnosis.[1] They present as several entities, each of which has its own pattern of expression, treatment, and natural

POORLY DIFFERENTIATED NEOPLASMS AND TUMORS OF UNKNOWN ORIGIN   ISBN 0-8089-1755-2

Table 4-1

Presentations and Clinical Syndromes of Tumors of Unknown Origin

Location of Unknown Primary	% of All TUO	Predominant Histological Types
Lymph node metastases[3]	31%	
Cervical[3]	15%	Squamous cell carcinoma
		Undifferentiated carcinoma
		Adenocarcinoma
Supraclavicular[3]	9%	Adenocarcinoma
		Undifferentiated carcinoma
		Squamous cell carcinoma
Axillary[3]	4%	Adenocarcinoma
Inguinal[3]	3%	Melanoma
		Undifferentiated carcinoma
		Squamous cell carcinoma
Liver metastases[30]	20%	Adenocarcinoma
Bone metastases[3,35]	16%	Adenocarcinoma
Brain metastases[54,56,57]	10%	Adenocarcinoma
Lung metastases[3]	12%	Adenocarcinoma
Skin metastases[3]	7%	See text
Pericardial effusion[60,61]	1%	Adenocarcinoma

The histological types and approximate percent of all TUOs presenting at each location are obtained from multiple references cited. Where differences of incidence were encountered, the preponderant view was used and cited.

history. TUOs are commonly discussed by their histological types, i.e., adenocarcinoma, epidermoid carcinoma, etc. This classification is useful, but it is equally important to consider the clinical presentation. A number of clinical syndromes emerge when one examines the location of the unknown primary as well as the histological type, and the differential diagnosis can be more limited. These presentations are shown in Table 4-1.

Cervical Node Presentations of Tumors of Unknown Origin

Cervical nodes are the most common nodal presentation of TUOs.[2,3] It is useful to distinguish cervical from supraclavicular presentation because the origins of the metastases can be different. Cervical nodes are the third most common location of TUOs, but they are the most common sites for

Table 4-2
Cervical Node Presentations of Tumors of Unknown Origin:
Frequency of Histological Types

Year/Author	Number of Cases	Squamous Cell Carcinoma	Undifferentiated Carcinoma	Adeno-carcinoma	Other
1957 Comess[7]	58	30	6	17	5
1963 France[8]	43	19	11	8	5
1966 Jesse[9]	127	60	27	20	20
1967 Smith[10]	33	7	17	3	1
1970 Barrie[11]	123	104	3	11	5
1970 Probert[12]	61	16	19	12	13
1971 Pico[13]	80	42	27	5	6
1974 Fitzpatrick[14]	108	50	54	1	3
1977 Coker[15]	64	39	17	2	6
Total	697	367 (53%)	181 (26%)	79 (11%)	64 (9%)

the presentation of squamous and undifferentiated cell types.[4] Three to nine percent of all cervical metastases are TUOs.[5]

These tumors usually present as firm, painless, unilateral, often solitary, neck masses. Patients who present with soft, pliable, and multiple nodes more commonly have lymphoma. Two-thirds of cervical TUOs are 5 cm or greater, and patients often delay consulting a physician for many months after the first appearance of the mass.[6] The tumors occur with equal frequency on the left and right sides of the neck. Men are afflicted more commonly than women, possibly due to the higher frequency of tobacco and alcohol abuse among men.

As shown in Table 4-2, squamous cell carcinoma predominates with 53 percent of the cases, followed in frequency by undifferentiated carcinoma (26 percent). Adenocarcinomas average 11 percent of cases when considering all reports, but some reports exclude from their analyses those adenocarcinomas which later prove to be of thyroid origin. Other tumors (clear cell carcinoma, melanoma, and undifferentiated cancers later found to be lymphoma) account for 9 percent of cases.

Squamous Cell Tumors of Unknown Origin in
Cervical Nodes

Squamous cell TUOs in cervical nodes present a significant diagnostic and therapeutic dilemma to otorhinolaryngologists. The approach to any solitary mass in the neck should be dictated by the concern that it may be the presentation of an occult squamous cell carcinoma of the head and neck. Many solitary cervical node cancers are squamous cell carcinoma, and often the primary tumors can be found by thorough examination; in others, a head and neck cancer is often found later.

Accepted surgical therapy of head and neck cancer dictates the approach. Many believe that an inopportune biopsy of a neck mass, later found to be a squamous cell tumor, may reduce the cure rate if the primary site is in the head and neck. Therefore, many measures are taken to identify any primary cancer including endoscopic examination of the nasal passages, oropharynx, upper esophagus and trachea, blind biopsies of the oropharynx and computed tomography. Only after the otorhinolaryngologist has completely evaluated the head and neck region thoroughly for an occult primary and has not found one, is the neck mass approached for biopsy.

The histological identification of squamous cell carcinoma of cervical nodes rarely presents a diagnostic problem to pathologists, provided adequate tissue is sampled. Uncommonly, electron microscopic studies are necessary to document desmosomes and intercellular bridging. Needle aspiration has been advocated in order to decrease the risk of seeding of tumor which could occur with biopsy. Unfortunately, tissue obtained by needle aspirate is not always adequate to differentiate squamous cell carcinoma from other histological types. Recently, however, the use of thin needle biopsy has increased substantially and in some centers is the procedure of choice following endoscopy.

Like most TUOs, the primary tumor is found at a later time in a minority of patients. Table 4-3 shows that the primary sites were ultimately discovered in only one-third of cervical squamous cell TUOs. This is slightly below the average of 40 percent reported from a review of over 1000 cases of cervical node TUOs of all histological types.[16] When the primary is ultimately found, oropharyngeal and nasopharyngeal occult tumors predominate (40 percent). Advances in fiberoptic examinations and the routine evaluation of patients with solitary neck masses where squamous cell carcinoma is suspected have not seemed to alter the incidence of this occult tumor. Larynx, tongue, and tonsillar cancers are of lesser frequency. Twenty-five percent of squamous cell TUOs of the cervical nodes arise outside the head and neck.

Autopsy series of metastatic carcinoma of the head and neck as well as clinical experience of head and neck surgeons demonstrate that squamous cell cancers of the neck show a predictable correlation between the site of nodal metastases and the primary site. Cervical node metastases from occult tumors of the head and neck fail to demonstrate this close relation-

Table 4-3
Cervical Node Presentions of Squamous Cell Tumors of
Unknown Origin. Chances of Finding the Primary Tumor:
Location of Primary When Found

Year/Author	Number of Cases	Cases Where Primary Found	ORO/N*	Larynx	Tongue	Tonsil	Other
1957 Comess[7]	42	17	7	1	2	2	5
1963 France[8]	19	2	1	0	0	0	1
1963 Marchetta[6]	27	8	5	0	0	0	3
1966 Jesse[9]	60	20	11	4	0	0	5
1970 Barrie[11]	104	31	8	9	5	4	5
1971 Pico[13]	42	7	2	0	3	0	2
Total	294	85 (29%)	34 (12%)	14 (5%)	10 (3%)	6 (2%)	21 (7%)

* Oropharyngeal and nasopharyngeal cancer

ship when the site of the node is later correlated with the site of the occult primary.

Undifferentiated Tumors of Unknown Origin in Cervical Nodes

The second most common histological type of cervical node TUO is undifferentiated cancer with the average incidence in several large series being 26 percent (Table 4-2). In many series the primary site of this tumor is not stated. When it is mentioned,[7,10,17] there are many primary tumor locations including nasopharynx, esophagus, tonsil, lung, stomach, prostate, ovary, skin, and an occasional case of lymphoma initially misclassified as an undifferentiated carcinoma. Clearly, these undifferentiated neoplasms represent a heterogeneous group of tumors, some of which are more responsive to therapy than others. This is discussed in detail in several other chapters of this book.

Adenocarcinoma of Unknown Origin in Cervical Nodes

Adenocarcinoma accounts for 11 percent of TUOs in cervical nodes (Table 4-2). This figure is low because it represents only those cases which present with cervical nodes as the only manifestation. Autopsies on patients with widespread carcinoma have revealed that the carcinoma often spread to cervical nodes. In contrast to adenocarcinomatous TUOs which present in other locations, cervical TUOs eventually manifest the primary tumor in the majority of cases. In 46 percent of these patients, when the primary tumor is found, it is located in the thyroid (Table 4-4). Other adenocarcinomatous TUOs of the neck arise from primary sites below the clavicle. Infradiaphragmatic primaries represent 42 percent of cases (mostly colon and stomach). Supradiaphragmatic primaries (excluding thyroid cancer) represent 12 percent, nearly equally divided between lung, breast, and other head and neck sites (salivary glands, parotid, etc.—Table 4-4).

Supraclavicular Node Presentations of Tumors of Unknown Origin

The supraclavicular nodes are often not distinguished from cervical nodes in reports of neck cancer of unknown origin, but it is useful to do so. Supraclavicular nodes represent 9 percent of all nodal TUOs (Table 4-1). Whereas cervical TUOs are predominately squamous cell cancers, supraclavicular TUOs are more evenly distributed between the three histological types (Table 4-5). Lung cancer is not the most common TUO in supraclavicular nodes as one might expect. This is probably explained by the relatively low incidence of the lung as the primary site of TUOs, due to the ability of chest radiographs to detect lung cancer.

From autopsy and anatomic studies, the supraclavicular nodes (notably the left supraclavicular or Virchow's node) are an important site for metastases.[18] Classically, we have believed that the left side was especially prone to manifest metastases from gastrointestinal cancer. However, the left supraclavicular fossa is only slightly more involved (55 percent) with metastatic tumor than the right (45 percent), and there is very little difference in the sites of origin of metastases to the left and right supraclavicular nodes. In 1447 cases of metastatic cancer to the supraclavicular nodes, over two-thirds of the tumors originated from four primary sites: lung (23 percent), breast (22 percent), stomach (15 percent), and prostate (9 percent).[18]

Adenocarcinomas represent 39 percent of TUOs presenting in supraclavicular nodes (Table 4-5). The primary sites for these neoplasms are often not reported, but appear to be similar to those in the cervical region with the exception of thyroid cancer. Squamous cell TUOs of supraclavicular nodes are least common (26 percent) in contrast to their incidence in

Table 4-4

Cervical Node Presentions of Adenocarcinoma of Unknown Origin: Location of Primary Tumor, When Found

Year/Author	Cases Where Primary Found	Thyroid	Stomach & Colon	Pancreas	Lung	Kidney	Head & Neck	Breast	Prostate
1957 Comess[7]	16	11	1	1	0	0	2	1	0
1963 France[8]	6	3	0	0	1	1	0	0	1
1966 Jesse[9]	11	6	5	0	0	0	0	0	0
1967 Smith[10]	3	0	1	0	1	1	0	0	0
1970 Barrie[11]	5	0	4	1	0	0	0	0	0
1971 Pico[13]	1	0	1	0	0	0	0	0	0
1977 Coker[15]	1	0	0	1	0	0	0	0	0
Total	43	20 (46%)	12 (28%)	3 (7%)	2 (5%)	2 (5%)	2 (5%)	1 (2%)	1 (2%)

Table 4-5
Supraclavicular Node Presentations of Tumors of Unknown
Origin: Frequency of Histological Types

Year/Author	Number of Cases	Adeno–Carcinoma	Undifferentiated Carcinoma	Squamous Cell Carcinoma
1963 France[8]	5	1	2	2
1974 Fitzpatrick[14]	35	15	12	8
1977 Coker[15]	6	2	2	2
Total	46	18 (39%)	16 (35%)	12 (26%)

cervical nodes. The likely sites of the occult primary are lung and head and neck cancers. Undifferentiated cancer represents 35 percent of TUOs in the supraclavicular nodes (Table 4-5). Undifferentiated TUOs of the supraclavicular nodes commonly represent an occult primary lung cancer which later becomes clinically evident. Tumors more responsive to current therapy should also be considered, as discussed at great length in other chapters of this book. These may include the intermediate subtype of small cell lung cancer, germinal neoplasms, undifferentiated lymphomas, and breast cancer.

Axillary Node Presentations of Tumors of Unknown Primary

Although uncommon, these tumors usually present as a painless, palpable lumps (85 percent); occasionally they are painful (15 percent).[19] Most solitary axillary nodes are benign. Pierce reported a series of 72 patients with solitary enlarged axillary lymph nodes with no other signs of malignancy.[20] Biopsies of these patients revealed malignancy in only 17 of the 72. Lymphoma was seen in 10, adenocarcinoma in 5, melanoma in 1, and squamous cell cancer in 1. An occult breast cancer was detected in all 5 women with adenocarcinoma.[20] Since two-thirds of patients with axillary node TUOs are women, the most common histological type is adenocarcinoma, and when the origin of this histological type is found, it is breast cancer in over 50 percent of the women[21] (Table 4-6).

The importance of occult breast cancer presenting as axillary adenopathy was recognized as early as 1907 by Halsted[22], and thereafter surgeons have approached adenocarcinoma of the axillary nodes as an

Table 4-6
Axillary Node Presentations of Tumors of Unknown Origin:
Sites of Primary in Cases Where Primary Found

Year/Author	Number of Cases	Breast	Lung	Pancreas	Stomach	Colon	Primary Not Found
1954 Owen[23]	27	20	0	0	0	0	7
1962 Feuerman[21]	21	7	5	1	2	1	5
1972 Copeland[19]	60	19	0	0	0	0	41
1976 Feigenberg[24]	7	3	0	0	0	0	4
Total	115	49	5	1	2	1	57 (50%)

indication of occult breast cancer. Mastectomy is often recommended. Due to the small number of patients in these studies and the lack of long-term follow up, the prognosis of women with axillary presentation of cancers of unknown primary treated with mastectomy is unknown. Biopsy specimens which reveal adenocarcinoma should be sent for estrogen receptors. Following histological diagnosis, reexamination of both breasts should be performed. Bilateral mammograms should be obtained, and any suspicious lesion biopsied. If no tumor is found, some advise mastectomy with careful sectioning of the breast tissue, in an effort to locate an occult primary.[21]

Little is known about undifferentiated or unclassifiable carcinomas of unknown origin presenting as axillary masses. In one report,[19] 8 cases of undifferentiated or unclassified cancers of unknown origin of the axillary nodes were reported. All patients underwent complete resection of the nodes. All the patients were alive and free of disease 2 to 10 years after surgery or local radiotherapy. Selection factors may have influenced the outcome in this limited retrospective series.

Inguinal Node Presentations of Tumors of Unknown Origin

Inguinal node metastases are an uncommon presentation of TUOs. Very few series have been reported. Inguinal node metastases of known primary origin are predominately melanoma and squamous cell carcinoma.[25] Papillary or serous adenocarcinoma and transitional cell carcinoma are less common.[25] Reflecting these histological types, the common primary tumors are melanoma and squamous cell cancer of the trunk and lower extremities, squamous cell carcinomas of the cervix, rectum and external genitalia, and ovarian and rectal adenocarcinomas.

Inguinal node metastases of unknown origin occur as 1 percent of all inguinal node metastases. They commonly present as painless masses in the groin, the left side being slightly more common than the right.[25] Unlike inguinal node metastases from known primary sites, melanoma is uncommon as a presentation of inguinal node TUOs.[25] Melanomatous TUOs are uncommon (only 2.5 percent of all melanomas) and most often present in axillary and cervical nodes. Only one-fourth of melanomatous TUOs present in inguinal nodes.[26,27,28,29] In the largest reported series of inguinal node presentations of TUOs, undifferentiated carcinomas represented 14 of the 22 cases, with 6 squamous cell carcinomas and 2 adenocarcinomas.[25] Similar to the experience in undifferentiated carcinomas presenting in an axillary node, the 14 cases of undifferentiated carcinomas of unknown origin which presented in the inguinal nodes had a relatively good prognosis. Following resection, a 50 percent survival was observed.

Hepatic Presentations of Tumors of Unknown Origin

Liver metastases represent the second most common presentation of TUOs with 20 percent of TUOs presenting as solitary or multiple liver metastases[30] (Table 4-1). Common symptoms which lead to the discovery of these hepatic metastases include right upper quadrant and epigastric abdominal pain, weight loss, and hepatomegaly. The laboratory abnormality most often found is an elevated alkaline phosphatase. The bilirubin and transaminases are usually normal.

Multiple metastases virtually exclude hepatoma. Documentation of the histology is possible in nearly every case by transcutaneous needle biopsy with very little morbidity and rare mortality. The histological type is nearly always found to be adenocarcinoma with occasional small cell carcinoma, squamous cell carcinoma or undifferentiated carcinoma.[31]

The primary will be found in 8 to 19 percent of cases, depending upon the intensity of the evaluation.[30,31,32] Because therapy of liver metastases is relatively ineffective, very few measures are usually taken to discover the primary. When a more intensive search is initiated, the primary cancer may be found in two-thirds of patients, and even higher rates are reported if the evaluation includes an exploratory laparotomy.[30]

It appears that patients with liver metastases detected by radiographic methods, should undergo percutaneous liver biopsy to confirm the histological type. If the tissue shows adenocarcinoma, only a limited search for the primary site should be undertaken, including thorough physical examination (especially of thyroid, rectum, and breast), three serial stool hemoccults, chest x-ray, proctoscopy and abdominal CT scan. Upper GI series, barium enema or colonoscopy should be reserved for those patients with symptoms of recent change in bowel habits, tenesmus or bowel obstruction. Small cell carcinomas and certain undifferentiated carcinomas may require other approaches, as discussed in other chapters.

Bone Presentations of Tumors of Unknown Origin

The data on TUOs presenting in bone are scanty. As in the case with liver, metastatic carcinoma is more common in bone, even with a solitary location, than is primary cancer. When multiple bone lesions are found, as is very often the case, primary bone cancer is virtually excluded. The radiological appearance of the tumor may be helpful in establishing a differential diagnosis. Tumors which are purely blastic are likely to arise from prostate, cancer, Hodgkin's disease, ovarian cancer, or carcinoid tumors. Tumors which are mixed blastic and lytic are often of breast origin, whereas purely lytic tumors are often myeloma.[33]

There are very few reports in which skeletal metastases are the sole sign of TUOs.[34,35] Skeletal metastases of unknown origin often present with involvement of other sites, such as lymph nodes and liver, which may lead the physician to a diagnostic biopsy of a site other than the bone. Simon reported 14 patients presenting with bone pain who on scan or x-ray were found to have bone metastases.[34] Of these, three were diagnosed as renal cell carcinoma, two as lung cancer, two as myeloma, and one as hepatoma. In the remaining six patients, the primary tumor was never detected during life. In the cases where a postmortem examination was performed, renal cell carcinoma was found in one case.[34]

The histology serves as a guide to the search for the primary. In the majority of cases, the histological type will be adenocarcinoma. Repeat physical examination of the breast, thyroid, and prostate are indicated. Simon routinely performs serum protein electrophoresis, acid phosphatase, chest x-ray, and intravenous pyelography to search for the most common tumors.[34] If this evaluation does not disclose a primary site, other studies such as barium enema and upper GI series may be performed as clinical symptoms indicate, but routine examination of these sites is unlikely to lead to a diagnosis of the primary. In women with metastatic adenocarcinoma, tissue should be collected for estrogen receptor assays.

Pulmonary Presentations of Tumors of Unknown Origin

Pulmonary metastases represent 12 percent of TUOs (Table 4-1). The cited incidence varies because of the difficulty in differentiating metastatic tumor from a primary bronchogenic carcinoma. Nystrom described 64 cases of TUOs presenting with pulmonary lesions. He identified several types of clinical presentation of these pulmonary lesions, including: solitary coin lesions, multiple nodules, and pleural effusions.[36]

Solitary Pulmonary Nodule as a Presentation of Tumor of Unknown Origin

The literature contains many excellent reviews on the solitary pulmonary nodule.[37,38,39,40,41] In general, these studies do not describe these tumors as being "of unknown primary site." This is not to suggest that TUOs presenting in the lung do not exist. Pathologists have tried to distinguish primary from metastatic lung cancer on the basis of hyperplastic changes surrounding the site of malignancy and by identification of adjacent areas of carcinoma-in-situ. Despite these efforts, Sherwin has stated that the majority of lung cancers cannot be identified conclusively as primary or metastatic tumors.[42] Until the controversies are resolved, clinicians will continue to identify a solitary nodule of the common histological types as a primary bronchogenic carcinoma when no obvious primary site exists.

Multiple Pulmonary Nodules as a Presentation of Tumors of Unknown Origin

Patients who present with multiple pulmonary nodules are generally assumed to have metastatic carcinoma.[43] When there is no previous history of malignancy, a limited search is usually instituted to look for signs of the primary. Bronchoscopy or chest computed tomography may reveal an endobronchial tumor and an assumption is usually made that the tumor is bronchogenic in origin. This is probably correct in the majority of cases, but numerous cases of endobronchial metastases have been reported.[36] Several tumors are common sites of origin for multiple lung metastases. One autopsy series has identified the following tumors which, when metastatic, spread to the lung in over half of the cases: melanoma (80 percent), testis (80 percent), osteosarcoma (75 percent), choriocarcinoma (70 percent), kidney (70 percent), thyroid (65 percent), and breast (60 percent).[44] Most of these are morphologically distinct from bronchogenic carcinoma, and diagnostic difficulties should be limited in scope.

Malignant Pleural Effusion as a Presentation of Tumor of Unknown Origin

Six to 15 percent of all malignant pleural effusions will be TUOs.[45,46,47] The histological diagnosis is adenocarcinoma in nearly all cases.[48] Analysis of data on malignant pleural effusions where the primary tumor is known leads one to suspect that the most likely sites of occult primary cancer would be lung cancer in men and lung, breast, and ovarian cancer in women.[46]

If the cytological diagnosis is adenocarcinoma, evaluation should include chest x-ray and breast examination, as well as bilateral mammography and pelvic examination in women. Following the removal of the pleural effusion, repeat chest x-ray, lung tomography, or CT scan may reveal the occult primary. If these fail to reveal the primary, further work-up is unlikely to be revealing. An exception might be ovarian cancer, although a malignant pleural effusion alone is rare without ascites. If the physical examination is positive or equivocal for the presence of ascites, laparoscopy and peritoneal lavage for cytology may be useful.

Brain Presentations of Tumors of Unknown Origin

About one-fifth of all brain tumors are TUOs, based on several large neurosurgical series[49] (Table 4-7). In most instances the histological type is adenocarcinoma.[51] When the primary is eventually found, lung cancer is the most common.[52,54]

Much has been written about the indications for resection of solitary brain metastases. In the case of cancer of unknown origin, resection has been advocated. Unfortunately, most patients with a TUO metastatic to the brain will die within one year, either from the appearance of the primary tumor, recurrence of brain metastases, or the appearance of other metastases. In several reports, the median survival following resection ranged from 4 to 16 months, with 11 to 16 percent of patients alive at one year.[51,54,55–57] Since a small number of patients are long-term disease-free survivors, resection of a solitary brain TUO may be desirable.

Skin Presentations of Tumors of Unknown Origin

Little is known about skin metastases as the presenting site of a TUO. Two review articles on metastatic tumors to the skin[58,59] fail to identify any cases of skin TUOs. A review of the data included in these articles suggests

Table 4-7
Brain Presentations of Tumors of Unknown Origin: Frequency
of Tumor of Unknown Origin Compared to Cases Where
Primary is Found

Year/Author	Number of Cases Primary is Found	Number of Cases of Tumors of Unknown Origin
1954 Stortebecker[51]	158	51
1960 Simionescu[50]	195	23
1963 Richards[53]	389	66
1964 Lang[55]	284	36
1975 Ransohoff[49]	100	22
1981 Zimm[52]	191	16
1982 Chann[54]	57	20
Total	1374	234 (17%)

some possible explanations. First, skin presentations of TUOs may be rare because of the ease of detection of the primary tumors that commonly metastasize to the skin (lung, melanoma). Second, TUOs metastatic to skin may have other sites of metastatic disease, allowing the skin tumors to be overlooked. Finally, since skin metastases occur in about 5 percent of cancers, and since TUOs represent less than 10 percent of all reported cancers, the incidence of TUOs presenting as skin metastases is low. Chloromas representing involvement by leukemic infiltration should be considered when dealing with an unclassified neoplasm in the skin or subcutaneous tissue, along with solid tumors.

Malignant Pericardial Effusion as a Presentation of Tumor of Unknown Origin

Malignant pericardial effusions are infrequently reported as a presentation of tumors of unknown origin. A review of the literature by Frazer in 1980 disclosed 22 cases, of which 14 were lung cancer.[60] In eleven of Frazer's cases, plus two additional cases[61] 9 of 13 had an adenocarcinoma. In all but two cases, the primary cancer was found to arise from the lung. Four of the eleven lung cancer patients presented with mass lesions on chest radiograph and would be excluded as a TUO by our definition. In the remaining seven cases, however, the chest radiograph was nondiagnostic, and bronchoscopy or autopsy revealed the diagnosis.

The increasing incidence of bronchogenic carcinoma as well as the capability of the echocardiogram to detect pericardial effusions should increase the frequency of presentation of TUOs as pericardial effusions. From these data, it is clear that a patient with malignant pericardial effusion of unknown origin should be fully evaluated for lung cancer. If the chest x-ray reveals no mass lesions, computed tomography of the chest and sputum cytology should prove useful. If these tests are negative, bronchoscopy should be considered, especially if dyspnea persists following removal of the pericardial effusion or if hemoptysis is present. It may be unwise to perform bronchoscopy routinely, since adenocarcinomas of the lung are relatively refractory to chemotherapy, and the presence of the pericardial effusion indicates lack of resectability as well as a poor chance of survival.

Summary

Tumors of unknown origin represent a constellation of several clinical syndromes. Each of these can be defined in terms of the location of the tumor at presentation and the histological type. These two features, histology and location, might allow one to predict the site of the occult primary tumor.

A summary of the association between histology and site of presentation is shown in Tables 4-8 and 4-9, from data reported by Greager.[3] TUOs presenting in cervical nodes are most often squamous cell carcinomas or undifferentiated carcinomas, and the most common site of presentation of squamous cell TUOs is the cervical and supraclavicular nodes.

Overall, adenocarcinomas are the most common histological type of TUO and may present in a wide variety of locations, predominately intra-abdominal. Chest masses, which are most often adenocarcinomas, are often reported as bronchogenic carcinomas with intrapulmonary metastases. For this reason, it is not known if adenocarcinomatous TUO presenting as lung masses are being under- or over-reported. Across the board, bronchogenic carcinoma is generally the principal site of origin of adenocarcinomatous TUO presenting in the bone, CNS, or as pleural and pericardial effusions. Breast cancer is the origin of most adenocarcinomatous axillary adenopathy.

Many cases of undifferentiated cancers have been described, in the abdomen, cervical nodes, or bone. Several chapters in this book will specifically address this topic, from clinical, pathological, and experimental perspectives. An interesting feature common to several classical reports of nodal metastases of this type of TUO is the long relapse-free survival following resection of the tumor. Advancing knowledge in clinical and

Table 4-8
Tumor of Unknown Origin: Site of Presentation vs. Histological Types

	Cervical Node	Supraclavicular Node	Axilary Node	Inguinal Node	Chest Mass	Abdominal Mass	Skin Nodule	Bone Lesion	Brain Mass	Total
Adenocarcinoma	4	7	2	3	13	49	11	11	5	105
Squamous Cell Carcinoma	17	5	0	1	3	1	3	5	0	35
Undifferentiated Carcinoma	15	9	1	2	4	16	3	13	1	64
Malignant Tumor—not otherwise specified	5	4	3	1	13	14	2	12	0	54
Other Tumor (lymphoma, melanoma, sarcoma)	2	1	6	1	1	8	1	4	3	27
Total	43	26	12	8	34	88	20	45	9	285

Adapted from Greager JA, Wood D, DasGupta TK, et al. Metastatic cancer from an undetermined primary site. J Surg Oncol 23:73–76, 1983

Table 4-9

Tumor of Unknown Origin: Frequency of Various Sites of
Presentation by Histological Type

Adenocarcinoma		Undifferentiated Carcinoma		Squamous Cell Carcinoma	
Cases (N = 105)	%	Cases (N = 64)	%	Cases (N = 35)	%
Abdominal mass	47	Abdominal mass	25	Cervical node	50
Chest mass	12	Cervical node	23	Supraclavicular node	14
Skin nodule	10	Bone lesion	20	Bone lesion	14
Bone leslion	10	Supraclavicular node	14	Skin nodule	8
Supraclavicular node	7	Chest mass	6	Chest mass	8
Cervical node	4	Skin nodule	5	Abdominal mass	3
Brain mass	4	Inguinal node	3	Inguinal node	3
Inguinal node	3	Brain mass	2	Brain mass	0
Axillary node	2	Axillary node	2	Axillary node	0

Adapted from Greager JA, Wood D, DasGupta TK, et al. Metastatic cancer from an undetermined primary site. J Surg Oncol 23:73–76, 1983

laboratory disciplines, however, may now allow us to dissect various subsets within these groups, as discussed extensively in this book. Thus, generalities based on earlier series may need to be closely scrutinized in the future.

References

1. Batsakis JG: The pathology of head and neck tumors: The occult primary and metastases to the head and neck, part 10. Head and Neck Surgery 3:409–423, 1981
2. Richardson RG, Parker RG: Metastases from undetected primary cancers. West J Med 123:337–339, 1975
3. Greager JA, Wood D, Das Gupta TK, et al: Metastatic cancer from an undetermined primary site. J Surg Oncol 23:73–76, 1983
4. Holmes FF, Fouts, TL: Metastatic cancer of unknown primary site. Cancer 26:816–820, 1970
5. Richard JM, Micheau C: Malignant cervical adenopathies. Tumori 63:249–258, 1977
6. Marchetta FC, Murphy WT, Kovaric JJ, et al: Carcinoma of the neck. Am J Surg 106:974–979, 1963
7. Comess MS, Beahrs OH, Dockerty MB, et al: Cervical metastasis from occult carcinoma. Surg Gyn Obst 104:607–617, 1957

8. France CJ, Lucas R: The management and prognosis of metastatic neoplasms of the neck with an unknown primary. Am J Surg 106:835–839, 1963

9. Jesse RJ, Neff LE: Metastatic carcinoma in cervical nodes with an unknown primary site. Am J Surg 112:547–553, 1966

10. Smith PE, Krementz ET, Chapman W, et al: Metastatic cancer without a detectable primary site. Am J Surg 113:633–637, 1967

11. Barrie JR, Knapper WH, Strong EW, et al: Cervical nodal metastases of unknown origin. Am J Surg 120:466–470, 1970

12. Probert JC: Secondary carcinoma in cervical lymph nodes with an occult primary tumor: A review of 61 patients including their response to radiotherapy. Clin Radiol 21:211–218, 1970

13. Pico J, Zenaida F, Bosch A, et al: Cervical lymph node metastases from carcinoma of undetermined origin. Am J Roent 111:95–102, 1971

14. Fitzpatrick PJ, Kotalik JF: Cervical metastases from an unknown primary tumor. Radiol 110:659–663, 1974

15. Coker DD, Casterline PF, Chambers RG, et al: Metastases to lymph nodes of the head and neck from an unknown primary site. Am J Surg 134:517–522, 1977

16. Nussbaum M: Carcinoma of prostatic origin metastatic to cervical lymph nodes. NY St J Med 73:2050–2054, 1973

17. Snyder RD, Mavligit GM, Valdivieso M, et al: Adenocarcinoma of unknown primary site: A Clinico-pathological study. Med Ped Oncol 6:289–294, 1979

18. Berge T, and Toremalm NG: Cervical and mediastinal lymph node metastases as an otorhinolaryngic problem. Ann Otol 78:663–670, 1969

19. Copeland EM, McBride CM: Axillary metastases from unknown primary sites. Ann Surg 178:25–27, 1973

20. Pierce EH, Gray HK, Dockerty MB, et al: Surgical significance of isolated axillary adenopathy. Ann Surg 145:104–107, 1957

21. Feuerman L, Attie JN, Rosenberg B, et al: Carcinoma in axillary lymph nodes as an indicator of breast cancer. Surg Gyn Obst 114:5–8, 1962

22. Halsted WS: The results of radical operations for the cure of carcinoma of the breast. Ann Surg 46:1–19, 1907

23. Owen HW: Occult carcinoma of the breast. Surg Gyn Obst 98:302–308, 1954

24. Feigenberg Z, Zer M, Dintsman M, et al: Axillary Metastases from an unknown primary source. Isr J Med Sci 12:1153–1158, 1976

25. Zaren HA, Copeland EM: Inguinal node metastases. Cancer 41:919–923, 1978

26. Baab GH, McBride CM: Malignant melanoma: The patient with an unknown site of primary origin. Arch Surg 110:896–900, 1975

27. Das Gupta T, Bowden L, Berg JW, et al: Malignant melanoma of unknown primary origin. Surg Gyn & Obst 117:341–345, 1963

28. Panagopoulos E, Murray D: Metastatic malignant melanoma of unknown primary origin: A study of 30 cases. J Surg Oncol 23:8–10, 1983

29. Giuliano AE, Moseley HS, Morton DL, et al: Clinical aspects of unknown primary melanoma. Ann Surg 191:98–104, 1980

30. Douglass HO: Liver metastasis from occult primary tumors, in Weiss L, Gilbert HA (eds): Liver Metastases. Boston, G. K. Hall & Co., 1982

31. Nesbit RA, Tattersall MHN, Fox RM, et al: Presentation of unknown primary cancer with metastatic liver disease—management and natural history. Aust NZ J Med 11:16–19, 1981

32. Fenster LF, Klatskin G: Manifestations of metastatic tumours of the liver. Am J Med 31:238–48, 1961

33. Mauch PM: Treatment of metastatic cancer to bone, in DeVita V, et al. (ed) Cancer: Principles and Practice of Oncology. Philadelphia, Lippincott, Harper Inc., 1982

34. Simon MA, Karluk MB: Skeletal metastases of unknown origin. Clin Orthop 166:96–103, 1982

35. Schwinn CP: The pathologist and the diagnosis of bone metastasis, in Weiss L, Gilbert HA (eds): Bone Metastases. Boston, G.K. Hall & Co., 1981

36. Nystrom JS, Weiner JM, Wolf RM, et al: Identifying the primary site in metastatic cancer of unknown origin. JAMA 241:381–383, 1979

37. Higgins GA, Shields TW, Keehn RJ, et al: The solitary pulmonary nodule. Arch Surg 110:570–575, 1975

38. Cahan WG, Shah JP, Castro EB, et al: Benign solitary lung lesions in patients with cancer. Ann Surg 187:241–244, 1978

39. Ray FJ, Magnin GE, Smullen WA, et al: The coin lesion story: Update 1976. Chest 70:332–336, 1976

40. Steele JD: The solitary pulmonary nodule. J Thorac Cardiovasc Surg 46:21–39, 1963

41. Toomes H, Delphendahl A, Manke H, et al: The coin lesion of the lung: A review of 955 resected coin lesions. Cancer 51:534–537, 1983

42. Sherwin RP: The differentiation of primary lung cancer from metastatic disease, in Weiss L, Gilbert HA (eds): Pulmonary Metastases. G.K. Hall, 1978

43. McCormack PM, Bains MS, Beattie EJ, et al: Pulmonary resection in metastatic carcinoma, Chest 73:163, 1978

44. Weiss L, Gilbert HA: Patterns of pulmonary metastases—Introduc-

tion, in Weiss L, Gilbert HA (eds): Pulmonary Metastases: Boston, G.K. Hall, 1978

45. Tinney WS, Olsen AM: The significance of fluid in the pleural space: A study of 274 cases. J Thorac Surg 14:248–242, 1945

46. Chernow B, Sahn SA: Carcinomatous involvement of the pleura: An analysis of 96 patients. Am J Med 63:695–702, 1977

47. Anderson CB, Philpott GW, Ferguson TB, et al: The treatment of malignant pleural effusions. Cancer 33:916–922, 1974

48. Hirsch A, Ruffie P, Nebut M, et al: Pleural effusion: Laboratory tests in 300 cases. Thorax 34:106–112, 1979

49. Ransohoff J: Surgical management of metastatic tumors. Sem Onc 2:21–27, 1975

50. Simionescu MD: Metastatic tumors of the brain. J Neurosurg 17:361–373, 1960

51. Stortebecker TP: Metastatic tumors of the brain from a neurosurgical point of view. J Neurosurg 11:84–111, 1954

52. Zimm S, Wampler GL, Stablein D, et al: Intracerebral metastases in solid-tumor patients: Natural history and results of treatment. Cancer 48:384–394, 1981

53. Richards P, McKissock W: Intracranial metastases. Br Med J 1:15–18, 1963

54. Chan RC, Steinbok P: Solitary cerebral metastases: The effects of craniotomy on the quality and the duration of survival. Neurosurg 11:254–257, 1982

55. Lang EF, Slater J: Metastatic brain tumors: Results of surgical and nonsurgical treatment. Surg Clin NA 44:865–872, 1964

56. Ebels EJ, van der Meulen JDM: Cerebral metastases without known primary tumor, Clin Neurol Neurosurg 80:195–197, 1978

57. Ransohoff J: Surgical therapy of brain metastases in Weiss L, et al. (ed): Brain Metastases. Boston, G.K. Hall & Co., 1980

58. Brady LW, O'Neill EA, Farber SH, et al: Unusual sites of metastases. Sem Onc 4:59–64, 1977

59. Brownstein MH, Helwig EB: Metastatic tumors of the skin. Cancer 29:1298–1307, 1972

60. Fraser RS, Viloria JB, Wang N, et al: Cardiac tamponade as a presentation of extracardiac malignancy. Cancer 45:1697–1704, 1980

61. Sulkes A, Wieshler Z, Kopolovic Y, et al: Pericardial effusion as first evidence of malignancy in bronchogenic carcinoma. J Surg Oncol 20:71–74, 1982

5

ADENOCARCINOMA OF UNKNOWN ANATOMIC ORIGIN: EVALUATION AND THERAPY

Matthew L. Sherman
Marc B. Garnick

Metastatic adenocarcinoma of an unknown primary anatomic site is a frequent and frustrating diagnosis in oncologic practice. No definition of this syndrome is widely accepted, and some define cases only when the primary site remains elusive even after autopsy.[1] The initial diagnosis is made when the histologic diagnosis of adenocarcinoma is given, but the anatomic site of origin is not known. Alternatively, one may be faced with a poorly-differentiated or undifferentiated carcinoma whose histogenesis is uncertain.

For the purposes of this chapter, we shall define the syndrome of "adenocarcinoma of unknown origin" as applying to patients who present with histologically confirmed metastatic adenocarcinoma which is not felt to originate from the anatomic biopsy site and where the history, physical examination, laboratory testing, or chest radiograph fail to reveal the anatomic site of origin. This chapter will review the natural history and clinical features of this syndrome, critically assess the utility of an extensive radiologic evaluation, provide feasible diagnostic guidelines, report the therapeutic modalities, and offer suggestions for future developments.

POORLY DIFFERENTIATED NEOPLASMS AND TUMORS OF UNKNOWN ORIGIN   ISBN 0-8089-1755-2

General Considerations

Taxonomy

Traditionally, nonhematologic malignant neoplasms have been broadly divided into those arising from epithelial cells (carcinomas) and those from mesenchymal cells (sarcomas). Malignant disease has been categorized by the primary organ or tissue of origin (breast, lung, cervix) and subtyped by the cellular features expressed within that primary site (adenocarcinoma, squamous, adenosquamous). At the time of diagnosis, the tumor may be localized or sites of metastatic dissemination may be determined by staging procedures. Sometimes, however, a diagnosis of a malignant neoplasm is made from a metastatic site prior to knowing the anatomic location of the primary site.

Incidence and Clinical Features

The incidence of metastatic adenocarcinoma of unknown primary site has been reported to range from 0.5 to 6.7 percent in large university-based oncologic practices.[2–4] When only solid tumors are considered, the incidence is estimated to be as high as 15 percent.[5] Other series which include both adenocarcinomas and undifferentiated carcinomas indicate a similar incidence of 2.3 to 9.6 percent.[1,6–10]

The mean age at the time of diagnosis is 60 years.[1,2,11] Men predominate slightly, comprising 54 to 62 percent of the patient population.[1,2,5] The majority of patients are usually symptomatic of their metastatic disease at the time of presentation (Table 5-1).[12,13] The most frequent presenting sign is palpable lymphadenopathy with an incidence of 26 percent. Patients may present with hepatomegaly (25 percent), pulmonary symptoms (19 percent), or bone pain (19 percent). A palpable abdominal mass or ascites (8 percent), soft tissue mass (7 percent), or neurologic symptoms or signs (6 percent) are infrequent. In one series, weight loss was seen in 35 percent of the patients, but less than 5 percent had anemia, jaundice, or fever at presentation.[2]

The median survival for untreated patients with adenocarcinoma of unknown origin is two to six months.[2,14,15,16]

Primary Site

The anatomical site of origin can be determined either antemortem or postmortem. The primary site was diagnosed in 16 percent of patients overall (Table 5-2); the range was 4 to 67 percent. The frequency of

Table 5-1

Frequency of Predominant Symptoms and Signs at Presentation in Metastatic Carcinoma of Unknown Origin

Presenting Signs and Symptoms	N (%)							
	1972[5]* N = 162	1975[12]† N = 86	1977[2] N = 254	1978[13] N = 67	1979[3] N = 87	1983[11] N = 106	1983[4] N = 75	Total N = 837
Lymphadenopathy	24 (15)	27 (31)	125 (49)	11 (16)	13 (15)	14 (13)	4 (5)	218 (26)
above clavicle	—	24 (28)	92 (36)	11 (16)	—	—	—	127 (15)
below clavicle	—	3 (3)	33 (13)	—	—	—	—	36 (4)
Hepatomegaly/Hepatic pain	113 (70)	—	31 (12)	13 (19)	15 (17)	16 (15)	23 (31)	211 (25)
Pulmonary	24 (15)	4 (5)	99 (39)	—	22 (25)	—	14 (19)	163 (19)
Bone pain	10 (6)	33 (38)	53 (21)	18 (27)	5 (6)	28 (26)	16 (21)	163 (19)
Other abdominal mass/ascites	23 (14)	—	29 (11)	—	16 (18)	—	—	68 (8)
Soft tissue mass	14 (9)	11 (13)	29 (11)	—	5 (6)	—	—	59 (7)
Neurologic	—	11 (13)	—	5 (7)	7 (8)	24 (23)	6 (8)	53 (6)

* Patients referred to center specializing in gastrointestinal cancer
† Series limited to patients referred to radiation therapy center for palliation

Table 5-2
The Frequency of Ante- and Postmortem Diagnoses in
Metastatic Carcinoma of Unknown Primary Sites

Year and Reference	N	Histology (%)	Ante-mortem Diagnoses		Post-mortem Diagnoses		Total	
			N	(%)	N	(%)	N	(%)
1977[2]	254	Adenocarcinoma (41) Undifferentiated (34) Squamous (15)	6	(2)	71	(28)	77	(30)
1977[7]	1568	Adenocarcinoma (37) Undifferentiated (30) Squamous (10)	13	(0.8)	43	(3)	56	(4)
1978[13]	67	N/A	38	(57)	7	(10)	45	(67)
1979[3]	87	Adenocarcinoma (100)	23	(26)	10	(11)	33	(38)
1979[10]	266	Adenocarcinoma (78) Undifferentiated (18)	22	(8)	107	(40)	129	(48)
1983[11]	106	Adenocarcinoma (63) Undifferentiated (29)	33	(31)	7	(7)	40	(38)
Total	2348		135	(6)	245	(10)	380	(16)

identifying the primary site during the patient's life was only 6 percent. Although previous reviews had emphasized the notion that the primary site is usually not found even with autopsy,[17–25] careful analysis of these data makes this a misleading statement. Not only is the origin of the primary tumor in the majority of patients established by autopsy, but also, when the total number of autopsies performed was reported in five series, 78 percent of the postmortem examinations yielded the primary site (Table 5-3). Thus, the origin is usually not cryptogenic when the search includes an autopsy.

Where, then, is the most likely anatomic origin? In general, the most common primary sites are either lung or pancreas. Of 432 patients combined from several series in which the primary site was eventually diagnosed (Table 5-4), 108 patients (25 percent) had lung cancer, and 74 (17 percent) had pancreatic cancer. Less common sites were colon, hepatobiliary system and stomach. Also listed in Table 5-4 is the estimated 1984 incidence of cancer by site.[26] Lung cancer is somewhat over-represented as an unknown primary site, but even more so is pancreatic

Table 5-3
The Yield of Postmortem Examinations to Determine the
Primary Site of Metastatic Carcinoma of Unknown Origin

Year and Reference	Postmortem Diagnosis/Total Autopsies	Percent
1977[2]	71/78	91
1978[13]	17/20	85
1979[14]	0/25	0
1979[3]	14/16	88
1979[10]	107/130	82
Total	209/269	78

cancer (17 percent compared to 3 percent expected incidence). This can be most easily explained by the location and the relative lack of symptoms in early pancreatic cancer, leading to difficulty in diagnosis. Gastric and hepatobiliary system cancer are also infrequent in the general cancer population, but are often seen as occult primaries. Surprisingly, common tumors such as breast and prostate cancer are not often seen as cancer of unknown primary site. The superficial location of the breast, mammography, and self-examination may all lead to earlier detection of breast cancer. Similarly, the unique location of the prostate within reach of the examining digit makes physical detection easier.

There are conflicting conclusions concerning the accuracy in the clinical diagnosis of bronchogenic carcinoma.[27] The incidence of overdiagnosis of lung cancer[28] (i.e., clinical diagnoses not confirmed at autopsies) and underdiagnosis[29,30] (i.e., confirmed autopsy findings not suspected or diagnosed incorrectly clinically) varies greatly among series. "Detection bias" will also contribute to the clinical misdiagnosis of lung cancer. Patients who smoke or have a severe cough may have a higher rate of surveillance and be diagnosed and misdiagnosed more frequently as having bronchogenic cancer.[31] In a series of 387 autopsied patients with primary lung cancer, 28 (7.2 percent) were clinically misdiagnosed. Similar to patients presenting with adenocarcinoma of unknown origin, the mean age was 60 years with a predominance of males. Histologically, 65 percent of the undiagnosed tumors were adenocarinoma (more than twice the incidence in the remaining patients diagnosed antemortem), and the mean survival was only 3.5 months.[32]

On the other hand, although the lung is the most frequently diagnosed primary site in carcinoma of unknown origin, pulmonary metastases

Table 5-4

Comparison of the Frequency of Diagnosed Primary Sites in Metastatic Carcinoma of Unknown Origin with the 1984 Cancer Incidence by Site

Primary Site	1972[5] N = 42	1977[2] N = 77	1977[7] N = 56	1978[13] N = 55	1979[3] N = 33	1979[10] N = 129	1983[11] N = 40	Total N = 432	1984 Cancer Incidence[26] (%)
				N (%)					
Lung	1 (2)	31 (40)	7 (13)	18 (33)	7 (21)	28 (22)	16 (40)	108 (25)	22M, 10F
Pancreas	16 (38)	5 (6)	10 (18)	6 (11)	1 (3)	30 (23)	6 (15)	74 (17)	3
Colorectal	5 (12)	3 (4)	3 (5)	5 (9)	5 (15)	15 (12)	—	36 (8)	15
Hepatobiliary	7 (17)	2 (3)	6 (11)	2 (4)	2 (6)	16 (12)	—	35 (8)	2
Stomach	5 (12)	5 (6)	7 (13)	2 (4)	3 (9)	12 (9)	—	34 (8)	3
Ovary	—	3 (4)	4 (7)	5 (9)	4 (12)	4 (3)	5 (13)	25 (6)	4
Kidney	2 (5)	4 (5)	2 (4)	2 (4)	2 (6)	9 (7)	—	19 (4)	2
Prostate	1 (2)	—	1 (2)	4 (7)	2 (6)	4 (3)	3 (8)	15 (3)	18M
Breast	2 (5)	—	1 (2)	3 (5)	—	3 (2)	3 (8)	12 (3)	26F

M = male; F = female.

126

can mimic primary bronchogenic cancer.[33] In 46 percent of 1000 autopsied cases of carcinoma, the lungs were involved with metastases.[34] Pancreatic carcinoma, particularly of the body and tail, not infrequently presents as primary lung cancer.[35] In a study of 294 patients with biopsy-proven adenocarcinoma of the pancreas, 10 patients (3.4 percent) initially were thought to have lung cancer (all of whom were cigarette smokers). The usual chest radiograph finding was a unilateral hilar mass.[36]

Several reasons may account for the reported infrequency in detecting the primary site.[37] These include spontaneous regression of the primary tumor through immunologic mechanisms, inadvertent removal of the primary site, such as by skin biopsy or dilatation and curettage without careful histologic examination of the extirpated tissue, and even spontaneous expulsion of an adenocarcinoma arising in a colonic polyp.[38] While the frequency is unknown, the relative rarity of reported cases make them unlikely to be of significance in the majority of cases of adenocarcinoma of unknown origin. Moreover, greater than 75 percent of autopsy examinations will reveal the primary site. A primary tumor which is too small to be detected clinically or radiologically is the most probable explanation for failure in detecting a primary anatomic site.

Nystrom[39] conducted a careful search for the primary site in 264 patients with metastatic adenocarcinoma or undifferentiated carcinoma of unknown primary origin. Whether the diagnosis was made antemortem or postmortem was determined in 125 of these cases. Diagnoses were grouped to include those located above the diaphragm (supradiaphragmatic, especially lung and breast) and below the diaphragm (subdiaphragmatic, especially pancreas, liver, colorectal), and sites of metastatic disease were scored accordingly. The presence of lung or brain metastases was associated with a primary site above the diaphragm, while the presence of bone or liver metastases or a pelvic or rectal mass was correlated with an origin below the diaphragm. Using a statistical approach assigning a numerical weight to each metastatic site, the authors were able to locate the primary anatomic location correctly in 91 percent of the patients with supradiaphragmatic origin and 75 percent of subdiaphragmatic origin. In addition, they noted the metastatic patterns were unusual when compared to those where the primary site is obvious. For example, while the incidence of bone metastases from lung cancer at autopsy is 30–50 percent, in patients with adenocarcinoma of unknown origin and eventually diagnosed lung cancer, bone involvement at postmortem examination was 11 percent. Their autopsy rate of only 50 percent, however, could bias this type of analysis.

Evaluation

Pathology

An open channel for communication between the clinician and the pathologist is of utmost importance once the diagnosis of a cancer of unknown origin is entertained. The pathologist will be the first to indicate a tumor to be metastatic adenocarcinoma based on its histologic appearance under the light microscope. Histologic staining for mucin with mucicarmine or alcian blue may be needed to confirm that the tumor is of epithelial origin. Cytoplasmic glycogen will be stained using the periodic-acid-Shiff method and may suggest a renal cell adenocarcinoma.

Immunocytochemical techniques may further classify neoplasms based on tissue markers. Staining for carcinoembryonic antigen indicates, in most situations, an anatomic site in the gastrointestinal tract, lung, breast, urothelium, ovarian, uterine, or cervix.[40,41] Thyroglobulin is specific for thyroid carcinoma, while immunoperoxidase staining for prostate-specific antigen[42] and prostatic acid phosphatase[43-45] indicates a prostate primary. Immunoperoxidase staining for alpha fetoprotein and human chorionic gonadotropin should be performed to evaluate for an occult germ cell origin of the tumor. Lastly, features seen on transmission electron microscopy (EM) may also identify the site of the primary tumor.[46] Tissue from a lymph node or other biopsy suspected to be metastatic carcinoma should be promptly and carefully fixed in glutaraldehyde for EM study. This will obviate the need for a second biopsy if the original histologic diagnosis is in question. The terminal web of the brush border of intestinal epithelial cells can be identified by EM as apical cytoplasm containing filaments and microvilli projecting into acini. These terminal webs are not seen in adenocarcinomas of the lung, breast, ovary, uterus, kidney, and prostate, and are thus specific for a gastrointestinal primary. To help further classify tumors, the microvilli from breast adenocarcinoma are short and stubby, and from renal adenocarcinoma markedly elongated. Also useful in EM is the presence of lamellar bodies (surfactant bodies) in broncho-alveolar cell carcinoma of the lung, multiple lysosomes in prostate adenocarcinoma, and numerous mitochondria in thyroid adenocarcinoma. In actuality, however, the diagnosis of metastatic poorly differentiated adenocarcinoma is often made with the primary site still unknown. Several other methods which may assist in the classification of such neoplasms are discussed extensively in other chapters of this book.

Clinical Evaluation

Once faced with a patient with metastatic adenocarcinoma of an unknown primary site, the clinician is responsible for directing the laboratory and radiologic evaluation of the patient. Since the oncologist usually bases therapy on the site of origin of a known cancer, many investigators have conducted a comprehensive and excessive search for a primary site.[47] More recently, common sense, clinical judgment, and a limited workup based on the likely primary site have been recommended.[48-50]

The early literature on the diagnostic workup of unknown primary cancer focused on cervical lymph node metastases.[51-53] Extensive and repetitive head and neck evaluations, including random biopsies of apparently normal mucosa, were suggested. A "timely" lymph node biopsy was recommended only if the initial evaluation was unrewarding.[54] The predominant histologic diagnosis was epidermoid carcinoma. The primary lesion was eventually found in only 30 - 45 percent of patients having cervical lymph node metastases and an occult primary site. Even in the absence of a documented primary site, however, curative radical neck surgery and radiotherapy were attempted with surprisingly good long-term results. The 3-year survival rate has been significant, ranging from 30 to 40 percent, after surgery, radiation therapy, or a combination of treatments.[55-57]

When the histologic diagnosis is unknown and the primary site not clear, the clinician is tempted to uncover a curable tumor, i.e., lymphoma, small cell of the lung, germ cell. With confirmation of adenocarcinoma as the histologic diagnosis, however, the presence of a more treatable cancer is less likely. The goal of the clinical and radiologic evaluation is primarily two-fold; first, to establish the anatomic origin during life, and second, to establish the extent of metastatic disease. The former goal may alleviate some psychologic burden for the patient, provide prognostic information, and guide therapy. The latter may also predict prognosis and provide early detection of potential morbidity, such as central nervous system metastases or lytic erosions of weight-bearing bones, allowing the initiation of appropriate palliative therapy.

History and Physical

Of primary importance in the workup of the newly diagnosed patient is the history-taking and physical examination. Particular emphasis should be placed on careful inspection of the head and neck region, including indirect laryngoscopy, palpation of the breasts, thyroid, lymph nodes, and prostate gland, a complete genital and pelvic examination, and testing of the stool and urine for blood. A thorough examination should be periodically repeated; the primary site may eventually be found.

Lab and Tumor Markers

Laboratory analysis should include a urinalysis to screen for microscopic hematuria, a complete blood count to evaluate for iron deficiency, and liver function tests. The tumor marker carcinoembryonic antigen (CEA) has been well-studied and is useful in the diagnosis, treatment, and follow-up of patients with adenocarcinoma of epithelial origin. In 32 patients with metastatic disease of intially unknown primary site,[58] a plasma CEA level of higher than 10 ng/ml occurred in 10. Of these, the anatomic origin was determined to be lung in 5, pancreas in 2, ovary in 2, and biliary duct in 1. Total acid phosphatase can be fractionated to determine the specific prostate portion, indicating primary prostate pathology.[59] Alpha-fetoprotein (AFP) and human chorionic gonadotropin (hCG) are of value in the diagnosis of germ cell tumors.[60]

Newer tumor markers have been reported. High serum levels of des-gamma-carboxyprothrombin, an abnormal prothrombin in patients with biopsy-confirmed hepatocellular carcinoma, have been described.[61] When used together with AFP, 84 percent of patients with hepatocellular carcinoma were identified. The course of epithelial ovarian carcinomas has been monitored using a radioimmunometric assay to detect serum levels of the antigen CA 125, derived from a human ovarian cancer cell line.[62] Antigen was detected in 82 percent of patients with surgically proven disease.

Estrogen Receptor

Estrogen receptor protein (ERP) assayed in a metastatic adenocarcinoma of unknown origin can be useful.[63,64] Approximately 50 percent of all breast carcinomas are ERP-positive. ERP may also be present, however, in cancer of the uterus, ovary, kidney, prostate, melanoma, and their metastases. A positive ERP value would be useful if present on a biopsy of an axillary lymph node in the absence of a primary breast lesion. Furthermore, a high level (greater than 100 fmoles/milligram cytosol protein)[65,66] of a biopsied lesion in a patient with metastatic adenocarcinoma of unknown primary site could very likely respond to hormonal manipulation and/or breast cancer specific chemotherapy.

Radiology

Chest Radiograph

The chest radiograph (CXR) is the single-most utilized radiologic examination in the workup of patients with adenocarcinoma of unknown origin. The CXR may establish the primary site, provide information about the extent of metastatic disease, or indicate other, unsuspected cardiopulmonary processes. In one study, however, primary carcinoma of the lung could not be distinguished from metastatic disease by chest radiograph.[10] Although five CXR patterns were identified (single mass lesion, multiple nodules, nodal disease, malignant effusion, or infiltrative lesions), none was able to distinguish primary lung cancer from metastatic cancer to the lung. However, the clinical features of bronchogenic carcinoma must be interpreted appropriately. The presence of a single large mass and mediastinal adenopathy suggests lung cancer. Since the lung is the most common primary anatomic site diagnosed in this syndrome, the CXR is obviously justified.

Dye–Contrast Radiologic Studies

Dye–contrast radiologic studies, such as upper gastrointestinal series (UGI), barium enemas (BaE), and intravenous pyelogram (IVP), are often performed in patients with cancer of an unknown origin. In over 200 examinations each, only 7.4 percent, 11 percent, and 8 percent of UGI, BaE, and IVP, respectively, were positive.[3,10] Of these, the number of true positive studies (as determined by biopsy results or eventual autopsies) was approximated or exceeded by the number of falsely positive tests (Table 5-5). The sensitivity of these examinations was correspondingly low. A high predictive value of a positive test is essential, because a false-positive result will lead to time-consuming, invasive, and expensive investigations or inappropriate therapy. These studies and others[13] indicate that, in the absence of symptoms and signs referrable to an organ system, routine dye-contrast studies are of low yield, infrequently establishing the anatomic primary site.

Computed Tomography

On the other hand, computed tomography (CT) has been found to be superior compared with radiologic contrast studies of the gastrointestinal tract and genitourinary system in demonstrating the primary organ in metastatic adenocarcinoma from an unknown primary site. In one study,[67]

Table 5-5
Sensitivity, Specificity, and Positive Predictive Value of Dye-Contrast Radiologic Studies

	Upper GI Series			Barium Enema			Intravenous Pyelogram		
	1979[3]	1979[10]	Total	1979[3]	1979[10]	Total	1979[3]	1979[10]	Total
Total No.	24	218	242	27	198	225	35	187	222
No. positive	4	14	18	7	17	24	2	16	18
TP	1	8	9	4	9	13	0	5	5
FP	3	6	9	3	8	11	2	11	13
FN	1	4	5	0	6	6	1	4	5
TN	19	200	219	20	175	195	32	167	199
Sensitivity			64%			68%			50%
Specificity			96%			95%			94%
PPV			50%			54%			28%

Adapted from Ultmann JE, Phillips TL: Management of patient with cancer of unknown primary site, in Devita VJ Jr, Hellman S, Rosenberg SA (eds): Cancer Principles and Practice of Oncology (ed 2). Philadelphia, J. P. Lippincott, 1985, p 1846, with permission.
TP = true–positive; FP = false-positive; FN = false-negative; TN = true-negative; PPV = positive predictive value
Sensitivity = TP/(TP + FN); Specificity = TN/(FP + FN); Positive predictive value = TP/(TP + FP)

132

Table 5-6
A Comparison of the Yield of Dye–Contrast Roentography and
Computed Tomography in the Diagnosis of the Primary Site

	Conventional (UGI, BaE, IVP)		CT (Abdomen, Pelvic, Chest)	
	1979[10]	1979[3]	1982[67]	1982[68]
Total Patients	266	87	46	98
No. Radiologic Diagnosis	22	8	16	31
Percent yield	8	9	35	32

CT detected the primary site (6 pancreas, 2 ovary, 2 hepatoma, 2 kidney, 1 lung, 1 adrenal, 1 gallbladder and 1 stomach) in 16 of 46 patients (35 percent). (In this study, 99 UGI, BaE, and IVP examinations revealed only 1 colon cancer.) In another series,[68] the primary site was demonstrated in 31 cases of clinically occult tumor (11 pancreas, 5 kidney, 5 lung, 4 hepatobiliary, 3 lymphoma, 1 ovary, 1 colon, and 1 germ cell) out of 98 patients (32 percent) using CT scanning. Interestingly, in 13 CT examinations which were falsely negative, the primary site was overlooked but demonstrated retrospectively. The diagnostic yield of CT is three to four times greater than that of conventional radiologic investigations (Table 5-6).

The role of chest CT in detecting the primary site is less clear. Conventional chest radiography and whole lung tomography (WLT) have been the standard in screening for pulmonary metastases. In several studies,[69–71] however, the chest CT has been found superior to whole lung tomography in detecting metastatic pulmonary nodules. CT can define smaller parenchymal lesions as well as pleural-based nodules not detected by CXR or WLT. When pathologic correlation is obtained, however, 60 percent of the additional lesions documented by CT were not malignant. The mediastinum may be better evaluated with chest CT.[72] Of the 144 patients undergoing CT scanning to locate the primary site, only 20 chest CT examinations were performed. Six primary lung cancers however, were identified (30 percent). As previously shown, the lung is the anatomic primary site in 25 percent of patients eventually diagnosed.

Evaluation of the pancreas can be best performed with ultrasonography or CT scanning. In a retrospective study,[73] 102 patients suspected of having pancreatic pathology were examined by both ultrasonography and computed tomography. Forty-one of those patients had a final histologic diagnosis of pancreatic cancer. Using ultrasound, only 64 patients (65 percent) had technically satisfactory studies. Of these, 54 patients were diagnosed correctly, yielding an overall accuracy rate of 54 percent (54 of 102). When computed tomography was used, 96 correct diagnoses were obtained in 100 technically adequate studies, giving an overall accuracy rate of 95 percent (96/102). Both modalities failed to detect pancreatic lesions less than 3 cm in size.

Clinically suspected pelvic masses have been prospectively evaluated with computed tomography and ultrasonography.[74] Of 24 patients with gynecologic pelvic masses, useful clinical information was provided by ultrasound in 71 percent and by CT scanning in 63 percent. Recurrent tumor was not detected in three patients by either method of evaluation. Ultrasonography, however, appeared to be advantageous over pelvic CT in the diagnosis of ovarian or cervical cancer. If the abdominal CT scan is negative in women with adenocarcinoma of unknown origin and subdiaphragmatic disease, a pelvic CT scan or ultrasound is indicated.

Radionuclide Imaging

Radionuclide imaging is unlikely to be of value in diagnosing the primary site in metastatic adenocarcinoma of unknown origin, but may be useful in staging the extent of the disease. The liver is the most common metastatic site of disease in autopsied patients with carcinoma. Although the accuracy of liver radionuclide scanning is approximately 80 percent,[75–78] an increased accuracy of hepatic CT scanning was noted, especially in detecting lesions less than 3 cm in diameter.[79,80] If an abdominal CT scan is being performed to search for the primary site, a liver radionuclide scan will generally add little other information and is not necessary.

Similarly, bone scanning is highly sensitive in identifying skeletal metastases.[81–83] The bone scan was productive as a screening procedure for metastases in 50–80 percent of patients with carcinoma of unknown primary site, even in patients who had no symptoms referrable to bone.[2,13] Thyroid cancer is often pursued, but is uncommon as the primary site. In 51 patients who underwent radionuclide thyroid scanning, none was positive.[2] Other radioisotopic scans (renal, brain) are likely to be of low yield in asymptomatic patients.

Mammography

The value of bilateral mammography in the early detection for breast cancer has been established by the randomized trial of the Health Insurance Plan of New York.[84] Screening mammography and physical examination reduced breast cancer mortality. Mammograms are also frequently recommended to detect an occult lesion in the presence of axillary adenopathy or disseminated adenocarcinoma of unknown origin.[85] Stewart[3] reported no cases of breast cancer in 14 women who underwent mammography in the evaluation of unknown primary adenocarcinoma. Didolkar[2] noted 6 out of 45 mammograms which were positive (13.3 percent). The low yield of mammography is probably a reflection of the low incidence of the breast as the primary site. Still, the relatively high response rate of breast cancer to chemotherapy and hormonal manipulation justifies a mammographic evaluation.

Therapy

Surgery

While surgery has a central role in the diagnosis of adenocarcinoma of unknown origin, there are few patients with this syndrome who can be cured by surgical resection of their metastatic disease, as most will have multiple metastases. In general, a solitary or small number of metastases to the liver, lung, or brain may be surgically resected for cure. However, the poor prognosis and short survival of patients with metastatic adenocarcinoma of unknown primary must be considered. Surgery for palliation of pain or prevention of damage to contiguous structures may be necessary. If the primary site is the ovary, then cytoreductive surgery for stage III disease may be required. The role of surgery as the primary therapy for possible breast cancer with isolated axillary adenopathy is discussed later in this chapter.

Radiation Therapy

While radiation therapy (RT) may be of value in the treatment of epidermoid carcinoma of an occult primary site metastatic to cervical lymph nodes, it is of limited usefulness in the therapy of adenocarcinoma of unknown origin. The patient may receive RT for palliation of symptomatic metastases, especially bone lesions. Of 86 patients with metastatic carcinoma of unknown origin referred to a radiation oncology center (many of whom also received chemotherapy), the mean survival was 3 months.[12] All long-term survivors in this study had cervical adenopathy and were treated with high doses for cure.

For a solitary site of metastatic disease, excision followed by localized high dose radiotherapy may be justified. This would be most appropriate for isolated lymphadenopathy or a soft tissue mass if the remainder of the metastatic workup was negative. Women presenting with isolated metastatic adenocarcinoma in the axillary region may have breast cancer and demand special consideration (vide infra).

Whole brain radiotherapy is the principal treatment for most patients with brain metastases and an unknown primary site. The recommended schedule is 3000 rad in 2 weeks. For selected patients with a solitary cerebral metastasis, however, surgery is indicated.

Chemotherapy

The role of chemotherapy in metastatic adenocarcinoma of unknown primary site is decidedly unclear.[86,87] The general experience at several institutions has been reported. In a retrospective analysis of 245 patients with metastatic adenocarcinoma of unknown primary site, the mean survival was 3.1 months.[16] Patients treated with chemotherapy had a similar mean survival (4.2 months) compared to untreated patients or those treated with local radiation therapy (2.6 months). A small number of patients receiving cyclophosphamide and/or doxorubicin had a mean survival of 9.4 months compared to 3.2 months for those patients given 5-fluorouracil. In a series of 77 patients with adenocarcinoma of unknown origin, the median survival of the whole group was 31 weeks.[15] Patients receiving chemotherapy survived 41 weeks, and responses were common with combination chemotherapy, especially cyclophosphamide-*adriamycin* containing regimens.

A retrospective evaluation of 20 patients with adenocarcinoma of unknown origin treated at the Dana-Farber Cancer Institute is summarized in Table 5-7. The "broad-spectrum" combination of cyclophosphamide and adriamycin was widely used. Responses were few. Many patients received only one cycle of chemotherapy prior to death. The mean survival of 7.5 months was not substantially different when compared to a randomly selected group of untreated patients.

In the last 20 years, there have been only 10 reports of trials using systemic chemotherapy in metastatic adenocarcinoma for an unknown primary site, only two of which were randomized (Table 5-8). In one study over a six-year period, 185 patients at The University of Wisconsin Medical Center had primary unknown cancers.[6] The most frequent type of tumor histologically was adenocarcinoma (43 percent). Of the 185 patients, 65 were treated with 5-fluorouracil (5-FU) alone. Four objective responses were seen; 2 were in patients with adenocarcinoma, producing a response rate of 6.2 percent. Eight patients were treated with 5-fluoro-2'-

Table 5-7

Chemotherapy of Metastatic Adenocarcinoma of Unknown
Primary Site at the Dana-Farber Cancer Institite

Regimen	# Pts*	# Cycles	Response CR	PR	NR
CTX	2	9	—	—	2
CTX/ADR	6	32	—	1	5
CTX/ADR/CDDP	2	4	—	—	2
5-FU	2	2	—	—	2
5-FU/ADR/MITO	5	8	—	—	5
5-FU/ADR/CDDP	1	2	1	—	—
CTX/ADR/MTX/5-FU	1	1	—	—	1
CDDP	1	1	—	—	1
HD-MTX	1	1	—	—	1
NCS	2	3	—	—	2
DAD	1	4	—	—	1
AD 32	1	4	—	—	1
PALA	1	5	—	—	1
Hepatic arterial infusion (BCNU, FUdR)	1	2	—	—	1

Total patients: 20
Cycles chemo: 78 (Mean 3.9)
Mean survival (diagnosis to death): 7.5 months

* Several patients received more than one regimen
CTX = Cyclophosphamide; ADR = Adriamycin; CDDP = Cisplatin; 5-FU = 5-Fluorouracil;
MITO = Mitomycin-C; MTX = Methotrexate; HD-MTX = High dose Methotrexate; NCS =
Neocarcinostatin; DAD = Dihydroxyanthracenedione (Mitoxantrone); AD 32 = N-trifluoroa-
cetyladriamycin-14-valerate; PALA = N-(phosphonacetyl)-L-aspartate; BCNU = bis-chlor-
oethylnitrosourea (Carmustine); FUdR = 5-Fluoro-2'-deoxyuridine
CR = complete response; PR = partial response; NR = no response

deoxyuridine (5-FUdR), and one objective response was seen (also in a
patient with adenocarcinoma). Moertel[5] treated 162 patients with adenocarcinoma of unknown origin with several chemotherapeutic regimens.
Three regimens yielded response rates of greater than 10 percent. A total
of 108 patients were given 5-FU, 5-FU and BCNU, or mitomycin-C, and
objective responses of 16 percent, 18 percent and 22 percent, respectively,
were observed. The median survival of the patients with an objective
response was 11.7 months, but the median survival of the entire group
overall was only 4 months.

Didolkar[2] reported 254 patients with histologically-proven metastatic
cancer from an unknown primary site, of which 103 (40.5 percent) were
adenocarcinoma. 5-FU, cyclophosphamide, vincristine, methotrexate, and

Table 5-8
Systemic Chemotherapy Trials in Metastatic Carcinoma of
Unknown Origin

Year and Reference	Regimen	N	Response	Survival All Patients/ Responders
1964[6]	5-FU	65	4 RR (6.2%)	—
1972[5]	5-FU	88	14 RR (16%)	4 months (M)/11.7 M
	5-FU/BCNU	11	2 RR (18%)	
	MITO	9	2 RR (22%)	
1977[2]	5-FU/CTX/VCR/MTX N MUST	103	4 CR (3.1%) 4 PR (3.1%)	6 M/24 M
1979[89]	CTX/ADR/5-FU	14	2 PR (14%)	7+ M/15+ M
	BLEO/VBL	2	1 PR (50%)	
1980[90]	CTX/MTX/5-FU versus	22	1 PR (5%)	7 weeks (W)/—
	ADR/MITO	25	1 CR (4%) 8 PR (32%)	18 W/28+ W
1980[91]	5-FU/ADR/MITO	28	3 CR (11%) 3 PR (11%) 8 SD (29%) 14 NR (50%)	4 M/11 M 4 M/12 M 4 M/11 M 4 M/—
1981[92]	5-FU/ADR/MITO or 5-FU/MITO versus	15	—	100 days (D)
	CONTROL	14	—	90 D
1983[93]	5-FU versus	20	0	105 D
	CTX/ADR/5-FU	16	0	95 D
1983[94]	CTX/ADR/VCR	20	4 CR (20%) 6 PR (30%)	8 M/8 M
1983[95]	TEGAFUR	17	1 CR (6%) 3 PR (18%)	18 W/18 W
	CTX/ADR/CDDP	9	2 PR (22%)	

5–FU = 5-Fluorouracil; BCNU = bis–chloroethylnitrosourea (Carmustine); MITO = Mitomycin-C; CTX = Cyclophosphamide; VCR = Vincristine; MTX = Methotrexate; N MUST = Nitrogen Mustard; ADR = Doxorubicin hydrochloride; BLEO = Bleomycin; VBL = Vinblastine; TEGAFUR = Ftorafur; CDDP = Cisplatin; RR = response rate; CR = complete response; PR = partial response; NR = no response; SD = stable disease nitrogen mustard were used alone or in combination; the exact regimens were not stated. Of the total group, 130 were treated with chemotherapy. The overall response rate was 6.2 percent with 4 complete responses and 4 partial responses seen. Survival data showed a median survival of 24 months for chemotherapy responders and 5 months for nonresponders, which is similar to Moertel's data.

Subsequent series report on the use of combination chemotherapy. With few exceptions, treatment with single agent chemotherapy cannot produce significant and lasting remissions nor cure patients with cancer. Based on the principles of combination chemotherapy and the development of the MOPP program as a curative program for Hodgkin's disease, most treatments for advanced cancer have been of combination chemotherapeutic regimens. Valentine[88,89] noted the limited response rates of 5-FU only and treated 14 patients with cycloposphamide, adriamycin, and 5-FU. Two patients obtained objective responses (14 percent). Of 2 patients given vinblastine and bleomycin after failing to respond to CAF, one additional partial response was obtained. The median survival of 14 patients was 7+ months. Responders to chemotherapy or patients who remained stable had a longer median survival of 15+ months, while nonresponders had a median survival of only 3 months.

In 1980, Woods[90] reported the first randomized study of patients with the histologic diagnosis of undifferentiated carcinoma or adenocarcinoma from an unknown primary site using two combination chemotherapy regimens. Patients were randomized to cyclophosphamide, methotrexate and 5-FU (CMF), or to doxorubicin (Adriamycin,® Adria) and mitomycin-C (DM). Nine of 25 patients (36 percent) receiving DM responded to therapy, while only one of 22 patients (5 percent) receiving CMF responded. Of five patients crossed-over to the alternative regimen, none responded. After discontinuing the randomized study, another 16 patients were treated with DM, and 6 responses were obtained. As in previous studies, life-table data analysis demonstrated greater survival in responders compared to nonresponders. They conclude that DM is a useful empirical treatment for symptomatic patients.

McKeen[91] reported on the use of the Georgetown FAM regimen (5-FU, Adriamycin, mitomycin-C) in 28 patients with adenocarcinoma of unknown origin, after noting the effectiveness of this regimen for pulmonary, pancreatic and gastric carcinomas. An overall complete and partial response rate of 21 percent was observed with a mean survival of responders of 11.5+ months versus 4 months for nonresponders.

Subsequent studies using an adriamycin containing regimen, however, have shown no responses or survival benefit. Rudnick[92] reported a nonrandomized study of FAM or 5-FU and mitomycin-C (Adriamycin was not given when contraindicated), compared to group not treated but matched for age, sex, performance status, and number of metastatic sites. Response rates were not mentioned, but survival of the treated and untreated groups did not differ statistically (100 days and 90 days respectively).

The Southwest Oncology Group[93] reported the second randomized study of 36 patients with metastatic adenocarcinoma of unknown primary site. Patients were randomized to receive either 5-FU or the combination of 5-FU, doxorubicin and cyclophosphamide. No objective responses were seen in either group. The median survival was 105 days for patients given the single agent chemotherapy and 95 days for the combination chemotherapy.

Anderson[94] studied 20 patients with metastatic carcinoma of unknown primary site. Histologic diagnoses were anaplastic carcinoma or poorly differentiated adenocarcinoma. Patients were treated with cyclophosphamide, doxorubicin and vincristine. An overall response rate of 50 percent (20 percent complete responders and 30 percent partial responders) was observed with lymph node metastases having the highest response rate. The median survival of all patients was eight months with no difference in survival between responders and nonresponders.

Bedikian[95] reported on patients with metastatic adenocarcinoma of unknown primary origin who were treated initially with oral tegafur. Of 17 patients evaluated for response, 1 complete response and 3 partial responses were seen. Nine patients failing to respond to tegafur were then given cyclophosphamide, doxorubicin, and cisplatin. Two additional partial responses were obtained. While responders survived longer than nonresponders, the median survival of all patients was only 18 weeks.

Several issues deserve further discussion. Although some studies have demonstrated an improved survival in responders, it does not necessarily follow that the success was due to the treatment. One may be selecting a group of patients who have a better prognosis and more indolent disease. The more important question is whether any therapy is better than no treatment at all. There is questionable evidence for improved survival in patients with non-small cell lung cancer or pancreatic cancer given chemotherapy when analyzed as a treatment group compared with an untreated group. In the situation such as in advanced testicular germ cell tumors of a high response rate when treated with combination chemotherapy, an untreated control group is neither statistically nor ethically necessary. However, when the existing response rates are low, the potential side effects from combination chemotherapy great, and overall survival rate short, a nontreatment control group is warranted in evaluating chemotherapeutic regimens in patients with adenocarcinoma of unknown origin.

A striking consistency of a median survival of between 3 to 8 months is seen in all reported series. This poor prognosis is understandably a reflection of the disseminated metastatic disease, and is not dissimilar for the survival seen in patients with either metastatic lung cancer or pancreatic cancer. Since the majority of patients with metastatic adenocarcinoma of unknown origin represents these two primary sites, we can compare their response to chemotherapy. Combination chemotherapy with cyclophosphamide, doxorubicin, and cisplatin (CAP) in non-small cell lung cancer in multiple trials yielded overall response rates of 25–40 percent and a complete response rate of 5–10 percent. Median survival of all patients was 5–10 months, and median survival of responders was 12 months. In pancreatic cancer, the FAM regimen has produced an overall objective response rate of 40 percent. Similar to lung cancer and not unlike patients with metastatic adenocarcinoma of unknown primary treated with FAM, median survival for responders was 8 months and only 3 months for nonresponders.

Special Considerations

Extragonadal Germ Cell Cancer Syndrome

Although a typical patient with adenocarcinoma of unknown origin is an older male with a history of weight loss, hepatomegaly, and bone pain secondary to metastatic disease, other clinical subsets deserve mention. A young male (or rarely female) with a rapidly growing midline tumor, central lymphadenopathy and/or pulmonary metastases may have an occult testicular carcinoma or the extragonadal germ cell cancer syndrome.[96–99] Serum levels should be assayed for beta-human chorionic gonadotropin and alpha fetoprotein, and immunocytochemical staining for hCG and AFP should be performed on the biopsy specimen. The initial histologic diagnosis in this syndrome has been misread as poorly differentiated adenocarcinoma or undifferentiated carcinoma. In one series of 12 patients, 5 were given the initial histologic diagnosis of metastatic adenocarcinoma.[99] Common sites of disease were the mediastinum, lungs, and retroperitoneum. As with known metastatic testicular carcinoma, treat-

ment with combination chemotherapy cisplatin, vinblastine, and bleomycin can be curative.

Isolated Axillary Lymphadenopathy

When biopsy of a lymph node in isolated axillary adenopathy reveals
metastatic adenocarcinoma, the most likely primary site is the ipsilateral
breast. Pierce[100] reviewed the pathologic diagnosis made on examination of
biopsy specimens from unilaterally enlarged axillary lymph nodes. In 50 of
the 72 specimens (69.5 percent), nonspecific changes were seen.
Lymphoma was the next most frequent finding, accounting for 13.9
percent of the specimens. Adenocarcinoma was diagnosed in 5 nodes,
metastatic from the ipsilateral breast in 3 patients and from an unknown
source in two patients. Feuerman[101] reported 14 females in whom axillary
node biopsy was the first documentation of carcinoma. Ten underwent
ipsilateral mastectomy in the absence of a breast mass, and primary breast
carcinoma was found in seven. The prognosis of patients with clinically
occult breast carcinoma presenting as isolated axillary metastases has been
compared favorably to palpable breast cancer with axillary metastases.[102–105] Ashikari reported a 79 percent five-year survival in 19 patients
after radical mastectomy.[105] A disease-free survival period of four years
between the axillary dissection and the appearance of the primary breast
lesion has been reported.[106] Assuming the diagnosis of metastatic adenocarcinoma after axillary biopsy with a negative physical breast examination
and mammography, attention should be directed toward primary staging
with a chest radiograph, liver function tests, CEA, and bone scanning. In
the absence of distant metastases, the primary therapy of ipsilateral
modified radical mastectomy has been recommended.[104,105,107,108] The more
conservative approach of diagnostic sector mastectomy of the upper, outer
quandrant and/or radiation therapy needs to be studied further.[109,110]

Inglehart reported 5 patients who presented with axillary lymphadenopathy.[111] Electron microscopy established the diagnosis of adenocarcinoma in all five after initial histology revealed undifferentiated carcinoma
(in 2 patients), poorly differentiated squamous cell carcinoma, lymphoma,
and melanoma (1 patient each). Excluding the original biopsied node, none
of the patients had other axillary nodal involvement. After ipsilateral
modified mastectomy, all 5 mastectomy specimens was found to contain a
primary breast tumor ranging in size from 0.2 to 1.4 cm. The histology of
the breast primary was infiltrating ductal in 4 and infiltrating lobular in
one. This emphasizes the need for accurate histologic diagnoses, especially
in establishing the diagnosis of isolated axillary metastatic adenocarcinoma.

Solitary CNS Metastasis

The brain is a frequent site of metastatic disease; 18 percent of autopsy examinations in patients with carcinoma reveal central nervous system (CNS) metastases.[34] For patients with CNS metastases, the median survival ranges from 3 to 12 months.[112] Lung cancer is most frequent in patients with a past history of cancer who develop intracranial metastases during life.[113–115] Carcinoma of unknown primary site frequently is seen as the second most common tumor, accounting for 8 to 12 percent of patients at the time of diagnosis;[114,115] however, lung cancer will often be subsequently diagnosed.[116] In one study of 16 patients with unknown primaries metastatic to brain, the lung was diagnosed as the primary in 6 postoperatively.[114] Of the remaining 10, an autopsy done in 2 also revealed lung cancer.

Patients presenting with a solitary cerebral tumor should undergo investigative studies, as previously outlined. Chest tomography and CT scanning may be particularly helpful. If no evidence of a primary site or other systemic metastatic disease is found, then total excision should be followed by radiation therapy. Longer survival for patients with an unknown primary site is seen, compared to other tumors. This may be due to the combined therapy of surgery and RT.

Conclusions

Future Developments

Future developments can be pursued in the evaluation and therapy of adenocarcinoma of unknown origin. The characterization of tumor-associated antigens, hormones, products of abnormal metabolism, and other biologic markers will increase the specificity of diagnosis. Improved radiologic testing may increase the diagnostic accuracy antemortem. Nuclear magnetic resonance imaging may emerge to replace CT scanning for detecting the anatomic location of tumors.[117]

Improved treatment will result from the development of more effective chemotherapeutic agents, as well as a better understanding of tumor heterogeneity and drug sensitivity. Autologous bone marrow transplantation following high dose combination chemotherapy may overcome the limitations of dose-related toxicities. Immunomodulation with interferon or tumor-specific monoclonal antibodies have therapeutic potential. Inducers of differentiation of tumor cells in vitro (cytosine arabinoside, DMSO)

Table 5-9
Pertinent Evaluation for Patients with Metastatic
Adenocarcinoma of Unknown Anatomic Origin

Complete history and physical with careful examination of the head and neck,
  breasts, thyroid, prostate, and genital region.
Laboratory testing, including CEA, AFP, hCG, and acid phosphatase (in men).
Immunocytochemical staining and electron microscopy of biopsied specimen.
Estrogen receptor protein analysis (female patients).
CXR, abdominal CT scan, and bone scan. Mammography and pelvic ultransound
  (in women).
Dye-contrast radiologic studies (UGI, BaE, IVP) for specific organ dysfunction.

may help control abnormal proliferation and allow the expression of
mature phenotypes.

Summary

In summary, the evaluation of a patient with adenocarcinoma of an
unknown primary site should be carefully planned after the initial histologic confirmation of the diagnosis (Table 5-9). Immunocytochemical
staining and electron microscopy may identify the anatomic origin. Serum
levels of the tumor markers CEA, AFP, hCG and acid phosphatase (in
men) should be measured. Immediate attention should be given to the
history, physical examination, and laboratory testing. Diagnostic radiologic
exams should be directed toward any organ dysfunction, as suggested by
presenting signs and symptoms. Routine dye contrast studies, such as
upper and lower GI series and IVP in asymptomatic patients who have no
blood in the stool or urine, are of low yield and should not be routinely
performed. The lung is the most common primary anatomic site, and the
CXR is thus justified. The presence of lung or brain metastases suggests a
supradiaphragmatic primary, and a chest CT scan may yield further
information. If a subdiaphragmatic primary is suggested by liver or bone
metastases, an abdominal CT scan is indicated. A pelvic ultrasonogram or
CT scan is useful for gynecologic pathology. Bilateral mammography
should be included for female patients. Although the breast is not a
frequent site of metastatic adenocarcinoma of unknown primary, metastatic breast cancer is both chemotherapeutically and hormonally responsive. Bone scanning can provide sites of metastatic disease, but routine
radionuclide liver scans do not provide additional information from that of
the abdominal CT scan.

Unfortunately, after the above studies have been made, two-thirds of patients will still have undiagnosed primary sites. Because of the limited survival in the majority of patients, those with a poor performance status should not be given chemotherapy routinely. No standard chemotherapy regimen can be recommended. If a supradiaphragmatic primary is suggested, the patient can be treated with cyclophosphamide, doxorubicin and cisplatin for assumed lung cancer. Otherwise, a subdiaphragmatic primary is suggested, and a doxorubicin–containing regimen may be useful. If one assumes an occult pancreatic malignancy, then 5-fluorouracil, doxorubicin and mitomycin-C (FAM) or streptozotocin, mitomycin-C and 5-fluorouracil (SMF) may improve survival for responders. Phase I testing of investigational agents can be offered when available. Since there is limited effectiveness of current combination chemotherapy for highly aggressive adenocarcinoma, other modalities should be considered. Differentiation induction of tumor cells and tumor-specific monoclonal antibodies both have therapeutic potential.

References

1. Holmes FF, Fouts TL: Metastatic cancer of unknown primary site. Cancer 26:816–820, 1970
2. Didolkar MS, Fanous N, Elias EG, et al: Metastatic carcinoma from occult primary tumors: a study of 254 patients. Ann Surg 186:625–630, 1977
3. Stewart JF, Tattersall MHN, Woods RL, et al: Unknown primary adenocarcinoma: incidence of over investigation and natural history. Brit Med J 1:1530–1533, 1979
4. Neilan BA: Adenocarcinoma of unknown origin. CA—A Cancer Journal for Clinicians 33:237–241, 1983
5. Moertel CG, Reitemeier RJ, Schutt AJ, et al: Treatment of the patient with adenocarcinoma of unknown origin. Cancer 30:1469–1472, 1972
6. Johnson RO, Castro R, Ansfield FJ: Response of primary unknown cancers to treatment with 5-fluorouracil. Cancer Chem Rep 38:63–64, 1964
7. Krementz ET, Cerise EJ, Ciaravella JM, et al: Metastases of undetermined source. CA—A Cancer Journal for Clinicians 27:289–300, 1977
8. Krementz ET, Cerise EJ, Foster DS, et al: Metastases of undetermined source. Curr Prob Cancer 4:1–37, 1979
9. Lleander VC, Goldstein G, Horsley JS III: Chemotherapy in the management of metastatic cancer of unknown primary site. Oncology 26:265–270, 1972

10. Nystrom JS, Weiner JM, Wolf RM, et al: Identifying the primary site in metastatic cancer of unknown origin. J Amer Med Assoc 241:381–383, 1979

11. Gaber AO, Rice P, Eaton C, et al: Metastatic malignant disease of unknown origin. Am J Surg 145:493–497, 1983

12. Richardson RG, Parker RG: Metastases from undetected primary cancers: clinical experience at a radiation oncology center. West J Med 123:337–339, 1975

13. Osteen RT, Kopf G, Wilson RE: In pursuit of the unknown primary. Am J Surg 135:494–498, 1978

14. Snyder RD, Mavligit GM, Valdivieso M: Adenocarcinoma of unknown primary site: a clinico-pathological study. Med Ped Onc 6:289–294, 1979

15. Indupalli SR, Bedikian AY, Bodey GP: Adenocarcinoma of unknown primary origin: impact of chemotherapy on survival. Southern Med J 74:1431–1435, 1981

16. Markman M: Metastatic adenocarcinoma of unknown primary site: analysis of 245 patients seen at the Johns Hopkins Hospital from 1965–1979. Med Ped Onc 10:569–574, 1982

17. Nissenblatt MJ: The CUP syndrome (carcinoma unknown primary). Cancer Treat Rev 8:211–224, 1981

18. Nissenblatt MJ: Carcinoma with unknown primary tumor (CUP syndrome). Southern Med J 74:1497–1502, 1981

19. Fischer DS: Management of cancer of unknown primary. Conn Med 39:205–208, 1975

20. Kennedy PS, Luedke DW: Adenocarcinoma of unknown origin. Postgrad Med 65:151–160, 1979

21. Stephens DS, Greco A: Carcinoma of unknown primary site. J Tenn Med Assoc 72:834–836, 1979

22. Grosbach AB: Carcinoma of unknown primary site: a clinical enigma. Arch Int Med 142:357–359, 1982

23. Greenberg BR: The problem of the unknown primary carcinoma. Arizona Med 39:787–791, 1982

24. Kelley SL, Meyer TJ: Carcinoma of unknown primary site: a prudent approach. Postgrad Med 74:269–280, 1983

25. Gilman A, Fordham E, Wiley E, et al: Metastatic carcinoma with an unknown primary. Med Ped Onc 12:59–63, 1984

26. Silverberg E: Cancer statistics, 1984. CA—A Cancer Journal for Clinicians 34:7–23, 1984

27. Cechner RL, Chamberlain W, Carter JR, et al: Misdiagnosis of bronchogenic carcinoma. Cancer 46:190–199, 1980

28. Rosenblatt MB, Teng PK, Kerpe S, et al: Causes of death in 1000 consecutive autopsies. NY State Journal of Medicine 71:2189–2193, 1971

29. Bauer FW, Robbins SL: An autopsy study of cancer patients. J Amer Med Assoc 221:1471–1474, 1972

30. Ehrlich D, Li-Sik M, Modan B: Some factors affecting the accuracy of cancer diagnosis. J Chron Dis 28:359–364, 1975

31. Feinstein AR, Wells CK: Cigarette smoking and lung cancer: the problems of detection bias: in epidemiologic rates of disease. Trans Assoc Am Phys 87:180–185, 1974

32. Clary CF, Michel RP, Wang N-S, et al: Metastatic carcinoma: the lung as the site for the clinically undiagnosed primary. Cancer 51:362–366, 1983

33. Sherwin RP: The differentiation of primary lung cancer from metastatic disease, in Weiss L and Gilbert HA (eds): Pulmonary Metastases. Boston, G. K. Hall, 1978, pp 91–98

34. Abrams HL, Spiro R, Goldstein N: Metastases in carcinoma: analysis of 1000 autopsied cases. Cancer 3:74–85, 1950

35. Rosenblatt MB, Lisa JR, Trinidad S: Metastatic lung cancer masquerading as bronchogenic carcinoma. Geriatrics 21:139–145, 1966

36. Cassiere SG, McLain DA, Emory WB, et al: Metastatic carcinoma of the pancreas simulating primary bronchogenic carcinoma. Cancer 46:2319–2321, 1980

37. Gikas PW, Labow SS, DiGiulio W, et al: Occult metastasis from occult papillary carcinoma of the thyroid. Cancer 20:2100–2104, 1967

38. Dye KR, Pattison CR, Fiore JP, et al: Spontaneous eradication of adenocarcinoma arising in a colonic polyp. J Amer Med Assoc 251:1162, 1984

39. Nystrom JS, Weiner JM, Heffelfinger-Juttner J, et al: Metastatic and histologic presentations in unknown primary cancer. Sem Onc 4:53–58, 1977

40. Goldenberg DM, Sharkey RM, Primus FJ: Immunocytochemical detection of carcinoembryonic antigen in conventional histopathology specimens. Cancer 42:1546–1553, 1978

41. van Nagell JR, Donaldson ES, Gay EC, et al: Carcinoembryonic antigen in carcinoma of the uterine cervix. Cancer 44:944–948, 1979

42. Nadji M, Tabei SZ, Castro A, et al: Prostate-specific antigen: an immunohistologic marker for prostatic neoplasms. Cancer 48:1229–1232, 1981

43. Jobsis AC, DeVries GP, Anholt RRH, et al: Demonstration of the

prostatic origin of metastases: an immunohistochemical method for formalin fixed embedded tissue. Cancer 41:1788–1793, 1978

44. Nadji M, Tabei Z, Castro A, et al: Immunohistological demonstration of prostatic origin of malignant neoplasms. Lancet 1:671–672, 1979
45. Li C-Y, Lam WKW, Yam LT: Immunohistochemical diagnosis of prostatic cancer with metastasis. Cancer 46:706–712, 1980
46. Dvorak AM, Monahan RA: Metastatic adenocarcinoma of unknown primary site: diagnostic electron microscopy to determine the site of tumor origin. Arch Pathol Lab Med 106:21–24, 1982
47. Steckel RJ, Kagan AR: Diagnostic persistence in working up metastatic cancer with an unknown primary site. Radiology 134:367–369, 1980
48. Moertel, CG: Adenocarcinoma of unknown origin. Ann Int Med 91:646–647, 1979
49. Steckel RJ, Kagan AR: Evaluation of the unknown primary neoplasm. Radiologic Clin North Am 20:601–605, 1982
50. Jochelson MS, Balikian JP: The work–up of the unknown primary. Postgrad Rad 3:203–211, 1983
51. Jesse RH, Neff LE: Metastatic carcinoma in cervical nodes with an unknown primary lesion. Am J Surg 112:547–553, 1966
52. Smith PE, Krementz ET, Chapman W: Metastatic cancer without a detectable primary site. Am J Surg 113:633–637, 1967
53. Barrie JR, Knapper WH, Strong EW: Cervical nodal metastases of unknown origin. Am J Surg 120:466–470, 1970
54. Martin H: Untimely lymph node biopsy. Am J Surg 102:17–18, 1961
55. Jesse RH, Perez CA, Fletcher GH: Cervical lymph node metastasis: unknown primary cancer. Cancer 31:854–859, 1973
56. Coker DD, Casterline PF, Chambers RG, et al: Metastases to lymph nodes of the head and neck from an unknown primary site. Am J Surg 134:517–522, 1977
57. Devine KD: Cancer in the neck without obvious source. Mayo Clin Proc 53:644–650, 1978
58. Koch M, McPherson TA: Carcinoembryonic antigen levels as an indicator of the primary site in metastatic disease of unknown origin. Cancer 48:1242–1244, 1981
59. Foti AG, Cooper JF, Herschman H, et al: Detection of prostatic cancer by solid-phase radioimmunoassay of serum prostatic acid phosphatase. N Engl J Med 297:1357–1361, 1977
60. Lange PH, McIntire KR, Waldmann TA, et al: Serum alpha fetoprotein and human chorionic gonadotropin in the diagnosis and

management of nonseminomatous germ–cell testicular cancer. N Engl J Med 295:1237–1239, 1976

61. Liebman HA, Furie BC, Tong MJ, et al: Des-gamma-carboxy (abnormal) prothrombin as a serum marker of primary hepatocellular carcinoma. N Engl J Med 310:1427–1431, 1984

62. Bast RC Jr, Klug TL, St. John E, et al: A radioimmunoassay using a monocolonal antibody to monitor the course of epithelial ovarian cancer. N Engl J Med 309:883–887, 1983

63. Golomb HM, Thomsen S: Estrogen receptor: therapeutic guide to undifferentiated metastatic carcinoma in women. Arch Intern Med 135:942–945, 1975

64. Kiang DT, Kennedy BJ: Estrogen receptor assay in the differential diagnosis of adenocarcinomas. J Amer Med Assoc 238:32–34, 1977

65. McGuire WL, Horwitz KB, Zava DT, et al: Hormones in breast cancer: update 1978. Metabolism 27:487–501, 1978

66. Lippman ME, Allegra JC: Quantitative estrogen receptor analyses. Cancer 46:2829–2834, 1980

67. McMillan JH, Levine E, Stephens RH: Computed tomography in the evaluation of metastatic adenocarcinoma from an unknown primary site. Radiology 143:143–146, 1982

68. Karsell PR, Sheedy PF II, O'Connell MJ: Computed tomography in search of cancer of unknown origin. J Amer Med Assoc 248:340–343, 1982

69. Muhm JR, Brown LR, Crowe JK: Use of computed tomography in the detection of pulmonary nodules. Mayo Clin Proc 52:345–348, 1977

70. Schaner EG, Chang AE, Doppman JL, et al: Comparison of computed and conventional whole lung tomography in detecting pulmonary nodules: a prospective radiologic-pathologic study. Am J Roentgenol 131:51–54, 1978

71. Muhm JR, Brown LR, Crowe JK, et al: Comparison of whole lung tomography and computed tomography for detecting pulmonary nodules. Am J Roentgenol 131:981–984, 1978

72. Heitzman ER: Computed tomography of the thorax. AJR 136:2–12, 1981

73. Kamin PD, Bernardino ME, Wallace S, et al: Comparison of ultrasound and computed tomography in the detection of pancreatic malignancy. Cancer 46:2410–2412, 1980

74. Walsh JW, Rosenfield AT, Jaffe CC, et al: Prospective comparison of ultrasound and computed tomography in the evaluation of gynecologic pelvic masses. Am J Roentgenol 131:955–960, 1978

75. Rosenthal S, Kaufman S: The liver scan in metastatic disease. Arch
     Surg 106:656–659, 1973
76. Lunia S, Parthasarathy KL, Bakskis S, et al: An evaluation of
     ^{99m}Tc-sulfur colloid liver scintiscans and their usefulness in meta-
     static workup: a review of 1424 studies. J Nucl Med 16:62–65, 1975
77. Drum DE: Optimizing the clinical value of hepatic scintiphotogra-
     phy. Semin Nuc Med 8:346–357, 1978
78. Smith TJ, Kemeny MM, Sugarbaker PH, et al: A prospective study of
     hepatic imaging in the detection of metastatic disease. Ann Surg
     195:486–491, 1982
79. Ucherer U, Rothe R, Eisenburg J., et al: Diagnostic accuracy of CT in
     circumscript liver disease. Am J Roentgeonol 130:711–714, 1978
80. Snow JH, Goldstein HM, Wallace S: Comparison of scintigraphy,
     sonography, and computed tomography in the evaluation of hepatic
     neoplasms. AJR 132:915–918, 1979
81. Shirazi PH, Stein AJ, Sidell MS, et al: Bone scanning in the staging
     and management of bronchogenic carcinoma: review of 206 cases. J
     Nuc Med 14:451, 1973
82. Felix EL, Sindelar WF, Bagley DH, et al: The use of bone and brain
     scans as screening procedures in patients with malignant lesions.
     Surg Gynecol Obstet 141:867–869, 1975
83. Tofe AJ, Francis MD, Harvey WJ: Correlation of neoplasms with
     incidence and localization of skeletal metastases. J Nuc Med
     16:986–989, 1975
84. Shapiro S: Evidence on screening for breast cancer from a random-
     ized trial. Cancer 39:2772–2782, 1977
85. Sadowsky NL, Kalisher L, White G, et al: Radiologic detection of
     breast cancer: review and recommendations. New Eng J Med
     294:370–373, 1976
86. Lleander VC, Goldstein G, Horsley JS III: Chemotherapy in the
     management of metastatic cancer of unknown primary site.
     Oncology 26:265–270, 1972
87. Feleppa VB, Leman HM: The therapeutic dilemma of carcinomas of
     unknown origin. J Surg Onc 9:453–462, 1977
88. Valentine J, Rosenthal S, Arseneau JC: Combination chemotherapy
     for adenocarcinoma of unknown primary origin (abstract). Proc
     Amer Soc Clin Oncol 20:349, 1979
89. Valentine J, Rosenthal S, Arseneau JC: Combination chemotherapy
     for adenocarcinoma of unknown primary origin. Cancer Clin Trials
     2:265–268, 1979
90. Woods RL, Fox RM, Tattersall MHN, et al: Metastatic adenocarci-

noma of unknown primary site: a randomized study of two combination–chemotherapy regimen. N Engl J Med 303:87–89, 1980

91. McKeen E, Smith F, Haidak D, et al: Fluorouracil (F), Adriamycin (A), and mitomycin-C (M), FAM, for adenocarcinoma of unknown origin (AUO) (abstract). Proc Amer Soc Clin Oncol 21:358, 1980

92. Rudnick S, Tremont S, Staab E, et al: Evaluation and therapy of adenocarcinoma of unknown primary (ACUP) (abstract). Proc Amer Soc Clin Oncol 22:379, 1981

93. Shildt RA, Kennedy PS, Chen TT, et al: Management of patients with metastatic adenocarcinoma of unknown origin: a Southwest Oncology Group study. Cancer Treat Rep 67:77–79, 1983

94. Anderson H, Thatcher N, Rankin E, et al: VAC (Vincristine, Adriamycin, Cyclophosphamide) chemotherapy for metastatic carcinoma from an unknown primary site. Eur J Cancer Clin Oncol 19:49–52, 1983

95. Bedikian AY, Bodey GP, Valdivieso M, Burgess MA: Sequential chemotherapy for adenocarcinoma of unknown primary. Am J Clin Oncol (CCT) 6:219–224, 1983

96. Richardson RI, Greco FA, Wolff S, et al: Extragonadal germ cell malignancy: value of tumor markers in metastatic carcinoma in young males (abstract). Proceedings of the American Association for Cancer Research 20:204, 1979

97. Greco FA, Fer MF, Richardson RL, et al: The unrecognized extragonadal germ cell cancer syndrome (abstract). Proceedings of the American Association for Cancer Research. 21:149, 1980

98. Fox RM, Woods RL, Tattersall MHN: Undifferentiated carcinoma in young men: the atypical teratoma syndrome. Lancet 1:1316–1318, 1979

99. Richardson RL, Schoumacher RA, Fer MF, et al: The unrecognized extragonadal germ cell syndrome. Ann Intern Med 94:181–186, 1981

100. Pierce EH, Gray HK, Dockerty MB: Surgical significance of isolated axillary adenopathy. Ann Surg 145:104–107, 1957

101. Feuerman L, Attie JN, Rosenberg B: Carcinoma in axillary lymph nodes as an indicator of breast cancer. Surg Gynecol Obst 114:5–8, 1962

102. Fitts WT JR, Steiner GC, Enterline HT: Prognosis of occult carcinoma of the breast. Amer J Surg 106:460–463, 1963

103. Owen HW, Dockerty MB, Gray HK: Occult carcinoma of the breast. Surg Gynecol Obstet 98:302–308, 1954

104. Westbrook KC, Gallagher HS: Breast carcinoma presenting as an axillary mass. Am J Surg 122:607–611, 1971

105.   Ashikari R, Rosen PP, Urban JA, et al: Breast cancer presenting as an axillary mass. Ann Surg 183:415–417, 1976
106.   Klopp CT: Metastatic cancer of axillary lymph node without a demonstrable primary lesion. Ann Surg 131:437–439, 1950
107.   Jackson AS: Carcinoma of the breast in the absence of clinical breast findings. Ann Surg 127:177–179, 1948
108.   Patel J, Nemoto T, Rosner D, et al: Axillary lymph node metastasis from an occult breast cancer. Cancer 47:2923–2927, 1981
109.   Copeland EM, McBride CM: Axillary metastases from unknown primary sites. Ann Surg 178:25–27, 1973
110.   Feigenberg Z, Zer M, Dintsman M: Axillary metastases from an unknown primary source: a diagnostic and therapeutic approach. Isr J Med Sci 12:1153–1158, 1976
111.   Iglehart JD, Ferguson BJ, Shingleton WW, et al: An ultrastructural analysis of breast carcinoma presenting as isolated axillary adenopathy. Ann Surg 196:8–13, 1982
112.   Lokich JJ: The management of cerebral metastasis. J Amer Med Assoc 234:748–751, 1975
113.   Voorhies RM, Sundaresan N, Thaler HT: The single supratentorial lesion: an evaluation of preoperative diagnostic tests. J Neurosurg 53:364–368, 1980
114.   Zimm S, Wampler GL, Stablein D, et al: Intracerebral metastases in solid tumor patients: natural history and results of treatment. Cancer 48:384–394, 1981
115.   Chan RC, Steinbok P: Solitary cerebral metastasis: the effect of craniotomy on the quality and the duration of survival. Neurosurgery 11:254–257, 1982
116.   Ebels EJ, van der Meulen JDM: Cerebral metastasis without known primary tumor: a retrospective study. Clin Neurol Neurosurg 80:195–197, 1978
117.   Koutcher JA, Burt CT: Principles of imaging of nuclear magnetic resonance. J Nucl Med 25:371–382, 1984

6

EPIDERMOID AND UNDIFFERENTIATED CARCINOMA OF UNKNOWN ORIGIN

Craig L. Silverman
James E. Marks

Metastatic epidermoid or undifferentiated carcinoma presenting with no obvious primary site often poses a number of difficult and challenging clinical problems. What workup is warranted to determine the site of the primary and other metastatic sites after a complete history and physical examination and routine workup have been performed? What is the proper treatment of the presenting site, and what effect will local treatment have on the patient's ultimate prognosis? Would prophylactic treatment of possible sites of origin of the primary tumor increase the likelihood of long-term survival or prevent local problems that could result from the eventual appearance of the primary tumor?

For the clinician who sees patients with an epidermoid or undifferentiated carcinoma from an unknown primary site, it is important to understand the biologic course of these tumors. Histology, site of presentation, and tumor burden are critical factors in the selection of an optimal and cost-efficient workup and treatment regimen. Management of these patients can cross several subspecialty lines: pathology, diagnostic radiology, otolaryngology, general surgery, medical oncology, and radiation

POORLY DIFFERENTIATED NEOPLASMS AND TUMORS OF UNKNOWN ORIGIN   ISBN 0-8089-1755-2
© 1986 by Grune & Stratton.   All rights of reproduction in any form reserved.

oncology. Each subspecialist can help the clinician determine the appropriate workup and treatment regimen.

Incidence

For most patients who present with an epidermoid or undifferentiated carcinoma, the origin of the primary tumor is apparent after a careful history and a complete physical examination, including inspection of the skin and the mucosal surfaces of likely primary sites. A more thorough workup of the most likely sites of origin will often yield the primary tumor. In a series of 404 patients admitted to the Mayo Clinic with the presumptive diagnosis of an unknown primary, the primary site was found in 35 percent of patients after a more comprehensive history, physical examination, panendoscopy, and bronchoscopy.[1]

The discrete population of patients who do undergo such a complete workup without discovery of the primary tumor site can truly be classified as having a metastatic tumor from an occult primary site. The reported incidence of true occult primary cancers has ranged from 0.5 percent to 3 percent of the total oncological population, although some authors have reported higher percentages.[2–7] In a detailed analysis by Holmes and Fouts,[8] the yearly incidence at a major medical center was unchanged or even rose slightly in the years 1950 to 1967 (Table 6-1). One might expect the incidence of occult primaries to slowly decrease as technological developments in diagnostic radiology (computed tomography and magnetic resonance imaging), pathology (radioimmune assays, specific tumor markers, monoclonal antibody histochemical staining techniques, cytology, and electron microscopy), and fiberoptic endoscopy are introduced and have more widespread usage, but this has not yet been substantiated.

The distribution of unknown primary patients by site and histology is seen in Table 6-2. Cervical lymph nodes are the most common single anatomical site for epidermoid or undifferentiated carcinoma, followed in frequency by all bone sites, lung or pleura, multiple lymph node involvement, and brain.

Pathology

The pathologist is an important member of the management team for these patients. After the biopsy of the involved lymph node or organ, the pathologist, using a variety of new techniques of histochemical staining,

Table 6-1

Percent of Patients Diagnosed per Year as Having Metastatic
Cancer of Unknown Primary Site

Year	Percent
1950	2.9
1951	2.1
1952	2.1
1953	2.3
1954	2.1
1955	3.0
1956	3.0
1957	3.1
1958	4.0
1959	3.1
1960	3.0
1961	3.0
1962	3.2
1963	2.9
1964	4.5
1965	4.2
1966	4.6
1967	2.8

* The incidence figures reflect all histologies. Based on the data that 152/617 patients had epidermoid or undifferentiated histology, the estimated incidence for those histologies only would be approximately ¼ the overall yearly figure.

Table 6-2

Presenting Sites for Epidermoid Carcinoma and
Undifferentiated Carcinomas from Occult Primaries

Anatomic Site	No. of Patients/Total with Epidermoid or Undifferentiated Carcinoma Metastatic from an Unknown Primary	
	U. of Kansas (8) (%)	Washington U. (22) (%)
Cervical lymph nodes	34/152 (22)	90/162 (56)
Bone	25/152 (16)	19/162 (12)
Lungs/pleura	23/152 (15)	—
Multiple lymph nodes	19/152 (13)	—
CNS	12/152 (8)	11/162 (7)
Inguinal lymph nodes	3/152 (2)	1/162 (1)
Supraclavicular lymph nodes	2/152 (1)	22/162 (14)
Axillary lymph nodes	1/152 (1)	11/162 (7)
Gastrointestinal	33/152 (22)	7/162 (4)

155

immunocytochemical assays, and electron microscopy,[9-12] can often properly classify what was thought to be, by light microscopy, an undifferentiated or anaplastic carcinoma, or even a carcinoma not otherwise specified (NOS), as epidermoid carcinoma, adenocarcinoma, melanoma, sarcoma or lymphoma. Most of these new techniques in histochemical staining use monoclonal antibodies and are useful in differentiating lymphomas from epithelial or sarcomatous tumors, but provide little help in determining likely primary sites for epidermoid carcinomas.[13] Occasionally, the pathologist may be able to recommend a likely site for the primary tumor after reviewing the histological pattern, but the reproducibility and accuracy of such recommendations are suspect. This should not detract from the important role the pathologist has in directing the clinician to the area of the body that is the most likely site of origin of an occult primary, thereby targeting the workup and directing the management of the patient.

Diagnostic Workup

When complete history and physical examination, routine radiographic studies, and pathological studies of the tissue have proven unsuccessful in determining the possible origin of the tumor, the clinician may be tempted to do a more extensive workup to determine the primary site and other metastatic sites as well. The two most important factors that must be considered before the initiation of such a workup are the presenting site of the disease and the histology. Knowledge of the relationship of the presenting site and the histology to the biologic behavior of the tumor can reduce costly workups by eliminating evaluation of unlikely sites of the primary or metastatic tumor, and can direct a workup to those anatomical areas that are most likely to be the origin of the occult tumor. For example, for the patient who presents with epidermoid carcinoma in a supraclavicular node, the most likely sites for the primary tumor are the mucosal surfaces of the head and neck, esophagus, and the lung; there would be little advantage to investigating subdiaphragmatic organs in this specific case.

In today's cost-conscious society, the clinician must select those tests which yield the most information for the least money. Table 6-3 lists commonly used diagnostic tests with their 1984 price lists (Evanston Hospital). Nuclear medicine scans, for instance, can be sensitive tests in detecting sites of metastatic involvement, but can offer little, if any, information in determining a primary site.[14-17] In several large stud-

Table 6-3
Cost (See also text) and sensitivity of commonly used
Diagnostic Tests

Test	$ Cost*	Sensitivity in Locating Occult Primary[1,15,17–21]
Soft tissue film	42	very low
Abdominal x–ray–KUB	44	very low
Chest x–ray	44	moderate
Sinus series	75	low
Skull x–ray	89	very low
Barium swallow	92	low–moderate
Thyroid scan	126	low
Upper GI	140	very low
Barium enema (BE)	140	very low
Air contrast BE	180	low
Liver spleen scan	201	low
Gallium scan (organ)	289	very low
Gallium scan (multiple views)	389	very low
Bone scan	326	very low
Mammogram	115	moderate–good
Skeletal Survey	169	very low
Bronchogram	175	low
Upper abdominal ultrasound	180	low
Laryngography	186	low
Sialography	190	very low
Nephrotomogram	219	very low
CT abd + contrast	480	moderate–good
CT chest + contrast	420	moderate–good

* Cost—1984—Tertiary Care Community Hospital

ies,[1,18–20] the efficacy of subdiaphragmatic tests in detection of the primary site for undifferentiated or adenocarcinomas was extremely limited (less than 10 percent true positive rate). In fact, Nystrom et al.[19] obtained as many false-negative and false-positive results as true-positive results, negating the value of the exam. The role of the CT scan for the chest and abdomen is being investigated and has been shown to be more sensitive than routine radiographic studies in detecting tumors of the kidney, pancreas, and lung.[21] Since these various approaches are discussed at length in other chapters, the scope of this section will be largely concerned with epidermoid and certain undifferentiated neoplasms.

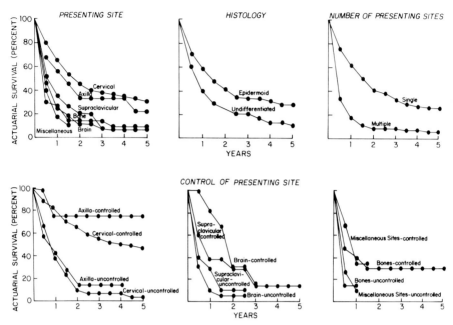

Figure 6-1. *Survival of patients with unknown primary as a function of presenting site, histology, number of presenting sites (tumor burden), and tumor control of the presenting site. Local control of the presenting site prolongs survival for patients with cervical and axillary lymph node presentations.*

Prognostic Factors

In this follow-up study and in our previous analysis,[22] we included nonkeratinizing undifferentiated epidermoid carcinomas in addition to keratinizing epidermoid carcinomas. We excluded undifferentiated carcinomas with any semblance of gland formation as well as other chemoresponsive undifferentiated tumors, such as lymphomas, germ cell tumors, and small cell carcinomas. These patients were pathologically classified and treated before we had monoclonal antibody techniques available to differentiate epithelial, sarcomatous, and lymphomatous tumors from one another. Moreover, they were, by and large, treated by surgery and radiation without the benefit of chemotherapy. The overall prognosis was worse for the undifferentiated carcinomas than for the epidermoid (Fig. 6-1); in the cervical lymph node group, the only group with adequate numbers for comparison of the two histologies, the undifferentiated carcinomas were more easily controlled (Table 6-4) and more

Table 6-4

Control of Ipsilateral Cervical Lymph Nodes as a Function of Size of Node, Dose of Radiation, Type of Surgery, and Histology

	Epidermoid				Undifferentiated				Totals
	Surgery* + XRT		Biopsy† + XRT		Surgery* + XRT		Biopsy† + XRT		
	<3 cm	≥3 cm	<3 cm	≥3 cm	<3 cm	≥3 cm	<3 cm	≥3 cm	
≥60 Gy	9/11	5/8	7/9	9/18	3/3	0/0	3/5	6/10	42/64 (66%)
<60 Gy	2/3	2/3	1/3	2/7	1/1	3/3	1/2	2/4	14/26 (53%)
Total	18/25 (72%)		19/37 (51%)		7/7 (100%)		12/21 (57%)		

* Excision of lymph node or neck dissection
† Incisional biopsy

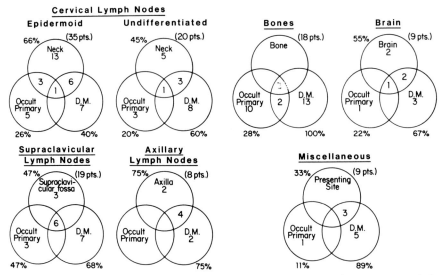

Figure 6-2. *Sites of failure for patients with unknown primary after treatment of the presenting site. Note the high proportion of patients with cervical or axillary lymph node presentation who fail with only local or loco-regional disease, while the overwhelming majority of patients with other presenting sites fail with systemic disease.*

often metastasized distantly (Fig. 6-2). We recognize that patients with undifferentiated tumors may represent a heterogeneous group and may include tumors of nonsquamous origin. For practical purposes however, we have analyzed them as a group, separate from the patients with squamous carcinomas.

In our previously reported series,[22] we subdivided our patients into various subsets in search of possible factors that might help predict more favorable outcomes. Treatment was excluded as a prognostic variable, since the more favorable groups of patients were arbitrarily selected for more aggressive and potentially curative treatment. The more favorable prognostic factors that seemed independent of treatment included epidermoid carcinoma, a single presenting site, male sex, longer duration of signs and symptoms prior to diagnosis, local control of the tumor at its presenting site, and cervical or axillary lymph node presentation (Fig. 6-1). Unknown primary tumors metastatic to inguinal nodes may also have a better prognosis.[23] The less favorable factors, independent of treatment, included female sex, anaplastic or undifferentiated histology, bone, brain or supraclavicular presentations, short duration of signs and symptoms before detection, and multiple sites of disease.

It is important to determine the effect of treatment on outcome for patients with favorable and unfavorable prognostic factors. Knowledge of the ultimate sites of failure and disease status can direct the clinician to a more rational diagnostic workup and management approach. Patients destined to die quickly of generalized disease do not need an expensive workup, but merely palliation, or systemic therapy, if it is available. Patients destined to die from the eventual manifestation of their primary tumor may need a more aggressive investigation for the primary site and/or prophylactic treatment of the probable primary site. Patients destined to succumb from local-regional disease need more aggressive local-regional treatment of the presenting site, as with cervical lumph node presentations.

Sites of failure and treatment outcome as a function of presenting site and histology for our patients are shown respectively in Figures 6-2 and 6-3. The remainder of the chapter will deal with a site-by-site discussion of metastatic epidermoid and undifferentiated carcinomas from occult primary sites as well as our recommendations for workup and treatment, based on an updated analysis of our own experience as well as the experience reported by others.

Cervical Lymph Node Presentations

In the analyses by Holmes and Fouts[8] and Silverman and Marks,[22] cervical lymph nodes as a single anatomical site was the second most commonly involved site for metastatic tumor and was also the most common site for squamous or anaplastic carcinoma from an unknown primary (Table 6–2). It is by far the one site most discussed in the literature and poses challenging problems of management. For these reasons, we will devote an extensive discussion to unknown primaries metastatic to cervical lymph nodes.

Workup for the primary site is important, since it can change both management and prognosis. It begins with a careful history, a careful head and neck examination, and endoscopy with blind biopsies of the nasopharynx, oropharynx, base of tongue and laryngopharynx, as well as esophagoscopy. It has been noted that 15 to 40 percent of these patients may eventually manifest a primary tumor,[3,4,24] and that the percentage of these primaries occurring above the clavicle is extremely high. Fitzpatrick and Kotalik[25] found that when only those patients with cervical metastases

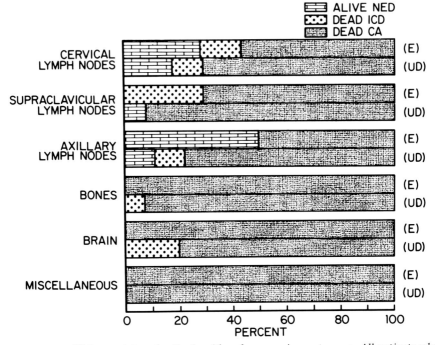

Figure 6-3. *Ultimate status of patients with unknown primary tumors. All patients who presented in bones, brain, or miscellaneous sites died of cancer regardless of histology (E = epidermoid, UD = undifferentiated). Patients who presented in supraclavicular lymph nodes fared slightly better, while a significant proportion of patients with cervical or axillary lymph node presentations were rendered free of disease and became long-term survivors.*

from an unknown primary were considered (eliminating those with metastases to a supraclavicular lymph node), eleven of fourteen (79 percent) of patients who eventually manifested a primary did so above the clavicles. In the series reported by Coker et al.,[24] only one–half of the manifested primaries were found to originate in the upper aerodigestive tract (though four tumors were later interpreted as a lymphoma in a head and neck site), while an additional three developed primaries in the lung. In the series reported by Barrie,[26] 38 of 123 patients eventually manifested a primary (31 percent) and of those 38 patients, 31 (81 percent) manifested a primary in the head and neck area. Because of the high percentage of patients with a cervical node presentation who then do develop a primary in the head and neck area or lungs, subdiaphragmatic workup is rarely justified in view of its low yield and high cost. Additional workup has also included diagnostic tests, such as thyroid scan and sinus x-rays, but their yield is low in the absence of symptoms (Table 6-3). The role of CT, however, may be increasing. Mancuso and Hanafee[27,28] have demonstrated the value of CT in detection of gross submucosal disease not found at panendoscopy or on routine radiography.

The pathologist can occasionally assist in finding an occult primary. A diagnosis of lymphoepithelioma in a lymph node will direct the clinician to search for the primary tumor in the nasopharynx or tonsil. Occasionally, the morphological appearance of the tumor will be indicative of a tonsillar cancer, which on biopsy, has been confirmed.[29] Coates has described a serological assay of antibodies to Epstein–Barr virus that is specific for nasopharyngeal cancer.[30] Of four previously untreated metastatic epidermoid carcinomas to the cervical lymph nodes, the Epstein-Barr virus titer in one patient was compatible with a nasopharyngeal tumor which, on later blind biopsy of the area, was positive for tumor.

The distribution of regional lymph node metastases from known head and neck primaries has been well-described by Lindberg.[31] Using that data as a starting point, Molinari, et al.[32] analyzed their experience from Italy and developed a statistical approach to the detection of the primary cancer based on the site and distribution of lymph node metastases in the neck. Their method gives the most likely primary sites in order of frequency, based on the anatomical location of the node and multiplicity of nodes involved. Unfortunately, no one has yet tested the accuracy of this method in detecting occult primaries metastatic to cervical lymph nodes.

Treatment of the Cervical Lymph Nodes and the Primary Site

A review of the ultimate sites of failure (Fig. 6-2) illustrates the high frequency of failure in the presenting site and/or the occult primary in these patients. Fifty-three percent of patients (29/55) with carcinomas presenting in the cervical nodes failed in the neck or in the occult head and neck primary site only (Fig. 6-2). Based on that data, treatment goals should include: 1) better control of the presenting lymph nodes in the neck, 2) *ultimate* control of a subsequent primary appearing in the head and neck area, and 3) control of the contralateral lymph nodes.

Most series that have dealt with this group of patients report only 2-, 3-, or 5-year survival data.[3,4,24,25,33–37] In our view, survival is a crude endpoint and a poor measure of treatment success. Better measures of treatment success are tumor control and patterns of failure. These parameters provide a rational basis for altering treatment strategies to improve results. Using these particular endpoints, we analyzed our experience of patients with occult primaries that presented in a cervical lymph node.

Control of the Presenting Cervical Lymph Nodes

Our series consisted of a group of ninety patients with epidermoid carcinoma (62 patients) or undifferentiated carcinoma (28 patients) who had presented with single, multiple, or bilateral cervical lymph nodes. Since control of the lymph nodes is a function of tumor burden, we divided the patients into those with small neck nodes less than 3 cm and those with neck nodes greater than 3 cm. The radiation only and combined radiation and surgery treatment groups were not comparable because those patients who had small neck nodes tended to be treated with radical neck dissection or total excisional biopsy in addition to radiation therapy, whereas those with larger neck nodes tended to receive incisional biopsy only, plus radiation. Table 6-4 gives the control of the presenting cervical lymph node by size of neck node, dose, and treatment method. There appears to be a definite advantage of combined radiation and surgical treatment over radiation alone for the larger neck nodes. There is the factor of radiation dose that must be considered as well. Probert[37] noted an ipsilateral neck failure of 50 percent with doses of less than 55 Gy, but only 14 percent with doses above 55 Gy (1 Gy = 100 rad).

For our patients, the effect of dose was less pronounced. For all patients who received greater than 60 Gy, tumor control in the ipsilateral neck was 66 percent, but for those who had received less than 60 Gy, tumor control was 53 percent. When the data was reanalyzed, however, to take into account the surgical procedure and size of node, there was little effect of radiation dose on neck control for those who had undergone a total excisional biopsy or radical neck dissection, but there was an effect of dose on neck control for those patients who had had a biopsy only (Table 6-4). In that group of patients, tumor control was improved in the ipsilateral neck for patients who received 60 Gy or more to the neck, especially for smaller neck nodes. Overall, 25 percent of patients with small neck nodes developed recurrent disease in the ipsilateral neck, compared to 53 percent for those patients with larger neck nodes. These results are comparable to those reported by other authors[3,24,37,38] (Table 6-5).

Contralateral Neck Control

The appearance of asynchronous lymph node metastases in the opposite neck is not an uncommon occurrence. Barrie et al.[26] reported contralateral neck metastases in 9 of 123 patients (8 percent), and Jessie et

Table 6-5

Regrowth of Tumor in the Ipsilateral or Contralateral Neck as a
Function of Treatment

		No. of Neck Recurrences/Total Treated	
	Reference	Ipsilateral (%)	Contralateral (%)
Surgery Alone	24	2/26 (8)	1/26 (4)
Surgery Alone	26	N/A*	9/123 (8)
Surgery Alone	38	25/90 (28)	16/97 (16)
Radiation Alone	22	27/58 (47)	0/58
Radiation Alone	24	5/16 (31)	0/58
Radiation Alone	38	11/52 (21)	0/39
Radiation Alone	37	20/61 (33)	0/61
Radiation + Surgery	22	7/32 (23)	0/32
Radiation + Surgery	24	3/14 (21)	0/14
Radiation + Surgery	38	5/28 (18)	0/28

* N/A = Not Available

al.[38] reported contralateral neck metastases in 16 percent of patients (Table
6-5). For patients treated with radiation alone to both necks, or with
radiation plus a neck dissection, no contralateral recurrences were noted in
248 patients from a variety of series.[22,24,37,38] In view of this low incidence
of contralateral neck metastases, we wonder if treatment of the contralateral neck is necessary, since treatment is not without morbidity. Though
the effectiveness of prophylactic contralateral neck irradiation is excellent,
an alternative approach would be to observe the contralateral neck closely
and treat only those 10 to 15 percent of patients who do fail, since salvage
therapy is reasonably effective.[39]

Subsequent Appearance of the Primary in the Head and Neck Area

Approximately 20–25 percent of patients who present with a cervical
node from an unknown primary eventually manifest the occult primary
tumor in the head and neck area after radical neck dissection of the affected
neck.[24,26,38] As reported by Barrie et al.,[26] the most frequent sites of the
occult primary were in the supraglottic larynx, nasopharynx, base of
tongue, tonsil, and pharyngeal wall. This distribution has been confirmed
by other authors.[3,4,24,38,40] Based on this anatomical distribution, it became

Table 6-6
Appearance of an Occult Primary Tumor Metastatic to Cervical
Lymph Nodes after Treatment of the Lymph Nodes ±
Prophylactic Irradiation of the Possible Sites of Origin

| | | No. Occult Primaries Discovered/ Total Treated | |
| | | Prophylactic Irradiation of NP, OP, | No Prophylactic Irradiation of NP, OP, LP |
	Reference	LP* (%)	(%)
Surgery Alone	24	—	4/17 (23)
Surgery Alone	26	—	31/125 (25)
Surgery Alone	38	—	21/104 (20)
Radiation Alone	22	7/44 (16)	2/14 (14)
Radiation Alone	24	0/8	—
Radiation Alone	38	3/52 (6)	—
Radiation Alone	37	8/61 (13)	—
Radiation + Surgery	22	4/25 (16)	0/7
Radiation + Surgery	24	3/8	—
Radiation + surgery	38	4/28 (16)	—

* Nasopharynx (NP), Oropharynx (OP), Laryngopharynx (LP)

reasonable to prophylactically irradiate these sites which are likely to harbor an occult primary utilizing doses of 50 to 60 Gy, which theoretically should control subclinical disease.[41] A review of the literature does demonstrate a small decrease in the incidence of subsequent primaries in the head and neck area with prophylactic irradiation (Table 6-6). For surgery only series, the reported incidence of later primaries in the head and neck areas has ranged from 20 to 25 percent, with an average incidence of 23 percent (56/246). The results for series using prophylactic irradiation range from 6 to 16 percent, with an average incidence of 13 percent (29/226).

In our own series, the incidence of subsequent head and neck primaries did not differ between those patients who had received prophylactic irradiation of the nasopharynx, oropharynx, and laryngopharynx and those patients who had received only local irradiation of the neck (16 percent vs. 14 percent—Table 6-6).[22]

It is difficult to theorize as to the possible reasons for this very small, if any, effect of such large doses of irradiation on the later development of cancer in the head and neck area. One possible reason is that the subsequent head and neck tumor represents a new primary and has no relationship to the previous metastatic disease. Another possible reason is that the occult primary is present and has significant tumor bulk, but it is entirely submucosal and undetectable with routine physical examination. Mancuso and Hanafee have used a CT scanner to locate submucosal disease in the nasopharynx and pharynx previously undetected by triple endoscopy and routine x-rays.[27,28] Such gross disease may have 10 to 100 times more tumor cells than subclinical disease and would need even higher doses of irradiation for eradication of disease.

This then leads us to consider the detrimental effects of such prophylactic radiation to the pharynx, since there is significant morbidity associated with irradiation of such a large volume. Patients routinely develop an acute mucositis, odynophagia, and weight loss, and may develop the late effects of permanent xerostomia, possible radiation caries, and numerous other potential complications.[42–44]

Also, if radiation therapy is used prophylactically to such high doses, as is the present practice, additional radiation is usually not possible for those patients who do indeed manifest a primary or fail locally in the neck. Post-radiation surgical salvage is difficult and not often successful;[44] only 4 of 13 patients were surgically rendered free of disease after appearance of the occult primary.

Conclusions: Cervical Lymph Node Presentations

Based on our review of cervical lymph node presentations and therapies, we conclude that:

- A significant percentage of patients who present in cervical lymph nodes eventually succumb to the persistent local neck disease and/or the appearance of the primary disease (Fig. 6-2).
- Local control is beneficial and has a positive prognostic impact on survival (Fig. 6-1).
- Local control is dependent on the initial size of the lesion as well as the aggressiveness of local treatment, with better control in patients who either undergo surgery (either a total excisional biopsy of all gross tumor or a radical neck dissection) or who have higher doses of radiation to the neck in excess of 60 Gy (Table 6-4).
- Contralateral neck metastases are low and range from 10 to 15 percent for patients who undergo surgery only; they are reduced to nearly 0 percent if prophylactic radiation is delivered to the opposite neck (Table 6-5).

- The subsequent appearance of the primary in the head and neck area does not seem to be dramatically affected with prophylactic radiation to the nasopharynx, oropharynx, or laryngopharynx with doses considered to be effective for subclinical disease (Table 6-6).
- The morbidity of prophylactic radiation of the pharynx can be considerable.
- Subsequent salvage treatment can be limited if the occult primary does indeed appear after high dose irradiation (50–60 Gy).

Taking these conclusions together, we generally recommend aggressive management of the presenting neck with either radiation only for small neck nodes, or in conjunction with surgery for larger lesions. Doses of 60 Gy or more should be delivered to the ipsilateral neck. We question the effectiveness of prophylactically irradiating the possible anatomical sites that may harbor the occult primary and believe that observation of the contralateral neck may be all that is indicated in view of the low incidence of contralateral neck metastases. Electron-beam irradiation of the ipsilateral neck to spare the opposite parotid would alleviate the chronic xerostomia and nutritional problems that result from bilateral photon irradiation of both parotids and the anatomical areas thought to harbor the occult primary tumor. This approach should reduce the recurrence rate in the ipsilateral neck and spare the patient the morbidity that results from irradiation of the contralateral neck and possible sites of origin.

Axillary Lymph Node Presentations

For the patient who presents with an undifferentiated or epidermoid carcinoma of the axilla, a thorough examination of the breast and the trunk for a primary skin cancer or a connective tissue tumor should be done. A mammogram is also recommended, since the breast is the most likely site for the occult primary in this group of patients.[45] Also, since the lung can be a possible site of the primary tumor,[46] a chest x-ray and sputum analysis should be performed. With such a workup, Copeland found the primary site in 29 percent (18/60) of patients with axillary metastases with no apparent primary.[45] If the workup is negative, the primary is seldom found afterward. Copeland and McBride[45] could find the primary antemortem in only 3 of their remaining 42 patients. Montague found 9 primary tumors in 48 patients,[47] and the primary was later found in only 1 of 11 patients in our experience.[22]

We recommend an aggressive attempt at local-regional control using radiation therapy alone for small lesions and a combination of radiation therapy and surgery for larger masses, since those patients who achieved local control had a much higher survival than those who were not controlled (Fig. 6-1). Similar results were obtained by Copeland and McBride[45] with 9 of 42 patients eventually rendered free of disease with long–term survival, most having been treated with radical axillary dissection and radiation or local excision, plus high-dose radiotherapy.

Inguinal Lymph Node Presentations

In a large series reported by Zaren and Copeland,[23] there were only 22 patients out of a total population of 2232 patients who had an unknown primary presenting in inguinal lymph nodes. Most were either undifferentiated or squamous cell carcinomas. Previous diagnostic workup had included an exhaustive examination of the perineum, rectum, genitourinary system, and vulva. Seven of the patients underwent a radical inguinal node dissection, while the remaining 15 patients had excisional biopsy only; 4 of these patients had adjuvant therapy after the excisional biopsy. All 7 patients who had had the radical node dissection were free of tumor 2 to 18 years later, while 5 of the 15 patients (33 percent) treated with excisional biopsy were free of disease 2 to 10 years later. Only 15 percent of the 22 patients subsequently developed recurrent nodal disease and, overall, there was a 50 percent two-year survival. Our own experience is extremely limited; only two patients presented with an occult primary metastatic to the inguinal lymph nodes, and both developed disseminated disease and died. Based on Zaren and Copeland's experience, these patients seem to be in a better prognostic group and should be treated aggressively, if possible, with an aim towards local control. There seems to be no advantage to treating the possible primary sites prophylactically, since no primary site developed after local treatment in any of their 22 patients.

Supraclavicular Lymph Node Presentations

Because of their unique location in the body, the supraclavicular lymph nodes can be the site of metastases from above, as well as from below, the diaphragm.[48] It is probably in this group of patients that questions concerning the diagnostic workup most often arise. In our analysis, if the histology was epidermoid carcinoma, the lung was the anatomical location of the primary in all three patients who eventually manifested a primary site. Similarly, if it was an undifferentiated tumor, the primary site eventually manifested itself in the lung over half the time with a small number of primary sites appearing in the head and neck area and in the subdiaphragmatic region, as others have reported.[1,19,25,33] When analyzed for treatment outcome, patients with supraclavicular nodes did exceedingly poor, with only a 10 percent survival (Fig. 6-3). Most patients died from tumor; a significant number died directly due to the manifestation of the primary site, while the rest died from disseminated disease (Fig. 6-2). Survival was not positively affected for those patients who achieved local control over those who did not achieve local control (Fig. 6-1).

Since the lung is the most common site of the occult primary for these patients, regardless of histology,[1,19,20,49] we feel that it is the organ that should be targeted during the workup with bronchoscopy, sputum analysis, tomography, and chest CT. In the absence of histological evidence for a subdiaphragmatic primary, we do not recommend a blind search for the primary below the diaphragm because of its low yield, high cost, and the dismal final outcome. Abdominal CT may be the best diagnostic test to evaluate the subdiaphragmatic area.

Because of the high incidence of later lung primaries, prophylactic irradiation of the mediastinum and hilum of the lung and possibly the apices of the lung, is recommended, since these areas are the common locations of the primary and are easily encompassed in the treatment portals. Chemotherapy has unquestionably improved prognosis for small cell undifferentiated carcinomas of the lung, but is as yet less effective for epidermoid and other non-oat cell carcinomas.

Bone, Brain, and Miscellaneous Site Presentations

This is a mixed group of patients. The more frequent histology in all the studies was undifferentiated carcinoma, especially for patients with brain presentations. Our analysis, and the analysis of others,[8,50–52] demonstrate that the life expectancy for these patients is so poor that the cost of an extensive workup is hard to justify. The primary site was eventually found in 26 percent of these patients (Fig. 6-2), most often in the lungs. Therefore, we would recommend routine chest x-rays and sputum cytologies as the only tests necessary for these patients.

Few, if any, of patients who present with sites in the brain, bone, or in miscellaneous sites are ever rendered free of tumor, and most quickly develop widely disseminated tumor and die in a short period of time of cancer (Figs. 6-1 and 6-3). Based on these observations, we recommend that the presenting site be irradiated with palliative intent only, and that the patient be observed for other symptomatic sites that may require palliative therapy. Patients with multiple sites on initial presentation should be considered for systemic therapy, since a proportion of patients may actually have chemoresponsive neoplasms, such as small cell carcinoma, lymphoma, or germinal cell tumors whose prognosis is much improved compared to patients with disseminated squamous cell carcinoma.

Conclusion

The management of this small but challenging group of oncologic patients with squamous cell or undifferentiated tumors must be individualized based on presenting site, histology, and tumor extent. The patients with the best prognosis and the ones who seem to benefit from local control of the presenting site should be treated aggressively with curative intent. These patients include those who present with cervical lymph nodes, axillary lymph nodes, and possibly inguinal lymph nodes. Survival in these patients depends on local control. Patients with extremely poor prognosis include those whose presenting sites are in the supraclavicular lymph nodes, bone, brain, or miscellaneous sites. Treatment for those patients should be limited to palliation of symptoms and signs and possible consideration of systemic therapy. The search for the occult primary tumor should usually be limited to investigation of the chest, since the lungs are the most common site for the occult primary for most noncervical lymph node presentation sites.[49] Additional workup is, for the most part, expensive and unproductive.

References

1. Didlolker MS, Fanous N, Elias EG, et al: Metastatic carcinomas from occult primary tumors; a study of 254 patients. Ann Surg 186:628–630, 1977
2. Mayo CW, Lee MJ: Significance of a tumor in the neck. Lancet 70:420–428, 1950
3. Martin H, Morfitt HM: Cervical lymph node metastases as the first symptom of cancer. Surg Gynec Obstet 78:113–159, 1944

4. Comess MS: Cervical metastases from occult carcinoma. Surg Gynec Obstet 104:607–617, 1957
5. France CJ, Lucas R: The management and prognosis of metastatic neoplasms of the neck with unknown primary. Am J Surg 106:835–839, 1963
6. Moertel CG, Reitemeier RJ, Schutt AJ, et al: Treatment of the patient with adenocarcinoma of unknown origin. Cancer 30:1469–1472, 1972
7. Nystrom JS, Weiner JM, Heffelfinger-Juttner J: Metastatic and histologic presentation in unknown primary cancers. Sem in Oncol 4:53–59, 1977
8. Holmes FF, Fouts TL: Metastatic cancer of unknown primary site. Cancer 26:816–820, 1970
9. Bosman FT, Silverberg SG: Differential diagnosis of metastatic tumors, in Silverberg, SG (ed): Principles and Practice of Surgical Pathology. New York, J. Wiley and Sons, 1983, pp 154–161
10. Ioachim HL: Metastatic tumors, in Ioachim HL (ed): Lymph Nodes in Lymph Node Biopsy, Philadelphia, J.B. Lippincott Company, 1982, pp 16–19
11. Fallini, B, Taylor CR: New developments in immunoperoxidase techniques and their application. Arch Path Lab Med 107:105, 1983
12. DeLellis RA: Immunoperoxidase techniques in diagnostic pathology. Report of a workshop sponsored by the NCI. Am J Clin Path 71:483, 1979
13. Battifora H, Trowbridge IS: A monoclonal antibody useful for the differential diagnosis between malignant lymphoma and nonhematopoietic neoplasms. Cancer 51:816, 1983
14. Felix EL: The use of bone and brain scanning as screening procedures in patients with malignant tumors. Surg Gynecol Obstet 141:867–869, 1975
15. Greenberg EJ, Weber DA, Pochaczevsky R, et al: Detection of neoplastic bone lesions by quantitative scanning and radiography. J Nuc Med 9:613–620, 1968
16. Langhammer H, Glaubitt G, Hampe JF, et al: Gallium–67 for tumor scanning. J Nuc Med 13:25–30, 1972
17. Teates CD, Bray ST, Williamson RJ: Tumor detection with Gallium–67 Citrate—A literature survey 1970–1978. Clin Nuc Med 3:456–460, 1978
18. Steckel RT, Kagan R: Diagnostic persistence in working up metastatic cancer with an unknown primary site. Radiology 134:367–369, 1980
19. Nystrom JS, Weiner JM, Wolf RM, et al: Identifying the primary site in metastatic cancer of unknown origin—inadequacy of roentgenographic procedures. JAMA 241:381–383, 1979

20. Osteen RT, Lopf G, Wilson RE: In pursuit of the unknown primary site. Am J Surg 135:494–498, 1978

21. McMillan JH, Levine E, Stephens RH: CT in the evaluation of metastatic adenocarcinoma from an unknown primary site. Radiology 143:143–146, 1982

22. Silverman CL, Marks JE: Metastatic cancer of unknown origin: Epidermoid and undifferentiated carcinomas. Sem in Oncol 9:435–441, 1982

23. Zaren HA, Copeland MM: Inguinal node metastases. Cancer 41:919–923, 1978

24. Coker DO, Casterline PF, Chambers RG, et al: Metastases to lymph nodes of the head and neck from an unknown primary site. Am J Surg 134:517–522, 1977

25. Fitzpatrick PJ, Kotalik JF: Cervical metastases from an unknown primary tumor. Radiology 110:659–663, 1974

26. Barrie JR, Knapper WH, Strong EW: Cervical nodal metastases of unknown origin. Am J Surg 120:466–470, 1970

27. Mancuso AA, Hanafee WN: Elusive head and neck carcinomas beneath intact mucosa. Laryngoscope 93:133–139, 1983

28. Mancuso AA, and Hanafee WN (eds): Computed Tomography of the Head and Neck. Baltimore, Williams and Wilkins, 1982

29. Micheau C, Cachin Y, Casilou B: Cystic metastases in the neck revealing occult carcinoma of the tonsil. Cancer 33:228–233, 1974

30. Coates HK: Immunological basis of detection of head and neck tumors. Cancer 41:912–916, 1978

31. Lindberg RD: Distribution of cervical lymph node metastases from squamous cell carcinoma of the upper respiratory and digestive tracts. Cancer 29:1446–1450, 1972

32. Molinari R, Cantu G, Chiesa F, et al: Statistical approach to detection of primary cancer based on the site of neck lymph node metastasis. Tumori 63:267–280, 1977

33. Acquarelli MJ, Matsunaga RS, Cruze K: Metastatic carcinoma of the neck of unknown primary origin. Laryngoscope 71:962–974, 1961

34. Nordstrom DG, Tewfik HH, Latourette HB: Cervical lymph node metastases from an unknown primary. Int J Rad Oncol Biol Phys 5:73–77, 1979

35. Fried MP, Diehl WH, Brownson RJ, et al: Cervical metastases from an unknown primary. Ann Otol 84:152–157, 1975

36. Winegar LK, Griffin W: The occult primary tumor. Arch Otol 98:159–163, 1973

37. Probert JC: Secondary carcinoma in cervical lymph nodes with an

occult primary tumor—a review of 61 patients. Clin Radiol 21:211–218, 1970

38. Jessie RH, Perez CA, Fletcher GH: Cervical lymph node metastases—unknown primary cancer. Cancer 31:354–361, 1973

39. Vandenbrouck C, Sancho–Garnier H, Chassagne D, et al: Elective vs. therapeutic radical neck dissection in epidermoid carcinoma of the oral cavity. Cancer 46:386–390, 1980

40. Batsakis JG: The pathology of head and neck tumors: The occult primary and metastases to the head and neck, Part 10. Head and Neck Surg 3:409–423, 1981

41. Fletcher GH: Elective irradiation of subclinical disease in cancers of the head and neck. Cancer 15:1085–1099, 1972

42. Dreizen S, Brown CR, Handler S, et al: Radiation induced xerostomia in cancer patients. Cancer 38:273–278, 1976

43. Daly TE, Drane JB: The management of teeth related to the treatment of oral cancer, Proceedings of the 7th National Cancer Conference 7:904–913, 1973

44. Fletcher GH: Oral cavity and oropharynx, in Fletcher GH (ed): Textbook of Radiotherapy (ed 2). Philadelphia, Lea & Febiger, 1973, pp 212–254

45. Copeland EM, McBride CM: Axillary metastases from unknown primary sites. Ann Surg 178:25–27, 1973

46. Feverman L, Attie JN, Rosenberg B: Carcinoma in axillary lymph nodes. Surg Gynecol Obstet 114:5–8, 1962

47. Montague E: Axillary metastases from unknown primary sites, in Fletcher GH (ed): Textbook of Radiotherapy. Philadelphia, Lea and Febiger, 1980

48. Berge T, Toremalm NG: Cervical and mediastinal lymph node metastases as an otorhinolaryngic problem. Ann Otol 78:663–670, 1969

49. Clary CF, Michel RP, Wang NS, et al: Metastatic carcinoma—the lung as the site for the clinically undiagnosed primary. Cancer 51:362–367, 1983

50. Copeland MM: Metastasis to bone from primary tumors in other sites. Proceedings of the National Cancer Conference 6:743–756, 1970

51. Ebels EJ, VanderMeulen JD: Cerebral metastases without a known primary tumor. Clin Neuro and Neurosurg 80:195–197, 1978

52. Lang EF, Slaton J: Metastatic brain tumors; results of surgical and nonsurgical treatment. Surg Clin of N Amer 44:865, 1964

7

MELANOMA WITH AN UNKNOWN PRIMARY SITE AND AMELANOTIC MELANOMA

Armando E. Giuliano
Alistair J. Cochran
Donald L. Morton

Unknown Primary Melanoma

Patients with an unknown primary melanoma present to the oncologist after biopsy of an enlarged lymph node or resection of a metastatic nodule. On physical examination, there is no detectable primary skin lesion. Typically, there is no history suggestive of a primary lesion; however, a small group of patients may describe a mole that has long since regressed and is undetectable. By definition, the patient with unknown primary melanoma can have no evidence of a primary skin lesion either at the time of diagnosis or previously. The criteria described by Das Gupta[1] remain the standard by which physicians should diagnose an unknown primary melanoma. Patients with orbital exenteration or enucleation should not be diagnosed as having an unknown primary melanoma, since the eye surgery may have been for melanoma, or the specimen may have contained a missed ocular melanoma.

Those patients having a history of a mole or other skin lesion

POORLY DIFFERENTIATED NEOPLASMS AND TUMORS OF UNKNOWN ORIGIN   ISBN 0-8089-1755-2

cauterized or removed should not be considered as having an unknown primary melanoma, unless the histologic material can be reviewed and the block carefully examined microscopically. Similarly, a surgical scar found in the drainage area of diseased lymph nodes must be assumed to result from excision of the primary lesion, unless the slides are available. Obviously, complete physical examination, including ophthalmoscopy and otolaryngologic assessment, must be done prior to considering that a metastatic melanoma is a tumor from an unknown primary site of origin.

Occurrence

The incidence of unknown primary melanoma varies from 2 to 16 percent of patients with malignant melanoma.[1–3] Most authorities find the incidence to be around 5 percent when strict criteria are used for diagnosis. Das Gupta[1] reported 37 (3.7 percent) cases of unknown primary melanoma from among 992 melanoma patients. Baab and McBride also found a 4 percent incidence of unknown primary melanoma in their series of patients.[3] Similarly, Chang and Knapper[4] noted a 4.4 percent incidence. At UCLA, of 980 melanoma patients seen during a 7-year-period, 55 (5.6 percent) had metastatic melanoma without an identifiable primary lesion.[5]

Unknown primary melanoma appears to be more common in men than in women. These tumors may become apparent at any age, but the peak incidence in most studies is in the fourth and fifth decades. In the UCLA experience, 18 of the 55 patients were in their forties. Less than 10 percent were older than 60.

Etiology

The etiology of the absence of a detectable primary melanoma is unknown. Numerous theories have been offered to explain this unusual phenomenon. Melanoma could conceivably arise de novo in lymph nodes or visceral organs. The lymph nodes of patients who have undergone lymphadenectomy for diseases other than melanoma occasionally have contained nevus cells. McCarthy et al.[6] found such cells in 8/129 axillary lymph node dissections. These cells are typically located in the capsule of the lymph node and only in nodes draining skin. A melanoma arising from these nevus cells would appear as an apparent lymph node metastasis with no obvious primary tumor.

Melanoma has been reported to arise in visceral organs. Melanomas of the mucous membranes and unusual locations are well-recognized.[7,8] Melanocytes are found in mucous membranes, and aberrant migration of neuroectodermal cells could account for visceral primaries. Most authorities, however, feel that visceral melanoma, even without obvious coexistent lesions, represents a metastatic tumor. Accidental trauma to a skin lesion may also account for a missing primary lesion when the patient presents with metastases. Patients often sustain minor skin injuries that could abrade or even avulse a small segment of skin. The resulting scar and inflammatory response could conceivably lead to the destruction of a small primary cutaneous melanoma. Over-the-counter medications, for example, are commonly used to treat "warts." Patients may medicate a small raised lesion that is actually a melanoma, causing chemical destruction of the skin primary, and fail to remember this minor incident when giving a history.

The most commonly accepted explanation for unknown primary melanoma is that an inapparent cutaneous lesion has undergone spontaneous regression. This phenomenon has been extensively documented.[9] Partial regression of malignant melanoma has been observed and the histologic appearances well-described by McGovern.[10] In his series, changes of regression were seen in 12.3 percent of 437 primary cutaneous melanomas, suggesting that this phenomenon is more common than usually expected. In our series, 5/55 patients gave histories of spontaneous regression of pigmented lesions that indeed may have been the missing primary.

The mechanism of spontaneous regression has not been demonstrated, but is believed to be mediated by the immune system. In numerous case reports, augmented tumor immunity has been associated with spontaneous regression of melanoma.[11,12] Sumner and Foraker[13] have shown that serum from a patient who had experienced a spontaneous regression of metastatic melanoma induced regression in another patient. Maurer, McIntire, and Rueckert[14] demonstrated that circulating factors from sera of a patient with regressing melanoma were capable of augmenting lymphocyte cytotoxicity in vitro. However, these isolated case reports do not prove that the immune system is responsible for the missing tumor in patients with an unknown primary.

Giuliano et al.[15] studied the immune responses of 36 patients with Stage II melanoma and an unknown primary and compared them to those of 83 Stage II patients with a known primary melanoma. The patients in each group were similar in age, sex, and extent of disease. There were no discernible differences in delayed cutaneous hypersensitivity to DNCB, lymphocyte blastogenesis, or antitumor antibody response in patients with unknown primary melanoma when compared to those with a known primary melanoma and similar extent of disease.

Table 7-1
Sites of Metastatic Spread of Unknown Primary Melanoma at
Presentation to UCLA (55 patients)

Site	Number of Patients
Lymph nodes	36
axillary	17
cervical	11
ingrimal	8
Skin and subcutaneous	9
Lungs	6
Brain	6
Bowel	2
Liver	2
Bone	2

Sites of Metastases and Stage of Disease

The lymph nodes are the most common site of presentation for metastatic melanoma from an unknown primary. Approximately 2/3 of such melanoma patients present with their disease confined to the lymph nodes, whereas 1/3 have extralymphatic spread. There is no site of lymph node metastases more common than another, according to most large series.[1-4] However, when we compared the site of lymph node metastases in unknown primary patients to that in patients with a known primary and clinically palpable diseased lymph nodes, we found a higher incidence of metastases to the cervical lymph nodes among patients with an unknown primary. The most common sites for nonlymphatic metastases are the skin and subcutaneous tissue. Table 7-1 shows the sites of presentation of metastatic melanoma among patients with an unknown primary treated at UCLA.

Evaluation and Treatment

The initial evaluation of the patient with a metastatic melanoma and no obvious primary lesion should begin with a careful examination of the skin. A knowledge of the regional lymphatic drainage permits a concentrated search in the area most likely to harbor the primary when the patient presents with lymph node metastases. An ultraviolet light is useful for detecting halo nevi or regressing primaries. Suspicious pigmented lesions and wholly or partially depigmented lesions should be excised and examined histologically. The pathologist should be informed of the clinical situation so that he may examine representative sections of several areas of each lesion.

The patient with lymph node metastases must undergo a thorough search for visceral tumor spread. A complete physical examination (including ophthalmoscopy and otolaryngoscopy), chest x-ray, liver function tests, liver scan, and brain CT scan for patients with palpable lymph node metastases from an unknown primary melanoma should be performed to accurately assess the extent of disease. If no disseminated disease is found, then a radical lymphadenectomy of the affected nodal group should be performed.

If the patient develops a second lymph node metastasis, a repeat search for visceral disease should be undertaken and, if none can be detected, a second lymphadenectomy should be performed. The involvement of multiple nodal groups is not necessarily an indication of disseminated disease because melanomas of the trunk often metastasize to bilateral or multiple nodal groups. Three patients in our series[5] underwent resection of several lymph node groups. One patient developed metastases in four regional node groups, all of which were resected.

Patients with disseminated melanoma from an unknown primary site should be treated with chemotherapy or in experimental protocols. Selected patients with an isolated visceral lesion may benefit from resection. Several patients in our series whose disease was diagnosed at thoracotomy or craniotomy have survived five years. These patients, however, are extremely unusual and were not identified and diagnosed preoperatively. If the diagnosis of metastatic melanoma has previously been made, an operative approach to visceral metastases should generally not be undertaken.

Prognosis

Some investigators speculate that patients with an unknown primary have a more favorable prognosis than those with a known primary melanoma.[3] It has been postulated that these patients have augmented tumor immunity, and micrometastases are destroyed by the immune system. Other investigators believe that patients with an unknown primary fare worse than those with a known primary.[1,2]

In order to determine the prognostic significance of the unknown primary melanoma, we compared the clinical course of these patients to that of patients with a known primary melanoma and similar extent of disease.[5] The clinical course of 36 patients with unknown primary melanoma metastatic to regional lymph nodes and no detectable visceral metastases was compared to that of 84 patients with a known primary melanoma and palpable regional lymph node metastases. The extent of the disease was documented at lymphadenectomy for patients in both groups. Sex and age distribution were similar. The number of involved lymph nodes at operation was similar, although the patients with an unknown primary had slightly more diseased nodes. The total number of lymph nodes resected per patient was similar for each group. Despite the slightly larger number of involved lymph nodes in the unknown primary group, the recurrence rate between the groups was nearly identical.

Because prognosis was nearly the same for the two groups of patients, we advocate the same aggressive surgical management for patients with unknown primary melanoma as for those with a known primary.

Amelanotic Melanoma

Primary cutaneous melanomas that are totally devoid of pigment on visual inspection do occur, though comparatively few are truly amelanotic if the inspection includes assessment of any surrounding radial growth phase. Much of the difficulty in diagnosing melanomas comes from the incorrect belief that some or all are "black." In fact, melanoma displays a range of brown colors, which may be admixed with the red of a prominent dermal vascular pattern and the blues of the hemosiderin detritus of previous hemorrhage and the whites of regression.[16] If primary melanomas are examined with the light microscope, virtually all contain some melanin. Truly amelanotic primaries are exceedingly rare and are mainly nodular or indeterminate in type; amelanotic lentigo maligna melanoma and superficial spreading melanoma are very unusual. Amelanotic metastases are rather more common than primary amelanotic tumors. Ultrastructural demonstration of characteristic premelanosomes, melanosomes, or parallel tubular arrays is the ultimate proof that a tumor is melanocytic.[17-19] Fortunately, these organelles are comparatively durable and are often still recognizable in tissues fixed in formalin or other conventional fixatives.[20] The demonstration of minor degrees of melanogenesis by electron microscopy and by other novel approaches noted below further reduces the frequency of truly amelanotic tumors.

Incidence

Table 7-2 shows the reported incidence of amelanotic melanoma in several large series. The precise incidence, however, is nearly impossible to determine, because most series do not clearly define what is meant by an

Table 7-2
Incidence of Amelanotic Melanomas in Selected Series

Study	Reported Incidence
Huvos et al.[21]	28/1483 (1.9%)
Clark et al.[22]	16/197 (8.1%)
Ariel[23]	6/332 (1.9%)
Balch[24]	35/238 (14.7%)

amelanotic melanoma. Furthermore, the reported incidence will vary greatly depending on whether only the primary tumor is considered or whether its metastases are also evaluated for the absence of pigment. Many lesions present as a pigmented skin primary and yet develop amelanotic metastases. It is striking that about 30 percent of amelanotic melanomas present as metastases from an occult primary tumor,[21] while few melanized metastatic malignant melanomas arise from an occult primary tumor.[25]

UCLA Experience

Of 2881 patients with cutaneous malignant melanoma seen at UCLA during the past 25 years, 50 (1.8 percent) had either an amelanotic primary tumor or amelanotic metastases. Of these 50 patients, 29 presented with an amelanotic primary tumor, and 21 had amelanotic metastases from a melanotic primary. In only three patients was there absence of pigment in both the primary tumor and its metastases to lymph nodes. Although most amelanotic primaries were located on the lower extremities, amelanotic primary tumors were found in many different locations. Twenty-eight (56 percent) of these patients had metastases to regional nodes. Six patients had lymph node metastases from an unknown primary.

Establishing that an Amelanotic Tumor is a Malignant Melanoma

Diligent and, often, protracted examination of thin, adequately fixed hematoxylin and eosin-stained sections from different areas of the tumor will reveal melanin deposits in most cases. Coarse granules of pigment (aggregates of fully melanized melanosomes) in intratumoral or peritumoral macrophages are often the first clue to the presence of significant melanogenesis. Such a finding by itself, however, can never be diagnostic of melanoma. To establish that a tumor is melanogenic, it is necessary to demonstrate fine granules of intracytoplasmic melanin (partly or wholly melanized individual melanosomes) in tumor cells and to demonstrate the nature of the pigment by a melanin stain, its removal by bleaching agents, and the absence of positive reactions to stains for iron or lipid. In minimally melanized tumors, a melanin stain may speed up the detection of the pigment if only an occasional cell or focus of cells is positive. It has been our experience, however, that melanin demonstrated in this manner is almost always visible on re-examination of the hematoxylin and eosin section. If doubt still remains after an adequate light microscopic assessment of the material, electron microscopy will usually settle the matter, even if only formalin-fixed tissues are available. Premelanosomes and melanosomes are comparatively durable organelles. Recently, it has been reported that some melanomas may be devoid of recognizable classical premelanosomes and that in such tumors, the diagnosis may be made by demonstrating "parallel tubular assays."[20]

A further possibility, if fresh tumor tissue is available, is to demonstrate in the tumor cells the presence of melanoma-associated enzymes, such as DOPA-hydroxylase, tyrosinase, leucine aminopeptidase and β–glycuronidase.[26] The DOPA reaction, the best known of these techniques, has been employed usefully for many years.[27] Recently, it has proved possible to combine ultrastructural examination and the DOPA technique.[28,29]

S-100 Staining

We have recently applied a new approach to confirming the melanocytic nature of amelanotic tumors. This method exploits the observation that S-100 protein is present in malignant melanoma tissue culture lines and biopsies of melanocytic tumors.[30,31]

S-100 protein is an acidic protein of unknown function named from its solubility in saturated ammonium sulfate at neutral pH.[32] This protein has been demonstrated in glial cells in the brain,[33] Schwann cells in the peripheral nervous system, and satellite cells in the peripheral ganglia.[34] It exhibits a strong serologic cross-reactivity among a variety of vertebrate species.[35]

After demonstrating that S-100 protein is present in melanoma cells, we indicated that to be of the most practical use as a histological marker, S-100 protein should be detectable in melanoma cells in formalin-fixed, paraffin-embedded tissue. We now routinely employ an immunoperoxidase assay for this purpose.[36]

Others have also reported that melanocytic tumors contain S-100 protein. Nakajima et al.[37] found S-100 protein in 39 of 41 melanomas and also in nevocytic nevi. They reported that the content of S-100 protein varied according to the histogenetic type of the melanoma (the least being found in melanomas of lentigo maligna type), a finding supported by others.[38,39] On the basis of these and similar studies, the detection of S-100 protein is now used by many pathology laboratories as part of the workup of tumors of debatable histogenesis. It is particularly useful in the assessment of amelanotic tumors and can be applied to primary and metastatic cutaneous and ocular melanomas.[40]

The S-100 protein approach cannot, however, be applied uncritically, as a variety of other, nonmelanocytic tumors contain this material. This includes neural tumors, such as gliomas, Schwannian tumors, including granular cell myoblastoma, and some neurogenic sarcomas. Separation of neurogenic sarcomas from spindle celled malignant melanoma is probably impossible on the basis of S-100 protein alone. Recent studies indicate that melanoma cells contain both a and b subunits of S-100 protein, while Schwannian tumors contain only b subunits. It has been possible to raise antibodies to these separate subunits, and this will certainly facilitate the separation of the different types of S-100 protein-containing tumors.[41]

A variety of other, non-neural, nonmelanocytic tumors reportedly contain S-100 protein, including chondrosarcomas, liposarcomas, a few myoepithelium-related tumors, pleomorphic adenomas and "histiocytic" tumors derived from dendritic cells of the lymphoid tissues.[42] While these lesions may potentially be confused with malignant melanoma, on the basis of their S-100 protein content, a consideration of the clinical history and the presence of other tissue markers, such as cytokeratins and leukocyte antigens, will usually permit these different classes of tumors to be separated.

As alternatives or supplements to the S-100 protein approach, melanoma-directed monoclonal antibodies are of considerable interest. Unfortunately, most are useful only when frozen sections are available, and they react poorly with formalin-fixed material. An exception to this is the monoclonal antibody NKl/C-3 from the Netherlands Cancer Institute, which reacts with an antigen which is not denatured during formalin-fixation.[43]

Prognosis

The prognostic significance of amelanotic melanoma has been controversial. Several authorities suggest that the absence of pigment production is associated with an adverse effect on survival. Melanogenesis is certainly a differentiated function, but there is no evidence that it is either directly correlated with morphologic differentiation or negatively correlated with the malignant phenotype. Thus, relatively well-differentiated malignant melanomas often show little or no pigment production, while relatively anaplastic melanomas may be highly melanized.

Huvos[21] found that only 15 percent of patients with Stage II amelanotic melanoma survived five years compared to a 42 percent five-year survival obtained in patients with State II pigmented melanoma. Similarly, Ariel[23] and Veronesi[44] suggested that patients with amelanotic lesions had a far worse prognosis than others. Most studies, however, have suggested that the pigment content of melanoma does not relate to prognosis.[45–48] McGovern[10] studied 202 melanoma patients and found no relationship between pigment production and prognosis. The survival of 19 of our patients with amelanotic melanoma metastatic to regional lymph nodes (Stage II) was compared to the survival of 121 patients with Stage II pigmented melanoma. All patients underwent regional lymph node dissection to confirm the presence of metastatic melanoma in the regional nodes. The number of positive lymph nodes in each group was similar. There was no apparent difference in survival between the two groups of patients. Although the number of patients with amelanotic melanoma was small, it would appear that the absence of pigment production does not relate to survival.

Conclusion

Both amelanotic melanoma and unknown primary melanoma are unusual variants of malignant melanoma. These lesions are often difficult to diagnose, and patients are often mismanaged due to confusion concerning the significance of the histologic findings. In our experience, however, neither unknown primary melanoma nor amelanotic melanoma implies a favorable or unfavorable prognosis. Diagnosis is often difficult in both situations. The special studies described, however, may be beneficial.

Once diagnosis is made, therapy should proceed on the basis of clinical stage, rather than the histologic absence of pigment or the absence of a primary tumor. These patients should be managed similarly to other patients with the more common types of melanoma. Localized and regional disease should be treated surgically. Systemic metastases are usually best treated with chemotherapy; however, immunotherapy, radiation, and surgical excision may also play a role.

References

1. Das Gupta T, Bowden T, Berg J: Malignant melanoma of unknown primary origin. Surg Gynecol Obstet 117:341–345, 1963
2. Milton GW, Lane–Brown MM, Gilder M: Malignant melanoma with an occult primary lesion. Br J Surg 54:651–658, 1967
3. Baab GH, McBride CM: Malignant melanoma—the patient with an unknown site of primary origin. Arch Surg 110:896–900, 1975
4. Chang P, Knapper WH: Metastatic melanoma of unknown primary. Cancer 49:1106–1111, 1982
5. Giuliano AE, Moseley HS, Morton DL: Clinical aspects of unknown primary melanoma. Ann Surg 191:98–104, 1981
6. McCarthy SW, Palmer AA, Bale PA, et al: Nevus cells in lymph nodes. Pathology 6:351–358, 1974
7. Das Gupta TK, Brasfield RD, Paglia MA: Primary melanomas in unusual sites. Surg Gynecol Obstet 128:841–848, 1969
8. Wanebo HJ, Woodruff JM, Farr GH, et al: Anorectal melanoma. Cancer 47:1891–1900, 1981
9. Everson TC, Cole WH: Spontaneous Regression of Cancer. Philadelphia, W.B. Saunders, 1966
10. McGovern VJ: Spontaneous regression of melanoma. Pathology 7:91–99, 1975
11. Bodurtha AJ, Berkelhammer J, Kim YH, et al: A clinical histologic and immunologic study of a case of metastatic malignant melanoma undergoing spontaneous remission. Cancer 37:735–742, 1965
12. Bulkley GB, Cohen MH, Banks PM, et al: Long-term spontaneous regression of malignant melanoma with visceral metastases. Report of a case with immunologic profile. Cancer 36:485–494, 1975
13. Sumner WC, Foraker AG: Spontaneous regression of human melanoma: Clinical and experimental study. Cancer 13:79–84, 1960
14. Maurer HL, McIntyre OR, Rueckert F: Spontaneous regression of malignant melanoma: Pathologic and immunologic study in a ten-year survivor. Am J Surg 127:397, 1974
15. Giuliano AE, Moseley HS, Irie RF, et al: Immunological aspects of unknown primary melanoma. Surgery 87:101–105, 1980
16. Mihm MC Jr, Fitzpatrick TB, Lane–Brown MM, et al: Early detection of primary cutaneous malignant melanoma: A color atlas. N Engl J Med 289:989–996, 1973
17. McKay B, and Osborne BM: The contribution of electron microscopy to the diagnosis of tumors. Patho Biol Annual 8:539–546, 1978
18. Hunter JAA, Zaynoun S, Paterson WD, et al: Cellular fine structure in

the invasive nodules of different histogenetic types of malignant melanoma. Brit J Derm 98:255–272, 1978

19. Mishima Y: Melanosis circumscripta praecancerosa (Subreuilh)-arnon-nevoid premelanoma distinct from junction nevus. J Invest Derm 34:361–367, 1960

20. MacKay B, Silva EG: Diagnostic electron microscopy in oncology, in: Sommers, SC and Rosen, PP (eds): Pathology Annual, part 2, vol. 15, New York, Appleton-Century-Crofts, p. 241, 1980

21. Huvos AG, Shaw JP, Goldsmith HS: A clinicopathologic study of amelanotic melanoma. Surg Gynecol Obstet 135:917–920, 1972

22. Clark WH, From L, Bernadino EA, et al: The histogenesis and biological behavior of primary human malignant melanomas of the skin. Cancer Res 29:705–720, 1969

23. Ariel IM: Malignant melanoma of the upper extremities. J Surg Oncol 16:125–143, 1981

24. Balch CM, Soong SJ, Murad TM, et al: A multi-factorial analysis of melanoma. Ann Surg 193:377–388, 1981

25. Giuliano AE, Gochran AC, Morton DL: Melanoma from an unknown primary site and amelanotic melanoma. Semin Oncol 9:442–447, 1982

26. Rouge F, Subert C: A new approach to the differential diagnosis of human malignant melanoma. Cancer 44:199–209, 1979

27. Milne JA: An Introduction to the Diagnostic Histopathology of the Skin. London, Edward Arnold, 1972, pp 254–355

28. Hunter JAA, Paterson WD, Fairley DJ: Human malignant melanoma: Melanosomal polymorphism and the ultrastructural DOPA reaction. Brit J Derm 98:381–387, 1978

29. Anderson CW, Stevens MH, Moatamed F: Electron microscopy and α-DOPA reaction in the evaluation of an unusual amelanotic malignant melanoma of the neck. Otolaryngol Head Neck Surg 89:594–598, 1981

30. Gaynor R, Irie RF, Morton DL, Herschman HR, S-100 protein in cultured human malignant melanomas. Nature (Lond), 286:400–401, 1980

31. Gaynor R, Herschman HR, Irie R, et al: S-100 protein: A marker for human malignant melanomas? Lancet 1:869–871, 1981

32. Moore BW, MacGregor D: Chromatographic and electrophoretic fractionation of soluble proteins of brain and liver. J Biol Chem 240:1647–1653, 1965

33. Ludwin SK, Kosek JC, Eng LF: The topographical distribution of S-100 and GFA proteins in adult rat brain. I Comp Neurol 165:197–208, 1976

34. Eng LF, Kosek JC, Forno L, et al: Immunohistochemistry of brain

protein in fixed paraffin embedded tissues. Trans Amer Soc Neurochem 7:211, 1976

35. Kessler D, Levine L, Fassman G: Some conformation and immunological properties of bovine brain acidic protein. Biochem 7:758–764, 1968

36. Cochran AJ, Wen DR, Herschman HR, et al: Detection of S-100 protein as an aid to the identification of melanocytic tumors. Int J Cancer 30:295–297, 1982

37. Nakajima T, Watanabe S, Sato Y, et al: Immunohistochemical demonstrations of S-100 protein in human malignant melanoma and pigmented nevi. Gann, 72:335–336, 1981

38. Dabbs DJ, Bolen JW: Superficial spreading malignant melanoma with neurosarcomatous metastases. Am J Clin Pathol, 82:109–114, 1984

39. Springall DR, Gu J, Cocchia D, et al: The values of S-100 immunostaining as a diagnostic tool in human malignant melanomas. Virchows Arch (A) (Pathol Anak) 400:331–343, 1983

40. Cochran AJ, Holland GN, Wen D-R, et al: Detection of cytoplasmic S-100 protein in primary and metastatic intraocular melanomas. Invest Ophthal & Vis Sci 24:1153–1155, 1983

41. Akagi T, Takahashi K, Ohtsuki Y: Immunohistochemical localization of S-100 protein subunits in the human lymphoreticular system. J Leuk Biol 36:181, 1984b.

42. Ide F, Iwase T, Saito I, et al: Immunohistochemical and ultrastructural analysis of the proliferating cells in histiocytosis-X. Cancer 53: 917–921, 1984

43. Mackie RM, Campbell I, Turbitt ML: Use of NKlC3 monoclonal antibody in the assessment of benign and malignant melanocytic lesions. J Clin Pathol 37:367–372, 1984

44. Veronesi U, Cascinelli N, Preda F: Prognosis of malignant melanoma according to regional metastasis. Am J Roentgenol Radium Ther Nucl Med 11:301–309, 1971

45. Wright CJE: Prognosis in cutaneous and ocular malignant melanoma. J Pat Bact 61:507–525, 1949

46. Wright RB, Clark DH, Milne JA: Malignant cutaneous melanoma—A review. Br J Surg 150:360–368, 1953

47. Mason M, Friedmann I: Melanoma of the nose and ear. J Laryng 69:98–107, 1955

48. Allen AC, Spitz S: Malignant melanoma. A clinicopathological analysis of the criteria for diagnosis and prognosis. Cancer 6:1–45, 1953

8

ADVANCED POORLY DIFFERENTIATED CARCINOMA OF UNKNOWN PRIMARY SITE: CLINICAL CHARACTERISTICS AND TREATMENT RESULTS

John D. Hainsworth
F. Anthony Greco

In managing the patient with neoplastic disease, the clinician depends upon the histopathologic diagnosis when making therapeutic decisions. The need for guidance by the pathologist is greatest in the patient who has no obvious primary site at the time of diagnosis. Unfortunately, pathologic features which pinpoint the primary site are often not present; hence, treatment decisions become very difficult. Patients with poorly differentiated or undifferentiated carcinomas of unknown primary site have been frustrating for both the pathologist and the clinician. Although recognized to be a heterogeneous group, including patients with neoplasms arising at a variety of primary sites, these tumors often elude more precise characterization by the pathologist, even when specialized techniques such as electron microscopy are employed. Likewise, treatment attempts in patients with advanced disease have been disheartening. Patients with carcinoma of unknown primary site have been treated with a variety of

POORLY DIFFERENTIATED NEOPLASMS AND TUMORS OF UNKNOWN ORIGIN   ISBN 0-8089-1755-2

outpatient chemotherapeutic regimens; results have been dismal; median
survival is three to four months, with no long-term disease-free survivors.[1,2] Most trials have included patients with adenocarcinoma of unknown primary site as well as those with poorly differentiated carcinomas.
Because of these discouraging results, the patient with carcinoma of
unknown primary site often receives little or no therapy.

In 1976, two patients were seen with poorly differentiated carcinomas
of unknown primary site who had experienced dramatic tumor responses
to systemic chemotherapy.

The first patient was a 27-year-old man who developed superior vena cava
syndrome in 1974 and was found to have a huge mediastinal tumor. He initially
received mediastinal irradiation with a good tumor response, but quickly developed recurrence in cervical lymph nodes. He received several courses of chemotherapy with cyclophosphamide, adriamycin, bleomycin, and vincristine. He had a
complete response to chemotherapy, and is currently disease-free nearly ten years
after initial treatment.

The second patient was a 43-year-old man who developed cough, hemoptysis,
right hemiparesis, and seizures. He was first seen in a hospital in Washington, DC,
where a chest roentgenogram showed a right upper lobe lung mass, and a
computed tomographic scan of the brain showed a left parietal mass. The parietal
lesion was removed at craniotomy, and was interpreted as an ''undifferentiated
carcinoma, favor adenocarcinoma.'' He received radiotherapy to both the whole
brain and the lung lesion, followed by chemotherapy with procarbazine and
CCNU. Three months later, bilateral pulmonary nodules developed, and urinary
HCG levels were found to be markedly elevated at 306 mIU/ml (normal less than 25
mIU/ml). He was treated with bleomycin, cyclophosphamide, vinblastine, dactinomycin, cisplatin, and chlorambucil (VAB III regimen) for a suspected germinal
neoplasm. Pulmonary nodules regressed, but HCG remained slightly elevated at
2.2 ng/ml. He was transferred to Vanderbilt for further management, but pulmonary nodules soon recurred and HCG serum level rose to 130 ng/ml. His pulmonary
nodules again responded to treatment with cisplatin, bleomycin, and etoposide
(VP-16), but HCG levels remained elevated at 45 ng/ml. His neurologic symptoms
recurred four months later, and he was found to have progressive brain metastases.
He died shortly thereafter and an autopsy was not permitted. Immunoperoxidase
staining for HCG staining was positive in the cytoplasm of tumor cells from the
original metastatic brain lesion.

The highly responsive tumors in these two young men stimulated our
interest in patients with poorly differentiated carcinomas, and suggested
the possibility that some of these patients may have had either atypical
extragonadal germ cell neoplasms or another responsive, but unknown
type of neoplasm. Beginning in 1976, the Vanderbilt group began to
consider the diagnosis of atypical germ cell neoplasm or another responsive tumor of unknown type in all young men with poorly differentiated or
undifferentiated carcinomas. In 1981, the same group reported successful

treatment of 12 patients with poorly differentiated carcinomas of unknown primary.[3] Eleven patients were treated with chemotherapy effective in the treatment of germinal tumors, and one received radiotherapy following the excision of a mediastinal tumor. All patients responded to therapy, and seven of 12 had complete remissions. Although two of these seven patients subsequently relapsed, five patients are currently disease-free, and are considered cured of their malignancy. Two of these 12 patients were later recognized to have metastatic testicular neoplasms, but no primary sites were identified in the other ten patients. Fox et al. have also reported five patients with "undifferentiated" carcinoma whose clinical findings and responses to systemic chemotherapy were suggestive of germinal tumors.[4]

These observations strengthened the hypothesis of the Vanderbilt group that these tumors may have been histologically atypical extragonadal germ cell neoplasms or another unrecognized tumor type with similar clinical and biologic features. Based on these initial observations, this group defined several criteria of potential utility in identifying a subset of patients with poorly differentiated carcinomas likely to respond to systemic chemotherapy. These features included

1. Patients under the age of 50 years (particularly men)
2. A tumor involving primarily midline structures, (i.e., mediastinum, retroperitoneum), lungs (in the form of multiple pulmonary nodules), or lymph nodes
3. Elevated serum levels of HCG or alpha-fetoprotein
4. HCG or alpha-fetoprotein demonstrated in tumor cells by immunocytochemical methods
5. Clinical evidence of rapid tumor growth
6. A tumor very responsive to previously administered chemotherapy or radiotherapy.

This constellation of clinical features was termed the "extragonadal germ cell cancer syndrome."

In order to better define the utility of these clinical features in identifying patients with poorly differentiated carcinomas responsive to systemic chemotherapy, we have continued to consider all patients with poorly differentiated carcinomas of unknown primary site for intensive treatment with chemotherapeutic agents proven effective in germinal tumors. Patients with poorly differentiated carcinoma who have one or more features of the extragonadal germ cell cancer syndrome (defined above) have been treated with cisplatin, vinblastine, and bleomycin (PVB). In this chapter, we outline the clinical characteristics, pathologic features, and response to treatment of the first 40 patients with this syndrome treated at Vanderbilt University Medical Center.

Patients and Methods

Forty patients seen at Vanderbilt Medical Center between 1976 and 1982 are reported here. All patients had either poorly differentiated carcinoma or pooly differentiated adenocarcinoma of unknown primary site. In addition, each patient had one or more features of the extragonadal germ cell cancer syndrome. Patients with well-differentiated adenocarcinomas of unknown primary site were not included in this patient group.

Serum levels of HCG and alpha-fetoprotein were measured by radio-immunoassay. When tissue was available, detailed pathologic evaluation including cytochemical staining and electron microscopy was performed. In addition, immunoperoxidase staining for HCG and alpha-fetoprotein using a modification of the Sternberger technique[5] was performed.

Because of the great variability in clinical presentations, diagnostic and staging procedures were not uniform in these patients. All patients, however, were evaluated with routine laboratory studies (hemogram, electrolytes, SMA-12, and chest roentgenogram). Additional radiologic evaluation was dependent on clinical presentation; most of the patients seen since 1978 had computerized tomography of the chest and/or the abdomen.

During the first two years when we were recognizing and defining this syndrome, patients were not treated in a standard fashion. In 1979, however, we began to treat all patients with combination chemotherapy known to be effective against germinal tumors. Twenty-six patients received cisplatin, vinblastine, and bleomycin (PVB) as described by Einhorn,[6] but with a total dose of vinblastine of 0.3 mg/kg per course. Six others received an adriamycin containing modification of this regimen.[7] Three patients received other cisplatin-containing regimens (cyclophosphamide/adriamycin/cisplatin (CAP), two; VAB III, one), while three patients received other chemotherapeutic regimens (cyclophosphamide/adriamycin/vincristine/prednisone (CHOP), two; vinblastine/bleomycin, one). Two patients were treated with surgical resection and radiotherapy, and received no chemotherapy.

Following three or four cycles of chemotherapy, complete restaging was performed. Response to treatment was defined using standard definitions. A complete response required normal physical examination,

Table 8-1
Sites of Tumor Involvement

Location	Number of Patients
Mediastinum	17
Retroperitoneum	8
Other lymph node areas	19
Lung	12
Pleura	5
Bone	4
Brain	3
Liver	2
Subcutaneous mass	2
Skin	1
Pericardium	1
Adrenal	1
Jejunum	1

radiographic studies, and laboratory parameters, including serum HCG and alpha-fetoprotein levels. Partial response required at least a 50 percent reduction in tumor measurements. Patients with tumor shrinkage of less than 50 percent, those with stable disease, and those with progressive disease are grouped together as nonresponders.

Results

Clinical Characteristics

Our series included 35 men and 5 women, with ages ranging from 18 to 61 years (median 36 years). Thirty-two of 40 patients (80 percent) had tumor involvement at more than one location at diagnosis. Seventeen patients had mediastinal masses, and eight had retroperitoneal masses; however, only four patients had tumor confined to these areas. Other lymph node areas were involved in 19 patients, but only three patients had tumor involving only lymph nodes. Lung involvement was also common (12 patients); six patients had single lung masses, three had multiple pulmonary nodules, and three had lung involvement from local extension of tumor. Multiple other metastatic sites were observed less frequently, as summarized in Table 8-1.

Pretreatment serum levels of HCG and alpha-fetoprotein were measured by radioimmunoassay in 35 of 40 patients. Five patients (14 percent) had elevated serum levels of HCG, while four patients (11 percent) had

Table 8-2
Initial Light Microscopic Diagnoses (40 Patients)

Diagnosis	Number of Patients
Poorly differentiated carcinoma	20 (50%)
Poorly differentiated adenocarcinoma	11 (28%)
Poorly differentiated large cell carcinoma	9 (22%)

elevated alpha-fetoprotein levels. One patient had elevated levels of both markers. Two of the patients with elevated tumor marker levels were later recognized to have germinal tumors (see below). Thirty-two of 40 patients (80 percent) had normal serum levels of both HCG and alpha-fetoprotein.

Two of our patients later developed testicular masses, and at rebiopsy and reexamination of the original pathologic material were recognized to have testicular neoplasms. In none of the other patients did the primary site become obvious during the clinical course.

Pathology

Biopsy specimens were examined using light microscopy in all patients. Cytology specimens alone were not considered adequate for diagnosis in these patients; many patients had material available for examination from more than one metastatic site. The initial light microscopic diagnoses in our 40 patients were either poorly differentiated carcinoma, poorly differentiated adenocarcinoma, or poorly differentiated large cell carcinoma, as shown in Table 8-2. In two patients with poorly differentiated carcinoma, the diagnosis of malignant melanoma was "favored"; germ cell tumor was "favored" in one patient with poorly differentiated adenocarcinoma.

Ten patients were later assigned more specific diagnoses, usually following pathologic examination of additional biopsy material. These diagnoses are summarized in Table 8-3. Two previously mentioned patients developed testicular masses, and reexamination of all pathologic material made it clear that they had metastatic testicular germinal neoplasms. These two patients are included in this series only to illustrate the difficulty which is sometimes encountered with histologic diagnosis in this clinical setting; they are not included in the analysis of treatment results. Three other patients later had a diagnosis of extragonadal germ cell tumor made after reexamination of initial slides and examination of subsequent biopsy specimens. The single patient who had a poorly differentiated

Table 8-3
Final Diagnoses in 40 Patients

Diagnosis*	Number of Patients
Poorly differentiated carcinoma or adenocarcinoma (diagnosis unchanged)	30
Testicular germinal neoplasm (testicular mass developed)	2
Extragonadal germinal neoplasm (repeat biopsy, reexamination of slides)	3
Lymphoma (electron microscopy)	1
Adenocarcinoma, lung (repeat biopsy 1, autopsy 1)	2
Adenocarcinoma, pancreas (autopsy)	1
Carcinoid tumor, lung (autopsy)	1

* Method of specific diagnosis indicated in parentheses

adenocarcinoma, "favor germ cell tumor," was later thought to have a "papillary adenocarcinoma of the lung" after thoracotomy was done for a removal of a lung mass. Three patients were reclassified on the basis of autopsy results as shown in Table 8-3.

Electron microscopy was performed on biopsy specimens from 12 patients. One patient was found to have a large transformed cell lymphoma on the basis of electron microscopic findings. No specific diagnoses could be made, however, in the other 11 patients. Two patients had ultrastructural features of poorly differentiated adenocarcinoma, and one had findings consistent with a neuroendocrine tumor, but no specific diagnoses could be assigned. Eight patients were considered to have poorly differentiated carcinomas, even after electron microscopy was performed.

In summary, 30 patients had poorly differentiated tumors which could not be classified further in spite of the frequent use of electron microscopy and the examination of multiple biopsies in many patients.

Response to Therapy and Survival

Thirty-seven patients received at least two courses of chemotherapy, and were evaluable for response to therapy. Both patients with testicular neoplasms had complete responses to therapy, but are excluded from analysis. In addition, the single patient with malignant lymphoma was treated appropriately for that diagnosis, and is also excluded.

Fourteen patients (38 percent) had complete responses to therapy, 14 (38 percent) had partial responses, and 9 (24 percent) had no response. After exclusion of patients with a subsequent specific diagnosis, the response rates are, complete response, 12 (40 percent); partial response, 10 (33 percent); no response, 8 (27 percent).

Patients who had no response or partial response to therapy did very poorly. All patients in this group are dead. The median survival was six months following diagnosis of malignancy, and only five of 23 patients survived longer than one year after diagnosis.

In contrast, patients achieving complete remissions with therapy have done very well. Nine of 14 patients who achieved complete remission remain continuously disease-free two to eight years following completion of treatment. Five patients relapsed and died 5–23 months (median 17 months) following diagnosis.

The case histories of four representative patients are now presented in detail to better illustrate this syndrome.

Patient Reports

Patient 1

This 56-year-old man developed rapidly enlarging cervical and supraclavicular lymph nodes in August of 1980. Physical examination was otherwise normal. Cervical lymph node biopsy showed poorly differentiated carcinoma. An abdominal CT scan revealed bilateral adrenal masses, large periaortic masses, left hydronephrosis, and left ureteral obstruction. He was initially treated with radiotherapy to his neck and experienced complete resolution of his large cervical lymph nodes. Serum HCG and alpha-fetoprotein levels were normal. During radiotherapy, he developed increasing abdominal pain; repeat abdominal CT scan revealed massive retroperitoneal disease, and a new right pleural effusion. He was treated with four cycles of PVB, and had complete resolution of all his abdominal disease except for a small mass in the area of his right adrenal. In February of 1981, he underwent an exploratory laparotomy, and no evidence of disease was found in his abdomen or retroperitoneum. He received no further chemotherapy, and did well until October of 1981 when he became confused and ataxic. A CT scan of his brain showed metastatic disease in both cerebral hemispheres, particularly around the ventricles. CT scans of his chest and abdomen were normal; serum alpha-fetoprotein and HCG levels also remained normal. He received radiotherapy to his whole brain, and repeat CT scan of the brain after 2000 rads showed complete resolution of his brain metastases. He developed leg weakness, however, and lumbar puncture revealed the presence of malignant cells on cytologic examination. He was treated with craniospinal irradiation and intrathecal methotrexate, but responded poorly. A rapidly enlarging left cervical mass appeared after his CNS involvement had become severe. He died in January of 1982, 17 months after the diagnosis of the malignancy.

Electron microscopy of his original tumor showed a carcinoma with desmosomes and occasional cells with microvilli consistent with an adenocarcinoma. Immunoperoxidase stains revealed focal staining for both HCG and alpha-fetoprotein.

Patient 2

This 27-year-old man developed a rapidly enlarging left neck mass in January of 1982. He was otherwise asymptomatic, and physical examination was normal except for a 4 cm painless left cervical mass at the angle of his mandible. Biopsy of this mass showed a poorly differentiated carcinoma, "favor nasopharyngeal, melanoma, or poorly differentiated squamous." The following staging procedures were normal: chest roentgenogram, chest and abdominal CT scans, CT scan of the brain and paranasal sinuses, thyroid scan, upper GI series, intravenous pyelogram, direct and indirect laryngoscopy, and nasopharyngeal examination with blind nasopharyngeal biopsies. Serum levels of HCG and alpha-fetoprotein were normal. He received three cycles of PVB + adriamycin, with complete resolution of his left cervical mass. He completed therapy in April 1982, and has now been continuously disease-free for 27 months.

Electron microscopy performed on his original biopsy revealed numerous desmosomes, tonofilaments, neurosecretory granules, and microtubules felt to be compatible with a neuroendocrine tumor.

Patient 3

This 31-year-old man was seen at Vanderbilt University Medical Center with a three-month history of increasing productive cough. He had smoked one pack of cigarettes per day for 12 years. Physical examination was entirely normal, but a chest roentgenogram revealed left hilar and mediastinal masses. Computed tomography of the chest confirmed the presence of a 6×4 cm anterosuperior mediastinal mass, extending into the left hilar region. Screening chemistries revealed LDH 409 IU/ml, SGOT 53 IU/ml, and all other tests normal. Serum levels of HCG and alpha-fetoprotein were normal. Computed tomography of the abdomen showed a single lesion in the right lobe of the liver compatible with a metastasis. Radionuclide scans of the bones and liver were normal. CT scan of the head was also normal. A thoracotomy was performed, which revealed a large mediastinal mass and several left pleural implants. Biopsy of both the mediastinal mass and the pleural implants revealed a poorly differentiated carcinoma. In March of 1981, he began chemotherapy with PVB and received four cycles of this treatment. A follow-up CT scan of his chest in May of 1981 showed only slight decrease in the size of his mediastinal mass. He was given further chemotherapy with cyclophosphamide, adriamycin, DTIC, and vincristine, to which he had no response. He experienced tumor progression and died in August of 1981, five months after the diagnosis of his malignancy.

Electron microscopy of the initial biopsies showed infrequent desmosomes, microfilaments, and occasional granules "suggestive of stage II melanosomes." The official electron microscopic interpretation was "poorly differentiated carcinoma, favor malignant melanoma." Autopsy was performed, and revealed tumor involvement of the superior and middle mediastinum, pericardium, pleura, liver, adrenals, and periaortic lymph nodes. Pathologic evaluation (including electron microscopy) of autopsy material revealed poorly differentiated carcinoma, with no distinguishing features to allow a more specific diagnosis.

Patient 4

This 19-year-old woman was referred to Vanderbilt University Medical Center in January of 1980 for evaluation of inguinal adenopathy. She had developed severe back pain in November 1979, and was seen at a hospital in Louisiana. Physical examination was normal. An intravenous pyelogram showed right ureteral compression and partial right hydronephrosis. Computerized tomography of the abdomen showed retroperitoneal masses. An exploratory laparotomy was performed, and a large retroperitoneal tumor mass was found. The remainder of the abdominal cavity including the liver and ovaries was normal. Biopsies of the retroperitoneal mass showed a high-grade anaplastic undifferentiated carcinoma. She was treated with radiotherapy, to a dose of 4000 rads over five weeks to her retroperitoneal area. She had resolution of her back pain, but within six weeks noted the rapid appearance of a left inguinal mass.

When first evaluated at Vanderbilt, physical examination showed a 3×3 cm left inguinal lymph node. CT scan of the abdomen revealed a large tumor mass in the retroperitoneum, which extended superiorly to involve the periaortic lymph nodes. Chest roentgenogram was normal. Biopsy of the left inguinal lymph node again revealed an undifferentiated carcinoma. The large neoplastic cells did not type as T or B lymphocytes. Serum levels of HCG and alpha-fetoprotein were normal. She was treated with four courses of PVB. After one course, repeat CT scan of her abdomen was normal. A follow-up CT scan in December of 1980 again showed no evidence of retroperitoneal tumor. She remains continuously disease-free 44 months after completion of therapy.

Electron microscopy performed on the left inguinal node biopsy showed large neoplastic cells with hemidesmosome structures, with no other distinguishing features. The electron microscopic diagnosis was "poorly differentiated carcinoma." Immunoperoxidase staining tumor cells for alpha-fetoprotein cells was negative, and HCG staining revealed faint, focal areas of staining.

Discussion

The patient with advanced poorly differentiated carcinoma of unknown primary site presents a difficult clinical problem, and no concensus exists regarding the optimal treatment approach. Clinical oncologists understand the importance of identifying treatable neoplasms such as lymphoma, sarcoma, breast carcinoma, ovarian carcinoma, and prostatic carcinoma, in patients with poorly differentiated neoplasms. Empiric treatment is often administered if one of these treatable types of tumors is suspected.

Extragonadal germinal neoplasms are now recognized to be extremely responsive to chemotherapy. Treatment with intensive cisplatin-containing regimens effective against testicular germinal neoplasms has produced cure rates as high as 64 percent.[8] It is also well-known that metastatic germinal neoplasms can often appear as undifferentiated tumors by light microscopy, and that diagnosis of these tumors can at times be extremely difficult for the pathologist. Based on these observations, and also on our early clinical experience, we postulated that some patients with poorly differentiated carcinomas of unknown primary site may have unrecognized extragonadal germinal tumors. In defining the "extragonadal germ cell tumor syndrome," we have identified several clinical features of potential utility in identifying patients with responsive tumors, so that appropriate intensive chemotherapy can be administered.

The results reported here on the treatment of 40 patients with poorly differentiated carcinomas confirm the fact that some patients in this group have tumors which are extremely responsive to chemotherapy. In this group of patients, who all had advanced tumors at the time of diagnosis, a 38 percent complete response rate was achieved. More impressive is the fact that nine patients (24 percent) have remained in continuous complete remission following the completion of treatment. All of these patients have been followed for more than two years after completing treatment, and are considered extremely unlikely to relapse.

The original hypothesis that some patients with poorly differentiated carcinomas may have extragonadal germinal tumors is borne out by the experience reported here. Three patients in this series were later recognized histologically to have germinal tumors, based on examination of repeat biopsies and reexamination of original specimens. Two additional patients developed testicular masses later in their course, and were at that time recognized to have metastatic testicular cancer. The clinical features of other patients who had complete remissions to therapy, however, were not particularly consistent with the recognized clinical behavior of extragonadal germinal tumors. Three patients who had complete responses (including patient 4 described earlier) were women, a group in which extragonadal germinal tumors have been rarely reported. Patient 1 not only was older than most patients with germinal tumors, but also had tumor in atypical locations (cervical lymph nodes, bilateral adrenal masses). Several other complete responders to therapy also had tumor in atypical locations (cervical mass, one patient; axillary mass, two patients; multiple bone metastases, one patient). If these patients indeed had extragonadal germinal tumors, recognition based on clinical features would have been extremely difficult. We have not discounted the possibility, however, that some of these patients have a heretofore unrecognized type of carcinoma.

Conversely, some patients who had clinical features suggestive of extragonadal germinal tumors failed to respond to treatment. Patient 3 is an example. This 31-year-old presented with a large mediastinal mass and had a biopsy which revealed poorly differentiated carcinoma; however, intensive therapy with PVB produced only a minimal response, and he survived only five months. Even at autopsy, no primary tumor site was found, and no more specific diagnosis could be made.

The role of specialized pathologic methods (i.e., electron microscopy, immunocytochemical staining) in better defining this group of patients is unclear at present. Electron microscopy is quite reliable in distinguishing undifferentiated lymphoma from carcinoma, and should be used for this purpose. In our series, one patient was proven to have a transformed cell lymphoma but only after electron microscopy was performed. In the relatively small number of other patients who had electron microscopy, no specific diagnoses were made which were clinically helpful. The significance of a diagnosis of "adenocarcinoma" or "neuroendocrine tumor" by electron microscopy is undetermined; some patients with these electron microscopic "diagnoses" had responsive tumors, and experienced long-term survivals following chemotherapy. The role of immunoperoxidase staining for HCG and alpha-fetoprotein is also unclear. Some patients with normal serum levels of these markers had tumors which contained HCG and/or alpha-fetoprotein; we have not completed our analysis of this pathologic feature, and do not know yet whether it will be a predictor of responsiveness to chemotherapy.

It is clear that the patients in this series had a wide variety of tumor types. Ten patients actually had other diagnoses made at some time during their course, either with repeat biopsy or at autopsy. Since we only required one feature of the extragonadal germ cell cancer syndrome to be present for inclusion in this series, the diversity of patients is not surprising.

The demonstration that some advanced poorly differentiated carcinomas are responsive to chemotherapy is only an initial step in understanding these tumors. Although they are probably quite rare, the incidence of these tumors is unknown. Clinical and/or pathologic features which are predictive of chemotherapy responsiveness remain to be defined. Many questions remain on a more basic level. Are these responsive tumors actually germinal tumors which are unrecognizable by pathologic and often by clinical criteria? Do some of these patients have a different, previously unrecognized tumor type? Are occasional tumors of many sites, when poorly differentiated, responsive to intensive chemotherapy? Is there a relationship between HCG production by a neoplastic cell and its responsiveness to some forms of chemotherapy?

The answers to these questions would provide us with a better understanding of poorly differentiated carcinomas, and of tumor biology in general. Until these answers are available, the clinician should evaluate the patient with poorly differentiated carcinoma with special care. Pathologic examination of adequate biopsy material is essential; biopsies from multiple metastatic sites should be considered if technically feasible. Electron microscopy should be performed whenever possible, to help identify undifferentiated lymphomas. Serum levels of HCG and alpha-fetoprotein should be measured in all patients with poorly differentiated carcinoma. If lymphoma can be ruled out, intensive chemotherapy treatment with regimens effective in the treatment of germinal tumors should be seriously considered in these patients.

Acknowledgments

Supported in part by grants CA 27333-01 and CA 19429 from the National Cancer Institute.

References

1. Moertel CG, Reitemeier RJ, Schull AJ, et al: Treatment of the patient with adenocarcinoma of unknown origin. Cancer 30:1469–1472, 1972
2. Woods RL, Fox RM, Tattersall MHN, et al: Metastatic adenocarcinomas of unknown primary site: A randomized study of two combination-chemotherapy regimens. N Engl J Med 303:87–89, 1980
3. Richardson RL, Schoumacher RA, Fer MF, et al: The unrecognized extragonadal germ cell cancer syndrome. Ann Intern Med 94:181–186, 1981
4. Fox RM, Woods RL, Tattersall MHN: Undifferentiated carcinoma in young men: The atypical teratoma syndrome. Lancet 1:1316–1318, 1979
5. Sternberger LA: Immunocytochemistry (ed 2). New York, Wiley, 1979, pp 104–169
6. Einhorn LH, Donohue J: cis-Diamminedichloroplatinum, vinblastine,

and bleomycin combination chemotherapy in disseminated testicular cancer. Ann Intern Med 87:293–298, 1977

7. Einhorn LH, Williams SD: Chemotherapy of disseminated testicular cancer: A random prospective study. Cancer 46:1339–1344, 1980

8. Hainsworth JD, Einhorn LH, Williams SD, et al: Advanced extragonadal germ-cell tumors: Successful treatment with combination chemotherapy. Ann Intern Med 97:7–11, 1982

9

THE EXTRAGONADAL GERM CELL CANCER SYNDROME: THE MAYO CLINIC EXPERIENCE

Allan Jones
George Farrow
Ronald L. Richardson

Poorly differentiated carcinomas, including poorly differentiated large cell and adenocarcinomas, are a histologically heterogeneous collection of malignant epithelial tumors whose common clinical features have been poor response to therapy and dismal prognosis.[1,2] Because of the bleak prospect of response to treatment, clinicians have traditionally approached these patients with pessimism, often using therapies with modest toxicity, but little chance of producing meaningful response. However, recent reports[3-6] have provided increasing impetus to subdivide or further define subsets in this heterogeneous group of neoplasms. Aggressive cisplatin-based chemotherapy programs have been recommended for young cancer patients presenting with advanced disease occurring in a midline anatomic distribution associated with or without elevated serum levels of the beta subunit of human chorionic gonadotropin (β-HCG) and or alpha-fetoprotein (AFP). Proponents of these intensive programs have emphasized that this subset of undifferentiated cancers may contain either extragonadal germ cell elements or may behave biologically like a germinal

POORLY DIFFERENTIATED NEOPLASMS AND TUMORS OF UNKNOWN ORIGIN   ISBN 0-8089-1755-2
© 1986 by Grune & Stratton.   All rights of reproduction in any form reserved.

tumor. Therefore, these patients may not only be treatable but may also be curable by chemotherapy. Some authors[4] have recommended a trial of chemotherapy designed for germ cell malignancies for any patient who exhibits at least one element of the syndrome.

Since the diagnosis of this syndrome is based primarily on clinical grounds, less emphasis has been placed on the histopathologic features of this heterogeneous group of poorly differentiated malignancies. Furthermore, no retrospective analyses of pathologic features of these tumors and the response to treatment of these patients have been offered in previously reported series to allow an assessment of pathologic classification in this clinical syndrome. Because these chemotherapy regimens are associated with significant toxicity (intense nausea, vomiting, nephrotoxicity, pulmonary fibrosis, ototoxicity, neurotoxicity, myelosuppression, electrolyte imbalance, etc.) we wished to assess whether a clinical or pathologic classification of good and poor prognosis patients with this syndrome greatly differed, and if so which classification may be the more predictive of response.

Materials and Methods

Between May 1979 and February 1983, 35 patients with clinical findings compatible with the extragonadal germ cell cancer syndrome were evaluated by several medical oncologists at the Mayo Clinic. Our definition of this syndrome included patients with poorly differentiated carcinomas of unknown primary site, as diagnosed at the time of initial review at the Mayo Clinic, presenting with three or more of the following characteristics: (1) age less than 50 years; (2) advanced disease in the midline distribution (mediastinum or retroperitoneum), multiple pulmonary nodules or lymphadenopathy; (3) elevated serum levels of β-HCG or AFP; (4) clinical evidence of rapid tumor growth; (5) normal testicular or pelvic examination. Because it is likely that not all patients potentially fitting this syndrome were referred to us, these data cannot be interpreted as reflecting the frequency of this disorder at the Mayo Clinic over this time period. Based on clinical findings, 34 of the patients were treated aggressively with cytotoxic chemotherapy; one patient died prior to initiation of therapy. Twenty-six patients received a standard germ cell chemotherapy regimen consisting of vinblastine, bleomycin, cisplatin (VBP);[7] cyclophosphamide, vinblastine, dactinomycin D, bleomycin, cisplatin (VAB III),[8] or etoposide, bleomycin, continuous infusion cisplatin (BECIP).[9] Seven patients received a cisplatin-containing regimen consisting of cyclophosphamide, doxorubicin, and cisplatin (CAP)[10] or mitomycin C, doxorubicin, and cisplatin (MAP).[11] One patient received cyclophosphamide, doxorubicin, vincristine, and prednisone (CHOP).[12]

Response to therapy was determined by physical examination, serial assays of serum tumor markers, and appropriate radiologic studies. After three to four cycles of chemotherapy, patients underwent a complete reevaluation including repetition of previously abnormal roentgenograms and determination of β-HCG and α-fetoprotein levels if these were abnormal prior to therapy. Criteria for complete remission included the complete disappearance of all evidence of tumor and the normalization of serum tumor markers. Partial remission was defined as an objective decrease in tumor size of greater than 50 percent but failure to meet the criteria for complete remission.

Results

In keeping with the clinical criteria for the diagnosis of the extragonadal germ cell cancer syndrome, all 35 patients had tumor in a midline distribution (e.g., retroperitoneal, mediastinal, or supraclavicular lymph nodes) or had multiple pulmonary nodules, and all had demonstrated rapidly progressive disease. All patients had normal testicular or pelvic examinations prior to treatment. As might be predicted, there was a male predominance with men comprising 29 of the 35 patients. The median age was 38 years with a range of 20 to 67 years. Only four patients were older than 50 years of age. The oldest patient in this series, a 67-year-old man, is the only patient who was not treated with antineoplastic therapy. This patient sought medical attention because of a one-month history of progressive dyspnea. He was noted to have bilateral alveolar and reticulonodular infiltrates on chest x-ray. An open lung biopsy was interpreted as showing large cell carcinoma. Shortly after this his respiratory status deteriorated and he required mechanical ventilatory assistance. He died of progressive pulmonary failure a few days later. At postmortem examination he was found to have disseminated choriocarcinoma with the primary lesion located in the anterior mediastinum and with widespread metastatic disease involving the brain, liver, kidneys, lungs, and heart; the testes were not involved. Serum drawn shortly after admission showed a β-HCG level of 35,000 IU/L, and the lung biopsy specimen subsequently was found to stain strongly positive for β-HCG using immunoperoxidase technique. Despite the fact that this patient was not treated with chemotherapy, we have included him in this series because his rapid, catastrophic clinical course illustrates the aggressive potential of these neo-plasms and because he demonstrates that the extragonadal germ cell cancer syndrome can be found in patients greater than 50 years of age.

Thirty-four patients were treated with multiple agent chemotherapy regimens with 18 obtaining a complete response (53 percent) and three obtaining a partial response for an overall response rate of 62 percent. Thirteen patients had no response to treatment. Half of the 34 treated patients remain alive with survivals of 14 to 60 months and with 70 percent of these patients having no evidence of disease and requiring no chemo-therapy. Half of the patients have died, with 76 percent dying within a year of diagnosis.

Clinical Classification of Good and Poor Prognosis Patients

Retrospective analysis of the clinical characteristics and responses to treatment of these 34 patients allowed segregation into two groups based on biologic behavior, tumor markers, initial pathologic diagnosis, and response to therapy. Those patients whose clinical characteristics and therapeutic responses suggested cancers resembling the usual germ cell malignancies comprised the "typical" group while those whose character-istics and responses were considered less likely to be seen in germ cell cancers formed the "atypical" group.

The "typical" group consisted of 14 patients, 11 males and one female, whose ages ranged from 20 to 44 years with a median age of 27 years. β-HCG or AFP or both markers were elevated in the sera of 11 of the 14 patients. Twelve patients (86 percent) responded to treatment with 11 (79 percent) obtaining a complete response; two patients had no response to therapy. Twelve patients are alive with nine patients off therapy and free of disease 14 to 46 months after diagnosis. Two patients died at seven and 19 months and three continue to receive treatment 32, 49, and 60 months after diagnosis. Median survival for these 14 patients has not been reached.

The "atypical" group was comprised of 20 patients, 14 males and six females, whose ages ranged from 20 to 56 years with a median age of 40 years. Two patients had markedly elevated serum AFP levels (1600 and 3600 ng/ml; normal less than 15 ng/ml) and two patients had minimal elevation of serum β-HCG (3.6 and 5.0 IU/L; normal less than 2.0). Twelve patients had normal serum levels of these substances, and four patients did not have serum levels measured. Nine of the 20 patients (45 percent) responded to treatment with complete responses in six patients (30 percent) and partial responses in three patients.

Histopathologic Classification

The diagnostic pathologic specimens of the 34 treated patients were reviewed without knowledge of the clinical histories, results of serum assays for β-HCG or AFP, or responses to chemotherapy. This review was performed for the purposes of this study, after an initial diagnosis of a poorly differentiated carcinoma was made at the Mayo Clinic. Histopathologic criteria for the diagnosis of germ neoplasms are not absolute and hence our division of cases into three categories reflected one group of uncertain histogenesis. With the exception of typical seminoma and choriocarcinoma with unique histopathologic features which permit certain classification, the diagnosis of poorly differentiated germ cell neoplasms, i.e., embryonal carcinoma, may be based as much on features which the neoplasm lacks as those it possesses. In the embryonal carcinomas (Fig. 9-1) there is an absence of differentiated structures, although the neoplasms may resemble adenocarcinomas. The presence of mucus-containing cells would tend to exclude embryonal carcinoma. In the usual more solid type tumors the cells have an epithelial appearance and are often large with polyhedral shape. Elaboration of specialized proteins such as keratin is not a feature of embryonal carcinoma.

Immunohistochemical markers for specific substances such as AFP and β-HCG may be helpful in identifying germ cell neoplasms. AFP is useful in identifying germ cell neoplasms of the embryonal type (Fig. 9-2) particularly when there is an element of yoke sac tumor. β-HCG is present in large stainable quantities in trophoblastic cells of choriocarcinoma (Fig. 9-3) and in smaller quanitities in the tumor syncytial giant cells of some seminomas. Histochemical results do not always correlate well with the levels of these substances circulating in the blood or present in other body fluids. Immunoperoxidase stains for β-IICG and AFP were performed on slides from paraffin-embedded tissue specimens of 32 of the 34 patients.

Based on the above morphologic criteria, patients were categorized into three groups: group 1, high probability of germ cell cancer (Table 9-1); group 2, intermediate probability of germ cell cancer (Table 9-2); and group 3, low probability of germ cell cancer (Table 9-3). The eight patients in group 1 (high probability) had neoplasms with features characteristic of germ cell malignancies. Seven of the eight responded to treatment and remain alive from 27 to 60 months after diagnosis; five of these patients remain free of disease though two continue to receive treatment for disease in relapse at 32 and 60 months. One patient did not respond to treatment and died seven months after diagnosis.

The 12 patients in group 2 (intermediate probability) had malignancies

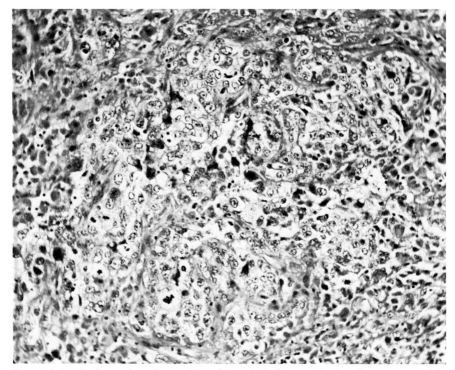

Figure 9-1. *Embryonal carcinoma. H and E × 160. The neoplastic cells are arranged in solid sheets without differentiation.*

with some histologic features compatible with germ cell cancers. Ten of the 12 responded to chemotherapy, but five have died of progressive disease. Seven remain alive 14 to 49 months after diagnosis, and five of these appear to be free of disease.

The 14 patients in group 3 (lower probability) had poorly differentiated tumors with little resemblance to germ cell cancers. Only four patients in this group responded to chemotherapy. These four survived for more than 18 months though only two remain clinically disease-free. Eleven patients have died, and the median survival for the patients in the low probability group is ten months.

Combining groups 1 and 2 (high and intermediate probabilities) and comparing the aggregate with the low probability group 3 patients provides a measure of the importance of differential histologic diagnosis in separating those patients with possible germ cell cancers from those whose

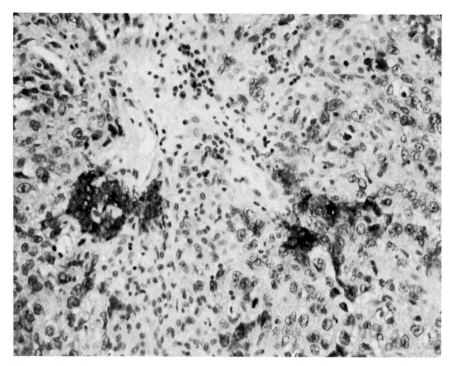

Figure 9-2. *Embryonal carcinoma. Immunoperoxidase × 250. The same case as Figure 9-1 stained for alpha-fetoprotein revealing the germ cell nature of an otherwise undifferentiated neoplasm.*

malignancies have few characteristics of germ cell cancers. By this classification the 20 patients in groups 1 and 2 have a response rate of 85 percent with 10 patients (50 percent) alive and free of disease; only 6 patients have died and median survival exceeds 27 months. In contrast, the 14 patients in group 3 had a response rate of 28 percent with only 2 patients (15 percent) alive without evidence of disease; 11 have died and the median survival for the group was 10 months. More importantly, combining the high and intermediate probability groups captured all of the clinically "typical" patients and nearly all of the long-term survivors. Only two of the low probability group appear to be disease-free; one patient had a remarkable response to chemotherapy for a pulmonary carcinosarcoma; the other patient had a malignancy involving mediastinal nodes that may be a thyroid carcinoma, a neoplasm that often follows a relatively indolent

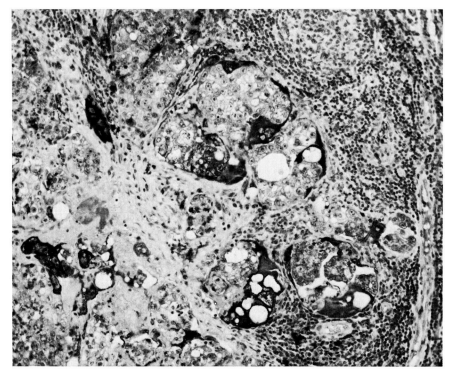

Figure 9-3.   *Choriocarcinoma. β-HCG immunoperoxidase stain. The darkly stained large multinucleated cells represent syncytiotrophoblasts.*

course. Careful histopathologic interpretation of adequate tissue specimens with recognition of the variable appearances of germ cell cancers thus appears to be an accurate indicator of prognosis in these patients.

Conclusion

Patients with poorly differentiated or undifferentiated carcinomas of uncertain etiology in a midline anatomic distribution are frequent problems for clinical oncologists and pathologists alike. Certainly some patients in this diverse group have tumors which may be very responsive to chemotherapy or radiotherapy and may resemble germ cell malignancies in their clinical behavior. Because of the potential for improved survival or even cure with appropriate treatment of these patients, it is important for both

Table 9-1
High Probability Germ Cell Origin

No.	Age	Sex	Disease Distribution	Markers Serum AFP	Serum β-HCG	Tissue AFP	Tissue β-HCG	Response	Survival	Final Pathology	Clinical Classification
1	21	M	Mediastinum; lungs	−	16,000	−	+	NR	7 Mo	Chorio- and Embryonal Carcinoma	T
2	43	M	Cervical, retroperitoneal nodes	−	−	−	−	CR	24 + Mo NED	Seminoma	T
3	41	M	Lungs, retroperitoneal, bilateral undescended testes	−	26	−	−	CR	27 + Mo NED	Seminoma	T
4	21	M	Mediastinum	96	150	−	−	PR	32 + Mo Act Dis	Ant Mediast Teratoma/ Embryonal Ca	T
5	26	M	Supraclavicular nodes	−	−	−	−	CR	39 + Mo NED	Embryonal Ca	T
6	20	M	Lumbar, epidural mass with cord compression, retroperitoneal nodes	−	−	−	−	CR	41 + Mo NED	Embryonal Ca	T
7	24	M	Mediastinum with caval obstruction; lung; pleura; bones	−	13.7	−	−	PR	60 + Mo Act Dis	Seminoma	T
8	44	M	Cervical, retroperitoneal nodes	−	33,000	+	+	CR	42 + Mo NED	Chorio- and Embryonal Carcinoma	T

NR: No response; PR: Partial Response; CR: Complete Response; T: "Typical" Group; A: "Atypical" Group

Table 9-2
Intermediate Probability Germ Cell Origin

No.	Age	Sex	Disease Distribution	Markers				Response	Survival	Final Pathology	Clinical Classification
				Serum		Tissue					
				AFP	β-HCG	AFP	β-HCG				
9	56	M	Liver; retroperitoneum	3600	–	–	–	PR	6 Mo	Germ Cell vs Epithelial Ca	A
10	47	M	Mediastinal nodes; lung	–	–	–	–	NR	8 Mo	Germ Cell vs Undiff Ca	A
11	41	M	Lung; liver; bone	–	–	–	–	PR	9 Mo	Adeno[4] vs Germ Cell Ca	A
12	29	M	Cervical, retroperitoneal nodes; liver	–	85,000	–	–	CR	14+ Mo Act Dis	Undiff Ca vs Chorio Ca	T
13	20	M	Thoracic epidural mass; lung nodules	–	–	–	–	NR	17 Mo	Undiff Sarc vs Embryonal	A
14	24	M	Cervical, retroperitoneal nodes; lung; pleura	2500	38	–	–	PR	19 Mo	Undiff Ca vs Embryonal	T
15	43	M	Cervical mass	–	–	–	–	CR	27+ Mo NED	Undiff Ca vs Embryonal	A
16	36	M	Cervical, axillary, retroperitoneal nodes; lung; liver	300	1800	+	–	CR	29+ Mo NED	Undiff Ca vs Embryonal	T
17	25	M	Mediastinum; retroperitoneal nodes	–	–	–	–	CR	33+ Mo NED	Embryonal vs Large Cell Lymphoma	A
18	31	F	Retroperitoneal nodes	–	900	–	+	CR	39+ Mo NED	Undiff Ca vs Dysgerminoma	T
19	25	M	Retroperitoneal nodes; lung	3000	89	+	–	CR	46+ Mo NED	Undiff Ca vs Germ Cell ca	T
20	43	M	Cervical, mediastinal nodes	4000	–	–	–	PR	49+ Mo Act Dis	Undiff Ca vs Embryonal	T

Undiff Ca: Undifferentiated Carcinoma; Adeno[4]: Grade 4 Adenocarcinoma; Undiff Sarc: Undifferentiated Sarcoma; NR: No Response; PR: Partial Response; CR: Complete Response; T: "Typical" Group; A: "Atypical" Group

Table 9-3
Low Probability Germ Cell Origin

No.	Age	Sex	Disease Distribution	Markers				Response	Survival	Final Pathology	Clinical Classification
				Serum		Tissue					
				AFP	β-HCG	AFP	β-HCG				
21	40	F	Mediastinum; lung	–	–	–	–	NR	2 Mo	LGC[4]	A
22	33	M	Mediastinum Cervical nodes; lung	–	–	–	–	NR	3 Mo	Thymic Carcinoma	A
23	27	F	Sacral mass; Para-aortic nodes; lung	–				NR	4 Mo	Melanoma	A
24	40	M	Cervical, mediastinal nodes	–			+	NR	4 Mo	LGC[4]	A
25	32	M	Mediastinal nodes; lung	–	–	–	–	NR	5 Mo	LGC[4], Giant Cell Type	A
26	55	M	Posterior mediastinum, pleura, ribs	–	–	–	–	NR	6 Mo	LGC[4]	A
27	45	M	Cervical, mediastinal, retroperitoneal nodes	–				NR	9 Mo	LGC[4]	A
28	57	F	Cervical nodes; bones; skin	–	3.6			NR	10 Mo	Adeno[4] w/ Giant Cell	A
29	26	M	Retroperitoneum; liver	1600				NR	10 Mo	Spindle Sarcoma	A
30	39	M	Lung nodules; pleura	–				Stable	14 Mo	Adeno[4]	A
31	31	M	Bilat lung hilum	–				CR-Surg	37+ Mo NED	Adeno[3]	A
32	46	F	Lung nodule; pleura	–				CR-Surg	38+ Mo	Adeno[4]	A
33	48	M	Rt thigh mass; bilat pulm nodules 10 Mo later	–				PR	41+ Mo Act Dis	Sarcoma	A
34	38	F	Hilar lung node; lung	ND	ND	–	–	CR	48+ Mo NED	Carcinosarcoma	A

Adeno[3]: Grade 3 Adenocarcinoma; Adeno[4]: Grade 4 Adenocarcinoma; NED: No Evidence of Disease; NR: No Response; PR: Partial Response; CR: Complete Response; LGC[4]: Grade 4 Large Cell Carcinoma; A: "Atypical" Group clinicians and pathologists to be able to identify these patients. Moreover, because of the potential for improved survival or cure with treatment, it has been argued that all patients fitting the definition of the extragonadal germ cell cancer syndrome should be treated with a regimen active in treatment of advanced germ cell cancers. While we cannot argue against the importance of considering this syndrome in some patients with poorly differentiated or undifferentiated carcinomas and of making an accurate diagnosis, we believe that applying cisplatin-based germinal cancer regimens to all patients with such tumors in a midline distribution may be inappropriate, resulting in costly inpatient therapy which may be associated with significant risks and adverse side effects and with little likelihood of benefit.

How should the clinical oncologist approach such patients? What factors appear to be important in diagnosing the extragonadal germ cell cancer syndrome? We believe that an accurate and complete history and a careful physical examination are essential in determining the pace of the disease and its distribution as well as the possible primary neoplasms to be considered in the differential diagnosis. Appropriate radiographic studies, including computerized tomography of the abdomen or chest, and determination of serum β-HCG and AFP levels can provide strong supporting evidence for this syndrome. Ultrasound examination of the testes may demonstrate clinically occult primary tumors in some patients, suggesting the germinal origin of their neoplasms. However, we believe that the histopathologic diagnosis remains critical to the management of these patients. Our experience shows that segregating these patients into high and intermediate probability versus low probability groups on the basis of cellular morphology may be a practical way of classifying these patients, rather than subjecting all patients to therapeutic trials. Careful histologic interpretation by a pathologist aware of the varying appearances of germ cell cancers coupled with close communication of clinical information by an oncologist with a high index of suspicion can form a sound basis for diagnosis of the extragonadal germ cell cancer syndrome.

References

1. Moertel CG, Reitemeier RJ, Schutt AJ, et al: Treatment of the patient with adenocarcinoma of unknown origin. Cancer 30:1469–72, 1972
2. Barrie JR, Knoppe WH, Strong CW: Cervical nodal metastasis of unknown origin. Am J Surg 120:466–70, 1970
3. Richardson RL, Schoumacher RA, Fer MF, et al: The unrecognized

extragonadal germ cell cancer syndrome. Ann Int Med 94:181–186, 1981

4. Greco FA, Oldham RK, Fer MF: The extragonadal germ cell cancer syndrome. Sem Oncol 9:448–455, 1982

5. Hainsworth J, Fer M, Oldham RK, et al: Advanced poorly differentiated carcinoma and adenocarcinoma. Further documentation of a treatable syndrome. Proc Am Soc Clin Oncol 2:138, 1983

6. Hainsworth JD, Einhorn LH, Williams SD, et al: Advanced extragonadal germ cell tumors—successful treatment with combination chemotherapy. Ann Int Med 97:7–11, 1982

7. Einhorn LH, Donahue JD, Cis-diammine dichloroplatinum, vinblastine and bleomycin combination chemotherapy in disseminated testicular cancer. Ann Int Med 87:293–298, 1977

8. Vugrin D, Herr HW, Whitmore WF Jr, et al: VAB 6 combination chemotherapy in disseminated cancer of the testis. Ann Int Med 95:59–61, 1981

9. Richardson RL, Hahn RG, Kvols LK, et al: Bleomycin (B), etoposide (E), and continuous-infusion cis-platin (P) [BECIP] in metastatic testicular cancer (MTC). Proceedings of the 1985 meeting of the American Society of Clinical Oncology, abstracted, vol 4, Houston, ASCO, 1985, p 105

10. Eagan RT, Ingle JN, Frytak S, et al: Platinum-based polychemotherapy versus dianhydrogalactitol in advanced non-small cell lung cancer. Cancer Treat Rep 61:1339–1345, 1977

11. Edmondson JH, Long HJ, Richardson RL, et al: Phase II study of a combination of mitomycin, doxorubicin, cisplatinum in advanced sarcomas. Cancer Chemother Pharmacol 15:181–182, 1985

12. McKelvey EM, Gottlieb JA, Wilson HE, et al: Hydroxyldaunomycin (adriamycin) combination chemotherapy in malignant lymphoma. Cancer 38:1484–1493, 1976

10

THE PROBLEM OF THE POORLY DIFFERENTIATED SARCOMA

Jon C. Ross
Michael R. Hendrickson
Norio Azumi
Richard L. Kempson

A frequent diagnostic problem is the investigation of a mass that has presented in the soft tissues and is light microscopically "poorly differentiated." Such lesions may also be encountered within most organs and, although the diagnostic strategies for dealing with poorly differentiated tumors in both the soft tissues and organs are generally parallel, those arising in organs pose some special problems. Some of these organ-specific differential diagnostic considerations are presented briefly in tabular form (Table 10-1).

The pathologist must address three key questions when confronted with a mass that arises in the soft tissues and light microscopically appears poorly differentiated.

Is the tumor a benign proliferation mimicking a sarcoma? A number of reactive, reparative, and benign idiopathic proliferations present as soft tissue masses and may resemble sarcomas clinically because of their rapid growth and microscopically because of their undifferentiated appearance

POORLY DIFFERENTIATED NEOPLASMS AND TUMORS OF UNKNOWN ORIGIN ISBN 0-8089-1755-2
© 1986 by Grune & Stratton.

Table 10-1

Lesions that May Resemble Pure Sarcomas in Whole or in Part
in Various Organs and Special Sites

Lung	Carcinoid tumors with spindled areas
	Carcinosarcoma
	Giant cell carcinoma[33,34]
	Pulmonary blastoma
Respiratory mucosa	Nasal polyps with stromal atypia[35,36]
	Myxomas arising in cranial bones and extending into paranasal sinuses[7]
Pharynx, larynx, and esophagus	Carcinoma with pseudosarcomatous sarcoma
Mediastinum	Sclerosing mediastinitis[37]
	Spindled carcinoid
	Spindled thymoma
Serous body cavities	Mesothelioma
	Metastatic carcinoma with marked stromal response
	Mesenteric fibromatosis and retractile mesenteritis
Thyroid	Giant cell and spindle cell carcinomas
	Medullary carcinoma with spindled areas
Skin and squamous mucosa	Spindled squamous carcinoma
	Desmoplastic melanoma
	Pyogenic granuloma
Kidney	Renal cell carcinoma, spindled anaplastic type
	Carcinosarcoma/carcinoma with mesenchymal metaplasia
	Wilms' tumor
Urethra and bladder	Postoperative spindle cell nodules of genitourinary tract[38]
Pancreas	Anaplastic spindled and pleomorphic carcinomas[39,40]
	Giant cell tumor[41]
Breast	Spindle cell carcinoma[42]
	Carcinosarcoma/carcinoma with mesenchymal metaplasia
	Cystosarcoma
Liver	Giant cell tumor[43]
	Hepatoblastoma
Vagina	Benign vaginal polyps with stromal atypia[44,45]
	Postoperative spindle cell nodules of genitourinary tract[38]
Uterus	Mixed mullerian tumors
	Anaplastic endometrial carcinoma (mistaken for stromal sarcoma and other sarcomas)

Table 10-1   *(continued)*

Ovary	Mixed mullerian tumors
	Immature teratoma
	Metastatic carcinoma simulating marked stromal hyperplasia e.g., Krukenberg tumors)
	Mucinous cystadenocarcinoma with pseudosarcomatous stromal reaction[46]
Salivary glands	Mixed tumor (pleomorphic adenoma)
	Spindled myoepithelial adenoma
Bone	Neuroblastoma(mistaken for Ewing's)
	Metastatic carcinoma with stromal response (simulating primary bone sarcoma)
Stomach and bowel	Poorly differentiated carcinoma
	Inflammatory fibrous polyps[47,48]
Paraganglia	Spindled paraganglioma

This table excludes lymphoreticular and hematopoietic neoplasms; see Table 10-5. Standard texts such as Rosai J: Surgical Pathology, (ed 6). CV Mosby, St. Louis, 1981, may be consulted for references pertaining to most of these lesions. Some rare entities are specifically annoted with pertinent sources.

and high mitotic counts. Distinguishing these proliferations from sarcoma is of obvious importance, and there are a number of simple strategies that insure the detection of most of these benign processes.

Assuming that the proliferation is malignant, is the tumor a primary soft tissue sarcoma or some other malignant neoplasm mimicking a sarcoma? Metastatic carcinoma and lymphoreticular malignancies may present initially in the soft tissues and, when poorly differentiated or spindled, may mimic sarcomas. These possibilities should be systematically excluded.

Assuming that the neoplasm is a soft tissue sarcoma, what prognostic and therapeutically relevant morphologic features should be noted? For example, which of the many morphologic distinctions made among soft tissue neoplasms currently make a therapeutic difference? An important preliminary to addressing these questions is a clear definition of the terms *anaplastic, undifferentiated,* and *high-grade*; too often they are used interchangably. Our use of these terms is detailed in Table 10-2.

Table 10-2
Definition of Terms

Anaplastic: We will use this term to denote the presence of most of the following nuclear features: marked pleomorphism (i.e., variation in size and shape of nuclei), nuclear hyperchromasia, striking irregularity of chromatin pattern, abnormal mitotic figures, and large numbers of mitotic figures.

Undifferentiated: This term denotes the absence of a distinctive tissue phenotype (cytoplasmic features, cell products, architectural patterns) as observed *using a particular technique of examination*. It is important to note that a neoplasm may be "undifferentiated" light microscopically but still show differentiated features when examined ultrastructurally, biochemically, or immunologically.

High-Grade: A grading scheme is the product of a clinicopathologic effort that attempts to relate variation in some morphologic feature (or features) with increasing clinical aggressiveness. Typically, grading schemes require an assessment of the architecture of a neoplasm, the nuclear features of its constituent cells, and/or the degree to which cytoplasmic differentiation is evident. "High-grade" thus may refer to architectural disarray, marked anaplasia, an absence of cytoplasmic differentiation, or some differentially weighted composite of these features. Grading criteria vary from organ to organ and there are a variety of competing grading schemes for most common malignancies. Obviously, "high-grade" is a meaningful term only with respect to a given grading system.

General Considerations

Many histopathologic diagnostic difficulties can be avoided if surgeon and pathologist give careful consideration to the appropriate type of biopsy and to careful processing of the resulting tissue. Moreover, many light microscopic diagnostic difficulties are resolved when the biopsy is interpreted in the clinical context with full knowledge of the operative findings.

The chances of correctly diagnosing a soft tissue tumor are greatly enhanced by intelligent and adequate sampling.[1] We do not believe in general that needle aspiration cytology or needle biopsy specimens provide adequate material for the proper classification of soft tissue tumors. Most soft tissue masses located entirely in the subcutaneous tissue can be removed by *excisional biopsy*. Should the neoplasm prove malignant, the re-excision of the tumor bed is usually not a technically difficult procedure. The majority of soft tissue sarcomas present clinically as deeply seated soft tissue masses. All such masses should be regarded as sarcomas until proven otherwise. *Incisional biopsy* is the diagnostic technique of choice for soft tissue masses in the deep soft tissues. When the skin incision is carefully planned and can be encompassed by the definitive resection, this biopsy technique is not known to be associated with an increased risk of either local recurrence or distant metastasis.[1,2] Frozen sections made at the time of biopsy can be used to assure the adequacy of the specimen but should not, in general, be used as a basis for undertaking definitive treatment of soft tissue masses. Fresh tissue can be obtained at the time of surgery and stored in the proper manner for possible subsequent ultrastructural and immunologic studies. We believe that the pathologist should be called to the operating room to receive the fresh specimen for every biopsy or resection of a soft tissue mass.

Unfortunately, all too often the pathologist is not consulted before the biopsy of a soft tissue tumor, and his first contact with the problem is with a distorted scrap of fixed tissue, sometimes partially necrotic, attached to wisps of "undifferentiated sarcoma." *Ex post facto* consultation with the surgeon then becomes mandatory to determine how representative the sample is and to intelligently plan the inevitable second biopsy. For example, ulcerated primary cutaneous neoplasms are sometimes biopsied centrally, and the resulting specimens often fail to reveal their epidermal origin, sometimes resulting in the misdiagnosis of sarcoma; a biopsy which samples the borders of the ulcer may disclose the junctional component of a spindled melanoma or features supporting a diagnosis of spindled squamous cell carcinoma.

Except for small amounts of material reserved for the special studies mentioned above, biopsy specimens should be entirely examined histologically. If a larger surgical specimen has been submitted to the pathologist, it is obviously wise to increase one's sample size by submitting additional blocks of any neoplasm which on initial examination appears undifferentiated. Deeper sections of the original blocks may also be required, but the pathologist should not hesitate to return to the gross specimen for additional material. These practical methods *very often* reveal a diagnostic differentiated focus. This examination of additional sections is often the most important aspect of the pathologist's work-up of the apparently poorly differentiated neoplasm. Careful gross examination of a large specimen may also allow directed sampling of regions likely to provide diagnostic information. For example, borders of a tumor are ideal samples to assess cellular cohesiveness. Degenerative changes which complicate interpretation can be minimized by selecting some sections from the better vascularized periphery of large tumors and from zones which do not appear grossly necrotic. (Note, however, the special significance of estimating the extent of necrosis in grading sarcomas, as discussed more thoroughly below.) When the gross appearance is heterogenous, samples should be taken from each distinct area. Myxoid or mucoid regions are particularly prone to be left behind on the cutting board, but may reveal important clues to the diagnosis.

Difficulties with the technical aspects of tissue handling, fixation, sectioning, and staining underlie a truly *startling* number of cases referred for consultation as diagnostic dilemmas. Correct morphologic diagnosis is utterly dependent on these mundane factors. The pathologist who neglects this aspect of his practice will be troubled by many more "poorly differentiated" neoplasms than his more meticulous colleagues.

The time and money spent on expensive special techniques and pathology consultants can also often be reduced by seeking the answers to a few cogent clinical questions. For example, the patient's age and the location of a soft tissue lesion are important features in the diagnosis of chordoma, sacrococcygeal teratoma, soft tissue Ewing's sarcoma and embryonal rhabdomyosarcoma. The radiographic assessment may show involvement of an underlying bone, increasing the likelihood of extension into soft tissues of a primary bone sarcoma, or it may show the pattern of soft tissue calcification of synovial sarcoma.[2a] An intravenous pyelogram may exclude the possibility of metastatic renal cell carcinoma, a frequent sarcoma mimic. A search for pigmented skin lesions and breast lumps may suggest an explanation of poorly differentiated inguinal or axillary tumors (and may considerably revitalize a pathologist's search for pigment or glandular differentiation in the poorly differentiated lesion.) Lymphadenopathy and hepatosplenomegaly may prompt reconsideration of the diagnosis of lymphoma, and blood or bone marrow smears may aid in the diagnosis of hematopoietic disorders such as granulocytic sarcoma. Obviously a patient's past medical history may be crucial in disclosing previous evidence of cancer, and biopsies of *any earlier lesions which might be pertinent* need to be reviewed in conjunction with current material.

With these considerations in mind, we will now examine the questions faced by the surgical pathologist when examining a poorly differentiated soft tissue lesion.

Is the Tumor a Benign Lesion Mimicking a Sarcoma?

A number of benign reactive, reparative, and idiopathic proliferations occur in the soft tissues and mimic sarcomas. They do so clinically because of their rapid growth; grossly, because they may infiltrate normal structures; and microscopically, because they may be cellular, cytologically atypical and mitotically active. The full range of nuclear alterations encountered in dividing and synthetically active cells may be seen in these benign soft tissue lesions. These include nuclear and nucleolar enlargement, coarsening of chromatin pattern, and some degree of nuclear pleomorphism. A small biopsy of such a lesion may easily be misconstrued as sarcoma. Table 10-3 presents a list of benign soft tissue lesions and the corresponding sarcoma patterns which they may mimic to variable extent.

The lesion most frequently misconstrued as undifferentiated sarcoma is *nodular fasciitis*, a benign mesenchymal proliferation of uncertain etiology.[21,22] This proliferation has all of the characteristics described above but in addition is composed of spindled cells without light microscopically distinctive differentiation. Ultrastructurally, the cells prove to be myofibroblastic.[23] There are a number of important, easily assessed features that serve to distinguish nodular fasciitis from sarcoma. Nodular fasciitis is generally small (less than 3.0 cm) and superficially located in the soft tissue. Most soft tissue sarcomas are deep seated and large (greater than 5.0 cm). However, deep location does not necessarily exclude the diagnosis of nodular fasciitis.[24] The cells of nodular fasciitis are relatively uniform, may be atypical, but lack the nuclear pleomorphism so common in soft tissue sarcomas. Usually the mitotic counts in the cellular phase of nodular fasciitis are in the range of only the most bizarre soft tissue sarcomas, and the combination of cytologically uniform cells and the high mitotic rate is striking.

Proliferative fasciitis and *proliferative myositis* are close relations of nodular fasciitis and feature a rather uniform population of plump ganglion-like cells set within an edematous stroma.[25,26] These proliferations are characteristically small and almost always less than 5 cm. The cases of proliferative fasciitis are characteristically superficial in location, in the subcutis or in association with superficial fascia. By definition proliferative myositis involves voluntary musculature, producing a "checkerboard" pattern as the lesion separates muscle bundles and individual fibers. Mitotic figures are common in both lesions. Awareness of these entities and the identification of the highly characteristic ganglion-like cells usually will avoid a misdiagnosis of sarcoma.

Other soft tissue tumors are misconstrued as sarcoma, not on the basis of nuclear abnormalities, cellularity, or mitotic activity, but simply because the abundant matrix they produce resembles that of some sarcomas. For example, until recently it was thought that all myxoid lesions of the soft tissues were malignant independent of their cytologic appearance.[27] Over recent years, however, a number of benign clinicopathologic entities in the myxoid group, such as intramuscular myxoma and some myxoid examples

Table 10-3
Benign and/or Reactive Lesions Mistaken for Sarcoma in the
Soft Tissue

Atypical fibroxanthoma* Nodular fasciitis Cranial fasciitis[3] Intravascular fasciitis[4] Proliferative fasciitis Proliferative myositis Neurofibroma with cellular atypia ("ancient neurofibroma") Malacoplakia[5] Silica reaction[6] Xanthogranulomatous inflammation Giant cell tumor tendon sheath Pigmented nodular tenosynovitis	Poorly differentiated sarcoma or MFH
Myxomas of facial bones extending into local soft tissues[7] Myxoma of muscle Myxoid neurofibroma	MFH or myxoid sarcomas
Lipoblastoma/lipoblastomatosis Pleomorphic lipoma[8,9] Atypical lipoma*[10] Spindle cell lipoma Intramuscular lipoma	Liposarcoma
Angiolipoma	Liposarcoma or leiomyosarcoma
Fibrous hamartoma Fibromatosis (many subtypes) Cellular blue nevus Congenital "fibrosarcoma-like" fibromatosis[11–13]*	Fibrosarcoma
Parosteal fasciitis[14–16] Myositis ossificans	MFH or osteosarcoma
Exuberant callus	Osteosarcoma, chondrosarcoma
Atypical papillary endothelial hyperplasia[17,18] Histiocytoid hemangioma[19] Epithelioid hemangioendothelioma (Benign form)[20]	Vascular sarcomas

Standard references such as Rosai J: Surgical Pathology, (ed 6). CV Mosby, St. Louis, 1981, may be consulted for literature pertaining to most of these lesions. Rarer entities are specifically annotated with pertinent sources.
* Rare tumors with this histologic appearance have metastasized, but the overwhelming majority are nonmetastasizing.

of nodular fasciitis, have been recognized.[28] Similarly, musculoaponeurotic fibromatosis with its abundant collagenous matrix is frequently misdiagnosed as sarcoma, although the constituent cells are bland and mitotically inactive. We suspect that the aggressive infiltration of normal tissues, which is characteristic of musculoaponeurotic fibromatosis, is the feature which often prompts its misclassification as a frank sarcoma.

Finally, there are lesions such as myositis ossificans, exuberant callus, and a variety of atypical vascular proliferations that combine atypical nuclear features with differentiated cytologic and architectural features or a specific type of matrix, suggesting the analogous type of differentiated sarcoma. A small biopsy sample of these lesions interpreted without the appropriate clinical, radiologic, and operative findings is easily misconstrued as sarcoma.

A further discussion of these benign proliferations which mimic sarcoma is outside the scope of this chapter; many of these are linked with references in Table 10-3. They must always be considered in the differential diagnosis of "poorly differentiated sarcoma", since any misdiagnosis of this type will lead to grave errors of treatment of the patient.

Assuming that the Lesion is Malignant, is the Tumor a Primary Soft Tissue Sarcoma or Some Other Malignant Tumor Mimicking Sarcoma?

The likelihood is great that an anaplastic and poorly differentiated neoplasm located in the soft tissues is a sarcoma, especially when there is no clinical evidence of lymphadenopathy, skin involvement, or organ-specific abnormalities. Nevertheless, the surgical pathologist must verify the diagnosis of sarcoma, since the less likely possibilities (e.g., pleomorphic lymphoma, soft tissue metastasis from occult poorly differentiated carcinoma, or melanoma) have very different prognostic and therapeutic implications. Although poorly differentiated anaplastic neoplasms, by definition, give little morphologic evidence of their resemblance to a normal tissue type, even routine methods, if applied properly, usually allow one to discover general differentiated features of these tumors sufficient to characterize them as mesenchymal, hematopoietic, or epithelial.

Light Microscopy

Table 10-4 presents some general light microscopic features useful in distinguishing soft tissue sarcomas from hematopoietic malignancies and from metastatic carcinoma. When poorly differentiated, these neoplasms

Table 10-4
Basic Light Microscopic Criteria for Recognizing Sarcomas in Contradistinction to Other Cancers

	Sarcoma	Lymphomas/Leukemia	Carcinoma
CYTOLOGIC FEATURES	Spindled cells the hall mark; epithelioid cells may occur. Pleomorphic sarcomas characterized by several or more cell types, i.e., marked variation in *both* nuclear and cytoplasmic appearance.	Cells generally have "family resemblance" to lymphoid cells in various stages of transformation. Exceptions: Signet ring lymphoma Lennert's lymphoma with epithelioid histiocytes Pleomorphic lymphoma	Epithelioid cells the hallmark; spindled cell may occur. Single characteristic cell type usually identifiable; pleomorphism tends to be more nuclear than cytoplasmic.
ARCHITECTURAL ORGANIZATION	1. Polarized sheets or bundles of spindled cells 2. Patterns dominated by matrix production (myxoid, fibrous, osseous, etc.) 3. Mixtures of 1 and 2	Structureless infiltration of pre-existing tissue Loose follicular or nodular aggregates (NSHD, follicular lymphomas)	Rich variety of highly organized patterns reflecting epithelial differentiation (glands, squamous sheets and eddies, trabeculae, etc.) Sheets supported by a scant fibrovascular stroma
		Rare compartmentalizing fibrosis	

226

	4. Organized epithelioid and biphasic sarcomas (alveolar rhabdomysarcoma, alveolar soft part sarcoma, clear cell and epithelioid sarcoma, synovial sarcoma)		Spindled patterns mimicking sarcoma may occur (e.g., spindled squamous and renal cellcarcinomas)*
CELL COHESION Nuclear molding	Absent in lesions with abundant matrix. Even in densely cellular sarcomas, cells tend to have shape independent of contact with adjoining cells and nuclear molding is absent.	Cells "fall apart" and show little nuclear molding except occasionally as they line up between preexisting connective tissue planes.	Cells are commonly cohesive, with adjoining cells molding each other's nuclear contours
Borders of tumor with surrounding tissue tissue	Vague, irregular borders most common although discrete or encapsulated tumors also occur; often entraps fat but does not generally infiltrate around and between individual fat cells	Diffuse infiltration around and between fat cells, muscle fibers, reflecting lack of cellular cohesiveness	Discrete borders most common, reflects cellular cohesiveness; obliterates fat and other connective tissue elements; less often entraps them.

(Continues)

227

Table 10-4 *(continued)*

	Sarcoma	Lymphomas/Leukemia	Carcinoma
INTERCELLULAR MATRIX PRODUCTION	Abundant matrix production by tumor cells characteristic of many types. Individual cells often separated by matrix material.	Matrix inconspicuous; or background stroma infiltrated by tumor; sclerosis in some subtypes (i.e., NSHD) and as a degenerative change.	Fibrovascular supporting stroma as opposed to matrix production by tumor cells; individual neoplastic cells tend to be closely opposed; sclerotic zones may occur as a degenerative change and be confused with sarcoma stroma.
RETICULIN	Most often abundant reticulin, often surrounding each individual tumor cell (exceptions among architectural organization 4, above)	Reticulin pattern variable; background stroma infiltrated by lymphoma/leukemia may contain abundant reticulium.	Often scant reticulin; pattern of reticulin fibers outlines sheets or nests or smaller groups of cells (but many exceptions).
SPECIAL STAINS FOR CYTOPLASMIC CONSTITUENTS[†] Nonspecific esterase; (will stain mast cells and cells of myelocytic series)	Absent in tumor cells	Present in granulocytic leukemic infiltrate (granulocytic sarcoma)	Absent in tumor cells

Stain for glycogen	Present in Ewing's sarcoma, clear cell sarcoma, leiomyosarcoma and rhabdomyosarcoma; absent or very scanty in MFH and many other sarcomas	Absent in any significant amount	Present in many carcinomas but particularly abundant in many spindled renal cell carcinomas and spindled squamous carcinomas; useful in distinguishing them from MFH and fibrosarcoma.
Stains for mucin	Acidic (sulfated and carboxylated) stromal mucosubstances stainable with alcian blue at pH 1.5, or 0.4 in some subtypes.[29] Epithelioid phase of synovial sarcoma may elaborate PAS+, diastase resistant, mucicarmine+, alcian blue+, hyaluronidase resistant mucosubstance which may be intracellular.[30]	Absent. PAS-positive diastase resistant material may be seen in signet ring lymphomas and as intranuclear inclusions in myeloma and macroglobulinemia (Dutcher bodies).	Neutral intracytoplasmic mucin seen in some poorly differentiated carcinomas. This stains with PAS after diastase, tol. blue, mucicarmine.

(Continues)

Table 10-4 *(continued)*

	Sarcoma	Lymphomas/Leukemia	Carcinoma
LYMPHOID INFILTRATE	Lymphoid infiltrate variable	Intimate admixture of normal lymphocytes in many extranodal lymphomas	Lymphoid infiltrate variable but often located at margin of tumor cell nests (reflecting cohesiveness of neoplastic cells in carcinoma)

* Spindle cells may also be seen in malignant melanoma (desmoplastic melanoma).

† Stains for melanin pigment (Fortana or FeFeCN) are also important for the diagnosis of malignant melanoma when it is predominantly amelanotic. But note that rare cases of certain sarcomas, including clear cell sarcoma of tendons and aponeuroses (see text), and mixed ectomesenchymal neoplasms with sarcomatous elements, may contain melanin.

Table 10-5
Hematopoietic and Lymphoreticular Neoplasms Misdiagnosed
as Soft Tissue Sarcomas

Hodgkin's disease
Lymphocyte depleted subtype
Nodular sclerosing subtype
Pleomorphic histiocytic lymphoma (Pleomorphic large lymphoid lymphoma)
Histiocytic lymphoma with compartmentalizing fibrosis[31]
Granulocytic sarcoma
Malignant histiocytosis[32]

may overlap to some degree in each of the listed morphologic respects so
that evaluation of a combination of these features is generally necessary in
order to properly classify a poorly differentiated tumor. Often the most
helpful approach when light microscopy appears to fail to resolve this
differential diagnosis is to submit more sections from histologic examination and obtain a more detailed clinical history as noted above. Many
diagnostic errors are also avoided if the histopathologist always remembers
to consider an appropriate differential diagnosis of sarcoma mimics as he
examines a putative sarcoma. A list of the hematopoietic and lymphoreticular malignancies most commonly misconstrued as sarcoma is found in
Table 10-5. Table 10-1 presented a differential diagnosis organized by site,
which lists various nonhematopoietic nonlymphoid lesions which may, in
whole or in part, resemble sarcoma in various organs or special locations.
Benign mimics of sarcoma located in soft tissue sites have already been
considered above and outlined in Table 10-3.

Electron Microscopy

Study of poorly differentiated soft tissue tumors with the electron
microscope complements light microscopic analysis, and in some instances
provides the only morphologic evidence upon which a classification can be
based.[49]

It has been suggested that electron microscopy may contribute to
diagnosis in one to eight percent of all tumors,[50-52] and this figure is likely
to be substantially higher when only light microscopically poorly differentiated tumors are considered. Of course, the increase in resolution which
one gains with electron microscopy—allowing examination of subcellular
organelles—comes at the expense of an enormous reduction in sample
size. This is a particular problem in the study of poorly differentiated

neoplasms which may show only focal differentiation. It underscores the importance of examining many 1 micron survey sections by light microscopy to choose those regions for ultrastructural study which are most likely to reveal diagnostic features and which are best preserved.

In general, the strategy for examining poorly differentiated neoplasms for ultrastructural evidence of sarcomatous differentiation involves looking for specialized structures which, if found, would count against the diagnosis of sarcoma (Table 10-6). Most important among these are specialized regions of the cell membrane which act as zones of intercellular attachment: desmosomes (maculae adherentes), intermediate junctions (zonulae adherentes), junctional complexes (an organized array of tight junction, intermediate junction, and desmosome), and other less well-formed caricatures of these intercellular attachments which are often termed "desmosome-like" junctions or simply poorly-formed cell attachment plaques. Morphologic variation in intercellular attachments is multiplied considerably in neoplastic tissues, and many of these attachments lose some of the detailing of the homologous normal structures. For example, the characteristic epithelial desmosome (with its slightly widened intercellular gap, intermediate line, and filaments radiating into the cytoplasm of adjoining cells from dense plaques in the cell membranes) may be scarce or absent in a poorly differentiated carcinoma, although a variety of aberrant intercellular attachments may be more easily located.[53] On the other hand, better differentiated carcinomas often contain numerous full-fledged desmosomes.

Classic well-formed desmosomes are *not* a feature of sarcomas.[52,54] Poorly formed cell junctions or "desmosome-like" attachments have been described in normal mesenchyme[55–58] and in several mesenchymal tumors, most notably in synovial sarcomas,[59] smooth muscle tumors,[54] schwannian tumors,[53,60] and hemangiopericytomas.[61] Arrays of intercellular attachments resembling the junctional complexes seen normally at the luminal aspects of many glandular epithelia, and commonly in adenocarcinomas, have also been observed in the epithelioid phase of synovial sarcoma.[62–64] Tight junctions and intermediate junctions have been observed in angiosarcomas.[61,65] It is thus apparent that the identification of a poorly formed cell attachment plaque in a light microscopically poorly differentiated neoplasm cannot reasonably *exclude* mesenchymal differentiation. Instead, one must rely upon the frequency of intercellular attachments and their degree and type of specialization in weighing the diagnosis of sarcoma. If such structures are frequently seen in the ultrastructural study of a poorly differentiated tumor located in the soft tissues, this is generally taken as evidence against the diagnosis of sarcoma and in favor of carcinoma. A search for a primary epithelial cancer is then in order. Importantly, any kind of cell attachment is vanishingly rare in hematopoietic tissues and lymphoreticular neoplasms, and therefore the presence of even rare, poorly formed junctions is against the diagnoses of lymphoma and leukemia and favors either sarcoma or carcinoma.[52–54]

The ultrastructural examination of neoplastic cells may also provide strong evidence of melanocytic differentiation, neuroepithelial differentiation, squamous or glandular differentiation and thus count *against* a competing diagnosis of sarcoma. The pleomorphic melanoma masquerading as a superficially located soft tissue sarcoma may contain scattered melanosomes ultrastructurally in the absence of light microscopically demonstrable pigment. The so-called desmoplastic melanoma, which is easily misdiagnosed light microscopically, has now been shown to contain melanosomes ultrastructurally, but few cases have been studied with the electron microscope, and finding melanosomes may not be possible in some cases.[66–69] On the other hand, malignancies other than the usual forms of melanoma may contain melanosomes, indicating their loose kinship with tissues derived from the neural crest; for example, melanosomes have been detected in lesions with the light microscopic appearance of clear cell sarcoma[70,71] and in ectomesenchymal sarcomas. Less ambiguously, bundles of tonofilaments serve to identify spindled squamous carcinoma and intracytoplasmic lumina may mark poorly differentiated and pleomorphic soft tissue metastases from an occult adenocarcinoma. Ultrastructural examination also plays an important role in the classification of childhood small round cell tumors. The presence of neurosecretory granules and neural processes, sometimes with synaptic complexes, will identify neuroblastoma and serve to separate it from Ewing's sarcoma and rhabdomyosarcoma, distinctions which may be difficult to make with the light microscope.

Electron microscopy may, then, provide good evidence that a neoplasm, poorly differentiated by light microscopy, is *not* a sarcoma (Table 10-6 provides a brief summary of this approach). Does this method often provide positive findings which suggest the diagnosis of sarcoma?

Certainly, the ultrastructural features of many forms of sarcoma have been fully described in the literature; the high resolution portraits which emerge are briefly sketched in Table 10-7. If the ultrastructural resemblance to a particular sarcoma subtype is strong, this may be useful evidence in excluding alternative diagnoses of pleomorphic lymphoma or soft tissue metastases of a poorly differentiated and occult carcinoma. More frequently, such data assists in subclassifying mesenchymal neoplasms which are confidently regarded as sarcomas on the basis of light microscopy.

Table 10-6
Basic Electron Microscopic Criteria Employed in the Recognition of Sarcomas

	Sarcomas	Lymphoma/ Leukemia	Melanoma	Carcinomas
Intercellular connections	Intermed. junctions (Zonulae adherentes) and various poorly formed cell interconnections may be present, although usually they are infrequent, rare or absent	Cell junctions absent	Cell junction very rare	Well-formed desmosomes (Maculae adherentes) and junctional complexes may be present; various other forms of intercellular attachments such as intermediate junctions (zonulae adherentes), desmosome-like, or poorly formed cell junctions are common and more easily found than in sarcomas
Basement lamina	External laminae may surround individual cells in some sarcoma types (for example, smooth muscle and schwannian tumors, see Table 10-7)	Absent	Absent	Basal laminae may be found surrounding groups of cells

Melanosomes	Clear cell sarcomas and rare extomesenchymal sarcoma may have melanosomes	Absent	Melanosomes present, although sometimes infrequent (melanosomes have been demonstrated in some desmoplastic melanomas, but not in all)	Absent
Intracellular lumina	Absent	Absent	Absent	Characteristic of adenocarcinoma
Bundles of tonofilaments	Absent	Absent	Absent	Characteristic of squamous carcinoma
Dense core granules	Absent	Absent	Absent	Present in various endocrine neoplasms, small cell carcinoma, and neuroblastoma

Table 10-7
Electron Microscopic Features of Some Sarcoma Subtypes

Fibrosarcoma	Fibroblastic cells predominate (spindle cells with prominent rough endoplasmic reticulum, often distended; collagenous interstitium with no external laminae); myofibroblastic cells may also be present (in addition to fibroblastic features these cells show bundles of thin myofilaments associated with focal densities, often arranged at the cell periphery).
Malignant fibrous histiocytoma	Mixtures of cell types, including fibroblastic, myofibroblastic, and histiocytic cells (the latter are rounded or irregular cells with variable numbers of cell processes, lysosomes, cytoplasmic vacuoles, and little rough endoplasmic reticulum).
Leiomyosarcoma	Smooth muscle differentiation characterized by pinocytotic vesicles, variable expression of external laminae, and cytoplasmic bundles of thin myofilaments associated with focal densities and dense plaques; some myofibroblastic cells may also be seen.
Rhabdomyosarcoma	Thick (15 nm) and thin myofilaments; often with identifiable Z band material.
Malignant Schwannoma	Elongated cytoplasmic processes, variable investment by external laminae, junctional complexes reported, long-spacing collagen.[60]
Hemangiopericytoma	Intermediate junctions (zonulae adherentes), poorly developed external laminae, fine cytoplasmic filaments, pinocytotic vessels; cells arranged around blood vessels.[61]
Angiosarcoma	Rare Weibel-Palade bodies, occasional poorly formed tight junctions, pinocytotic vesicles and fine cytoplasmic filaments may be found.[61]
Synovial sarcoma	Fibroblast-like cells compose the stromal component, zonulae adherentes have been observed between the spindle cells, which are not surrounded by an external laminae; epithelioid component shows microvilli lining tubular spaces, junctional complexes between cells and basal laminae.[59,62,63,72,73]

Table 10-7 *(continued)*

Liposarcoma	Intracytoplasmic lipid droplets (both membrane and nonmembrane bound), polymorphic mitochondria, fine cytoplasmic filaments, glycogen, variable external laminae, and pinocytotic vesicles, little intercellular collagen (multilayered basal laminae around the vessels of myxoid liposarcoma.[74-77]
Alveolar soft part sarcoma	Intracytoplasmic crystalline bodies, numerous mitochondria.

Specific references are cited for some subtypes. Further descriptions of these and of the remaining subtypes can be found in Ghadially[53] and Henderson and Papadimitriou[54]

However, a considerable lack of diagnostic specificity of individual ultrastructural features is rather common, a single example of which is Henderson and Papadimitriou's documentation of the long list of tumors which may contain myofibroblatic cells.[54] The prognostic importance of subclassifying poorly differentiated sarcomas will be considered subsequently.

Several practical and methodologic problems must be considered when using electron microscopy to subclassify poorly differentiated soft tissue neoplasms. First, poorly fixed and improperly prepared material is just as likely to yield ambiguous or even misleading information electron microscopically as it is in routine histology. It is for this reason that we advocate prompt placement in gluteradlehyde of 1 millimeter cubes of *all* soft tissue tumors. This of course presupposes a mechanism for insuring that fresh specimens are promptly submitted to the pathologist.

Secondly, benign mesenchymal cells are ubiquitous even in epithelial and hematopoietic neoplasms. This fact, combined with the notorious difficulty in distinguishing benign from malignant cells ultrastructurally, can lead to misconstruing of non-neoplastic mesenchymal cells of a supporting stroma as neoplastic cells, and to an erroneous inference of sarcomatous differentiation. Non-neoplastic endothelial cells, fibroblasts, and smooth muscle cells are especially liable to be inappropriately promoted to neoplastic status in this manner. Similarly, malignant tumors infiltrating muscle may contain remnants of skeletal muscle which, having been overrun by the neoplasm, are easily misconstrued as rhabdomyoblasts ultrastructurally. The best protection against these errors is to maintain as much "architectural" orientation as possible at high magnifications. This is done by having in mind the 1 micron survey section of the block from which the thin sections derive and by paying close attention to the low magnification (500–2000X) appearance of the grid being examined ultrastructurally. The ultrastructural nuclear features of the neoplastic cells may also be examined in order to assess whether or not a particular differentiated cell fits into the general nuclear pattern of the neoplastic cell population. It should be recognized, however, that nuclear irregularities are not invariably present ultrastructurally in neoplastic cells.[53,54]

A third and seldom discussed problem is fundamental to integration of ultrastructural data into clinical decision making. It is generally unrecognized that the diagnosis of a poorly differentiated tumor on the basis of electron microscopic findings often represents an expansion or redefinition of the morphologic (light microscopic) component of an earlier *clinicopathologic definition* of the disease entity. It may be a likely hypothesis that many lesions so diagnosed with electron microscopy will behave in a manner somewhat akin to their better differentiated counterparts diagnosed with routine light microscopy; but this hypothesis is generally assumed or implied to be true in the surgical pathology literature rather than having been explicitly tested. This hypothesis may be either extremely likely or quite unlikely to be true, depending upon the context. For example, the ultrastructural finding of several poorly formed intercellular attachments in a soft tissue neoplasm may suggest to a pathologist the diagnosis of poorly differentiated metastatic carcinoma; the clinician should be made aware, however, that such an assignment is based on very slender grounds, since some sarcomas have intercellular attachments. Careful statistical data relating *frequency* of cell attachments in a soft tissue mass to clinical outcomes, such as to the success of a search for an epithelial primary, is simply unavailable at this time. Another example is provided by the wide variation in light microscopic appearances and clinical behaviors of neoplasms that ultrastructurally contain dense core granules.

Immunopathologic Studies

The most important advance in diagnostic histopathology in recent years is undoubtedly the introduction of immunophenotyping reagents, and particularly monoclonal antibody preparations capable of recognizing antigenic determinants in routinely processed paraffin-embedded tissues. The importance of this methodology is evident in its impact on the new classifications of lymphomas and in its day-to-day utility as a diagnostic tool in hematopathology. We are beginning to find immunologic reagents similarly useful in diagnosing poorly differentiated sarcomas and their mimics. While immunologic methods are dealt with in detail elsewhere in this monograph, some specific information and caveats pertinent to the problems of sarcomas are presented here.

Summarized in Table 10-8 are antigens used in the diagnosis of sarcomas and their mimics. Only those antigens are included of which the immunologic recognition in routinely processed paraffin sections has been reasonably well-established. These are related in the table to the various lesions in which they are characteristically found. Where data is scanty, we have indicated this by listing the number of published cases which have been stained. References to specific methods are available in the papers cited in the table. As any user of these methods is already well aware, some antigens are more useful than others in specific diagnostic situations. We have attempted to convey this situation by highlighting those associations in the table which we find diagnostically very useful in our laboratory, or which our evaluation of the literature suggests may prove very useful in the near future as the reagents become more generally available.

In particular, we would like to draw attention to the following diagnostic decisions regularly faced by the surgical pathologist, in which immunophenotyping methods may prove quite helpful in refuting or confirming a sarcoma diagnosis.

Sarcoma versus carcinoma. Immunohistochemical demonstration of keratin proteins is very helpful in the diagnosis of carcinoma.[87,88,91,94,95] Carcinomas mimicking sarcoma may be detected in this manner. Various antibodies, including monoclonal and polyclonal types with varying specificities and sensitivities, are available. They may recognize keratins with different molecular properties e.g., different molecular weights, but a discussion of these differences is beyond the scope of this chapter.[92,93,93a,96] The demonstration of milk-fat globule protein has also been reported as a useful technique for recognizing epithelial differentiation in poorly differentiated lesions.[103,104]

Sarcomas with epithelial-like antigens (synovial sarcoma; epithelioid sarcoma) versus other sarcomas. The pathologist must be aware that keratin has also been demonstrated in several specific sarcomas, i.e., synovial sarcoma and epithelioid sarcoma.[89,90,120] Thus it is clearly necessary to narrow one's differential diagnosis by other methods before utilizing immunologic demonstration of keratin as a diagnostic method. For example, when a differential diagnosis includes both carcinoma *and* epithelioid sarcoma, a keratin stain is not helpful in separating these possibilities, since both may be positive. However, when confronted with a subclassification problem, where the possibilities include malignant fibrous histiocytoma, fibrosar-

Table 10-8 (Part A)
Antigens Useful for Diagnosing and/or Subclassifying Sarcomas

	S-100[80-86a]	"Keratins"[87-120]	"Panhematolymphoid" Antigen[98]	Fast Myosin[99]	Myoglobin[100-101a]
SARCOMAS					
Malignant schwannoma	±	–		–	–
Liposarcoma	±	–		–	–
Chondrosarcoma	±	–		–	–
Osteosarcoma	±	–		–	–
Leiomyosarcoma	–	–		–	–
MFH					
Fibrosarcoma		–	–		–
Rhabdomyosarcoma[99,113]			– (0/1)	+	±
Ewing's sarcoma[116]			–	+	
Synovial sarcoma[89,90]		+	–		
Angiosarcoma					
Kaposi's sarcoma	– (0/1)				
Epithelioid sarcoma[120]	– (0/1)	+			
Clear cell sarcoma[117-119]	+				
Alveolarsoftpartsarcoma[121,122]		– (0/1)			
Carcinoma		+	–		
Mesothelioma[93,97,123]		+			
Neuroblastoma	±				
Lymphoma/Leukemia		–	+		– (0/1)
Melanoma	+	–	–		
Desmoplastic melanoma[69]	+				
BENIGN LESIONS					
Neurilemmoma/Neurofibroma	+				
Fibromatosis					
DFSP# (Pigmented and nonpigmented)		– (0/1)			
Leiomyoma	– (0/1)				
Nodular faciitis					–

(Table continues in Parts B and C)

[†] Several different keratin-specific antigens have been described. Different preparations have slightly different reactivities.[87-97,120]

[‡] A "panhematolymphoid" antigen recognized in paraffin section by PD7/26 and 2B11 monoclonal antibodies.[98]

[#] DFSP is Dermatofibrosarcoma Protuberans.

240

Table 10-8 *(continued, Part B)*

	Alpha-1 Antitrypsin and Alpha-1 Antichymotrypsin[102]	Human Milk-fat Globule[103,104]	Desmin[87]	Vimentin[87,94,95]	Neuron-specific Enolase[105-107]
SARCOMAS					
Malignant schwannoma				+ (1/1)	+
Liposarcoma				+ (1/1)	
Chondrosarcoma	– (0/1)			+	
Osteosarcoma					
Leiomyosarcoma	–		+	+	
MFH	+		–	+	
Fibrosarcoma	–			+	
Rhabdomyosarcoma[99,113]	– (0/1)		+	+	
Ewing's sarcoma[116]	–	– (0/2)			
Synovial sarcoma[89,90]	–				
Angiosarcoma			–	+	
Kaposi's sarcoma					
Epithelioid sarcoma[120]					
Clear cell sarcoma[117-119]					
Alveolar soft part sarcoma[121,122]			– (0/1)		
Carcinoma	–	+	–	– *	+|
Mesothelioma[93,97,123]		–			
Neuroblastoma					+
Lymphoma/Leukemia	–			+	–
Melanoma				+	
Desmoplastic melanoma[69]					
BENIGN LESIONS					
Neurilemmoma/Neurofibroma					
Fibromatosis					
DFSP[#] (Pigmented and nonpigmented)	±			+ (0/1)	
Leiomyoma					
Nodular fasciitis					

(Table continues in Part C)

[#] DFSP is Dermatofibrosarcoma Protuberans.

* Merkel cell tumor and neuroendocrine carcinoma are positive.

241

Table 10-8 (continued, Part C)

	Factor VIII Associated Antigen[108,109]	Laminin[87,110,111]	Fibronectin[112]	Creatine Kinase (mm-isozyme)[113,114]	Lysozyme[115]
SARCOMAS					
Malignant schwannoma		–			
Liposarcoma	–	– (0/2)			–
Chondrosarcoma					
Osteosarcoma		+			– (0/1)
Leiomyosarcoma		–		+	–
MFH		±	+		±
Fibrosarcoma	–	±			–
Rhabdomyosarcoma[99,113]	±			+	– (0/1)
Ewing's sarcoma[116]	–	– (1/1)			–
Synovial sarcoma[89,90]	±		+		–
Angiosarcoma	±				
Kaposi's sarcoma	±				
Epithelioid sarcoma[120]					
Clear cell sarcoma[117–119]					
Alveolar soft part sarcoma[121,122]					
Carcinoma			±		
Mesothelioma[93,97,123]					
Neuroblastoma					
Lymphoma/Leukemia					
Melanoma					
Desmoplastic melanoma[69]		+			
BENIGN LESIONS					
Neurilemmoma/ Neurofibroma					
Fibromatosis					
DFSP[#] (Pigmented and nonpigmented)					+
Leiomyoma					
Nodular fasciitis					

Antigens are related in the table to specific pathologic lesions and the differential diagnosis of poorly differentiated sarcoma. The symbol ± indicates variable staining results (in the range less than or equal to 50 percent of the cases), while – indicates lesions that stain very rarely or not at all. Where no data is currently available in the literature, a blank appears, for future updates by the user. Where data is based on only one or several cases, this is indicated numerically. Those results of particular diagnostic value—whether positive or negative—are highlighted in bold print, and are further discussed in the text. References reporting immunodiagnosis utilizing a particular antigen are cited at the top of the table, beside the name of the antigen. Articles reporting immunophemotyping of a particular type of lesion are cited with the name of the lesion at the left of the table.

DFSP is Dermatofibrosarcoma Protuberans.[98]

coma, and synovial sarcoma, a positive keratin stain is very supportive of the latter diagnosis.

Lymphoma/leukemia versus other sarcomas.   In recent years, numerous studies have been reported concerning antigenic markers characteristic of lymphomas and leukemias. Many of these antigens are restricted in their distribution to specific types of lymphoma or leukemia, and many also require frozen section technique for their demonstration. These features make them less useful for distinguishing the broad category of lymphoma/leukemia from other sarcomas and also less practical for routine diagnostic surgical pathology. Discovery of so-called "panhemato-lymphoid markers" which can be demonstrated in regular paraffin sections, circumvent the shortcomings of these other reagents. Most notably, the antibodies PD7/26 and 2B11 have these desirable characteristics.[98] They recognize an antigen present on virtually all lymphomatous and leukemic cell lines and often are very helpful and reliable in distinguishing these lesions from other sarcomas and from carcinomas. Other antibodies, such as T29/33 (recognizing T200-like antigen) also have panhematolymphoid specificity, but frozen section technique is required for their utilization.[124]

Sarcoma versus melanoma.   The presence of S-100 protein, as demonstrated by immunostaining, is very characteristic of malignant melanoma, including amelanotic mimics of sarcoma.[81,84] Again, this method must be used with discretion because certain classes of sarcoma also stain positively with S-100 (as noted in the following section).

Sarcomas with neural supportive differentiation versus other sarcomas.   The separation from one another of malignant schwannoma, malignant melanoma, and clear cell sarcoma of tendon sheaths and aponeuroses must rely on morphologic and clinical features of the lesions, rather than solely on S-100 staining since all may contain this substance.[80,81,84,119] In our experience, we have not found the intensity of staining for S-100 a very reliable criterion for separating such categories. Some chondrosarcomas and liposarcomas may also bear this antigen, but these are not usually differential diagnostic problems.[82] A substantial fraction of the malignant schwannomas are reported to lack S-100 antigen.[80] Thus, a negative result for S-100 must be interpreted carefully in the context of other morphologic and clinical information. However, several benign proliferations with neural supportive tissue differentiation which contain S-100 antigen (neurilemmoma, neurofibroma) may be reliably distinguished from dermatofibrosarcoma protuberans (DFSP), from pigmented DFSP, from

fibrous histiocytoma, and from nodular fasciitis, as our experience and the
scanty published reports indicate.[80]

Sarcomas with skeletal muscle differentiation versus other sarcomas. Although the presence of myoglobin is characteristic of *normal* skeletal muscle
differentiation, it is our experience that myoglobin is not usually demonstrable in cases of poorly differentiated rhabdomyosarcomas for which a
definite diagnosis is difficult by light microscopy. This is compatible with
the recently published experience of De Jong et al., whose excellent study
has also shown that fast myosin is a better marker for skeletal muscle
differentiation in less differentiated rhabdomyosarcomas.[99] The immunophenotyping reagents used by those authors may find wide application, once they are generally available.

In addition to the many useful immunophenotyping methods listed in
Table 10-8, one should be aware that the pathology landscape is littered
with antibody reagents which now find little application because they are
diagnostically largely irrelevant. This can be expected at a time when a
major new technology is finding its application, and we should anticipate
rapid evolution in this field, rather than stability. Antibodies against
creatine kinase, factor VIII related antigen, lysozyme, fibronectin, laminin,
collagen subtypes,[126] and myoglobin are among the reagents which we
would currently classify as less useful diagnostically. These antigens are
either widely present in many tissue types (creatine kinase), uncommon in
all but the better differentiated tumors (myoglobin, factor VIII), or of little
consequence because more diagnostically relevant antigens are available in
the same range of tumors (lysozyme, laminin, collagen subtypes, and
fibronectin). Our current negative evaluation of these reagents as diagnostic aids does not preclude, however, the possibility of some future
diagnostically or therapeutically relevant use for them.

Several caveats are also important for pathologists who apply these
new immunologic diagnostic methods to cases which are difficult to
classify by ordinary light microscopy. First, we cannot overemphasize that
in the current state of the surgical pathologist's art, differential diagnostic
possibilities should be winnowed first by light microscopy, after which
specific immunophenotyping reagents can be employed intelligently.
These reagents should not be used as initial screening batteries in place of
thinking. The latter habit can lead to confusion rather than clarification of
difficult cases. When the immunoperoxidase result appears to contradict
other evidence of differentiation established by light microscopy or electron
microscopy, the immunopathologic result should not be accepted uncriti-

cally, as we have often found has become a current tendency among pathologists.

Another of the reasons for caution relates to the relative complexity of proper immunophenotyping methods. These methods require careful attention to numerous details of proper technique as well as performance of positive and negative control stains. Monoclonal and polyclonal antibodies have different sensitivities and specificities which add to the complexity; false-positive and false-negative results can only be interpreted by those with abundant experience and good awareness of light microscopic constraints on interpretation of each case.

These cautions notwithstanding, we believe that immunophenotyping will prove to occupy an increasingly prominent role in the pathologist's practice in general, and in the specific problem of poorly differentiated sarcomas. Not only will immunoperoxidase methods grow to be of major use in reaching specific diagnostic decisions related to pre-existing categories of sarcomas, but we may also anticipate that they may have an increasing role in *regrouping and reclassifying* what are now considered light microscopically distinctive entities. Examples of this process of reclassification are already available in the pathology literature and illustrate some of the pitfalls as well. For example, alveolar soft part sarcoma—a sarcoma of previously unknown histogenesis—was recently proposed to be reclassified as "angiorenioma," mainly based on the immunohistologic demonstration of renin in the cytoplasm.[122] A subsequent study by others, however, questioned the specificity of the antibodies used in this demonstration of renin and failed to confirm the presence of renin in the alveolar soft part sarcoma cells, both by biochemical and immunohistologic means.[121]

A more subtle difficulty of renaming entities is exemplified by the recent history of the entity "clear cell sarcoma of tendons and aponeuroses."[125] Because of the presence of melanin pigment and S-100 protein, this tumor was recently reclassified as "melanoma of soft parts,"[119] despite the fact that many of the morphologic and clinical features are quite distinct from ordinary malignant melanomas of skin. In appraising the merits of reclassifying "clear cell sarcoma" as "melanoma of soft parts," we must question whether this moniker is histogenically more accurate and whether the renaming will prove clinically useful. With regard to the first of these issues, we note that several recent studies have demonstrated some electron microscopic features of schwann cell-like differentiation, as well as melanocytic differentiation, in these clear cell sarcomas.[117,118] Does renaming them "melanomas" obscure this strange hybrid character of these lesions? With regard to the second question, we have encountered therapeutic indecision on the part of clinicians, related to the new name, "melanoma of soft parts." Specifically this has related to the utility of adjuvant therapy appropriate for sarcoma, on the one hand, versus treatment appropriate for ordinary melanoma on the other. Other questions are also raised. Do pigmented clear cell sarcomas behave differently than those which are not pigmented? Do those with S-100 antigen behave differently than those few without?

As in the case of electron microscopy, discussed earlier in this chapter, it is essential that new immunopathologic data be carefully integrated into the existing clinical and pathologic framework. The natural tendency is to propose a new partition of a group of neoplasms based upon recently developed technology before attention has been given to building the requisite clinicopathologic linkages that tie the new observations to clinical outcomes. In the interim, while the relevant clinicopathologic studies are being performed, it is reasonable to base clinical decisions on sensible expansions or alterations of previously defined clinicopathologic categories. A little skepticism is appropriate; we should not be so credulous as to believe that every straw in the pathologist's growing haystack is a clinically relevant needle.

Assuming that the Neoplasm is a Soft Tissue Sarcoma, what Prognostically and Therapeutically Relevant Morphologic Features Should Be Noted?

We have reached the final stage in the diagnostic investigation of the poorly differentiated soft tissue neoplasm. We have eliminated the benign and malignant mimics of sarcoma and are now left with a "poorly differentiated" sarcoma. What are the important prognostic and therapeutic decisions to be made?

In this regard, it is helpful to recognize that from the therapist's point of view, the current morphologic classificaton of the soft tissue neoplasms is probably overly complex for his purposes. In fact, the morphologic distinctions that have proliferated in classifications over recent years are, from a practical viewpoint, more finely drawn than either the natural histories of these neoplasms or their response to currently available therapies would necessarily warrant. The tendency of a more pragmatic clinicopathologic approach would be toward "lumping" of some categories. For example, after excision, soft tissue neoplasms generally exhibit one of five possible patterns of clinical behavior:

Clinical disease I	They neither recur nor metastasize.
Clinical disease II	They may on occasion recur (less than 10 percent of cases) but never metastasize
Clinical disease III	They frequently recur but never metastasize.
Clinical disease IV	They frequently recur and metastasize (often after local recurrence).
Clinical disease V	They metastasize with such regularity that they are usefully considered systemic diseases at the outset.

Taking a radical clinical view, soft tissue neoplasms could then be regarded for therapeutic purposes as though they were five clinical diseases. In the first case, nothing more need be done (the lesion is clinically benign). In the second case, either doing nothing or performing a wider local excision might be appropriate. In the third and fourth cases, definitive local therapy (usually surgical) is performed and adjuvant therapy is sometimes employed in the fourth category. In case five, therapy is systemic at the outset with some nonradical approach to the site of initial local presentation.

There may be some variation within a given clinical disease in the frequency with which the defining clinical events occur, but typically these differences are not sufficiently great to warrant alternative therapy at this time. Clinical diseases four and five are the ones most likely to be subdivided as new chemotherapeutic agents are developed, and the differential responses of morphologic variants are observed.

This underlying simplicity of the clinical choices need not always be recognized by the pathologist when he classifies a well-differentiated sarcoma, that is, a sarcoma which morphologically fits neatly into one of the myriad well-described categories. Nevertheless, in such easily classified cases, specific clinicopathologic studies are readily available to the clinician to tie the pathologist's morphologic diagnosis to knowledge about prognosis and therapy. On the other hand, when dealing with a *poorly differentiated* and difficult to classify sarcoma, the pathologist may be tempted to construct a lengthy report of morphologic distinctions which, in reality, make little or no clinical difference and which offer little guidance to the clinician in planning therapy. *In the process he may neglect consideration of some practical variables that should govern therapy and prognosis in these cases.* In fact this is a general problem with the classifications of soft tissue sarcomas, which are so heavily invested in histopathologic evidence of differentiation. One is left with only fragmentary data relating features other than differentiation to clinical outcomes, such variables as size, location, nuclear anaplasia, mitotic activity, etc. For example, the World Health Organization classification is a "splitter's" paradise including numerous types defined by differentiation and proposed histogenesis.[127]

The exigencies of therapy are more realistically addressed in the proposed AJC Grading-Staging scheme,[128–130] and NCI grading scheme[131] which employ a variety of variables in addition to differentiation in stratifying patient populations.

We employ the WHO scheme[127] in our morphologic distinction-making, but attempt to translate the significance of these distinctions into meaningful clinically directive diagnoses. Specifically, when we cannot arrive at an unequivocal histologic subclassification of a soft tissue tumor, we try to place the case into one of the five clinical disease groups defined above. Given the available evidence of prognostic indicators other than differentiation, we suggest that once a difficult-to-classify soft tissue neoplasm has been judged to be a sarcoma, answers to the following questions are the most relevant in guiding subsequent management.

Does the sarcoma involve the skin, the superfical or the deep soft tissues? In some differentiated types of soft tissue sarcomas the location of the neoplasm has been shown to be of considerable prognostic significance. This would appear to be true for some malignant fibrous histiocytomas[132] and may be true for well-differentiated fatty tumors.[10] For example, there is a neoplasm in the fibrous histiocytoma group, atypical fibroxanthoma, that is, in essential respects, histologically identical to a sarcoma in this group, malignant fibrous histiocytoma.[132] Atypical fibroxanthoma occurs, by definition, in the skin, while malignant fibrous histiocytomas are encountered instead in either the superficial or deep soft tissues. Atypical fibroxanthoma pursues a benign clinical course in the vast majority of cases, while malignant fibrous histiocytomas show an increasing tendency to metastasize depending upon whether they are superficially situated in the subcutaneous tissue and fascia or extend more deeply to involve muscle.[132] In this group of neoplasms, evaluation of histology alone provides much less prognostic insight than when histologic data is combined with a knowledge of the lesion's location. Similarly, the behavior of fatty tumors composed of atypical "adult" adipocytes varies depending upon location. These important clinical differences are embodied in the terms "atypical lipoma" or "pleomorphic lipoma" for superficially located fatty tumors with atypical lipoblasts,[8–10] while a histologically identical neoplasm located in the retroperitoneum is labeled "well-differentiated liposarcoma."[10] The latter designation is considered appropriate for retroperitoneal tumors both because local recurrence in this site is usual and often fatal, and because some authorities believe that well-differentiated fatty tumors in the retroperitoneum and deep soft tissues can metastasize. Similarly, Ranchod and Kempson found that all of the thirteen

retroperitoneal smooth muscle tumors which they studied behaved aggressively.[133] It is presumably such data that have led to the widely held
belief[134] that location of a sarcoma in superficial versus deep compartments
of the soft tissues (or in other specific sites such as the retroperitoneum)
may often be an important prognostic indicator independent of other
variables such as histologic type. Similarly, location of the neoplasm *may* be
an important variable for a sarcoma which is difficult to classify. Thus, we
advocate inclusion of this parameter in the assessment of the likelihood of
recurrence of such a poorly differentiated tumor and in treatment
decisions.

Is the margin of surgical excision adequate?   Adequate surgical excision is
an extremely important determinant of prognosis and bears directly on the
issue of local recurrence.[1,135] While seemingly adequate surgical margins
about a poorly differentiated sarcoma unfortunately are no guarantee that
the neoplasm will not recur, inadequate surgical margins, proven histologically, virtually guarantee recurrence in our experience. Oftentimes this
vitally important prognostic indicator is obscured in pathology reports by
extended discussions of histogenesis or speculation about differentiated
cell types of little or no clinical significance. Careful examination and
documentation of the surgical margins is essential.

What is the size of the sarcoma?   Several studies of specific types of soft
tissue sarcomas have shown the importance of tumor size in predicting
clinical outcome. For example, increasing size is correlated with increased
recurrence rate and metastatic rate in liposarcomas[136–138] and with metastatic rate in malignant fibrous histiocytomas.[132] Tumor size was also found
to be a helpful indicator of clinical aggressiveness in gastrointestinal
smooth muscle tumors.[133]

There are both theoretical reasons and experimental data in some
systems[139] to suggest that tumor doubling time is a better indicator of
prognosis than tumor size *per se*. A measurement of tumor doubling time
is not available clinically, however, in initial stages of management of a soft
tissue sarcomas, and is generally available only subsequently after metastases have occurred. Tumor size is also not independent of location since
sarcomas in the thigh, for example, typically attain a much larger size
before initial clinical presentation than those arising more distally in the
extremity. Nevertheless, a measurement of tumor size belongs in every
pathology report of such lesions, and may prove to be an independent
prognostic factor.

Since, by definition, cell type is ill-defined for poorly differentiated sarcomas, what other histopathologic features of the sarcoma might be related to prognosis and therapy? Although a lack of differentiation is often loosely equated with nuclear anaplasia, the two terms mean quite different things in surgical pathology (see Table 10-1). In actual fact, most poorly differentiated sarcomas are also anaplastic, but this is not always the case. Nuclear features and mitotic rate are easily evaluable, even in the absence of evidence of specific cytoplasmic or architectural differentiation. Other features, such as tumor necrosis and cellularity, are also evaluable. There are few studies of the relationship of nuclear anaplasia, cellularity, and mitotic rate to clinical outcomes for specific tumor subtypes among the sarcomas. Some work has been done with fibrosarcomas. For example, Van der Werf-Messing and Van Unnik[140] showed a direct relationship between mitotic rate and metastatic rate, and Pritchard et al.,[141] demonstrated a dependence of survival on "grade," a parameter that included nuclear features, cellularity, and mitotic rate in their study. An assessment of nuclear anaplasia and mitotic figure counts were also included in the earlier methods of grading soft tissue tumors in a large, cooperative study of sarcomas of the AJC.[128,129,130]

More recently, Costa et al. have subjected to more refined analysis the grading parameters used in earlier studies.[131] They relied on data derived from treating 163 sarcoma patients, according to defined protocol, at the National Cancer Institute (NCI). A broad range of sarcomas was analyzed, including 23 unclassifiable cases. The statistical analyses in this study were stratified to remove from consideration the effects of treatment and location of tumor on survival, and to focus on the effect of histopathologic variables. Mitotic activity was shown to have a statistically significant effect on overall survival, and some trend toward an effect on time to recurrence. Cellularity, pleomorphism, and matrix production by the sarcomatous cells could not be shown, however, to have an independent prognostic importance.

More importantly, the NCI study focused attention on necrosis, a histopathologic parameter which generally has been considered of minor importance in grading schemes. The results of this study emphasize the need for the pathologist to consider the following question in his evaluation of each sarcoma case, including poorly differentiated and unclassifiable lesions.

What evidence of necrosis is there in the sarcoma? Costa et al. have demonstrated a highly significant effect on overall patient survival and a significant effect on time to tumor recurrence of the finding of necrosis in sarcomas.[131] In this NCI study, the authors included all forms of necrosis in their category (whether inflammatory or ischemic, individual cell or geographic), as long as the necrosis was not clearly the result of previous surgery or ulceration. Tumors were divided into two groups: (1) those with absent or minimal necrosis (up to 15 percent of the sample), and (2) those with moderate to massive necrosis. These rules offer some guidelines for the practicing pathologist in applying this grading criterion. However, some questions remain.

As mentioned earlier in this chapter, the detection of differentiated cell types in a sarcoma often requires extensive sampling of the neoplasm for histopathologic examination. A natural and probably irrepressable tendency for the examining pathologist is to sample those regions which grossly appear most likely to be contributory in this regard, a practice which would naturally tend to steer one away from areas of obvious necrosis. Costa et al. give the following guidelines for adequate tumor sampling in their report: at least two sections in lesions up to 3 cm in size, at least five sections for lesions up to 10 cm in size, and up to 10 sections for lesions 20 cm or larger.[131] Unfortunately, these guidelines do not specifically address the issue of *directed sampling,* the process by which every pathologist selects his blocks for microscopic examination. We suspect that as the general awareness increases of the importance of necrosis as a variable for grading soft tissue sarcomas, there will be a subtle change towards examining microscopically more tissue from necrotic regions of neoplasms, since these can often be identified grossly. We should be cognizant that this type of directed sampling may represent an uncontrollable variable, tending to bias application of this grading scheme suggested by the NCI. Perhaps estimation of the amount of necrosis at the level of gross examination, and subsequent confirmation of necrosis by microscopic examination, would circumvent of this problem. Other strategies to avoid this bias might also be devised.

Grade I neoplasms in the NCI scheme are especially important to recognize because they probably do not need adjuvant therapy if excision has been complete. Moreover, if they do cause the patient further difficulty, it is usually by local recurrence. Metastases are unusual unless the tumors come back morphologically worse than they started. The grade II and grade III neoplasms are more aggressive, and metastases can be expected in a substantial proportion of cases. It should be noted that the rules for placing lesions in the grade I category in the NCI scheme are *type-specific,* putting a premium on distinguishing the form of cytoplasmic differentiation.[131] Fortunately for grade I lesions, this is seldom a problem because these lesions tend to be reasonably well-differentiated in terms of cytoplasmic and architectural phenotype, just as they tend to lack features of nuclear anaplasia and tumor necrosis. Several specific concerns may be raised, however, about grading assignments made in the NCI scheme.

First, no category of low-grade synovial sarcoma is recognized by the NCI group, which appears to be an error in light of the recently reported prognostically favorable category of extensively calcified synovial sarcoma.[2a] Secondly, the assignment of myxoid lesions in the NCI scheme differs somewhat from our experience. We agree that most myxoid malignant fibrous histiocytomas would be considered grade II (or even sometimes grade III) neoplasms on the basis of cytologic features, whereas myxoid liposarcomas are cytologically low-grade neoplasms. The classic myxoid malignant fibrous histiocytiocytoma demonstrates considerable cellular pleomorphism, contains bizarre giant cells at least focally, and often has a frankly sarcomatous stroma. These features are not present in myxoid liposarcoma. Myxoid liposarcoma generally demonstrates lipoblastic differentiation somewhere in the neoplasm and a characteristic plexiform vascular pattern. Bland myxoid malignant fibrous histiocytomas, however, indistinguishable from myxoid liposarcoma except for the absence of lipoblasts and the characteristic vasculature, do occur. Behavior of these low-grade neoplasms is identical, in our experience, to that of myxoid liposarcoma, i.e., they are recurring neoplasms; they do not metastasize unless they come back worse than they started.

We may summarize that, in our view, grading of sarcomas is extremely important. Largely by analogy to experience with neoplasms of various other organ systems, and partly in response to specific published pathologic data relating to sarcomas, it would appear useful to attempt *always* to define "grade" of soft tissue sarcomas, even if the specific cell type towards which the cells are differentiated is inapparent. Mitotic figure counts and necrosis should generally be included in this assessment. Whether the grading decision should rely as heavily upon necrosis as a single criterion, as does the distinction of grade II and grade III sarcomas in the NCI approach, or whether it should involve a multivariate approach, i.e., including assessment of mitotic rate, remains untested.

Histologic Distinctions Versus Clinical Differences

In contrast to the variables just outlined, some of the distinctions based on histogenesis or cellular differentiation drawn from soft tissue literature have less clinical significance whatever merit they may have on other scientific grounds. Recognition of this fact should serve to direct the surgical pathologist's efforts to extracting the most clinically relevant information from each case. This outlook will also serve to relieve the sometimes unwarranted pressure to find some grounds—no matter how slender, ambiguous or irreproducible—upon which to pidgeon-hole every sarcoma according to its putative differentiation. For example, let us examine a variety of histologic distinctions which can often pose a problem for the pathologist from the standpoint of their clinical significance.

Pleomorphic (Adult) Rhabdomyosarcoma Versus Pleomorphic Malignant Fibrous Histiocytoma Versus Pleomorphic Liposarcoma

Although pleomorphic rhabdomyosarcoma was a popular diagnosis some years ago for pleomorphic sarcomas occurring in adults, it has currently been defined almost out of existence. The insistence on evidence of skeletal muscle differentiation, such as cross striations by light micros-copy, or ultrastructural evidence of thick and thin filaments or Z band-like structures, has reduced the pleomorphic rhabdomyosarcoma ranks to a few collector's cases although this type of differentiation may be seen in nerve sheath sarcomas and Triton tumors.[142] Sarcomas containing large cells with eosinophilic cytoplasm that would have been categorized as pleomorphic rhabdomyosarcoma in the past are now classified among the pleomorphic malignant fibrous histiocytomas, because acceptable evidence of skeletal muscle differentiation cannot be demonstrated by light micros-copy or by electron microscopy. The renaming of this group of pleomor-phic sarcomas, although descriptively more accurate, has not changed their clinical behavior. Nor have those few pleomorphic sarcomas in adults which do demonstrate structural evidence of skeletal muscle differentiation been shown to have a behavior notably different from cases called pleomorphic malignant fibrous histiocytoma.

Recently, a few pleomorphic rhabdomyosarcomas in young patients have been shown by immunohistologic methods to contain myoglobin and fast myosin, features of a rhabdomyosarcoma immunophenotype.[99] What effect such methods will have on the classification of pleomorphic sarcomas in adults remains uncertain. A few malignant fibrous histiocytomas have been reported negative for myoglobin and fast myosin.[99] Considering the history of the reclassifications of these pleomorphic neoplasms, we would not be surprised to find a mixture of immunophenotypes in the currently defined categories. Whether investigation of immunophenotype will be-come a common definitional requirement in the work-up of pleomorphic sarcomas will surely depend in part on whether any clinical implications for positive or negative staining for these muscle-associated antigens can be demonstrated.

The distinction between pleomorphic liposarcoma and pleomorphic malignant fibrous histiocytoma is often difficult because the two tumors share many morphologic features and lipoblasts are often sparse and difficult to recognize in pleomorphic liposarcoma. Most of the available literature suggests pleomorphic liposarcoma and pleomorphic malignant fibrous histiocytoma have the same clinical behavior, although contrary claims have been made.[143]

Monomorphic Spindled Sarcomas

Monomorphic spindled sarcomas are often difficult for the pathologist to distinguish from one another. The clinical differences among these neoplasms include the following characteristics.

There is a greater predilection of synovial sarcoma to metastasize to lymph nodes. Ordinary biphasic synovial sarcoma by virtue of its biphasic pattern would seem to be a fairly tightly defined and easily recognized morphologic entity; its characteristic age and site predilection, radiologic appearance of calcified lesions, and tendency to metastasize to lymph nodes would seem to be real.[30,144] To our knowledge, these clinical observations have not led to the recommendation that lymph node dissections be employed in the management of synovial sarcomas. Whether these clinical differences between classic biphasic synovial sarcoma and other monomorphous spindled tumors, such as fibrosarcoma and the fibrous variant of malignant fibrous histiocytoma, are sufficiently distinct and important to lend much support to a category of *monophasic* synovial sarcoma is uncertain.[144,145] What is involved to establish the utility of such an entity is the demonstration of a monomorphous spindled cell neoplasm whose behavior resembles more that of classic biphasic synovial sarcoma than that of fibrosarcoma. One of the problems with evaluating the utility of a monophasic synovial sarcoma category has been the difficulty of crisply defining the category by light microscopy. In the absence of such well-defined criteria, clinicopathologic studies to demonstrate differences in clinical behavior become almost impossible. Recent studies utilizing keratin antibodies indicate that many light microscopically "monophasic" synovial sarcomas may contain keratin.[89] Thus it may now be possible to reliably separate a monophasic synovial sarcoma immunophenotype from other monophasic spindle cell sarcomas, recognizing that this has not yet proven to be a distinction with clinical importance for the monophasic lesions. Certainly at this time, in poorly differentiated and ambiguous cases, the distinction cannot be considered critical operationally.

The clinical differences among these spindled sarcomas also include the association of nerve sheath sarcoma with von Recklinghausen's disease. Only a small percentage of patients with nerve sheath sarcoma, even when strictly defined, have associated stigmata of von Recklinghausen's disease.[146,147] Obviously, this is an important clinical consideration to be raised when any monomorphous spindled neoplasm is encountered in association with a nerve. Even a biphasic neoplasm, ostensibly synovial sarcoma, may actually represent a neurofibrosarcoma with glandular differentiation, since such lesions have been reported, especially in von Recklinghausen's disease.[143] In this regard, the search for other stigmata of von Recklinghausen's disease including brain tumors and other maldevelopmental or neoplastic peripheral nerve lesions, is warranted.

The clinical differences among these monophasic sarcomas also include the claimed association of multiple leiomyosarcomas of the soft tissues with leiomyosarcoma of the retroperitoneum. Series of leiomyosarcomas from Scandinavia[148] have suggested an association between cutaneous smooth muscle neoplasms and retroperitoneal neoplasms. This association would seem to be real but extraordinarily infrequent and has not been confirmed by others.[149,150] Leiomyosarcomas of skin and soft tissue are, in our experience, uncommon lesions. They become less common as one's criteria for smooth muscle differentiation become stricter.

We would suggest that once these relatively minor clinical associations have been raised, the actual management of the various spindled sarcomas is *essentially the same* and depends on size, site, and grade (see earlier section on grading).

Myxoid Fibrous Histiocytoma and Myxoid Liposarcoma

In our experience there is some morphologic overlap between these two entities as noted above. The morphologic overlap is most apparent when the cytologically bland end of the spectrum of myxoid malignant fibrous histiocytomas is compared to lesions classified as myxoid liposarcoma. Nevertheless, in concert with our recurring theme, when deeply seated, both of these lesions have been reported to have very similar behaviors.[137,151] Myxoid fibrous histiocytoma may involve the superficial soft tissues (in which case its prognosis is good), whereas myxoid liposarcomas rarely develop in the subcutaneous tissues.[137]

Table 10-9
Small Blue Cell Neoplasms Primary in the Soft Tissues

Tumor treated on the IRS protocols
  Alveolar rhabdomyosarcoma
  Mixed alveolar and embryonal rhabdomyosarcoma
  Soft tissue Ewing's sarcoma—Small Cell (Undifferentiated—Type I)
  Soft tissue Ewing's sarcoma—Large Cell (Undifferentiated—Type II)
  Undifferentiated mesenchymal small cell tumor
Other small blue cell neoplasms, reported in small series
  Malignant small cell tumor of the thoracopulmonary region
  Chest wall sarcoma of childhood with a good prognosis, "Vasoformative small
    cell tumor"

Small Blue Cell Tumors

The differential diagnosis of the small blue cell tumor (SBCT)[152,153] is an important problem in pediatric pathology that has been recently reviewed.[153,154] Assuming that one has excluded presentation of lymphoma or leukemia as a soft tissue mass and excluded metastasis or extension from some other site such as bone (Ewing's sarcoma, small cell osteosarcoma, mesenchymal chondrosarcoma), adrenal (neuroblastoma), CNS (medulloblastoma) or orbit (retinoblastoma), the problem then becomes one of assigning the case to one of the existing clinicopathologic categories listed in Table 10-9.

This subclassification of differentiated forms of SBCT into the categories of Table 10-9 may be extremely difficult in some cases, if not impossible, for the surgical pathologist. Our assessment of the difficulties of this histologic differential diagnosis, however, may be considerably modified by some familiarity with clinical aspects of these childhood sarcomas. The best insights into the treatment and prognosis of SBCT of soft tissues have been provided by the ongoing Intergroup Rhabdomyosarcoma Study (IRS).[152,152a] An important observation of the IRS from the point of view of the practicing pathologist is that all of these neoplasms responded *in a similar fashion* to the therapies that were evaluated by the IRS with the exception of alveolar rhabdomyosarcoma which had a poorer prognosis than the others, independent of other features such as site of origin.[155] This has lead to the suggestion that alveolar rhabdomyosarcoma should be treated more aggressively than the other neoplasms in this group.[156] It would seem to follow that the pathologist's energies should be directed toward distinguishing alveolar rhabdomyosarcoma from the other neoplasms in this differential diagnosis. Unfortunately, alveolar rhabdomyosarcoma does not separate sharply from embryonal rhabdomyosarcoma morphologically. Many cases show both patterns, and evolution from one pattern to the other is frequently observed. While many cases are easily recognized as one or the other form of rhabdomyosarcoma, assignment of cases with overlapping features is fraught with many practical difficulties.

This has led to an attempt to evaluate the prognostic significance of individual histologic features, such as nuclear anaplasia.[157] Traditional morphologic syndromes (such as alveolar rhabdomyosarcoma) would thus be decomposed into their constituent cytologic and architectural components. Regression analysis would then be used to pinpoint favorable or unfavorable histologic features. This is the tack that has been pursued successfully in the Wilms' tumor studies,[158] and is similar in some respects to the approach of Costa in grading of adult soft tissue sarcomas at the NCI.[131] The pathologists reanalyzing the data derived from the IRS have identified anaplastic cytology and/or monomorphous round cell features as unfavorable histologic findings. These have been tested in logistic-regression models and are the second best predictors after stage. Interestingly, from the point of view of our thesis, the groups derived from an evaluation of individual cytologic features do not correspond to the groupings obtained by using the traditional rhabdomyosarcoma categories.

Several small series of patients with soft tissue SBCT have been published in which histologic and/or clinicopathologic features have been thought to be distinctive. Malignant small cell tumor of the thoracopulmonary region in childhood[153,159,161] and a chest wall sarcoma of childhood, "vasoformative tumor,"[160] are examples. It is difficult to interpret the therapeutic significance of findings in these studies of highly selected patients. These studies are certainly suggestive of some clinical differences and would lead one to search larger groups of unselected uniformly treated patients, such as those studied in the IRS protocols, to see if these groups still emerge.

Clear Cell Sarcoma, Epithelioid Sarcoma, and Synovial Sarcoma

Morphologic differences between classic examples of these three types are real and easily recognized by the expert pathologist, and immunophenotyping for keratin and S-100 may assist in these distinctions, as discussed earlier in this chapter. There are also minor clinical differences (such as the forearm site predilection and tendency to simulate an ulcerating inflammatory process of epithelioid sarcoma). We wish to point out, however, that a diagnostic error among these categories translates into no therapeutic difference. It will be interesting whether in future the melanogenic form of clear cell sarcoma shows any clinically important differences from other sarcomas in this group (including the nonmelanogenic clear cell sarcomas), especially in response to chemotherapy regimens. Similarly it will be interesting to note whether immunophenotype for keratin or S-100 is prognostically or therapeutically significant.

Conclusions

These are pragmatic views of sarcoma classification differing somewhat from the conventional belief in a pathologist's ability to segregate *each* case into distinct and reproducible histogenetic categories. These observations are not meant to suggest that an attempt to characterize the histologic type of a poorly differentiated soft tissue sarcoma is without clinical and scientific merit. Obviously, this exercise, at the very least, will serve to eliminate various mimics of sarcoma in the soft tissues, both benign and malignant, and will presumably result in the creation of relatively reproducible and homogeneous groups upon which to base clinical studies of new or revised treatment regimens. Thus, we strongly suggest an effort to characterize as many variables of cellular differentiation as possible in the assessment of soft tissue neoplasms. Such a process will also have scientific dividends as we learn more about the phenotypes expressed by neoplastic cells. However, if arbitrary distinctions based on minor histopathologic differences are to be employed in daily practice or in clinicopathologic studies, it is essential that the pathologic criteria used to segregate cases be spelled out in detail. We would prefer, as does Enterline, that tumors not be forced into categories on "shaky and slender grounds" and for little clinical purpose.[162]

References

1. Rosenberg SA, Glatstein E: The management of local and regional soft tissue sarcomas, in Principles of Cancer Treatment. New York, McGraw-Hill, 1982, pp 697–706
2. Lieberman Z, Ackerman LV: Principles in management of soft tissue

sarcomas: A clinical and pathologic review of one hundred cases. Surgery 35:350–365, 1954

2a. Varela-Duran J, Enzinger FM: Calcifying synovial sarcoma. Cancer 50:
345–352, 1982

3. Lauer DH, Enzinger FM: Cranial fasciitis of childhood. Cancer 45:401–406, 1980

4. Patchefsky AS, Enzinger FM: Intravascular fasciitis. A report of 17 cases. Am J Surg Pathol 5:29–36, 1981

5. Colby TV: Malakoplakia: Two unusual cases which presented diagnostic problems. Am J Surg Pathol 2:377–382, 1978

6. Weiss SW, Enzinger FM, Johnson FB: Silica reaction simulating fibrous histiocytoma. Cancer 42:2738–2743, 1978

7. Fu Y, Perzin KH: Non-epithelial tumors of the nasal cavity, paranasal sinuses and nasopharynx: A clinicopathologic study. VII. Myxomas. Cancer 39:195–203, 1977

8. Enzinger FM: Benign lipomatous tumors simulating sarcoma, in M. D. Anderson Tumor Institute (ed): Management of primary bone and soft tissue tumors. Chicago, Year Book Medical Publishers, 1977, pp 11–24

9. Shmookler BM, Enzinger FM: Pleomorphic Lipoma: a benign tumor simulating liposarcoma, a clinicopathologic analysis of 48 cases. Cancer 47:126–133, 1981

10. Evans HL, Soule EH, Winkelmann RK: Atypical lipoma, atypical intramuscular lipoma, and well differentiated retroperitoneal liposarcoma. Cancer 43:574–584, 1979

11. Allen PW: The fibromatoses: A clinicopathologic classification based on 140 cases. Am J Surg Pathol 1:255–270, 1977

12. Chung EB, Enzinger FM: Infantile fibrosarcoma. Cancer 38:729–739, 1976

13. Soule EH, Pritchard DJ: Fibrosarcoma in infants and children: A review of 110 cases. Cancer 40:1711–1721, 1977

14. Hutter RVP, Foote FW Jr, Francis KC, et al: Parosteal fasciitis: A self limited benign process that simulates a malignant neoplasm. Am J Surg 104:800–807, 1962

15. McCarthy EF, Ireland DCR, Sprague BL, et al: Parosteal (nodular) fasciitis of the hand. A case report. J Bone Joint Surg 58A:714–716, 1976

16. Spjut HJ, Dorfman HD: Florid reactive periostitis of the tubular bones of the hands and feet. A benign lesion which may simulate osteosarcoma. Am J Surg Pathol 5:423–433, 1981

17. Clearkin KP, Enzinger FM: Intravascular papillary endothelial hyperplasia. Arch Pathol Lab Med 100:441–444, 1976

18. Kuo TT, Sayers CP, Rosai J: Masson's "vegetant intravascular hemangioendothelioma": A lesion often mistaken for angiosarcoma. Study of seventeen cases located in the skin and soft tissues. Cancer 38:1227–1236, 1976

19. Rosai J, Gold J, Landy R: The histoiocytoid hemangiomas. A unifying concept embracing several previously described entities of skin, soft tissue, large vessels, bone and heart. Hum Pathol 10:707–730, 1979

20. Weiss SW, Enzinger FM: Epithelioid Hemangioendothelioma. A vascular tumor often mistaken for a carcinoma. Cancer 50:970–981, 1982

21. Allen PW: Nodular fasciitis. Pathol 4:9–26, 1972

22. Bernstein KE, Lattes R: Nodular (Pseudosarcomatous) fasciitis, a nonrecurrent lesion: clinicopathologic study of 134 cases. Cancer 49:1668–1678, 1982

23. Wirman JA: Nodular fasciitis, a lesion of myofibroblasts. An ultrastructural study. Cancer 38:2378–2389, 1976

24. Meister P, Buckmann FW, Konrad E: Nodular fasciitis. (Analysis of 100 cases and review of the literature) Path Res Pract 162:133–165, 1978

25. Chung EB, Enzinger FM: Proliferative fasciitis. Cancer 36:1450–1458, 1975

26. Enzinger FM, Dulcey F: Proliferative myositis. Report of 33 cases. Cancer 20:2213–2223, 1967

27. Allen PW: Myxoid tumors of soft tissues. Pathol Ann 15:133–192, 1980

28. Mackenzie DH: The myxoid tumors of somatic soft tissues. Am J Surg Pathol 5:443–458, 1981

29. Kindblom LG, Angervall L: Histochemical characterization of mucosubstances in bone and soft tissue tumors. Cancer 36:985–994, 1975

30. Evans HL: Synovial sarcoma: A study of 23 biphasic and 17 probable monophasic examples. Pathol Ann 15:309–331, 1980

31. Rosas-Uribe A, Rappaport H: Malignant lymphoma "histicytic" type with sclerosis (sclerosing reticulum cell sarcoma). Cancer 29:945–953, 1972

32. Turner RR, Wood GS, Beckstead JR, et al: Histiocytic malignancies morphologic, immunologic, and enzymatic heterogeneity. Am J Surg Pathol 8:485–500, 1984

33. Herman DL, Bullock WK, Waken JK: Giant cell adenocarcinoma of the lung. Cancer 19:1337–1346, 1966
34. Wang, NS, Seemayer TA, Ahmed MN, et al: Giant cell carcinoma of the lung: A light and electron microscopic study. Hum Pathol 7:3–16, 1976
35. Compagno J, Hyams VJ, Lepore ML: Nasal polyposis with stromal atypia: Review and follow-up study of 14 cases. Arch Pathol Lab Med 100:224–226, 1976
36. Smith CJH, Echavarria R, McLelland CA: Pseudosarcomatous changes in antrochoanal polyps. Arch Otolaryngol 99:228–230, 1974
37. Michinson MJ: Aortic disease in idiopathic retroperitoneal and mediastinal fibrosis. J Clin Pathol 25:287–293, 1972
38. Proppe KH, Scully RE, Rosai J: Postoperative spindle cell nodules of genitourinary tract resembling sarcomas. A report of eight cases. Am J Surg Pathol 8:101–108, 1984
39. Alguacil-Garcia A, Weiland LH: The histologic spectrum, prognosis and histogenesis of the sarcomatoid carcinoma of the pancreas. Cancer 36:1181–1189, 1977
40. Tschang RP, Garza-Garza R, Kissane JM: Pleomorphic carcinoma of the pancreas. An analysis of 15 cases. Cancer 39:2114–2126, 1977
41. Rosai J: Carcinoma of pancreas simulating giant cell tumor of bone; electron microscopic evidence of its acinar cell origin. Cancer 22:333–344, 1968
42. Gersell DJ, Katzenstein ALA: Spindle cell carcinoma of the breast: A clinicopathologic and ultrastructural study. Hum Pathol 12:550–561, 1981
43. Munoz PA, Rao MS, Reddy JK: Osteoclastoma-like giant cell tumor of the liver. Cancer 46:771–779, 1980
44. Chirayil SJ, Tobon H: Polyps of the vagina: A clinicopathologic study of 18 cases. Cancer 47:2904–2907, 1981
45. Norris JH, Taylor HB: Polyps of the vagina: A benign lesion resembling sarcoma botryoides. Cancer 19:227–232, 1966
46. Prat J, Scully RE: Ovarian mucinous tumors with sarcoma-like mural nodules: A report of seven cases. Cancer 44:2322–1344, 1979
47. Johnsone JM, Morson BC: Inflammatory fibroid polyp of the gastrointestinal tract. Histopathol 2:349–361, 1978
48. Suen KC, Burton JD: The spectrum of eosinophilic infiltration of the gastrointestinal tract and its relationship to other disorders of angitis granulomatosis. Hum Pathol 10:31–43, 1979
49. Bonikos DS, Bensch KG, Kempson RL: The contribution of electron

microscopy to the differential diagnosis of tumors. Beitr Path Bd 158:417–444, 1976

50. Carr I, Toner PG: Rapid electron microscopy in oncology. J Clin Pathol 30:13–15, 1977

51. Gyorkey F, Min KW, Krisdo I, et al: The usefulness of electron microscopy in the diagnosis of human tumors. Hum Pathol 6: 421–441, 1975

52. Johannessen JV: Use of paraffin material for electron microscopy. Pathol Ann 12:189–224, 1977

53. Ghadially FN: Diagnostic Electron Microscopy of Tumors. Butterworths, London, 1980

54. Henderson DW, Papadimitriou JM: Ultrastructural Appearances of Tumors: A Diagnostic Atlas. Churchill Livingston, Edinburgh, 1982

55. Palfrey AJ, Davis DV: The fine structure of chondrocytes. J Anat 100:213, 1966

56. Trelstad RL, Revel JP, Hay ED: Tight junctions between cells in the early chick embryo as visualized with the electron microscope. J Cell Biol 31:C6, 1966

57. Trelstad RL, Hay ED, Revel JP: Cell contact during early morphogenesis in the chick embryo. Devl Biol 16:78, 1967

58. Ross R, Greenlle TK: Electron microscopy: Attachments sites between connective tissue cells. Science 153:997, 1966

59. Kubo T: A note on fine structure of synovial sarcoma. Acta Pathol Jpn 24:163–168, 1974

60. Alvira MM, Mandybur TI, Menefee MG: Light microscopic and ultrastructural observations of a metastasizing malignant epithelioid schwannoma. Cancer 38:1977–1982, 1976

61. Waldo ED, Vuletin JC, Kaye GI: The ultrastructure of vascular tumors: Additional observations and a review of the literature. Pathol Ann 12:279–308, 1977

62. Dische FE, Darby AJ, Howard ER: Malignant synovioma: Electron microscopical findings in three patients and review of the literature. J Path 124:149–155, 1978

63. Gabbiani G, Kaye GI, Lattes R, et al: Synovial sarcoma: Electron microscopic study of a typical case. Cancer 28:1031–1039, 1971

64. Klein W, Huth F: The ultrastructure of malignant synovioma. Beitr Path Bd 153:194–202, 1974

65. Rosai J, Sumner HW, Kostianovsky M, et al: Angiosarcoma of the skin: A clinicopathologic and fine ultrastructural study. Hum Pathol 7:83, 1976

66. Labrecque PG, Hu CH, Winkelmann RK: On the nature of desmo-plastic melanoma. Cancer 38:1205–1213, 1976
67. Valensi QJ: Desmoplastic malignant melanoma: A light and electron microscopic study of two cases. Cancer 43:1148–1155, 1979
68. Bryant E, Ronan SG, Felix EL, et al: Desmoplastic malignant mela-noma. A study by conventional and electron microscopy. Am J Dermpathol 4:467–473, 1982
69. From L, Hanna W, Kahn HJ, et al: Origin of the desmoplasia in desmoplastic malignant melanoma. Hum Pathol 14:1072–1080, 1983
70. Bearman RM, Noe J, Kempson RL: Clear cell sarcoma with melanin pigment. Cancer 36:977–984, 1975
71. Tsuneyoshi M, Enjoji M, Kubo T: Clear cell sarcoma of tendons and aponeuroses: A comparative study of 13 cases with a provisional subgrouping into the melanotic and synovial types. Cancer 42: 243–252, 1978
72. Mickelson MR, Brown GA, Maynard JA, et al: Synovial sarcoma: An electron microscopic study of monophasic and biphasic forms. Cancer 45:2109–2118, 1980
73. Roth JA, Enzinger FM, Tannenbaum M: Synovial sarcoma of the neck: A follow-up study of 24 cases. Cancer 35:1243–1253, 1975
74. Desai U, Ramos CV, Taylor HB: Ultrastructural observations in pleomorphic liposarcoma. Cancer 43:1284–1290, 1978
75. Kindblom LG, Save-Soderbergh J: The ultrastructure of liposarcoma: A study of 10 cases. Acta Path Microbiol Scand (A) 87:109–121, 1979
76. Lagace R, Jacob S, Seemayer TA: Myxoid liposarcoma: An ultrastruc-tural study of two cases. Am J Clin Pathol 72:521–528, 1979
77. Wetzel W, Alexander R: Myxoid liposarcoma: An ultrastructural study of two cases. Am J Clin Pathol 72:521–528, 1979
78. Shipkey FH, Lieberman PH, Foote FN, et al: Ultrastructure of alveolar soft part sarcoma. Cancer 7:821–830, 1964
79. Unni KK, Soule EH: Alveolar soft part sarcoma: An electron micro-scope study. Mayo Clin Proc 50:591–598, 1975
80. Weiss SW, Langloss JM, Enzinger FM: Value of S-100 protein in the diagnosis of soft tissue tumors with particular reference to benign and malignant schwann cell tumors. Lab Invest 49:299–308, 1983
81. Nakajima T, Watanabe S, Sato Y, et al: An immunoperoxidase study of S-100 protein distribution in normal and neoplastic tissues. Am J Surg Pathol 6:715–727, 1982
82. Cocchia D, Lauriola L, Stolfi VM, et al: S-100 antigen labels neoplas-tic cells in liposarcoma and cartilaginous tumours. Virchows Arch (Pathol Anat) 402:139–145, 1983

83. Kahn HM, Marks A, Thom H, et al: Role of antibody to S100 protein in diagnostic pathology. Am J Clin Pathol 79:341–347, 1983

84. Nakajima T, Watanabe S, Sato Y, et al: Immunohistochemical demonstration of S100 protein in malignant melanoma and pigmented nevus, and its diagnostic application. Cancer 50:912–918, 1982

85. Nakamura Y, Becker LE, Marks A: S-100 protein in tumors of cartilage and bone: An immunohistochemical study. Cancer 52:1820–1824, 1983

86. Stefansson K, Wollmann R, Jerkovic M: S-100 protein in soft-tissue tumors derived from Schwann cells and melanocytes. Am J Pathol 106:261–268, 1982

86a. Cochran AJ, Wen D-R, Herschman HR, et al: Detection of S-100 protein as an aid to the identification of melanocytic tumors. Int J Cancer 30:295–297, 1982

87. Osborn M, Weber K: Biology of disease: tumor diagnosis by intermediate filament typing: a novel tool for surgical pathology. Lab Invest 48:372, 1983

88. Nagle RB, McDaniel KM, Clark VA, et al: The use of antikeratin antibodies in the diagnosis of human neoplasms. Am J Clin Pathol 79:458–466, 1983

89. Corson JM, Weiss LM, Banks-Schlegel SP, et al: Keratin proteins and carcinoembryonic antigen in synovial sarcomas: An immunohistochemical study of 24 cases. Hum Pathol 15:615–621, 1984

90. Miettinen M, Lehto V, Virtanen I: Keratin in the epithelial-like cells of classical biphasic synovial sarcoma. Virchows Arch (Cell Pathol) 40:157–161, 1982

91. Schlegel R, Banks-Schlegel S, Mcleod JA, et al: Immunoperoxidase localization of keratin in human neoplasms. Am J Pathol 101:41–48, 1980

92. Van Muijen GND, Ruiter DJ, Ponec M, et al: Monoclonal antibodies with different specificities against cytokeratins: An immunohistochemical study of normal tissues and tumors. Am J Pathol 114:9–17, 1984

93. Wu Y, Parker LM, Binder NE, et al: The mesothelial keratins: A new family of cytoskeletal proteins identified in cultured mesothelial cells and non-keratinizing epithelia. Cell 31:693–703, 1982

93a. Nelson WG, Battifora H, Santana H, et al: Specific keratins as molecular markers for neoplasms with a stratified epithelial origin. Cancer Res 44:1600–1603, 1984

94. Altmannsberger M, Osborn M, Holscher A, et al: The distribution of

keratin type intermediate filaments in human breast cancer: An immunohistological study. Virchows Arch (Cell Pathol) 37:277–284, 1981

95. Altmannsberger M, Osborn M, Schauer A, et al: Antibodies to different intermediate filament proteins. Cell type-specific markers on paraffin-embedded human tissues. Lab Invest 45:427–434, 1981

96. Hashimoto K, Eto H, Matsumoto M, et al: Anti-keratin monoclonal antibodies: production, specificities and applications. J Cutaneous Pathol 10:529–539, 1983

97. Corson J, Pinkus G: Mesothelioma: Profile of keratin proteins and carcinoembryonic antigen. An immunoperoxidase study of 20 cases and comparison with pulmonary adenocarcinomas. Am J Pathol 108:80–88, 1982

98. Warnke R, Gatter K, Falini B, et al: Diagnosis of human lymphoma with monoclonal antileukocyte antibodies. N Engl J Med 309: 1275–1281, 1983

99. de Jong ASH, van Raamsdonk W, van Vark M, et al: Myosin and myoglobin as tumor markers in the diagnosis of rhabdomaysarcoma: a comparative study. Am J Surg Pathol 8:521–528, 1984

100. Kagawa N, Sano T, Inaba H, et al: Immunohistochemistry of myoglobin in rhabdomyosarcomas. Acta Pathol Jpn 33:515–522, 1983

101. Brooks JJ: Immunohistochemistry of soft tissue tumors. Cancer 50:1757–1763, 1982

101a. Mukai K, Rosai J, Hallaway BE: Localization of myoglobin in normal and neoplastic human skeletal muscle cells using an immunoperoxidase method. Am J Surg Pathol 3:373–376, 1979

102. de Boulay CEH: Demonstration of alpha-I-antitrypsin and alpha-1-antichymotrypsin in fibrous histiocytomas using the immunoperoxidase technique. Am J Surg Pathol 6:559–564, 1982

103. Epenetos AA, Canti G, Taylor-Papadimitriou J, et al: Use of two epithelium-specific monoclonal antibodies for diagnosis of malignancy in serous effusions. Lancet 2:1004–1006, 1982

104. Gatter KC, Mason DY: The use of monoclonal antibodies for histopathologic diagnosis of human malignancy. Sem Oncol 9:517, 1982

105. Gu J, Polak JM, Noordan SV, et al: Immunostaining of neuron-specific enolase as a diagnostic tool for Merkel cell tumors. Cancer 52:1039–1043, 1983

106. Lloyd RU, Sisson JC, Marangos P: Calcitonin, carcinoembryonic antigen and neuron-specific enolase in medullary thyroid carcinoma. An immunohistochemical study. Cancer 51:2234–2239, 1983

107. Warner TF, Lloyd RU, Hafez GR, et al: Immunocytochemistry of neurotropic melanoma. Cancer 53:254–257, 1984

108. Mukai K, Rosai J, Burgdorf W: Localization of factor VIII-related antigen in vascular endothelial cells using an immunoperoxidase method. Am J Surg Pathol 4:273–276, 1980

109. Nadji M, Gonzalez MS, Castro A, et al: Factor VIII-related antigen: An endothelial cell marker. Lab Invest 42:139, 1980

110. Miettinen M, Foidart JM, Ekblom P: Immunohistochemical demonstration of laminin, the major glycoprotein of basement membranes, as an aid in the diagnosis of soft tissue tumors. Am J Clin Pathol 79:306–311, 1983

111. McCoy JP Jr, Lloyd RV, Wicha MS, et al: Identification of a laminin-like substance on the surface of high-malignant murine fibrosarcoma cells. J Cell Sci 65:139–151, 1984

112. de Boulay CEH: Demonstration of fibronectin in soft tissue tumours using the immunoperoxidase technique. Diagnos Histopath 5:283–289, 1982

113. Tsokos M, Howard R, Costa H: Immunohistochemical study of alveolar and embryonal rhabdomyosarcoma. Lab Invest 48:148, 1983

114. Wold LE, Li C-Y, Homburger HA: Localization of the B and M polypeptide subunits of creatinine kinase in normal and neoplastic human tissues by an immunoperoxidase technic. Am J Clin Pathol 75:327–332, 1981

115. Nakanishi S, Shinomiya S, Sano T, et al: Immunohistochemical observation of intracytoplasmic lysozyme in proliferative and neoplastic fibrohistiocytic lesions. Acta Pathol Jpn 32:949–959, 1982

116. Navas-Palacios JJ, Aparicio-Duque R, Valdes, MD: On the histogenesis of Ewing's s!rcoIa: an ultrastructural, immunohistochemical, and cytochemical study. Cancer 53:1882–1901, 1984

117. Kindblom LG, Lodding P, Angervall L: Clear-cell sarcoma of tendons and aponeuroses. Virchows Arch (Pathol Anat) 401:109–128, 1983

118. Azumi N, Turner R: Clear cell sarcoma of tendons and aponeuroses: Electron microscopic findings suggesting schwann cell differentiation. Hum Pathol 14:1084–1089, 1983

119. Chung EB, Enzinger FM: Malignant melanoma of soft parts: A reassessment of clear cell sarcoma. Am J Surg Pathol 7:405–413, 1983

120. Chase DR, Enzinger FM, Weiss SW, et al: Keratin in epithelioid sarcoma. An immunohistochemical study. Am J Surg Pathol 8:438–441, 1984

121. Mukai M, Iri H, Nakajima T, et al: Alveolar soft-part sarcoma. A

review on its histogenesis and further studies based on electron microscopy, immunohistochemistry, and biochemistry. Am J Surg Pathol 7:679–689, 1983

122. De Schryver-Kecskemeti K, Kraus FT, Engleman W: Alveolar soft part sarcoma—A malignant angioreninoma. Histochemical, immunohistochemical, and electron-microscopic study of four cases. Am J Surg Pathol 6:5–18, 1982

123. Holden J, Churg A: Immunohistochemical staining for keratin and carcinoembryonic antigen in the diagnosis of malignant mesothelioma. Am J Surg Pathol 8:277–279, 1984

124. Battifora H, Trowbridge IS: A monoclonal antibody useful for the differential diagnosis between malignant lymphoma and nonhematopoietic neoplasms. Cancer 51:816–821, 1983

125. Enzingher FM: Clear-cell sarcoma of tendons and aponeurosis. An analysis of 21 cases. Cancer 18:1163–1174, 1965

126. Stern R: Current concept in the diagnosis of human soft tissue sarcomas. Hum Pathol 12:777–781, 1981

127. Enzinger FM, Lattes R, Torloni H: Histologic typing of soft tissue tumors. Roto-Sadag SA, Geneva, 1969

128. Russel WO, Cohen J, Edmonson JH, et al: Staging system for soft tissue sarcoma. Sem Oncol 8:156–159, 1981

129. Russel WO, Cohen J, Enzinger F, et al: A clinical and pathological staging system for soft tissue sarcomas. Cancer 50:1562–1570, 1977

130. Suit HD, Russel WO, Martin RG: Sarcoma of soft tissue: Clinical and histopathologic parameters and response to treatment. Cancer 35:1478–1483, 1975

131. Costa J, Wesley RA, Glatstein E, et al: The grading of soft tissue sarcomas: results of a clinicohistopathologic correlation in a series of 163 cases. Cancer 53:530–541, 1984

132. Weiss SW, Enzinger FM: Malignant fibrous histiocytoma: An analysis of 200 cases. Cancer 41:2250–2266, 1978

133. Ranchod M, Kempson RL: Smooth muscle tumors of the gastrointestinal tract and retroperitoneum: A pathologic analysis of 100 cases. Cancer 39:255–262, 1977

134. Hadju SI: Pathology of Soft Tissue Tumors. Lea and Febiger, Philadelphia, 1979, p 45

135. Rosenberg SA, Glatstein EJ: Perspectives on the role of surgery and radiation therapy in the treatment of soft tissue sarcomas of the extremities. Sem Oncol 8:190–200, 1981

136. Allen PW: Tumors and Proliferations of Adipose Tissue: A clinicopathologic approach. Masson Publishing USA, New York, 1981

137. Evans HL: Liposarcoma: A study of 55 cases with a reassessment of its classification. Am J Surg Pathol 3:507–523, 1979

138. Kindblom LG, Angervall I, Svendson P: Liposarcoma: A clinico-pathologic, radiographic, and prognostic study. Acta Pathol Micro-biol Scand (A): Suppl 253, 1975

139. Joseph WL, Morton DL, Adkins PG: Variation in tumor doubling time in patients with pulmonary metastatic disease. J Surg Pathol 3:143, 1971

140. Van der Werf-Messing B, Van Unnik JAM: Fibrosarcoma of the soft tissues—a clinicopathologic study. Cancer 18:1113–1123, 1965

141. Pritchard DJ, Soule EH, Taylor WF, et al: Fibrosarcoma—a clinicopathologic statistical study of 199 tumors of the soft tissues of extremity and trunk. Cancer 33:888–897, 1974

142. Woodruff JM, Chernik NL, Smith MC, et al: Peripheral nerve tumors with rhabdomyosarcomatous differentiation (malignant "Triton" tumors). Cancer 32:426–439, 1973

143. Enzinger FM, Weiss SW: Soft Tissue Tumors. C V Mosby, St. Louis, 1983

144. Mackenzie DH: Synovial sarcoma: A review of 58 cases. Cancer 19:169–180, 1966

145. Mackenzie DH: Monophasic synovial sarcoma—a histologic entity? Histopathol 1:151–157, 1977

146. D'Agostino AN, Soule EH, Miller RH: Primary malignant neo-plasms of nerves (Malignant neurilemmomas) in patients without manifestations of multiple neurofibromatosis (von Recklinghausen's disease). Cancer 16:1003–1014, 1963

147. D'Agostino AN, Soule EH, Miller RH: Sarcomas of peripheral nerves and somatic soft tissues associated with multiple neurofibro-matosis (von Recklinghausen's disease). Cancer 16:1015–1027, 1963

148. Dahl I, Angervall L: Cutaneous and subcutaneous leiomyosarcoma: A clinicopathologic study of 47 patients. Path Europ 9:307–315, 1974

149. Fields SP, Helwig EB: Leiomyosarcoma of the skin and subcutaneous tissue. Cancer 47:156, 1981

150. Wile AG, Evans HL, Romsdahl MM: Leiomyosarcoma of soft tissue: A clinicopathologic study. Cancer 48:1022–1032, 1981

151. Weiss SW, Enzinger FM: Myxoid variant of malignant fibrous histiocytoma. Cancer 39:1672–1685, 1977

152. Gaiger AW, Soule EH, Newton WA: Pathology of rhabdomyosarcoma: Experience of the Intergroup Rhabdomyosarcoma Study 1972–1978. National Cancer Institute Monograph 56:19–27, 1981

152a. Maurer HM, Ragab AH: Rhabdomyosarcoma, in Sutow WW et al.

(eds): Clinical Pediatric Oncology (ed 3). Saint Louis: Mosby, 1984, pp 622–650

153. Dehner LP: Soft tissue sarcomas of childhood: the differential diagnostic dilemma of the small blue cell. National Cancer Institute Monograph 56:43–59, 1981

154. Triche T: Pathology of Cancer in the Young, in Levine A (ed): Cancer in the Young. Masson Publishing USA, New York, 1982, pp 119–180

155. Gehan EA, Glover FN, Maurer HM, et al: Prognostic factors in children with rhabdomyosarcoma. National Cancer Institute, Monograph 56:83–92, 1981

156. Hays DM, Newton Jr W, Soule EH, et al: Mortality among children with rhabdomyosarcomas of the alveolar histologic subtype. Journal Ped Surg 18:412–417, 1983

157. Palmer N, Sachs N, Foulkes M: Histopathology and prognosis in rhabdomyosarcoma (IRSI). ASCO Abstracts, No. C-660:170, 1982

158. Beckwith JB, Palmer NF: Histopathology and prognosis of Wilms' tumor: Results from the first National Wilms' Tumor Study. Cancer 41:1937–1948, 1978

159. Askin FB, Rosai J, Sibley RK, et al: Malignant small cell tumor of the thoracopulmonary region in childhood: a distinctive clinicopathologic entity of uncertain histogenesis. Cancer 43:2438–2451, 1979

160. Barson AJ, Ahmed A, Gibson AAM, et al: Chest wall sarcoma of childhood with a good prognosis. Archives of Disease in Childhood, 53:882–889, 1978

161. Newsbit Jr ME, Robison LL, Dehner LP: Round cell sarcoma of bone, in Sutow WW, et al. (eds): Clinical Pediatric Oncology (ed 3). Saint Louis: Mosby, 1984, pp 710–733

162. Enterline RT: Histopathology of sarcomas. Sem Oncol 8:133–155, 1981

11

POORLY DIFFERENTIATED LUNG CANCER

Mehmet F. Fer
Paul G. Abrams
Robert K. Oldham
Stephen A. Sherwin
James Mulshine
F. Anthony Greco
Mary J. Matthews

All too often, the physician will confront a mediastinal mass or a pulmonary nodule, the biopsy of which will show "poorly differentiated neoplasm," or "poorly differentiated carcinoma." Although the frequency of this diagnostic uncertainty is unclear, it probably varies in different settings based upon the patient population, the expertise of the pathologist, and the technology available. In most cases, an experienced pathologist can distinguish carcinomas from lymphomas and sarcomas, either by light microscopy or by performing lymphocyte marker studies and electron microscopy. This is important, since many lymphomas or sarcomas warrant different therapies from lung cancers. Once the diagnosis is narrowed down to a poorly differentiated carcinoma, the question becomes whether the primary site is in the lung or elsewhere.

While there are no definitive tests to determine this conclusively, for

POORLY DIFFERENTIATED NEOPLASMS AND TUMORS OF UNKNOWN ORIGIN   ISBN 0-8089-1755-2

practical purposes, endobronchial lesions have been generally considered to be primary lung cancers. In the absence of an endobronchial mass, most clinicians would still suspect the presence of a bronchogenic carcinoma, if an alternate primary site is not evident. The extent to which these patients should be evaluated for an occult primary site is discussed in depth in other chapters of this book; as a general rule, extensive radiographic and endoscopic searches have had a low yield and should not be performed routinely. In all cases, however, the question should be entertained if a highly responsive type of neoplasm may be the case. These possibilities include mediastinal germ cell tumors, particularly in younger patients, some of which are potentially curable even at advanced stages. Hainsworth and Greco discussed this topic in detail in Chapter 8.

Once these possibilities are eliminated to a reasonable degree, one is left with the preliminary diagnosis of a "poorly differentiated lung cancer" (PDLC). It is now clear that there are vast differences in the clinical behavior and appropriate therapy of small cell carcinomas of the lung as opposed to the non-small cell types (adenocarcinoma, squamous cell carcinoma, and large cell undifferentiated carcinoma).[1-3] The diagnostic abbreviation "PDLC" would refer to a malignant neoplasm in the lung that lacks readily apparent distinguishing features by light microscopy. While the use of this term may not pose a major problem in patients who are good surgical candidates or others who need supportive care alone, it may hamper significantly the recognition of small cell carcinoma which requires systemic therapy. This chapter will focus on problems associated with the use of this term as a diagnosis and will discuss some of the current and emerging methods which may be used in characterizing lung cancers in the future.

Historical Background and Classification Systems

The three major classification systems for lung cancers published within the past two decades are summarized in Table 11-1.[4-6] The first major classification system was proposed by the World Health Organization (WHO) in 1967,[4] dividing lung cancers into four major types: epidermoid (squamous) carcinoma, small cell carcinoma, adenocarcinoma, and large cell carcinoma. The small cell type was also divided into four subtypes, the lymphocyte-like (oat cell) subtype, fusiform, poligonal subtypes and "others." The large cell carcinoma was considered to be an anaplastic malignancy which lacked the distinct morphological criteria of squamous or glandular differentiation. It was recognized that the majority

Table 11-1

Classification Schemas for Lung Cancers

WHO (1967)	WP-L (1973)	WHO (1981)
I. Epidermoid carcinoma	10. Epidermoid carcinoma 11. Well-differentiated 12. Moderately differentiated 13. Poorly differentiated	1. Squamous cell carcinoma Spindle cell variant
II. Small cell carcinoma 1. Fusiform 2. Polygonal 3. Lymphocyte-like 4. Others	20. Small cell carcinoma 21. Lymphocyte-like (oat cell) 22. Intermediate cell	2. Small cell carcinoma Oat cell Intermediate cell Combined

III. Adenocarcinoma
1. Bronchogenic
  a. Acinar
  b. Papillary
2. Bronchioloalveolar
	30. Adenocarcinoma
	31. Well-differentiated
	32. Moderately differentiated
	33. Poorly differentiated
	34. Bronchiolopapillary
		3. Adenocarcinoma
		Acinar
		Papillary
		Bronchioloalveolar
		Solid tumor with mucin

IV. Large cell carcinoma 1. Solid tumor with mucin 2. Solid tumor without mucin 3. Giant cell 4. Clear cell	40. Large cell carcinoma 41. With stratification 42. Giant cell 43. With mucin formation 44. Clear cell	4. Large cell carcinoma Giant cell Clear cell
V. Combined epidermoid and adenocarcinoma		5. Adenosquamous carcinoma

of poorly differentiated squamous and glandular malignancies also lacked many of these distinguishing criteria. Subsequently, the Pathology Committee of the Working Party for the Therapy of Lung Cancer (WP-L) revised this classification to simplify the categories and define more precisely diagnostic criteria.[5] In this classification the lymphocyte-like (oat cell) subtype of small cell carcinoma (SCC) was separated from the other subtypes (fusiform, poligonal, and other subtypes) with the latter categories being grouped together as an "intermediate" subtype. It was not known at the time whether these two different subtypes represented different biological entities.

These classification systems were designed to help develop distinct light microscopic features that can be used consistently by pathologists, thereby minimizing interobserver variability. In fact, when the specific guidelines proposed in these classification systems are used, consistency in the diagnosis has been achieved by experienced pathologists in over 90 percent of the cases.[7] This degree of consistency contrasts sharply with earlier reports when discrepancies in the diagnosis could occur in up to 40 percent of poorly differentiated squamous carcinomas and adenocarcinomas.[8] All of the classification systems to date rely heavily on light microscopy, and none of them contain a type designated as PDLC.

The proponents of the term PDLC, on the other hand, prefer to rely on electron microscopy. Many of these pathologists in recent years have questioned whether a large cell undifferentiated carcinoma truly exists. Electron microscopists have often been successful in identifying ultrastructural characteristics in an anaplastic tumor which provides evidence of squamous, glandular, or even small cell characteristics.[9–13] Cytopathologists have also been able to distinguish squamous, glandular, or small cell features when the tissue biopsies are in fact inadequate or nonconclusive. Thus, these pathologists will often prefer to avoid the label large cell undifferentiated carcinoma and resort to the PDLC nomenclature as the light microscopic diagnosis. In a review of 28,119 lung cancers submitted to the Surveillance, Epidemiology and End Results Program of the WHO, 3500 cases (12 percent) were initially reported in nonspecific terms, such as bronchogenic carcinoma, lung cancer, or PDLC.[14]

Frequent Problems in the Classification of Lung Cancers

The problems that hamper the diagnosis of lung cancers can be either technical or interpretive in nature. Some of these technical problems that impede the accurate classification of lung cancers are listed below.

Instrumental crushing of biopsy samples
Poor fixation of tissues
Thick sectioning
Drying artifacts
Overstaining of tissues

Any of the factors tabulated may alter or distort nuclear and cytoplasmic detail, preventing a precise diagnosis. Whenever possible, an effort should be made to at least separate small cell carcinoma from large cell undifferentiated neoplasms, although even such broad distinctions can be difficult at times. In those situations, repeat biopsies should be obtained whenever possible. If SCC can be excluded with certainty, the use of the term, large cell anaplastic carcinoma, will assure the clinician that a small cell tumor has not been overlooked.

Interpretive problems in the classification of lung cancers may include the following. Fine needle aspirates of necrotic non-SCC may be misinterpreted as SCC if tumor cells have small round hyperchromatic nuclei and scanty cytoplasm. In some studies, however, there can be agreement between pathologists in as high as 80 percent of non-small cell carcinomas.[15] Tumors with mixed histology, i.e., with both small cell and large cell components, may cause problems, particularly when the biopsy samples are small. Small cell tumors which form tubules, squamous nests, or syncytial giant cell may be misinterpreted as non-small cell carcinomas. Finally, the intermediate subtype of small cell carcinoma (ICS-SCC) may at times be difficult to recognize. Although this tumor is biologically similar to the lymphocyte-like (oat cell) subtype of small cell (OCS-SCC) carcinoma, cells may have larger vesicular nuclei and more obvious cytoplasm (Fig. 11-1). If nuclear features are overlooked (i.e., the diffuse dispersion of nuclear chromatin and indistinct nucleoli), these tumors may be misinterpreted as PDLC. Experience in two series summarized below illustrate the difficulties in the recognition of the ICS-SCC.

At Vanderbilt University, of the 162 consecutive patients with SCC seen after January 1976, only 19 had the ICS-SCC subtype, compared to the expected number, which would be 81 patients, reflecting 50 percent of all patients with SCC.[16–17] Of the 19 patients with ICS-SCC, seven had an outside diagnosis of PDLC leading to a median of 10 weeks delay in their referral. This observation prompted a pathology review at Vanderbilt University where the slides from 101 consecutive unselected patients previously diagnosed as PDLC were reviewed by a pathologist in an effort to classify those tumors according to current terminology. Patient histories

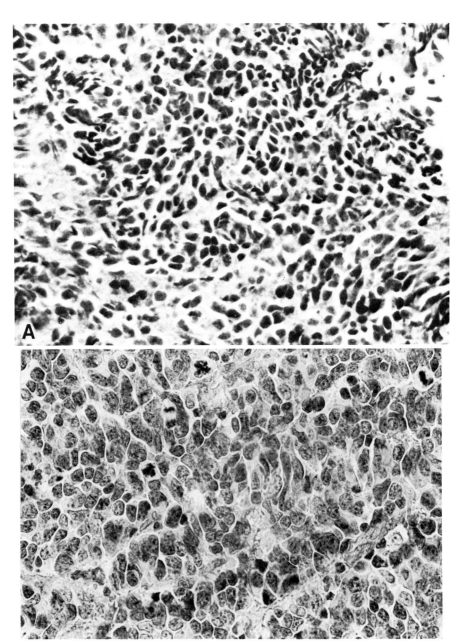

Figure 11-1. *A-Small cell carcinoma, oat cell subtype. Lymphocyte-like cells with scanty cytoplasm are seen. B-Small cell carcinoma, intermediate subtype. Cells are slightly larger with more prominent cytoplasm. This tumor was initially assessed as a poorly differentiated carcinoma of a non-small-cell type. The patient has had a complete response to combination chemotherapy. (original magnification × 400)*

were reviewed independently. Twenty-four patients were excluded from this study because of the uncertainty of the clinical diagnosis of lung cancer in 19 patients and the lack of evaluable pathologic material in five. Of the remaining 77 patients, 15 were felt to have small cell carcinomas, 12 of which were of the intermediate subtype. The initial diagnoses on these 12 patients were poorly differentiated epidermoid carcinoma in three, poorly differentiated adenocarcinoma in one, and PDLC in eight. The median survival for these 12 patients was 14 weeks. Only three had received a trial of chemotherapy with responses seen in all of these three patients, with one complete response.

A surgical series from the Veteran's Administration Surgical Oncology Group (VASOG) reveals similar findings. Of over 800 resected lung tumor samples reviewed by the VASOG between 1973 and 1980, only 35 (less than 4 percent) were small cell carcinomas. Of these 35 patients, however, 32 had the intermediate subtype. The remaining three cases in this group included one oat cell subtype and two mixed tumors with both SCC and non-SCC components. Thus, it appeared that the difficulty in recognizing the ICS-SCC led to thoracotomy in these 32 patients, while the great majority of OCS-SCCs were presumably diagnosed prior to surgery. Of these 35 patients, 15 (42 percent) had been originally submitted to the referral center with a non-small cell diagnosis. Eight cases were diagnosed as PDLC, four as poorly differentiated epidermoid carcinoma, one as poorly differentiated adenocarcinoma, and two as carcinoid tumors. Effective systemic therapy was unnecessarily delayed in these patients until postoperative recovery.

Thus, it appears that the majority of patients referred for the therapy of SCC in the community have the readily identified oat-cell subtype. Patients with the intermediate cell subtype are often at risk for receiving an incorrect diagnosis of PDLC, leading to the assumption that the tumor is of non-small cell type. This difficulty may result in unnecessary delays in appropriate therapy and sometimes unnecessary surgery. It is estimated tht 5–6 percent of patients with SCC have mixed small cell/non-small cell elements at diagnosis.[18] This group referred to as small cell lung cancer variants (SCC-V) have lower complete response rates and a shortened survival,[19] distinct biology,[20,21] and molecular genetics with the amplification of the c-myc oncogene.[22] This group of patients may represent a source of diagnostic confusion and more work is required to identify markers to routinely identify this subset. Candidates for this include reagents to monitor c-myc expression such as monoclonal antibodies with specificity for c-myc protein, or antibodies that recognize other antigens perturbed by the SCC-V phenotype such as glycolipid expression.[23]

Approaches to a Diagnosis of PDLC

Based on the significant differences in the therapeutic approaches to small cell and non-small cell carcinomas of the lung, a concerted effort is warranted in all patients with lung cancer to distinguish each tumor as either a small cell or a non-small cell carcinoma. The need for generous biopsy specimens fastidiously handled to ensure optimal pathologic evaluation cannot be overemphasized. Since it is unlikely that electron microscopy will become a routine diagnostic procedure in the near future, light microscopy should be employed whenever possible. Mucin, keratin, and other special stains should be considered within this context. Important features which may assist in distinguishing SCC from non-SCC types include diffuse dispersion of nuclear chromatin, indistinct nucleoli scanty cytoplasm, and nuclear molding of neoplastic cells. Whenever necessary, second opinions should be obtained as well as additional material, including cytology specimens. When available, electron microscopy may be very helpful. This is discussed in further detail in Chapter 2, by Drs. Ordonez and Mackay. In one study, Mackay et al. observed that of 20 patients with large cell anaplastic carcinoma by light microscopy, 12 showed evidence of differentiation either by the presence of desmosomes and tonofilaments, suggesting squamous histology, or by microvilli or microacini compatible with a glandular type.[9] Small cell carcinomas, regardless of their subtype, have oval or rounded nuclei with fine, diffusely distributed chromatin, scanty cytoplasm, and sparse organelles. Desmosomes may be present. Small membrane-bound neurosecretory-type granules may be present within the cytoplasmic processes. These neoplasms can be distinguished from carcinoid tumors, since the latter contain larger and more numerous neurosecretory granules.

Occasionally, clinical features that are highly suggestive of a certain form of lung cancer may provide clues.[1,2,24-26] For example, the presence of the neuromuscular disorder described by Eaton and Lambert is almost exclusively seen with small cell carcinoma.[27] Other paraneoplastic syndromes that are often associated with small cell carcinoma include the syndrome of inappropriate antidiuretic hormone secretion (SIADH), which is seen in 5–10 percent of patients with SCC and infrequently in non-SCC.[28-29] Alternately, hypercalcemia is rarely seen with SCC, but occurs in close to one-quarter of the patients with squamous carcinomas and in 13 percent of patients with large cell carcinomas.[30] Other clinical features associated with small cell carcinomas include proximal location of the tumor with early mediastinal involvement.[25-26] These features are in no way restricted to this tumor, however, since squamous carcinomas also arise frequently in proximal locations. Squamous carcinomas generally do not show early mediastinal involvement, but may manifest cavitation in as many as 20 percent of the cases, a feature that is rare in SCC.[31] Because of their early mediastinal spread, small cell carcinomas represent the most common cause of superior vena cava obstruction.[32] Radiologically, early lymphatic invasion by small cell carcinomas have been characterized as a "sunburst" appearance radiating from the tumor mass, a feature seen infrequently with other types of lung cancer. All of the characteristics discussed above are simply clinical clues and can in no way replace a definitive histologic diagnosis.

Experimental Approaches to the Characterization of Lung Cancers

Several experimental methods offer potential for the future development of lung cancer recognition methods. Among these are tumor marker studies, surface membrane receptors, chromosome abnormalities, and monoclonal antibody panels recognizing antigenic determinants on tumor cells. Although these techniques are currently far from consideration as diagnostic tools, they provide avenues for research and offer potential for future utility. It needs to be emphasized that much of the data regarding these investigational methods are derived from well-differentiated and well-characterized neoplasms, and their applicability to undifferentiated carcinomas is uncertain.

Small cell carcinoma of the lung has been associated with a variety of marker substances, including ADH, neurophysins, histaminase, calcitonin, and creatinine kinase (BB fraction), dopa-decarboxylase, neuron-specific enolase and bombesin.[28,29,33-39] While only 5–10 percent of patients with SCC will have SIADH, over 35 percent will have elevated serum levels of ADH.[28] An additional 20 percent of the patients may exhibit an inability to excrete maximally dilute urine when water loading tests are performed.[33] These patients are likely to have either normal basal ADH levels with an inability to suppress ADH secretion or have bio-chemically active analogues of ADH which are not recognized in the current assays. Neurophysins, which are binding proteins for ADH or oxytocin, have been detected in high levels in plasma from patients with SCC in approximately

65 percent of the cases studied.[34] North et al. have also associated neurophysin levels with tumor bulk during the course of therapy.[34]

A variety of hormones or their analogues (ACTH, calcitonin, PTH) have all been associated with carcinomas of the lung.[30,36,40–43] ACTH and calcitonin are more frequently associated with small cell carcinoma, and PTH-like substances with squamous carcinomas. When tumor cells are cultured in vitro, some of these products can be detected in the tissue culture medium.[44] All of these hormones associated with lung cancers, however, are far from being specific and cannot be used as diagnostic tests. Similarly, enzymes such as creatinine kinase-BB isoenzyme have been found in elevated levels in the serum of patients with small cell carcinoma, but again, this cannot be used as a diagnostic marker.[37] CK-BB isoenzyme is more often associated with extensive stage disease (39 percent), while it is infrequently elevated in limited stage small cell carcinoma.[37] This would reduce the value of markers such as CK-BB in the clinic since the impact of therapy is clearly greater in patients with less advanced disease.

Immunocytochemical staining techniques recognizing either marker substances within tumor tissues or tumor-associated antigens offer an important avenue in the recognition of lung cancers. Immunoperoxidase staining techniques have been described earlier in this book by Drs. Ordonez and Mackay. The advent of monoclonal antibody technology has further enhanced our ability to use these techniques in a more standardized fashion. As opposed to polyclonal heteroantisera which need to be harvested from immunized animals, monoclonal antibodies can be produced in much larger quantities by propagating the antibody-producing hybrid clone in tissue cultures or mouse ascites. These antibodies can then be used with much more reproducible results and on a broader scale. The use of monoclonal antibodies in histopathologic diagnosis is further discussed in Chapter 16 by Drs. Gatter and Mason.

In this chapter, we will focus on monoclonal antibodies against lung cancer which offer significant potential both in the diagnosis and therapy of these tumors. In certain respects, one could speculate that if a given antibody conjugated to drug or toxins ensures selective delivery of these toxic substances to the tumor site in vivo, with a subsequent response, the importance of a histopathologic diagnosis may then be confined to academic interest. In this setting, all that would matter would be whether a given tumor contains a certain antigen with which the immunotoxin reacts, irrespective of the tumor's cell of origin or appearance under the microscope. Such a hypothesis can be tested only after highly selective antibodies and immunotoxins are developed to achieve optimal delivery in tumor tissues with subsequent anti-tumor effects. While rapid progress continues in this area, further research is needed to validate such an approach.

At present, therapeutic considerations make the most critical distinction between small cell and non-small cell carcinomas. The most promising reagents in regards to separating these two major categories have been developed by Mulshine et al. using a large cell carcinoma line to immunize mice and screening hybridoma supernatants for positive reactions to the large cell and negative reactions to the small cell lines propagated in their laboratory.[45] The resulting 703 series antibodies recognize a 31,000 molecular weight internal antigen with very restricted normal tissue representation as assessed by immunoperoxidase staining of formalin-fixed histologic specimens (Table 11-2). Only three of 16 small cell tumors were positive in discrete focal areas that may represent transformation to large cell morphology. Twenty-three of 25 non-small cell tumors encompassing the major histologic subtypes were positive in a diffuse (all tumor cells positive) pattern. It will be interesting to see if focally positive small cell is equated with poor response to chemotherapy due to the emergence of resistant clones, and if positively staining poorly differentiated carcinomas as determined by light microscopy respond to chemotherapy similar to small cell carcinoma. Prospective evaluations of these questions are currently underway.

Both Abrams et al. (353 series) and Brenner et al. (922 series) have produced monoclonal antibodies which predominantly bind to squamous carcinomas of the lung and are negative when tested against normal tissues or small cell carcinomas (Table 11-2).[46-47] There are some other non-small cell carcinomas that express the 143 Kd cell surface antigen recognized by 353 H10, but this is an inconsistent finding. Used in conjunction with the 703 series of Mulshine, these antibodies may establish a squamous origin of a poorly differentiated carcinoma, or a squamous transformation in small cell tumors. An example of the positive staining of a squamous and negative staining of a small cell tumor by 353 H10 is shown in Figure 11-2. Since the antigen is expressed on cell surface membranes, the antibody appears to be promising as a vehicle to detect or treat squamous carcinomas in vivo. Other antibodies, such as the KS1/4 series may also be useful in in vivo applications.[48] These antibodies in the 534 F8 series developed by Cuttita et al. recognize the oligosaccharide lacto-N-fucopentose-III. This glycolipid antigen is expressed both on small cell and non-small cell tumors and thus adds little to the analysis of PDLCs.[49] The 604 A9 series, on the other hand, reacts more selectively with small cell carcinoma[50] and would be useful to confirm small cell origin of a poorly differentiated neoplasm of the lung, so categorized because of negative staining with the 703 series.

Table 11-2
Monoclonal Antibodies to Human Lung Cancer

Antibody	Source	SCLC/NSCLC	Antigen	Comments
Non-Small Cell				
353 H10 Series	Abrams, et al.	−/+	143 Kd Glycoprotein Cell Surface	Predominantly squamous. Some other non-small cell. No binding to normal tissues except very weak to kidney tubules.
703 D_4 Series	Mulshine, et al.	−/+	31 Kd Internal	All non-small cell. Rare small cell. No binding to normal tissues.
KS 1/4 Series	Varki, et al.	+/+	40 Kd Glycoprotein Cell Surface	Binds to all lung carcinomas and adenocarcinomas of breast, lung, pancreas, and colon. Weak binding to kidney, lung, and pancreas.
1680-25-35	Mazauric, et al.	−/+	149/119 Kd Glycoproteins	No histochemistry to define antigen distribution on normals.
9.2.2	Brenner, et al.	−/+	Unknown	Negative on normal tissues and small cell. Predominantly squamous carcinomas bind.
169 D_4 Series	Kasai, et al.	?/+	Unknown	Unknown
503 D_8	Abrams, et al.	−/+	15/69 Kd Glycoproteins	Secreted antigen. Present in lower but easily detectable quantities on normal tissues.
Small Cell				
534 F8 Series	Cuttita, et al.	+/+	Lacto-N-Fucopentose III	Glycolipid equivalent to SSEA. Binds to normal kidney and breast carcinoma, neuroblastom.
604 A9 Series	Rosen, et al.	+/+ (rare)	Glycolipid	More restricted to small cell.
2HH7	Minna, et al.	+/+	120 Kd Protein	Large cell converters from small cell.

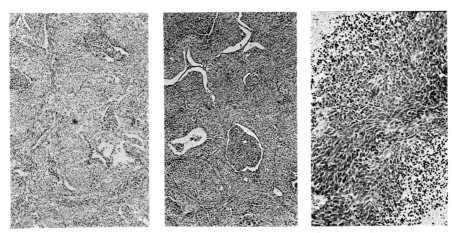

Figure 11-2. *Immunoperoxidase staining of lung cancers by the monoclonal antibody 353 H-10. A-Squamous carcinoma stained with 353 H-10. B-Section from the same squamous tumor stained with mouse immunoglobulin P-3 (negative control) C-Small cell carcinoma stained with 353 H-10. No staining is seen.*

Finally, antibodies recognizing certain non-lung carcinoma antigens such as leu-7 react with small cell but not with non-small cell carcinomas .[51] Also antibodies to the Type-I histocompatibility antigens such as HLA-mainframe or beta-2-microglobulin can distinguish small cell from non-small cell tumors, since SCCs have greatly reduced or absent expression of these antigens.[52]

Among the candidates for non-hormonal markers of lung cancers are growth factor receptors. Sherwin et al. have demonstrated that receptors for epidermal growth factor were lacking in eight cultured small cell carcinoma cell lines, but present in five of six non-small cell carcinoma cell lines studied.[53] Receptors for nerve growth factor were absent in all non-small cell carcinoma cell lines, but present in three of the eight small cell carcinoma cell lines. Of the three "converter" cell lines (small cell carcinomas which lost ultrastructural, biochemical, and morphological features of small cell carcinoma), one had receptors for EGF and three for NGF, at low levels.

Another investigational method that has been applied to lung cancers has been chromosome analyses by banding techniques. Whang-Peng et al. have described a chromosome abnormality specific for small cell carcinoma of the lung (deletion 3p [14-23]).[54] In their original article, these authors reported that all 12 small cell carcinoma cell lines studied manifested this deletion while five non-small cell carcinoma cell lines and lymphoblastoid cell lines cultured from small cell carcinoma patients did not exhibit the deletion.

Recent experimental and clinical experience has undermined the conventional notion that different lung cancer histologies arise from distinct cells of origin.[55] Examples exist of transitions or combinations of various types of lung cancers. For example, in approximately 6 percent of all small cell lung cancers, there is a non-small cell component.[5,18,56] It would be difficult to assume that these cells are independent of the small cell carcinoma. Thus, one would need to hypothesize a mechanism to explain the morphologic heterogeneity observed in those patients. Additionally, in several series of patients undergoing therapy for small cell carcinoma, relapsing patients have occasionally demonstrated a non-small cell type.[56–57] Whether these patients had separate clones in the beginning or the small cell carcinoma changed morphology during therapy remains unclear. On the other hand, when small cell carcinoma prolonged passage in vitro.[55] Some of these interrelationships between different types of lung cancer and time-dependent changes in human tumors are discussed at length by Drs. Mendelsohn and Baylin later in this book. The separating lines between different types of lung cancer may not be clearcut, and poorly differentiated neoplasms may prove difficult to categorize no matter how sophisticated our technology may eventually become.

The Clinical Approach to the Treatment of PDLC

Most experienced pathologists should be able to classify the majority of lung tumors at least as small cell or non-small cell types by light microscopy. Based on the technical and interpretive problems discussed above, it is often enough that the clinician will face a diagnosis of PDLC. Whenever possible, additional biopsies should be obtained in these cases and second opinions sought. In light of the increasing appreciation of coexistence of SCC and non·SCC histologies in a particular tumor, reliance on cytologic specimens for diagnosis may lead to misclassification errors and should be discouraged. When available, electron microscopy should be employed. When none of these options are helpful, the patients need to be approached in as rational a way as possible. A systematic approach to these patients is offered in Figure 11-3. If the tumor appears to be confined to the ipsilateral chest and if the patient is otherwise a good surgical candidate, a potentially curative resection should be performed. The

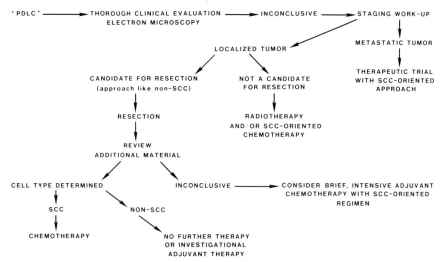

Figure 11-3. *A schematic approach to poorly differentiated lung cancer.*

resected sample will provide material for further histologic evaluation. If, based on this sample, the tumor proves to be a non-small cell carcinoma, no further therapy would be indicated, unless an investigational adjuvant therapy protocol is pursued. If mediastinal nodes, capsular invasion, or soft tissue extension are present, radiotherapy to the area should be considered. If the resected tumor proves to be a small cell carcinoma, the patient should then proceed with combination chemotherapy regardless of the extent of residual disease.

Although surgical resection is not routinely recommended for small cell carcinoma, it would not necessarily be a disservice to these patients who would then be left with microscopic disease alone and placed in a very favorable category with adjuvant chemotherapy.[58,59] Patients with apparently limited disease who are not candidates for surgery due to other medical reasons should receive radiotherapy in potentially curative doses (5-6,000 rads), but since they will most likely relapse, regardless of the cell type, the addition of a brief intensive course of SCC-oriented chemotherapy should be considered. Since the value of maintenance therapy in responding patients with any form of lung cancer remains controversial, this therapy could be stopped after a 4-6 cycle course. Patients with proven metastatic disease and a diagnosis of PDLC should be considered for a trial of SCC-oriented chemotherapy. Only the responding patients would be continued on therapy until either relapse, unacceptable toxicity, or complete remission occurs. Several regimens effective against small cell lung cancer have been recently reviewed elsewhere.[1,2,58,60] The use of chemotherapy oriented for small cell carcinoma should not be inappropriate in this setting for other histologic types since most of these drugs have some marginal activity against non-small cell carcinomas as well.[61,62] In some respects, response to a therapeutic trial could be considered an ultimate diagnostic tool that may distinguish patients with a favorable prognosis from others.

Summary and Conclusions

Given the current therapeutic options, all primary carcinomas of the lung must be classified at least into a small cell or non-small cell category. Most experienced pathologists can accomplish this by using the currently available guidelines. There may be, however, a variety of technical and interpretive problems, such as the adequacy of the biopsy sample, crush artifacts, small samples obtained by needle aspiration or bronchoscopy, and the presence of mixed histologies, or the intermediate type of small cell carcinoma. Electron microscopy will often provide useful clues for the recognition of various tumors, although the current classification systems have been based on light microscopy to facilitate their widespread use. While several investigational tools, including tumor marker and monoclonal antibody panels, may be of interest in the future, at this point their diagnostic utility is limited. In patients with "PDLC, not further classified", therapeutic trials should be offered to all patients who can tolerate it, according to the guidelines discussed above. It is possible that through advances in therapy, the need for classification by current methods may diminish. Until such treatment programs are developed, clinicians will need to rely on the currently available methods and insist on making optimal use of the existing guidelines.

References

1. Minna JD, Higgins GA, Glatstein EJ: Cancer of the lung, in DeVita VT, Hellman S, Rosenberg SA (eds): Cancer. Principles and Practice of Oncology. Philadelphia, Lippincott, 1982, pp 396–474
2. Greco FA, Oldham RK: Small cell lung cancer. N Engl J Med 301:355–358, 1979

3. Bergsagel D, Feld R: Small cell lung cancer is still a problem. J Clin Oncol 2:1189–1191, 1984

4. Yesner R, Sobel L: Histological typing of lung tumors. International histological classification of tumors. Geneva, World Health Organization, 1977

5. Matthews MJ: Morphological classification of bronchogenic carcinoma. Cancer Chemother Rep 4:299–301, 1973

6. Yesner R, Sobel L: Histological typing of lung tumors. International Histological Classification of Tumours. Geneva, World Health Organization, 1981

7. Stanley KE, Matthews MJ: Analysis of a pathology review of patients with lung tumors. J Natl Cancer Inst 66:989–992, 1981

8. Feinstein AR, Gelfman NA, Yesner R, et al: Observer variability in the histopathologic diagnosis of lung cancer. Am Rev Resp Dis 101:671–684, 1970

9. Mackay B, Osborne BM, Wilson RA: Ultrastructure of lung neoplasms, in Strauss MJ (ed): Lung Cancer. Clinical Diagnosis and Treatment. New York, Grune & Stratton, 1979, pp 71–84

10. Mennemeyer R, Hammar SP, Bauermeister DE, et al: Cytologic, histologic and electron microscopic correlations in poorly differentiated primary lung carcinoma. A study of 43 cases. Acta Cytologica 23:297–302, 1979

11. Churg A, Warnock ML: The fine structure of large cell undifferentiated carcinoma of the lung: Evidence for its relation to common adeno and squamous cell carcinoma. Lab Invest 36:334, 1977

12. Auerbach O, Frasca JM, Parks VR, et al: A comparison of World Health Organization (WHO) classification of lung tumors by light and electron microscopy. Cancer 50:2079–2088, 1982

13. Leong AS: The relevance of ultrastructural examination in the classification of primary lung tumours. Pathology 14:37–46, 1982

14. Percy C, Sobin L: Surveillance, epidemiology, and end results of lung cancer data applied to the World Health Organization's classification of lung tumors. JNCI 70:663–666, 1983

15. Taft PD, Szyfelbein WM, Greene R: A study of variability in cytologic diagnoses based on pulmonary aspiration specimens. Am J Clin Pathol 73:36–40, 1980

16. Fer MF, Rogers LW, Richardson RL, et al: The intermediate subtype of small cell lung cancer: A frequently unrecognized neoplasm. Clin Res 27:384A, 1979

17. Fer MF, Sherwin SA, Oldham RK, et al: Poorly differentiated lung cancer. Semin Oncol 1982, 9:456–466

18. Matthews MS, Gazdar AF: Pathology of small cell carcinoma of the lung and its subtypes. A clinicopathologic correlation, in Livingston RB (ed): Lung Cancer. The Hague, Martinus-Nijhoff, 1981, pp 283–306

19. Radice, PA, Matthews MJ, Ihde DC, et al: The clinical behavior of "mixed" small cell/large cell bronchogenic carcinoma compared to "pure" small cell subtypes. Cancer 15:2892–2902, 1982

20. Gazdar AF, Carney DN, Nau MM, et al: Characterization of variant subclasses of cell lines derived from small cell lung cancer having distinctive biochemical, morphological and growth properties. Cancer Res 45:2924–2930, 1985

21. Carney DN, Gazdar AF, Bepler G, et al: Establishment and identification of small cell lung cancer cell lines having classic and variant features. Cancer Res 45:2913–2923, 1985

22. Little CD, Nau MM, Carney DN, et al: Amplification and expression of the c-myc ocogene in human lung cancer cell lines. Nature 306:194–196, 1984

23. Mulshine J, Cuttita F, Rosen S, et al: Reduced expression of glycolipid antigens in small cell cancer variant cell lines (SCLC-V) as detected by a panel of monoclonal antibodies. Proc Am Soc Clin Oncol 3:C–64, 1984 (abstr)

24. Green H, Jurohara SS, George FW, et al: The biologic behavior of lung cancer according to histologic type. Radiol Clin Biol 42:160–170, 1972

25. Cohen MH, Matthews MJ: Small cell bronchogenic carcinoma: A distinct clinicopathologic entity. Semin Oncol 5234–343, 1978

26. Greco FA, Richardson RL, Snell JD, et al: Small cell lung cancer. Complete remissions and improved survival. Am J Med 66:625–630, 1979

27. Tyler HR: Paraneoplastic syndromes of nerve, muscle, and neuromuscular junction. Ann NY Acad Sci USA 230:348–357, 1974

28. Greco FA, Hainsworth J, Sismani A, et al: Hormone production and paraneoplastic syndromes, in Greco FA, Oldham RK, Bunn PA (eds): Small Cell Lung Cancer. New York, Grune & Stratton, 1981, pp 171–223

29. Gilby ED: Ectopic hormone products of bronchial neoplasms. Br J Dis Chest 70:282, 1976

30. Bender R, Hansen H: Hypercalcemia in bronchogenic carcinoma. Ann Intern Med 80:205–208, 1974

31. Chin FTS: Cavitation in lung cancers. Aust NZ J Med 5:523–530, 1975

32. Perez CA, Presant CA, Van Amburg AL: Management of superior vena cava syndrome. Semin Oncol 5:123–134, 1978

33. Gilby ED, Bondy PK, Fosling M: Impaired water excretion in oat-cell lung cancer. Br J Cancer 34:323–342, 1976

34. North WG, Maurer LH, Valtin H, et al: Human neurophysins as potential tumor markers for small-cell carcinoma of the lung: Application of specific radioimmunoassays. J Clin Endocrinol Metab 51:892–896, 1980

35. Baylin SB, Weisburger WR, Eggleston JC et al: Variable content of histaminase, l-dopa-decarboxylase, and calcitonin in small cell carcinoma of the lung. N Engl J Med 299:105–110, 1978

36. Schwartz KE, Wolfsen AR, Forster B, et al: Calcitonin in non-thyroid cancer. J Clin Endocrinol Metab 49:438–444, 1979

37. Gazdar AF, Zweig MH, Carney DN, et al: Levels of creatinine kinase and its BB isoenzyme in lung cancer specimens and cultures. Cancer Res 41:2773–2777, 1981

38. Sheppard MN, Corrin B, Bennett MH, et al: Immunocytochemical localization of neuron-specific enolase in small cell carcinomas and carcinoid tumors of the lung. Histopathology 8:171–181, 1984

39. Moody TW, Pert CB, Gazdar AF, et al: High levels of intracellular bombesin characterize human small cell lung carcinoma. Science 214:1246–1248, 1981

40. Yalow RS: Ectopic ACTH in carcinoma of the lung, in Muggia FM, Rosencweig M (eds): Lung Cancer: Progress in Therapeutic Research. New York, Raven Press, 1979, pp 209–216

41. Bloomfield GA, Holdaway IM, Corrin B, et al: Lung tumors and ACTH production. Clin Endocrinol 6:95–104, 1977

42. Silva OL, Broder LE, Doppman JL, et al: Calcitonin as a marker for bronchogenic cancer. 44:680–684, 1979

43. Hansen M, Hummer L: Ectopic hormone production in small cell carcinoma, in Muggia F, Rosencweig M (eds): Lung Cancer: Progress in Therapeutic Research. New York, Raven Press, 1979, pp 199–207

44. Sorenson GD, Pettengil OS, Brick-Johnson T, et al: Hormone production by cultures of small cell carcinoma of the lung. Cancer 47:1289–1296, 1981

45. Mulshine JL, Cuttitta F, Bibro M, et al: Monoclonal antibodies that distinguish non-small cell from small cell lung cancer. J Immunol 131:497–502, 1983

46. Abrams PG, Fer MF, Giardina S, et al: Monoclonal antibodies detecting antigens on squamous carcinoma of the lung. (submitted for publication)

47. Brenner BG, Jothy S, Shuster J, et al: Monoclonal antibodies to human

lung tumor antigens demonstrated by immunofluorescence and immunoprecipitation. Cancer Res 42:3187–3192, 1982

48. Varki NM, Reisfeld RA, Walker LE: Antigens associated with a human lung adenocarcinoma defined by monoclonal antibodies. Cancer Res 44:681–687, 1984

49. Cuttitta F, Rosen S, Gazdar AF, et al: Monoclonal antibodies that demonstrate specificity for several types of human lung cancer. Proc Natl Acad Sci USA 78:4591, 1981

50. Rosen ST, Mulshine JL, Cuttitta F, et al: Analysis of human non-small cell lung cancer differentiation antigens using a panel of rat monoclonal antibodies. Cancer Res 44:2052–2061, 1984

51. Bunn PA, Linnoila I, Minna JD, et al. Small cell lung cancer, endocrine cells of the fetal bronchus, and other neuroendocrine cells express the Leu-7 antigenic determinant present on natural killer cells. Blood 65:764–768, 1985

52. Doyle A, Martin WJ, Funa K, et al: Markedly decreased expression of Class I histocompatibility antigens, protein, and mRNA in human small cell lung cancer. J Exp Med 161:1135–1151, 1985

53. Sherwin SA, Minna JD, Gazdar AF, et al: Expression of epidermal and nerve growth factor receptors and soft agar growth factor production by human lung cancer cells. Cancer Res 41:3538–3542, 1981

54. Whang-Peng J, Kao-Shan CS, Lee EC, et al: Specific chromosome defect associated with human small cell lung cancer: Deletion 3 p (14–23). Science 215:181–182, 1982

55. Gazdar AF, Carney DN, Guccion JG, et al: Small cell carcinoma of the lung: Cellular origin and relationship to other pulmonary tumors, in Greco FA, Oldham RK, Bunn PA (eds): Small Cell Lung Cancer. New York, Grune & Stratton, 1981, pp 145–175

56. Abeloff MD, Eggleston JC, Mendelsohn G, et al: Changes in morphologic and biochemical characteristics of small cell carcinoma of the lung. Am J Med 66:757–764, 1979

57. Fer MF, Grosh WW, Greco FA: Morphologic changes in small cell lung cancer, in Greco FA (ed): Biology and Management of Lung Cancer. The Hague and Boston, Martinus-Nijhoff, 1983, pp 109–124

58. Greco FA, Oldham RK: Clinical management of patients with small cell lung cancer, in Greco FA, Oldham RK, Bunn PA (eds): Small Cell Lung Cancer, New York, Grune & Stratton, 1981, pp 353–379

59. Comis R, Meyer G, Ginsberg S, et al: Effectiveness of combination chemotherapy plus adjuvant surgery in small cell anaplastic lung cancer. Proc Am Soc Clin Oncol 22:509 (C–692), 1981

60. Ihde DC: Current status of therapy for small cell carcinoma of the lung. Cancer 54:2722–2728, 1984
61. Knost JA, Greco FA, Hande KR, et al: Cyclophosphamide, doxorubicin and cis-platin in the treatment of advanced non-small cell cancer. Cancer Treat Rep 65:941–945, 1981
62. Hoffman PC, Bitran JD, Golomb HM: Chemotherapy of metastatic non-small cell bronchogenic carcinoma. Semin Oncol 10:111–122, 1983

12

UNCLASSIFIED HEMATOPOIETIC AND LYMPHOID NEOPLASMS: CLINICOPATHOLOGIC FEATURES

Ellen P. Wright
Alan D. Glick
John C. York
Maria R. Baer
Robert D. Collins
John B. Cousar

The presumed cell of origin of most malignant neoplasms may be identified with the sophisticated methods currently available. Certain tumors, however, remain unclassified despite careful evaluation. These neoplasms are often designated as "undifferentiated", although it is likely that the problem lies in our inability to recognize their slight degree of differentiation. The recent development of techniques in the fields of molecular genetics and cell labeling by monoclonal antibodies has been especially helpful in precisely identifying neoplasms which previously would have been characterized as undifferentiated. These developments have been particularly useful in studying leukemias and lymphomas.

The pathologic and clinical features of unclassified leukemias and

POORLY DIFFERENTIATED NEOPLASMS AND TUMORS OF UNKNOWN ORIGIN   ISBN 0-8089-1755-2

lymphomas are not well-known, although most large studies of hematopoietic and lymphoid neoplasms list a number of "unclassified" or "undifferentiated" tumors. Direct comparison of these different series is
difficult since the thoroughness of the evaluation varied among the
reported studies, different classification schemes were used, the number of
unclassified cases was small, and the terminology used for unclassified
cases was often not defined. For example, the terms "acute undifferentiated leukemia" (AUL) and "null" are used frequently, but have not been
uniformly applied. York et al.[1] reviewed published series from 1975 to 1981
and found that an average of 4.7 percent and 10 percent, respectively, of
leukemias and lymphomas were unclassified. Several reviews including
unclassified hematopoietic and lymphoid tumors have emphasized the
benefit of electron microscopy (EM) as a diagnostic tool.[2–4] In these series,
the term "unclassified" has generally referred to lack of light microscopic
differentiation, sometimes accompanied by lack of diagnostic cytochemical
profiles. In contrast, other major studies of leukemia and/or lymphoma
generally relied on immunologic phenotyping to classify neoplasms.[5–10] A
few studies were noteworthy in using multiple diagnostic methods.[11–14]

At our hospital, a multiparameter approach has successfully classified
98–99 percent of leukemias and lymphomas. Cases were not considered
unclassified unless extensive evaluation including light microscopy (LM),
cytochemistry, immunologic phenotyping, and EM failed to identify evidence of differentiation. In this paper, the clinical and morphologic
findings in the cases remaining unclassified are briefly described in
relationship to the experience at other investigative centers.

Methods

The term *unclassified* will be used to describe tumors without recognizable defining features. In the case of marrow-based neoplasms (leukemias), the term refers to tumors composed of hematopoietic cells for which
a myeloid or lymphoid origin was not clearly established after
multiparameter analysis, including EM. In our experience, acute
lymphocytic leukemia (ALL) of various immunologic types has a distinctive EM appearance, different from lymphoma involving the bone marrow
or myeloid leukemias.[15–18] Therefore, cases of ALL are considered classified tumors, even though many are common ALL, and hence do not mark
as T or B cells. Lymphomas (peripheral lymphoid neoplasms) were

accepted as unclassified only if EM indicated lymphoid origin, immunologic studies did not show T or B characteristics, and the neoplasm lacked
definitive features of lymphoma by LM.

Unclassified cases were identified by reviewing the final diagnoses of
approximately 500 lymphomas and 400 leukemias evaluated in this institution over the past three and 10 years, respectively, and were included
only if they had been studied by LM, including appropriate cytochemical
stains, immunologic typing, and EM. All available materials were reviewed; cases lacking the original diagnostic material were excluded.
Charts were reviewed, and follow-up was obtained either from the patients
or from their referring physicians.

The English literature of the past ten years was selectively reviewed,
with emphasis placed on papers dealing specifically with unclassified
neoplasms or series including unclassified leukemias and lymphomas.
Papers detailing new diagnostic techniques were also included.

Fresh tissue on all patients with hematopoietic and lymphoid neoplasms was studied by protocol.[19] Fresh tissue for LM was fixed in B-5
fixative. A portion of the fresh tissue was reserved for EM and immunologic studies. Bone marrow particle smears were stained routinely with
Wright's stain, alpha naphthyl acetate esterase, naphthol ASD chloroacetate esterase, periodic acid Schiff-hematoxylin (PAS), and Sudan black B
(SB). Five cases were stained for acid phosphatase (AP). Paraffin-
embedded marrow particle sections and biopsies were cut at 3 microns and
stained with hematoxylin and eosin (H & E), PAS, and iron stain. All other
histologic sections were cut at 3 microns and routinely stained with H & E,
PAS, and methyl green pyronine (MGP). Immunologic studies were
performed on cell suspensions by direct and indirect immunofluorescence
for detection of immunoglobulin, B and T cell antigens, and terminal
deoxynucleotidyl transferase (TdT). Cells were evaluated for their ability to
form nonimmune sheep erythrocyte rosettes (ER). Since 1982, frozen
section immunoperoxidase (FSIP) has been used for typing when tissue for
cell suspensions was not available or the cell suspension data were
questionable. The standard FSIP battery included antisera to HLA-DR (Ia),
immunoglobulin heavy and light chains, T29/33 (marker for common
leukocyte antigen), pan-T markers (Leu 1 and 4) and markers for T helper
(Leu 3a + 3b) and suppressor (Leu 2) phenotypes. Paraffin immunoperoxidase (PIP) for cytoplasmic immunoglobulin (CIg) and lysozyme were
used to complement other typing studies. Tissue for electron microscopy
was fixed in glutaraldehyde and prepared by methods previously
described.[15]

Table 12-1
Unclassified Leukemia: Morphologic, Immunologic, Cytochemical, and Cytogenetic Features

Patient	Blood Involvement	Marrow Pattern	Blast Cytology	Immunochemical Findings	Cytochemical Profile	Karyotype
1	Yes	Extensive Involvement	↑N/C ratio, Dispersed chromatin, Prominent nucleoli, Vacuolated cytoplasm	ER 12% SIg—	PAS— SB— CE— AP granular +	47 X,Y + 21 t(12p13;20q12)
2	Yes	Extensive Involvement	↑ N/C ratio, Dispersed chromatin, Small nucleoli	ER 16% SIg 10% TdT—	PAS— SB— CE— AP—	Not done
3	Yes	Extensive Involvement	↑ N/C ratio, Dispersed chromatin, Inconspicuous nucleoli	Not done	PAS— SB— CE— AP—	Not done

4	No	Extensive Involvement	↑ N/C ratio, Dispersed chromatin, Prominent nucleoli, Vacuolated cytoplasm	ER 14% SIg— CIg— TdT—	PAS— SB— CE— AP granular +	46 X,Y
5	Yes	Extensive Involvement	↑ N/C ratio, Dispersed chromatin, Small nucleoli	ER 10% SIg 13%	PAS occ granular + SB— CE—	Not done
6	No	Focal Involvement	↑ N/C ratio, Dispersed chromatin, Prominent nucleoli	Indeterminate— low viability	PAS— SB— CE— AP—	Not done

↑ = increased; N/C = nuclear/cytoplasmic; PAS = periodic acid Schiff hematoxylin; SB = Sudan black; CE = combined esterase (alpha naphthyl acetate esterase + naphthol ASD chloroacetate esterase); AP = acid phosphatase

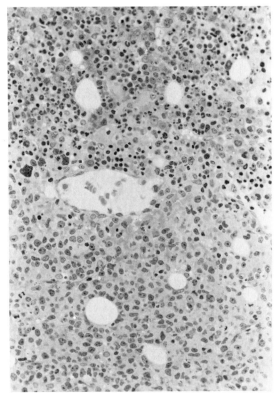

Figure 12-1. *Marrow biopsy from Case six demonstrating (bottom of panel) focal involvement by tumor, with (top) adjacent normal hematopoietic elements. (original magnification X 56.3)*

Unclassified Leukemias

Pathologic Findings

The morphologic features of our cases of unclassified leukemia are summarized in Table 12-1. By light microscopy, marrow sections from all cases were hypercellular. Case six showed only focal marrow involvement by the neoplasm (Fig. 12-1), while in the remaining five, there was extensive involvement (Fig. 12-2). In cases one and four, the cells had large, relatively round nuclei, dispersed chromatin, prominent nucleoli, and vacuolated cytoplasm, interpreted by LM as a large noncleaved cell

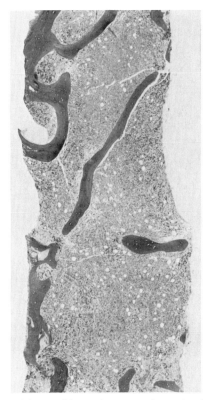

Figure 12-2. *Marrow biopsy demonstrating extensive involvement by tumor. (original magnification X 9)*

lymphoma (Fig. 12-3A & B). In contrast, in cases two, three, and five, the neoplastic cells were smaller, had relatively irregular nuclei, and lacked cytoplasmic vacuolation (Fig. 12-4A & B). Definite marking patterns were not seen with cytochemical stains. The pattern of acid phosphatase seen in cases one and four was not the focal positivity associated with T cells.[20]

Neoplastic cells of our unclassified leukemia patients were all similar by EM. Most were medium-sized to large with rounded or only slightly indented nuclei and dispersed chromatin with large nucleoli. Cytoplasm was abundant, contained very few or no granules, singly distributed ribosomes and sparse rough endoplasmic reticulum (Fig. 12-5). Only a few polyribosome clusters were seen. A few lipid droplets were occasionally encountered. Myeloperoxidase reaction (at the EM level) performed on

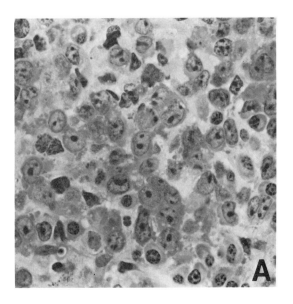

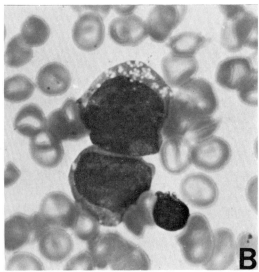

Figure 12-3. *(A) Marrow biopsy from Case four demonstrating large blasts with rounded nuclei and prominent nucleoli. (original magnification X 180) (B) Cytology of blasts on Wright's stained marrow smear from Case one demonstrating prominent cytoplasmic vacuolation. (original magnification X 225)*

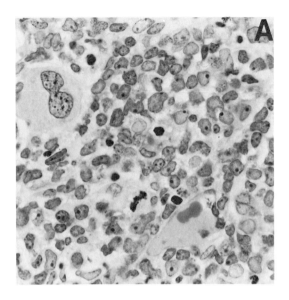

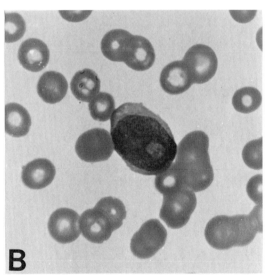

Figure 12-4. *(A) Marrow biopsy from Case three demonstrating irregular blasts with small nucleoli. (original magnification X 180) (B) Cytology of blasts on Wright's stained smear of peripheral blood from Case five demonstrating no granules or vacuoles. (original magnification X 225)*

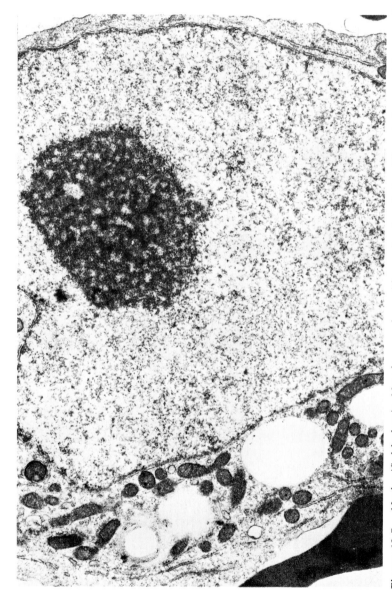

Figure 12-5. *Unclassified leukemia. Note large nucleus with prominent nucleolus. The cytoplasm contains several lipid droplets and mitochondria, but no granules. (X 20,700)*

case four demonstrated no conclusive positivity in tumor cells. By ultra-structural examination, the leukemic blasts in these cases did not resemble ALL blasts, in that they lacked the characteristic nuclear folding and marginated chromatin usually seen in ALL cells.[17] They differed from noncleaved lymphoma cells in that they lacked significant numbers of polyribosomes.[21]

The results of immunologic studies on our unclassified leukemias are also summarized in Table 12-1. In those cases in which cell suspensions were successfully studied, an average of 13 percent of cells formed ER, and six percent of cells displayed surface immunoglobulin (SIg). Cytocentrifuge preparations for CIg were performed in case four, and were negative.

TdT was negative in cases two and four.

Karyotypic analysis was performed on two cases of unclassified leukemia. In case four, a normal karyotype was found. Cells from case one, a child with Down's syndrome, showed trisomy 21 along with a 12;20 translocation.

Clinical Features

Clinical features of our patients with unclassified leukemia are given in Table 12-2. Five of the six were adults. All patients presented with constitutional symptoms, which varied in duration from three days to six weeks. Two patients had severe bone pain. Three patients had liver and/or splenic enlargement; none had a mediastinal mass. The periaortic and retroperitoneal adenopathy seen on CT scan in patient four was not confirmed at autopsy. Peripheral blood involvement was present in four patients. Only two patients had severe anemia, and one of these also had marked thrombocytopenia. Four patients were treated with ALL protocols. All achieved remission but relapsed on maintenance therapy at 15 to 31 months. Two achieved a second remission. Patient four received therapy for lymphoma and nonlymphoid leukemia, but never achieved remission. Patient six was treated palliatively. Patients two and three are still receiving chemotherapy.

Unclassified Lymphomas

Pathologic Findings

Morphologic and immunologic features of our unclassified lympho-mas are given in Table 12-3. In cases two and four, there was only partial nodal involvement, suggesting a nonlymphoid neoplasm (Fig. 12-6).

Table 12-2
Unclassified Leukemia Patient Population: Clinical Features

Patient	Age, Sex	Major Presenting Features	Organomegaly/ Adenopathy	Laboratory Data	Treatment	Follow-up
1	2, M	Petechiae X three days Fever	Hepatosplenomegaly	PCV 19% WBC 11,000/mm³ (13% blasts) Platelets 20,000/mm³	"Average risk" pediatric ALL protocol[37] Relapse: MTX/L-asp[38]	Relapsed on therapy 24 months after diagnosis; died three months later
2	26, F	Weakness, fatigue X one month Fever	None	PCV 14% WBC 2700/mm³ (41% blasts) Platelets 206,000/mm³	Adult ALL protocol[39,40] Relapse: Adult ALL protocol High dose Ara-C[41] MTX/L-asp	Relapsed in marrow & CNS on therapy 31 months after diagnosis; currently in remission six months after relapse
3	30, M	Bone pain X four weeks Fever Weight loss	None	PCV 35.7% WBC 2000/mm³ (6% blasts) Platelets 201,000/mm³	Adult ALL protocol mega-COMLA consolidation[23] Relapse: Adult ALL protocol	Relapsed on therapy 25 months after diagnosis; currently in remission two months after relapse
4	31, M	Bone pain X six weeks Fever Weight loss	Periaortic and retroperitoneal adenopathy by CT scan	PCV 38.4% WBC 13,900/mm³ Normal differential Platelets 238,000/mm³	COMLA[42] mega-COMLA Ara-C/DNR '7+3'[43] High dose Ara-C	Did not achieve remission. Died four months after diagnosis
5	66, M	Weakness, fatigue X two weeks	Hepatomegaly (mild)	PCV 36.7% WBC 1000/mm³ (10% blasts) Platelets 244,000/mm³	ALL protocol Relapse: no therapy	Relapsed on therapy 15 months after diagnosis; died one month later
6	85, F	Nausea, anorexia, malaise X three weeks	Splenomegaly (marked)	PCV 33.9% WBC 14,400/mm³ Normal differential Platelets 58,000/mm³	Prednisone Splenic irradiation	Died two months after diagnosis

PCV = packed cell volume; WBC = white blood cell count; MTX = methotrexate; L-asp = L-asparaginase; Ara-C = cytosine arabinoside; CNS = central nervous system; COMLA = cyclophosphamide, vincristine, methotrexate, leucovorin, cytarabine; DNR = daunorubicin

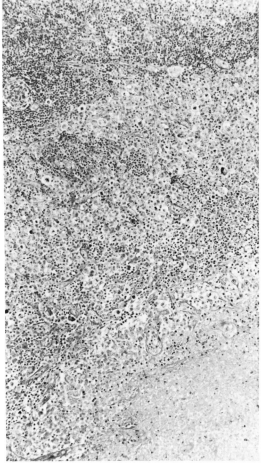

Figure 12-6. *Lymph node from Case four demonstrating partial nodal involvement. Note necrosis (lower right) surrounded by tumor and residual normal lymphoid tissue (upper left). (original magnification X 20.1)*

Partial sparing of thymus was seen in case three (Fig. 12-7). Nodularity was not seen in any case. Cases one and four contained variable amounts of fibrous connective tissue, prominent in case one (Fig. 12-8). Necrosis was not a conspicuous feature, except in case four. The cytology of the tumor cells was varied; however, all cases were composed almost exclusively of large cells (Fig. 12-9). The cells in case four were very large and bizarre,

Table 12-3
Unclassified Lymphoma: Morphologic and Immunologic Features

Patient	Growth Pattern (Biopsy Site)	Tumor Cell Population and Cytology	Special Stains	Immunologic Findings
1	Diffuse involvement with sclerosis (mediastinum)	Medium-large cells with ↑↑ N/C ratio Moderate nuclear irregularity with occasional multilobulated nuclei Finely dispersed chromatin Small nucleoli Occasional tumor giant cells Moderate mitotic rate	MGP + Mucicarmine— Lysozyme—	*Cell suspension:* SIg 18% kappa 8% lambda 2% *ER:* 34%-tumor cells not seen in rosettes *PIP:* IgM, IgG, IgA, kappa, lambda—
2	Partial nodal involvement Diffuse growth pattern Slight ↑ vascularity (inguinal lymph node)	Large cells with ↑ N/C ratio; moderate amount cytoplasm Moderate nuclear folding Partially dispersed chromatin 1–3 prominent nucleoli Numerous tingible body macrophages High mitotic rate	MGP + Mucicarmine—	*FSIP:* T29/33 + IgM, IgG, IgA, IgD, kappa, lambda— Leu 1,2,3a + 3b, 4—

306

3	Slight sparing of thymus (mediastinum); Diffuse growth pattern; Individual cell necrosis (mediastinum and ovary)	Small-medium cells with ↑ N/C ratio; moderate amount cytoplasm; Regular ovoid nuclei; Partially dispersed chromatin; Small nucleoli; Moderate mitotic rate	Weak MGP +	*FSIP:* T29/33 + Ia— IgM, IgG, IgA, IgD, kappa, lambda— Leu 1,2,3a + 3b, 4—
4	Partial nodal involvement with diffuse growth pattern, marked necrosis and focal fibrosis (scalene lymph node); deep dermal involvement, epidermal ulceration; no Pautrier's abscesses (skin)	Very large cells with ↑↑ N/C ratio; Pronounced nuclear folding; Partially dispersed chromatin; Multiple large nucleoli; Numerous multinucleated tumor cells; Numerous eosinophils; occasional plasma cells; High mitotic rate	MGP +	*FSIP (skin):* T29/33 + Ia— IgM, IgG, IgA, IgD, kappa, lambda— Leu 1,2,3a + 3b, 4—
5	Diffuse involvement (chest wall)	Large cells with ↑↑ N/C ratio; Slight nuclear irregularity; Vesiculated chromatin; 1–2 large nucleoli; Numerous tingible body macrophages; High mitotic rate	Not done	*FSIP:* T29/33— Ia focally + IgM, IgG, IgA, IgD, kappa, lambda— Leu 1,2,3a + 3b, 4—

MGP = methyl green pyronine

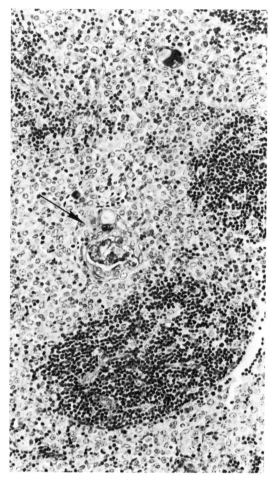

Figure 12-7. *Mediastinal mass from Case three showing partial sparing of thymus. Arrow marks a remaining Hassel's corpuscle. (original magnification X 50)*

with unusually irregular nuclear contours (Fig. 12-10). Numerous tumor giant cells were also seen. In all cases, nuclear chromatin was partially to finely dispersed. Nucleoli were easily found, and were prominent in three cases. The MGP positivity in four cases reflects the high ribosomal content typically seen in transformed lymphocytes. Mucicarmine stains were performed in cases one and two and were negative. Lysozyme was negative in case one.

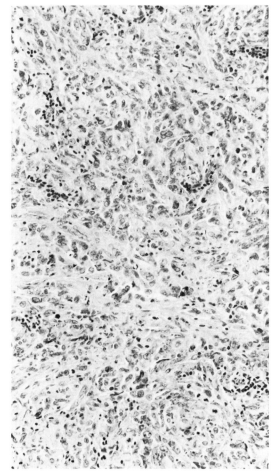

Figure 12-8. *Mediastinal lymph node from Case one demonstrating sclerosis. (original magnification X 40)*

The differential diagnosis in our cases of unclassified lymphoma included neoplasms of nonlymphoid origin. Ultrastructurally, the neoplastic cells demonstrated large nuclei, dispersed chromatin and prominent nucleoli. The cytoplasm was filled with polyribosome aggregates, a few mitochondria, and occasional rough endoplasmic reticulum profiles, features consistent with transformed lymphocytes (Fig. 12-11).[21,22] The

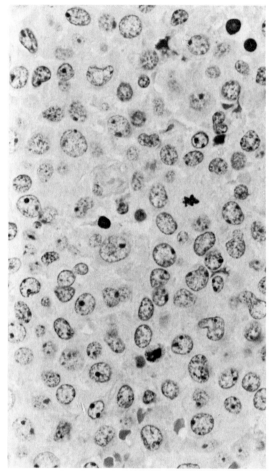

Figure 12-9. *Cytology of neoplastic cells in mediastinal mass from Case three. Note large cells with a moderate amount of cytoplasm, dispersed chromatin, and prominent nucleoli. (original magnification X 201)*

cells differed from leukemic blasts by the presence of more aggregated ribosomes and more abundant cytoplasm.

Case four demonstrated additional features, including multinucleation, very large nucleoli, and occasional cells with a few clusters of granules.

Using FSIP, three of four lymphomas tested showed positive tumor

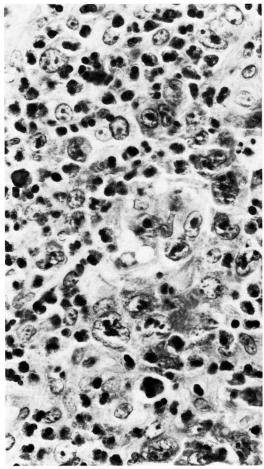

Figure 12-10. *Cytology of neoplastic cells in lymph node from Case four. Note large, pleomorphic and multinucleated cells. (original magnification X 160)*

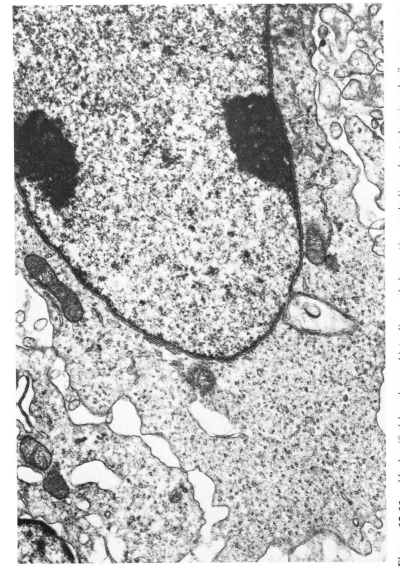

Figure 12-11. *Unclassified lymphoma. Note dispersed chromatin, nucleoli, and cytoplasmic polyribosome aggregates.* (X 19,000)

312

cell marking with T29/33. Case five failed to mark; however, it showed focal staining for Ia antigen. Eighteen percent of cells showed SIg in case one, but monoclonality was not demonstrated. In all other cases, surface immunoglobulins were not detected. A battery of monoclonal T cell antisera gave negative results.

Clinical Features

The clinical features of our patients with unclassified lymphomas are given in Table 12-4. Two of these patients had constitutional symptoms, which were of slightly longer duration than seen in the leukemia patients. One patient had stage III disease, and four had stage IV tumors. Three patients had a mediastinal mass. Four patients received mega-COMLA (see Table 12-4), an aggressive protocol designed at our institution.[23] Two patients who were treated initially with this protocol are in remission at 12 and 23 months follow-up, while the third had a CNS relapse 11 months after diagnosis. The two patients treated with other combination chemotherapy for lymphoma failed to respond to treatment.

Discussion

With careful multiparameter analysis, 98–99 percent of leukemias and lymphomas were successfully classified at our institution. We studied our unclassified cases in order to determine if they constituted a distinct clinicopathologic group.

York et al.[1] pointed out the heterogeneous light microscopic morphology of unclassified leukemias and lymphomas reported in the literature between 1975 and 1981. They attributed the varying appearances to different cells of origin. Our unclassified tumors were similarly varied. Morphologically, our leukemias were heterogeneous by LM (two resembled lymphomas) but were similar by EM. The lymphomas were all large cell neoplasms which were similar ultrastructurally but varied in their distribution within the biopsy and the connective tissue response. Clinically, the unclassified leukemia and lymphoma patients were a heterogeneous group. Ages varied considerably in the unclassified leukemia group; although all unclassified leukemia patients had constitutional symptoms, their specific complaints differed. The unclassified lymphoma patients all presented with advanced disease, although only two had constitutional symptoms. The number of patients in both groups is small, and follow-up is short for the lymphoma group. Nevertheless, there is considerable variation in both groups in response to therapy.

Table 12-4
Unclassified Lymphoma Patient Population: Clinical Features

Patient	Age, Sex	Major Presenting Features	Distribution of Disease	Lab Data	Treatment	Follow-up
1	31, M	Cough for three weeks	Mediastinal mass; splenomegaly and periaortic adenopathy by CT	PCV 45.3% WBC 6500/mm^3 Platelets 197,000/mm^3 LDH 244 IU/L	mega-COMLA MTX (intrathecal) Cranial irradiation CHOP consolidation[44]	Alive without disease 23 months after diagnosis
2	63, M	Left inguinal mass for three months Weight loss Anorexia	Generalized adenopathy Bone marrow involved	PCV 38.3% WBC 7400/mm^3 Platelets 358,000/mm^3 AST 55 IU/L LDH 2580 IU/L Alk phos 680 IU/L	mega-COMLA CHOP consolidation	Alive without disease 12 months after diagnosis

		Presenting symptoms	Findings	Laboratory values	Treatment	Outcome
3	26, F	Cough for several months Dyspnea/stridor Fever	Mediastinal mass Hepatosplenomegaly Pulmonary infiltrates Periaortic adenopathy, enlarged kidneys and ovaries by CT	PCV 26.0% WBC 11,800/mm³ Platelets 570,000/mm³ Alk phos 177 IU/L AST 85 IU/L LDH 1705 IU/L	mega-COMLA CHOP consolidation	Relapsed in CNS 11 months after diagnosis
4	62, F	20x30 cm ulcerated skin lesion, left thigh for six weeks	Skin of left thigh Right scalene lymph node Pulmonary nodules on CXR	Hgb 10.5 g/dl WBC 20,200/mm³ (57% eos) Platelets 393,000/mm³ LDH 255 IU/L	CHOP Ara-C Bleomycin Local irradiation mega-COMLA salvage	Died eight months after diagnosis
5	31, M	Sternal pain and swelling for eight weeks	Mediastinal mass Anterior chest wall mass Destructive sternal lesion on CXR	PCV 40.5% Hgb 13.4 g/dl WBC 7400/mm³ Platelets 390,000/mm³ LDH 680 IU/L	Adriamycin Vincristine Prednisone Ara-C (SEG protocol)	Alive with disease three months after diagnosis

LDH = lactate dehydrogenase; CHOP = Cytoxan, Adriamycin, vincristine, prednisone; AST = aspartate aminotransferase; Alk phos = alkaline phosphatase; CXR = chest x-ray; Hgb = hemoglobin; SEG = Southeastern Cancer Study Group

This group of unclassified neoplasms may be heterogeneous in appearance and clinical behavior for several reasons. The most likely explanation is that several slightly differentiated neoplasms are represented for which methods are not yet available to detect their degree of differentiation. Alternatively, some of these neoplasms may have arisen from a cell for which the phenotype is not yet recognized, or they may represent currently defined tumors which have lost their phenotypic expression. Lastly, some neoplasms may indeed represent neoplams of primitive, truly undifferentiated cells.

In general, the morphologic and clinical features of unclassified leukemias and lymphomas are not well described in the literature. Most laboratories have reported small numbers of unclassified lymphomas, with considerable morphologic heterogeneity. Our cases of unclassified lymphoma also showed varying histology, but were all large cell processes, in contrast to other reports of nonmarking diffuse poorly differentiated lymphocytic lymphoma (DPDLL)[12], anaplastic centrocytic lymphoma, Burkitt's lymphoma, and lymphoblastic lymphoma.[6,8] Although the undifferentiated leukemias of Youness et al.[2] were morphologically similar at the LM level, our cases of leukemia had differing LM appearances.

Most reported lymphomas are considered unclassified or undifferentiated on the basis of immunologic marking. Pinkus et al.[12] found four "null" cases out of 72 non-Hodgkin's lymphomas. One of the cases was a recurrence in a patient who originally had a follicular lymphoma, indicating the possibility of transformation of an underlying B cell neoplasm. Cleaved cells predominated in another two cases, suggesting B cell differentiation. The fourth was a large noncleaved cell tumor (diffuse histiocytic lymphoma). A more recent study of 257 non-Hodgkin's lymphomas using FSIP[9] contained no unclassified cases. In contrast, Pallesen et al.[8] identified nine cases (17 percent) of "O" type (nonexpressive) lymphoma among 53 cases of high grade lymphomas (Kiel classification). The different results in these two recent studies may be due to the inclusion in the Pallesen study of only high grade neoplasms. An intermediate figure, (11 percent or 9/78 undifferentiated high grade lymphomas) was found by Horning et al.,[10] while Watanabe et al.[6] found 14 percent nonmarking lymphomas, all of which had lymphoblastic/ALL type morphology.

Greaves et al.,[7] after detailed immunologic study, found only two undifferentiated leukemias in 594 cases; Marie et al.[14] found two "undifferentiated" leukemias among 16 cases studied with ultrastructural peroxidase and a battery of immunologic markers. Both nonmarking cases were TdT positive.

The value of electron microscopy in identifying differentiation in leukemias has been clearly established, especially in those cases of acute nonlymphoid leukemia where rudimentary granule formation leads to negative or equivocal cytochemical staining.[2,15,18] Youness et al.[2] found that 22/225 leukemias were "undifferentiated" by light microscopy. After ultrastructural examination, 16 of the 22 cases were successfully reclassified as acute myelogenous leukemia, acute monocytic leukemia, or malignant lymphoma. Another ultrastructural technique which may be useful in difficult cases is ultrastructural peroxidase staining.[2,14,24,25]

Ultrastructural examination is especially useful in distinguishing lymphomas from nonlymphoid neoplasms.[3,4] EM apparently does not distinguish B from T cells except in those cases containing Sezary cells or cells with plasmacytic differentiation.[13] Diagnostic difficulties are particularly noted in the case of the diffuse, large noncleaved cell lymphoma that does not mark immunologically. EM may only provide confirmation of the lymphoid origin in this instance, and will not provide the important immunologic data.

Due to the paucity of cases, there is little clinical information on unclassified leukemias. In the only report dealing solely with unclassified leukemias, Youness et al.[2] noted the lack of organomegaly and peripheral blood involvement in all six patients with unclassified leukemia.

Warnke et al.[26] studied thirty diffuse large cell lymphomas and found that immunoglobulin (Ig) negative patients (including two patients with nonmarking lymphomas) fared better than Ig positive patients. None of the cases marked as T cell lymphomas. In a more recent report from the same institution,[10] advanced age and stage proved to be the most important predictors of survival.

Recently developed techniques are likely to reduce the number of unclassified cases to a number approximating the truly unclassifiable figure. These methods include flow cytometry using monoclonal antibodies, biochemical markers, karyotypic analysis, and gene rearrangement.

Flow cytometry is particularly suited for examining hematopoietic and lymphoid neoplasms, whether in node, bone marrow, peripheral blood, CSF, or other body fluids.[27] Flow cytometry must be correlated with histopathologic analysis in order to avoid misdiagnoses of lymphomas. In particular, some B cell tumors contain a high percentage of intermixed T cells.[27]

Monoclonal antibodies that identify myeloid, megakaryocytic, and erythroid differentiation have recently been developed, and appear to be useful in classifying nonlymphoid leukemias.[7,28,29] The value of using multiple monoclonal antibodies (including markers for common ALL antigen (cALLA), M_1, M_2, Ig, TdT, glycophorin, glycoprotein I, Ia, and various T cell antigens) was reported by Greaves et al.,[7] who successfully classified 22/24 "undifferentiated" leukemias. Although 21/22 were lymphoid leukemias of various phenotypes, one case was shown to have myeloid differentiation.

TdT is the biochemical marker most extensively studied. Despite the recognition that TdT may be seen in occasional nonlymphoid cells,[5,24,30] many observers consider it a predictor of lymphoid differentiation. TdT may be particularly useful in identifying adult ALL, which is frequently cALLA negative.[20] Other biochemical markers have been studied less thoroughly than TdT, including hexosaminidase isoenzyme ratio, used to define common ALL, and adenosine deaminase levels.[20]

Characteristic karyotypic abnormalities have been described in hematopoietic lymphoid neoplasms[31,32]. The 8;14 translocation seen in small noncleaved B cell (both Burkitt's and non-Burkitt's) lymphoma and the 15;17 translocation found in acute promyelocytic leukemia[33] seem to be reproducible abnormalities. Numerous other chromosomal disorders, most of them complex structural rearrangements, have been described for a variety of leukemias and lymphomas. It is of interest that chromosome 14 is frequently abnormal in lymphoid neoplasms, but only rarely in myeloid tumors.[31] A wide variety of karyotypic abnormalities may be encountered in a given tumor, but each appears to be unique and thus a recognizable marker for that particular neoplasm.

Immunoglobulin gene rearrangement is a recently described marker of B cell neoplasms; it is highly sensitive and therefore may detect even small populations of monoclonal B cells.[34,35] Immunoglobulin gene rearrangement may allow definitive diagnosis in several otherwise difficult instances: identification of a malignant neoplasm arising in a reactive process, differentiation of lymphoid from nonlymphoid neoplasms, identifying a small population of neoplastic cells, and differentiating B from T cell lymphomas.[34] Although currently in use in only a few centers, immunoglobulin gene rearrangement holds much promise as a useful diagnostic tool in difficult cases.

A recently published abstract[36] shows the utility of performing a battery of marker studies (including common leukocyte antigen, Ia antigen, cALLA, TdT, B and T monoclonal antibodies, cytoplasmic mu heavy chains, and Ig gene rearrangement) in cases of non-Hodgkin's lymphoma which are SIg and ER negative. The authors successfully reclassified 17 nonmarking cases as B (13 cases) or T (four cases) cell neoplasms.

Experience with multiparameter analyses over the last ten years indicates that the majority of hematopoietic and lymphoid neoplasms may be categorized with reasonable assurance using currently available methods. Batteries of techniques must be used, as no single technique is sufficient for categorization of all cases. DNA characterization obviously has the greatest potential as the most sensitive and specific marker of differentiation, but wide application may be limited by the need for fresh tissue and the complexity of the procedure. Using these techniques, the present unclassified group may be reduced to a more homogeneous pathologic and clinical group. The number of cases is now so small their recognition may have more biologic than clinical significance.

Acknowledgments

We would like to thank Mrs. Constance Singleton and Ms. Yvette Adams for secretarial assistance, Mrs. Cheryl Marcum for technical assistance, and Drs. William Shasteen (Huntsville, Alabama) and Larry Vogler for case referral and patient information. This work was supported in part by NIH training Grant AMO 7186.

References

1. York JC, Glick AD, Collins RD: Unclassified leukemias and lymphomas. Semin Oncol 9:497–503, 1982
2. Youness E, Trujillo JM, Ahearn MJ, et al: Acute unclassified leukemia. A clinicopathologic study with diagnostic implications of electron microscopy. Am J Hematol 9:79–88, 1980
3. Azar HA, Espinoza CG, Richman AV, et al: "Undifferentiated" large cell malignancies: An ultrastructural and immunocytochemical study. Hum Pathol 13:323–333, 1982
4. Gillespie JJ: Ultrastructural diagnosis of large cell 'undifferentiated' neoplasia. Diag Histopathol 5:33–51, 1982
5. Janossy G, Bollum FJ, Bradstock KF, et al: Cellular phenotypes of normal and leukemic hemopoietic cells determined by analysis with selected antibody combinations. Blood 56:430–441, 1980
6. Watanabe S, Shimosato Y, Shimoyama M, et al: Studies with multiple markers on malignant lymphomas and lymphoid leukemias. Cancer 50:2372–2382, 1982
7. Greaves MF, Bell R, Amess J, et al: ALL masquerading as AUL. Leuk Res 7:735–746, 1983

8. Pallesen G, Madsen M, Schifter S: Immune marker expression in 53 lymphomas of high-grade malignancy. Histopathol 7:841–857, 1983

9. Tubbs RR, Fishleder A, Weiss RA, et al: Immunohistologic cellular phenotypes of lymphoproliferative disorders. Comprehensive evaluation of 564 cases including 257 non-Hodgkin's lymphomas classified by the international working formulation. Am J Pathol 113:207–221, 1983

10. Horning SJ, Doggett RS, Warnke RA, et al: Clinical relevance of immunologic phenotype in diffuse large cell lymphoma. Blood 63:1209–1215, 1984

11. Filippa DA, Lieberman PH, Erlandson RA, et al: A study of malignant lymphomas using light and ultramicroscopic, cytochemical and immunologic technics. Correlation with clinical features. Am J Med 64:259–268, 1978

12. Pinkus GS, Said JW: Characterization of non-Hodgkin's lymphomas using multiple cell markers. Immunologic, morphologic, and cytochemical studies of 72 cases. Am J Pathol 94:349–380, 1979

13. Said JW, Hargreaves HK, Pinkus GS: Non-Hodgkin's lymphomas: An ultrastructural study correlating morphology with immunologic cell type. Cancer 44:504–528, 1979

14. Marie JP, Perrot JY, Boucheix C, et al: Determination of ultrastructural peroxidases and immunologic membrane markers in the diagnosis of acute leukemias. Blood 59:270–276, 1982

15. Glick AD, Horn RG: Identification of promonocytes and monocytoid precursors in acute leukaemia of adults: Ultrastructural and cytochemical observations. Br J Haematol 26:395–403, 1974

16. Glick AD: Acute leukemia: Electron microscopic diagnosis. Semin Oncol 3:229–241, 1976

17. Glick AD, Vestal BK, Flexner JM, et al: Ultrastructural study of acute lymphocytic leukemia: Comparison with immunologic studies. Blood 52:311–322, 1978

18. Glick AD, Paniker K, Flexner JM, et al: Acute leukemia of adults: Ultrastructural, cytochemical and histologic observations in 100 cases. Am J Clin Pathol 73:459–470, 1980

19. Collins RD, Cousar JB, Russell WG, et al: Diagnosis of neoplasms of the immune system, in Rose NR, Friedman H (eds): Manual of Clinical Immunology. Washington, American Society for Microbiology, 1980, pp 84–101

20. Hoffbrand AV, Ganeshaguru K, Llewelin P, et al: Biochemical markers in leukaemia and lymphoma. Recent Results Cancer Res 69:25–36, 1979

21. Glick AD, Leech JH, Waldron JA, et al: Malignant lymphomas of follicular center cell origin in man. II. Ultrastructural and cytochemical studies. J Natl Cancer Inst 54:23–36, 1975

22. Glick AD, Leech JH, Flexner JM, et al: Ultrastructural study of Reed-Sternberg cells. Comparison with transformed lymphocytes and histiocytes. Am J Pathol 85:195–208, 1976

23. Hainsworth JD, Wolff SN, Stein RS, et al: Treatment of very poor prognosis lymphoid neoplasms with mega-COMLA, a high dose modification of the COMLA protocol: Preliminary results. (in preparation)

24. Catovsky D: Symposium: Classification of leukemia. 1. The classification of acute leukemia. Pathology 14:277–281, 1982

25. Jansson S-E, Gripenberg J, Vuopio P, et al: Classification of acute leukaemia by light and electron microscope cytochemistry. Scand J Haematol 25:412–416, 1980

26. Warnke R, Miller R, Grogan T, et al: Immunologic phenotype in 30 patients with diffuse large-cell lymphoma. N Engl J Med 303:293–300, 1980

27. Lovett EJ, Schnitzer B, Keren DF, et al: Application of flow cytometry to diagnostic pathology. Lab Invest 50:115–140, 1984

28. Foon KA, Schroff RW, Gale RP: Surface markers on leukemia and lymphoma cells: Recent advances. Blood 60:1–18, 1982

29. Shumak KH, Rachkewich RA: An antigen shared by human granulocytes, monocytes, marrow granulocyte precursors and leukemic blasts. Acta Haemat 69:164–170, 1983

30. Bollum FJ: Terminal deoxynucleotidyl transferase as a hematopoietic cell marker. Blood 54:1203–1215, 1979

31. Rowley JD, Fukuhara S: Chromosome studies in non-Hodgkin's lymphomas. Semin Oncol 7:255–266, 1980

32. Yunis JJ, Oken MM, Kaplan ME, et al: Distinctive chromosomal abnormalities in histologic subtypes of non-Hodgkin's lymphoma. N Engl J Med 307:1231–1236, 1982

33. Testa JR, Golomb HM, Rowley JD, et al: Hypergranular promyelocytic leukemia (APL): Cytogenetic and ultrastructural specificity. Blood 52:272–280, 1978

34. Arnold A, Cossman J, Bakhshi A, et al: Immunoglobulin-gene rearrangements as unique clonal markers in human lymphoid neoplasms. N Engl J Med 309:1593–1599, 1983

35. Cleary ML, Chao J, Warnke R, et al: Immunoglobulin gene rearrangement as a diagnostic criterion of B-cell lymphoma. Proc Natl Acad Sci USA 81:593–597, 1984

36. Knowles DM, Wang CY, Ault F, et al: Determination of the B or T cell lineage of SIg⁻E⁻ ("null cell") non-Hodgkin's lymphomas by multiparametric analysis. Lab Invest 50:31A, 1984

37. Coccia PF, Bleyer WA, Siegel SE, et al: Development and preliminary findings of children's cancer study group protocols (161, 162 and 163) for low-, average-, and high-risk acute lymphoblastic leukemia in children, in Murphy SB, Gilbert JR (eds): Leukemia Research: Advances in Cell Biology and Treatment. New York, Elsevier Biomedical, 1983, pp 241–250

38. Lobel JS, O'Brien RT, McIntosh S, et al: Methotrexate and asparaginase combination chemotherapy in refractory acute lymphoblastic leukemia of childhood. Cancer 43:1089–1094, 1979

39. Stein RS, Flexner JM, Collins RD: Effective multidrug, multimodality consolidation therapy of adult acute lymphocytic leukemia. A preliminary report. Cancer 49:846–849, 1982

40. Stein RS, Baer MR, Flexner JM: Improved survival in adult acute lymphoblastic leukemia: need for more effective CNS prophylaxis. Am J Clin Oncol (in press)

41. Herzig RH, Wolff SN, Lazarus HM, et al: High dose cytosine arabinoside therapy for refractory leukemia. Blood 62:361–369, 1983

42. Sweet DL, Golomb HM, Ultmann JE, et al: Cyclophosphamide, vincristine, methotrexate with leucovorin rescue, and cytarabine (COMLA) combination sequential chemotherapy for advanced diffuse histiocytic lymphoma. Ann Intern Med 92:785–790, 1980

43. Cassileth PA, Katz ME: Chemotherapy for adult acute nonlymphocytic leukemia with daunorubicin and cytosine arabinoside. Cancer Treat Rep 61:1441–1445, 1977

44. McKelvey EM, Gottlieb JA, Wilson HE, et al: Hydroxyldaunomycin (Adriamycin) combination chemotherapy in malignant lymphoma. Cancer 38:1484–1493, 1976

13

SMALL CELL CARCINOMAS OF EXTRAPULMONARY ORIGIN

Ronald L. Richardson

Small cell anaplastic carcinomas may be difficult diagnostic and therapeutic problems. Though the majority of small cell carcinomas (SCC) found outside the bronchial tree in adults are metastatic small cell lung cancers, clearly some small cell carcinomas originate in extrapulmonary sites such as the following.

Paranasal sinuses	Gallbladder
Major and minor salivary glands	Pancreas
Hypopharynx	Thymus
Larynx	Breast
Trachea	Prostate
Esophagus	Uterine corpus
Stomach	Uterine cervix
Small Intestine	Bladder
Colon	Skin

Despite this diversity of origins, SCCs from these sites share a number of histologic characteristics. By light microscopy the cells are two to three times the diameter of a small lymphocyte. The cells may be small and round, resembling pulmonary oat cell carcinoma, or may be somewhat

POORLY DIFFERENTIATED NEOPLASMS AND TUMORS OF UNKNOWN ORIGIN   ISBN 0-8089-1755-2
© 1986 by Grune & Stratton.

larger with polygonal, fusiform, or spindle shapes. Some cells may have finely dispersed "salt and pepper" nuclear chromatin with indistinct nucleoli, but others may have hyperchromatic nuclei with intense basophilia. Crush artifact may be prominent in some specimens. In areas adjacent to necrosis, basophilic material may be deposited in elastic fibrils in vessel walls. These cells tend to grow in sheets but other patterns such as ribbons, rosettes, and palisades may be seen. Occasionally they are arranged in tubular structures, sometimes with mucicarmine- or PAS-positive material between the cells. Intracytoplasmic PAS-positive material is uncommon though Matsusaka and associates[1] have reported PAS-positive cells in an esophageal SCC. Argyrophil stains by the Sevier-Munger or Grimelius methods are usually positive in some cells but argentaffin stains are negative.

The light microscopic features of the oat cell variant of SCC usually enable ready distinction from other poorly differentiated small cell malignancies such as those listed below.

Small cell carcinoma (lymphocyte-like (oat cell) and intermediate cell variants)
Carcinoid/islet cell carcinomas
Squamous carcinoma
Adenocarcinoma
Malignant melanoma
Lymphoma
Ewing's sarcoma
Neuroblastoma

Because of similar histologic characteristics, however, the separation of carcinoids from oat cell carcinomas may be difficult. Fisher and coworkers[2] compared light microscopic, histochemical, and electron microscopic features of bronchial carcinoids with those of pulmonary oat cell carcinomas. They found a ribbon-like arrangement of monomorphic cells of high (favorable) nuclear grade to be useful features in the diagnosis of carcinoid. Necrosis, mitotic figures, basophilic perivascular deposits, low (unfavorable) nuclear grade, and perineural invasion were seen only in oat cell carcinomas. Argyrophilic granules by light microscopy and "neurosecretory type" granules by electron microscopy were seen more often in cells of carcinoids.

The separation of the intermediate cell size variant of SCC from the other tumor types may be difficult with routine hematoxylin–eosin stained material alone. The recognition of this SCC variant is based primarily on appreciation of the slightly larger cell size in comparison to the lymphocyte-like variant and of the similar monomorphic pattern, often with necrosis, but clinical clues may also be helpful in suggesting the diagnosis.

Special staining techniques may be useful in the differential diagnosis of tumors of small cell size. Demonstration of glycogen granules by PAS staining before and after diastase digestion may suggest a diagnosis of Ewing's sarcoma. Immunofluorescence studies utilizing labeled antibodies to human immunoglobulin chains may demonstrate a monoclonal aggregation of malignant cells indicative of lymphoma.

Electron microscopy may be a useful adjunct to light microscopy in the diagnosis of small cell malignancies. A hallmark of SCC by electron microscopy is the presence of cytoplasmic electron dense neurosecretory granules. These granules may be bounded by a limiting membrane and vary in size from less than 100 to greater than 400 mμ in diameter. The fraction of tumor cells containing granules and the numbers of granules within these cells are variable, and in some SCCs granules may be difficult to find. Dense core granules are found in neuroblastoma cells, usually toward the ends of elongated cytoplasmic processes. Though some consider these granules diagnostic of a "neuroendocrine" malignancy, dense core granules have also been found in pulmonary large cell carcinomas. Other electron microscopic features of SCCs include occasional desmosomal attachments, cytoplasmic microfilaments, and in some instances, abundant free ribosomes. These ultrastructural features are useful in distinguishing the various types of small cell size neoplasms. The presence of well-developed desmosomes between cells indicates the neoplasm is a carcinoma rather than a lymphoma. Tonofibrils and cytoplasmic mucin granules suggest squamous carcinoma and adenocarcinoma respectively. Electron dense melanosomes are found in malignant melanoma, and glycogen granules may be seen in abundance in Ewing's sarcoma. Glutaraldehyde-fixed specimens are preferred in electron microscopy but Gyorkey and associates[3] have reported good preservation of cellular ultrastructural detail in tissues fixed in the 10 percent buffered formalin routinely used for light microscopic studies.

Clinical Factors

In contrast to pulmonary SCC, which comprises about 20 percent of all lung cancer, extrapulmonary SCCs are thought to be rare malignancies. In her 1952 report, generally regarded as the first description of extrapulmonary SCC, McKeown[4] found her two cases of oat cell carcinoma of the esophagus to be the only extrapulmonary small cell tumors in 9000 autopsies at her institution. More recently, Fer and colleagues[5] reviewed a combined series from two institutions of 400 patients with a histologic diagnosis of SCC seen in a six-year period. They found 20 patients (five percent) who had no detectable pulmonary lesions and who appeared to have SCC arising in extrapulmonary sites.

Extrapulmonary small cell carcinomas (ESCCs) have been observed in a variety of sites, and this number of sites is increasing. In fact, three additional sites (bladder, endometrium, and gallbladder) have been reported since the author reviewed this subject in 1982.[6] Though ESCCs are still regarded as interesting but uncommon anecdotes, it is likely that these tumors are more frequent than the case reports and small series may indicate. There is a paucity of information regarding the clinical behavior or responsiveness to treatment of this group of neoplasms. Hence, there has been little impetus to separate this group of malignancies from other poorly differentiated carcinomas arising in a given site because of a lack of information that such a distinction has clinical importance. As the number of case reports of ESCCs of a given site increases, however, there is growing evidence that such a distinction may be important for some types of ESCC.

Esophagus

Since McKeown's report[4] of esophageal SCC in 1952, others have reported single cases or small series of patients with this neoplasm. This malignancy appears to be rare in the United States and Western Europe but more common in Japan. Turnbull and associates[7] found only a single case of esophageal SCC among 1918 esophageal malignancies seen at Memorial Hospital from 1926 to 1968. Briggs and Ibrahim[8] found 23 cases of esophageal SCC in 955 cases of esophageal carcinoma seen over a 14-year span. Reyes and colleagues[9] reviewed 928 cases of primary esophageal cancers and found 16 cases of undifferentiated carcinomas defined as neuroendocrine carcinomas on the basis of neurosecretory granules by electron microscopy. Interestingly, four of the 16 cases displayed tonofilament bundles and keratohyalin granules; mucosubstance droplets were seen in others, suggesting that some of these malignancies are capable of multidirectional differentiation. Others[8,10,11] have reported light or electron microscopic features of squamous carcinoma in esophageal SCC.

The majority of patients with esophageal SCC are male, usually in their seventh decade. Surgery alone has yielded disappointing results with median survivals of about six months. Chemotherapy may be of benefit to some patients. Fer and coworkers[5] reported that a patient with supraclavicular nodal metastasis who was treated with multiple drug therapy achieved a complete remission; this patient died 11 months after diagnosis and had no evidence of malignancy at postmortem examination. They also reported that a patient treated with adjuvant chemotherapy remained free of disease more than six months following surgery. Rosenthal and Lemkin[12] treated a 74-year-old patient having multiple foci of esophageal SCC with a combination of cyclophosphamide, doxorubicin, and vincristine; this patient had a transient response, showing evidence of recurrence after five courses of chemotherapy. The author is aware of two cases (unpublished observations) treated with similar regimens (cyclophosphamide, doxorubicin, and etoposide), both of whom appeared to respond to chemotherapy. Both patients received radiotherapy to the mediastinum in an attempt to consolidate response; however, one patient developed progressive disease within the radiation port and died 15 months after diagnosis; the other patient developed hepatic metastases 10 months after diagnosis and remains alive with progressive disease.

The short survival with widespread metastasis at death in patients with esophageal SCC is similar to the clinical courses seen in patients with esophageal squamous and adenocarcinomas. Nevertheless, the responses noted in a small number of patients treated with multiple agent chemotherapy regimens suggest that these neoplasms may be more sensitive to drug therapy than squamous and adenocarcinomas of the esophagus.

Stomach

Gastric SCCs are rare. Matsusaka and associates[13] found only two cases in nearly 2000 gastric carcinomas. One patient had metastasis to the liver at the time of distal partial gastrectomy. He died one year later of tumor progression but his postsurgical treatment was not described. Their second patient was treated by partial gastrectomy for a mixed tumor composed of SCC, mucous cell carcinoma, and well differentiated adenocarcinoma; he remained disease-free five years later.

Eimoto and Hayakawa[14] reported findings in a 66-year-old man found to have an unresectable gastric SCC. This patient was treated with 5-fluorouracil and mitomycin C but had no response to treatment and died four months after diagnosis. At postmortem examination he had a large fungating tumor involving the anterior wall of the gastric cardia with tumor invading transmurally to involve the left lobe of the liver, peritoneal surface of the diaphragm, and perigastric lymph nodes. In addition, there were several separate tumor nodules in the liver suggesting hematogenous spread, although no tumor was found in the lungs, adrenals, or other organs.

Chejfec and Gould[15] described biochemical and histologic findings in two patients having undifferentiated gastric carcinomas with focal areas resembling oat cell carcinoma. Both patients had hepatic metastasis at time of diagnosis and had rapid downhill courses, dying four weeks and 10 weeks after admission. Tumor extracts contained vanillylmandelic acid and 5-hydroxy-3 indoleacetic acid. Electron microscopy demonstrated membrane-bound dense core granules in many tumor cells.

Fer and associates[5] described a 69-year-old patient with gastric SCC who was treated with chemotherapy alone. He had a partial response lasting seven months but died of progressive cancer 10 months later.

Bernatz[16] reviewed the Mayo Clinic experience with gastric SCC up to 1950. He found 72 patients with gastric SCC, but in three-fourths of these patients SCC was part of a mixed histologic pattern. Seventeen patients had only SCC without other histologic types; 16 of these patients were male, and the median age for these 17 patients was 49.5 years. Eleven of 16 patients (68.7 percent) with gastric SCC survived five years. Size of the primary neoplasm did not appear to affect prognosis as 50 percent of the five-year survivors had tumors greater than 8 cm in diameter. Bernatz stated that it may be difficult to distinguish between lymphoma and carcinoma by light microscopy. Indeed, it seems likely that some of the cases diagnosed as gastric SCC might be reclassified as lymphomas if examined with such diagnostic aids as electron microscopy and immunofluorescence stains for lymphocyte markers.

Small Intestine

Toker reported[17] findings in a 17-year-old woman who had a SCC in the upper jejunum. She was treated by surgical resection and appeared to be disease-free six years after her surgery.

Colon

Clery and coworkers[18] reviewed the colonic SCCs seen at the Mayo Clinic from 1907 to 1957. They found 28 small cell colonic cancers in 27 patients, a figure comprising 0.2 percent of all colonic malignancies seen at the institution during that 50-year period. The male/female ratio of these patients was two to one, and they ranged in age from 25 to 74 years (average 54 years). Depth of invasion was ascertained in 23 tumors: five were classified as Duke's B_1, six as Duke's B_2, and 12 as Duke's C lesions. Nineteen patients had attempts at curative surgery and could be followed for survival. Six died within 18 months, but six survived more than ten years; three lived more than 20 years after surgery.

More recently, Gould and Chejfec[19] reported histochemical and ultrastructural findings in four patients with undifferentiated colonic carcinomas which had neuroendocrine characteristics. Tumor extracts contained catecholamines and vanillylmandelic acid, and electron micros- copy showed dense core granules in tumor specimens from all four patients. All patients had widespread abdominal disease as well as involvement of lungs or distant lymph nodes at death. In three patients the diagnoses were made nine to 14 months prior to death, and in the remaining case the neoplasm was found at autopsy.

Mills and associates[20] reported five cases of colonic SCC, four of which arose within adenomas. One of the adenomas was a typical sessile villous adenoma and the remaining three lesions were composed of mixed tubular and villous elements. The junctions between the SCC components and the adenomas were distinct and abrupt with no transitional areas or blending into the undifferentiated components. In one case the primary tumor and the liver metastasis showed foci of squamous differentiation surrounded by SCC. Electron microscopy in three specimens showed dense core granules. Three of the five patients died of rapidly progressive malignancy; one patient died three weeks after seeking medical care and the diagnosis was made at autopsy; two patients died of widely disseminated malignancy one and three months after diagnosis. Petrelli and coworkers[21] and Damjanov and colleagues[22] described two additional patients with SCC of the colon whose tumors showed squamous, neuroendocrine, and exocrine differen- tiation. Both patients had very aggressive malignancies, dying nine days and four weeks after diagnosis. Schroeder and Snow[23] reported a case of a cloacogenic SCC associated with a villous adenoma. Their patient, a 33-year-old woman, underwent an abdominoperineal resection, left salpingo-oophorectomy, and partial resection of the vagina for SCC invading the pelvis and involving regional lymph nodes. She received two courses of cyclophosphamide, doxorubicin, and etoposide but developed progressive disease in the pelvis. Radiotherapy and additional chemother- apy with mitomycin C, 5-fluorouracil, and streptozotocin failed to halt the disease. She died seven months after diagnosis with widespread metastasis in the brain, chest, retroperitoneum, liver, and pelvis.

Although the number of patients in recent reports of colonic SCC is small, the aggressive behavior of the neoplasm and poor survival of these patients appear quite different from those reported by Clery and associ- ates.[18] Given the evolution of criteria for distinguishing SCC from carcinoid tumors, it is possible that Clery's series included patients with the less aggressive carcinoid tumors of the colon.

Gallbladder

Albores-Saavedra and colleagues[24] reported finding 19 oat cell carcinomas among 448 epithelial malignancies of the gallbladder (4.5 percent). These SCCs had typical oat cell appearance though four tumors contained areas of well-differentiated adenocarcinoma. Eighteen of the patients had cholelithiasis, and 17 of the patients were elderly women. The diagnosis was made at autopsy in 14 patients and during surgery in five patients. Only two patients were treated with chemotherapy (doxorubicin, vincristine, cyclophosphamide, and nitrosourea), and they survived 11 and 13 months though their responses were not reported.

Pancreas

SCC of the pancreas is uncommon. Reyes and Wang[25] found five cases of pancreatic SCC among 485 pancreatic cancers accumulated over 29 years. All five patients died within two months but treatment details were omitted. Cubilla and Fitzgerald[26] found seven cases of pancreatic SCC among 508 pancreatic cancers; no information on clinical behavior of these neoplasms or patients survival was given.

Fer and associates[5] included two patients with SCC of the pancreas in their review. Both patients responded to combination chemotherapy, and one patient had a complete response confirmed by "second look" laparotomy.

Corrin and colleagues[27] reported a patient with SCC of the pancreas and Cushing's syndrome due to ectopic ACTH production.

Salivary Glands

In 1965 Raychowdhuri[28] reported a patient who died of a frontal lobe abscess and purulent meningitis and who was found to have a SCC involving the ethmoid, nasal cavity, and sphenoid sinus. In a later report Koss and associates[29] reviewed 434 malignant tumors of minor salivary glands seen at Memorial Hospital between 1939 and 1963 and found 14 cases of SCC. These SCCs were seen in areas in which minor salivary glands are found (the hard and soft palate, base of tongue, tonsil, epiglottis, ethmoid, antrum, and nasal cavity), and in each case minor salivary gland tissue was the presumed site of origin of the neoplasm. Five of the 14 patients had cervical nodal metastasis at time of diagnosis, and two patients subsequently developed nodal involvement. Eight patients developed local recurrence despite surgery and/or radiotherapy. Four of the 14 patients lived five years or more but two of these five-year survivors later succumbed to progressive malignancy. Weiss and colleagues[30] described a case of SCC of the ethmoid sinus. Electron microscopy of the tumor showed dense core granules but no salivary gland tissue was seen in association with the neoplasm. The patient was treated with radiation but developed widespread metastasis in bone and in subcutaneous tissue on the chest and abdominal wall. She responded to combination chemotherapy consisting of cyclophosphamide, vincristine, methotrexate, and carmustine but subsequently died of disease progression 21 months after diagnosis. Leipzig and Gonzales-Vitale[31] reported findings in two cases of small cell malignancy of the parotid. In one case light microscopy suggested two populations of malignant cells. The first consisted of light cells with round or oval nuclei, finely granular chromatin, and scanty cytoplasm, and the second of dark cells with irregular, elongated nuclei, heavily clumped chromatin, and scanty cytoplasm. In the second case electron microscopy showed tonofilaments and desmosomes; neurosecretory granules were not seen. They interpreted these light and electron microscopic findings as showing epidermoid differentiation and concluded that SCCs of the salivary glands are a heterogeneous group. Kraemer and coworkers[32] presented clinical and histologic features of three SCCs of the parotid. They found dense core granules and cytoplasmic dendritic processes in two cases and mature desmosomes in the third case. They concluded that there are at least two types of SCC of salivary gland origin, a neuroendocrine type and a duct cell type. Ferlito and Polidoro[33] have reported a patient having a tumor of the hypopharynx with mixed small cell and squamous carcinoma features.

Nagao and associates[34] reported finding 12 cases of small cell undifferentiated carcinoma in 176 malignant parotid tumors. Electron microscopy showed abundant tonofilaments and desmosomes but no neurosecretory granules in all 12 cases.

Larynx

In 1972 Olofsson and Van Nostrand[35] reported a case of SCC of the larynx, and nearly 50 cases have been reported since then. Gnepp and associates[36] have reviewed findings in 18 cases from their institutions and in 25 cases from the literature. Like squamous carcinoma, SCC of the larynx is found predominantly among older men, usually in their sixth or seventh decades, with a history of tobacco use. Seventy-nine percent of the patients in Gnepp's review were male and at least 60 percent had a history of cigarette smoking. More than half of the patients initially presented with cervical nodal metastasis or were found to have nodal involvement at time of radical neck dissection. The most common site of laryngeal involvement by SCC was supraglottic; in contrast squamous carcinoma most often arises in a glottic location. Twenty-seven of 37 patients on whom follow-up data were available died from their laryngeal SCCs; average survival for this group was 9.8 months, ranging from 1 to 26 months. Thirty-four patients presented with metastatic disease or developed metastasis later. Excluding cervical nodes, the most common sites of spread were liver (13 patients), lung (11 patients), and bone (10 patients). Eight patients remained clinically disease-free with follow-up from 6 to 90 months. Though various combinations of surgery, radiation, and chemotherapy were tried in these patients, there were no substantive differences in survival between the various treatment modalities. Posner and colleagues[37] presented four cases of SCC of the larynx treated with combination chemotherapy (cyclophosphamide, doxorubicin, and vincristine). Three patients were assessable for response: two achieved partial responses, while a complete response was reached in the third patient. Based on their patients' responses and on the similarities in clinical behavior of this neoplasm and pulmonary SCC, they recommended combined modality treatment of this neoplasm using combination chemotherapy and radiation.

Medina and coworkers[38] reported a case of SCC of the larynx associated with the Eaton-Lambert syndrome. Thompson and associates[39] presented a case of laryngeal SCC associated with an IgD multiple myeloma.

Despite the relatively small number of reports of SCC of the larynx, it is clear that this neoplasm is clinically aggressive with rapid spread to regional nodes and extranodal dissemination. The poor prognosis associated with laryngeal SCC when managed only with local–regional treatment methods and its responsiveness to chemotherapy strongly recommend a combined modality strategy similar to that employed for pulmonary SCC.

Trachea

Primary carcinoma of the trachea is very uncommon: autopsy data from several large centers reported by Culp[40] and by Stenn[41] showed 11 cases in 87,663 autopsies. Most tracheal cancers are epidermoid carcinomas and Sweeney[42] has estimated that only one to four percent of primary tracheal cancers are SCCs. Like other respiratory tract cancers, SCC of the trachea tends to occur in older individuals; the median age of nine reported cases[43–49] was 60 years. Survival in these cases was poor with only one patient surviving more than a year. Though virtually all patients had distant spread at autopsy, in most cases death resulted from progression of local disease in the trachea. Two of the nine patients received chemotherapy including the longest survivor who lived 26 months after diagnosis.

Thymus

Rosai and associates[50] reported four patients with mediastinal SCC who had no detectable pulmonary primary tumors at autopsy and who, they felt, had SCC originating in the thymus. One patient died of an unrelated disorder five years after resection of his mediastinal SCC and had no evidence of residual SCC at autopsy. Details of the survivals, patterns of metastasis, or responses to therapy of the other three patients were not presented.

Breast

Cohle and colleagues[51] and Woodard and associates[52] have described two patients with adenocarcinomas of the breast and ectopic ACTH production. In both cases electron microscopy showed dense core granules, and immunoperoxidase staining of tumor specimens showed cytoplasmic ACTH though the histologic patterns of the two specimens were typical of lobular carcinoma[51] and of infiltrating ductal carcinoma.[52] Estrogen receptor assay of tumor in one case[52] showed a moderately high estrogen receptor value. Apart from the development of Cushing's syndrome, the distributions of disease, clinical courses, and responses to therapy of these two patients seemed comparable to those of other breast cancer patients.

Prostate

SCC of the prostate is uncommon though a number of investigators[53-55] have reported ectopic ACTH production in poorly differentiated adenocarcinomas of the prostate. Electron microscopy showed dense core granules in two cases, and ACTH assay or immunoperoxidase staining for ACTH was positive in four cases. Fer and associates[5] included a patient with prostatic SCC in their series. The author has seen two patients with SCC of the prostate at the Mayo Clinic in the last four years. In neither case nor in any of the reported cases does it appear that SCC of the prostate behaves differently from the behavioral spectrum seen in adenocarcinoma of the prostate. It is possible that there is a sizable subgroup of poorly differentiated prostatic cancers possessing neuroendocrine features but causing no ectopic hormone syndromes, but it remains unclear whether this subgroup has a unique clinical behavior or therapeutic response.

Bladder

Cramer and colleagues[56] reported the first case of SCC of the bladder in 1981. Their patient, a 69-year-old man, had hematuria, nocturia, and frequency for one month. Evaluation showed hypophosphatemia, and contrast radiograms of the bladder showed multiple diverticula. Cystoscopy showed white, irregular mucosa in one diverticulum, and biopsy of this area showed SCC. A partial cystectomy was performed with removal of the diverticulum and the associated mass. The patient appeared to be free of disease 14 months after surgery but was lost to follow-up. Microscopically the SCC invaded the submucosa and penetrated the thin wall of the diverticulum into the surrounding fat. At the periphery of the SCC lay larger tumor cells with eosinophilic cytoplasm compatible with transitional carcinoma. Electron microscopy of the SCC showed a small fraction of the cells having membrane-bound dense core granules.

Davis and coworkers[57] reported three cases of SCC of the bladder. Electron microscopy of tumor specimens from all three cases showed dense core neurosecretory granules. All three had tumor invading bladder muscle, and in one case tumor extended into perivesicular fat. Two of the patients received preoperative radiotherapy to the bladder followed by radical cystectomy, and the third was treated with radiotherapy alone. One patient developed bone marrow metastasis and carcinomatous meningitis three months after cystectomy. He had a transient response to chemotherapy and cranial radiation and died 11 months after diagnosis. The second patient developed a retroperitoneal recurrence 12 months after diagnosis; he was treated with chemotherapy and appeared to be in complete remission 23 months after diagnosis and 11 months after recurrence. The third patient remained alive and clinically disease-free 28 months after diagnosis and radiotherapy of SCC invading into perivesicular fat. Although meningeal carcinomatosis in bladder cancer is rare, the clinical behavior of these malignancies and their responses to treatment are within the spectrum of behavior seen with other histologic types of bladder cancer, and additional cases need to be examined to determine whether SCC of the bladder is unique in its behavior.

Uterine Cervix

Small cell nonkeratinizing carcinomas comprise less than 15 percent[58,59] of cervical carcinomas in the United States. Tumors of this type have been associated with ectopic ACTH production and Cushing's syndrome, and electron microscopy in these cases has shown cytoplasmic dense core granules. Since only about 10 percent of pulmonary SCCs are associated with clinically apparent ectopic hormone syndromes, it seems likely that there may be a larger population than previously reported of SCCs of the cervix with neuroendocrine properties among the heterogeneous group of nonkeratinizing carcinomas. Pazdur and associates[60] performed electron microscopic studies on five consecutive cases of SCC of the cervix and found neurosecretory granules in all five. In all five cases the malignancies disseminated rapidly in a manner similar to SCC of the lung. Despite the possible similarities in rates of growth and dissemination and sites of metastasis between cervical and pulmonary SCC, chemotherapy of cervical SCC with regimens used in treatment of bronchogenic SCC has had little success. Pazdur and associates treated four of their five patients with a combination of cyclophosphamide, doxorubicin, and vincristine and achieved a complete remission lasting 11 months in one patient; responses of the other three patients were not described. Fer and colleagues[5] saw no response to this same three-drug regimen in treating a 28-year-old patient with SCC of the cervix and Cushing's syndrome secondary to ectopic ACTH production. Jacobs and coworkers[61] saw no response to a single dose of cisplatin in a 25-year-old woman with a polypoid SCC of the cervix.

While SCC of the cervix may differ in its biologic behavior from other types of cervical carcinoma and may resemble SCC of the lung in this regard, there is little evidence suggesting a unique sensitivity to chemotherapy for this subtype when compared to other histologic types of cervical cancer.

Uterine Corpus

SCC with neuroendocrine features arising in the endometrium has been described only recently. Olson and associates[62] described findings in a 64-year-old woman with endometrial SCC and regional lymph node metastasis. Electron microscopy showed cytoplasmic dense core granules. Immunoperoxidase staining for ACTH and argyrophilic and argentaffin stains were negative. Kumar[63] reported a case of an endometrial SCC in a 23-year-old woman. No argyrophilic granules were demonstrated by light microscopy, but dense core granules were seen by electron microscopy.

Although argyrophilia by the Grimelius or Sevier-Munger techniques has been regarded as a property of cells with neuroendocrine differentiation, the clinicopathologic importance of this feature in endometrial carcinomas is doubtful. Bannatyne and associates[64] correlated the incidence and pattern of argyrophilia in 25 endometrial carcinomas with other pathologic features of these tumors. Seventeen of the 25 tumors showed some argyrophilia including 12 of 16 adenocarcinomas, three of four adenoacanthomas, and two of four adenosquamous carcinomas; argyrophilia was not seen in the single SCC in this series. They found no relationship between the presence or intensity of argyrophilia and either histologic type or grade of the neoplasm. Electron microscopic examination of seven tumors (four adenocarcinomas, one adenosquamous carcinoma, one adenoacanthoma, and one SCC) showed membrane-bound dense core granules in all seven. Immunoperoxidase staining for ACTH, calcitonin, somatostatin, and gastrin was performed on nine tumors; four were positive for ACTH and calcitonin (two adenosquamous carcinomas, one adenoacanthoma, and one adenocarcinoma). The adenoacanthoma was also weakly positive for somatostatin. The SCC was negative for all hormones examined. These authors concluded that argyrophilia in endometrial carcinomas has no clinicopathologic importance.

Skin

In 1972 Toker[65] described five patients with small cell tumors of the skin who had no evidence of other primary malignancies and who did not develop primary malignancies in other sites during follow-up periods. These neoplasms were composed of small cells having relatively uniform nuclei and scant cytoplasm. The cells were sometimes arranged in rosette-like clusters, and because these groups of cells were separated by thin connective tissue trabeculae, Toker called these neoplasms trabecular carcinomas. He believed these tumors represented a unique primary skin cancer. Electron microscopy of tumors from subsequent cases[66] has shown cytoplasmic dense core granules and intercellular junctions. Because of the presence of "neurosecretory" granules in these tumor cells, some investigators[66,67] have suggested that these malignancies arise by transformation of Merkel cells, epidermal cells that contain dense core granules and that may form part of the cutaneous mechanoreceptor complex. The recent report by Tang and coworkers,[68] however, of three cases of mixed SCC–squamous cell carcinoma suggests that the neuroendocrine or SCC pattern may represent a pathway of differentiation available to a cutaneous malignant stem cell.

Primary cutaneous SCC (PCSCC) occurs predominantly in older patients. Tang and Toker[66] found their 17 patients ranged in age from 46 to 92 years with a median of 69 years. Silva and Mackay[69] reported 11 cases whose age ranged from 56 to 84 years with a median of 69 years. These neoplasms seldom occur on the trunk but originate with equal frequency on the extremities and on the head and neck. Most patients have subcutaneous nodules but some may have flat, indurated lesions. These neoplasms may be present from a few weeks to a few years before diagnosis.

Most patients with PCSCC have been treated surgically. Fifteen of the 17 patients reported by Tang and Toker[66] had surgical resection of their tumors. Five patients had no evidence of local recurrence or distant spread at follow-up. Four patients developed local recurrence; one patient had re-excision of the recurrence and was free of disease several years later; two patients had surgery and radiotherapy and achieved prolonged disease-free survival. Nine patients had metastatic involvement of regional lymph nodes; these patients were treated by node dissection, in some cases with radiotherapy before or after surgery. Despite this regional involvement, several patients remained clinically free of disease at follow-up several years later. Five patients were evaluable for response to radiotherapy; two had regression of their tumors but three had no response. Regardless of treatment most patients were alive at the time of the report with six patients alive more than five years after diagnosis.

Silva and Mackay[69] reported findings in 11 patients. Three patients had local recurrence of disease and six developed regional nodal involvement. Details of therapy were not given but the authors felt that radiotherapy may help survival. Three patients died of metastatic disease within two years of diagnosis, but survival data of the other eight patients were not given.

Few patients with PCSCC have been treated with chemotherapy. Taxy and associates[70] treated a 74-year-old woman with recurrent PCSCC of the face with a combination of cyclophosphamide, vincristine, methotrexate, and carmustine. She had a transient response to the combination and again responded transiently when her treatment was switched to cyclophosphamide, doxorubicin, and etoposide. Sibley and coworkers[67] reported treatment of an 82-year-old man with PCSCC of the face. This patient developed local recurrence after radiotherapy and had partial responses to low-dose cyclophosphamide, vincristine, and prednisone; to vincristine, doxorubicin, bleomycin, cyclophosphamide, and methotrexate; and to vincristine, cyclophosphamide, doxorubicin, and prednisone. However, he died 35 months after diagnosis with massive local and regional disease. Fer and associates[5] included in their review three patients thought to have PCSCC. All were treated with chemotherapy with or without radiotherapy, and all responded. One patient achieved a complete remission lasting 17 months but relapsed with brain metastasis and died seven months later.

These reports suggest that the clinical behavior of PCSCC is quite variable with some patients having lengthy survival despite local recurrence or regional nodal metastasis and others having aggressive disease and short survival with only transient or no response to therapy.

Conclusions

Despite the growing number of case reports, extrapulmonary small cell carcinomas remain relatively uncommon malignancies. The majority of patients with SCC in extrapulmonary sites will prove to have SCC of the lung after careful evaluation. Some patients, however, clearly have SCCs arising in extrapulmonary locations, and appropriate management of such patients may pose difficult problems because of the paucity of information regarding natural history, modes of spread, and therapeutic responsiveness of these neoplasms. Nevertheless, some guidelines can be offered.

SCCs arising in the upper aerodigestive tract (pharynx, paranasal sinuses, larynx, trachea, and esophagus) appear to resemble pulmonary SCC in aggressive behavior, capacity for local growth and early regional and distant metastasis, and perhaps response to radiation and to chemotherapy. Because of this proclivity for early metastasis and encouraging reports of responses to chemotherapy, combined modality approaches utilizing chemotherapy and surgical resection or radiotherapy seem appropriate. SCCs arising in the gastrointestinal tract may have a natural history different from pulmonary SCC, and the efficacy of radiotherapy and chemotherapy in treatment of gastrointestinal SCCs remains uncertain. The aggressive behavior exhibited by some SCCs of the rectum and of the gallbladder suggests the need for close observation of such patients at a minimum.

The numbers of cases of SCCs of the breast and of the genitourinary tract (prostate, uterine cervix and endometrium, and bladder) are too few to make judgments regarding clinical behavior or responsiveness to therapy. There are few convincing data suggesting differences in response to treatment of such patients compared to patients with more common carcinomas in these locations.

Cutaneous SCC appears to follow a variable course with some patients dying rapidly of progressive disease and others having lengthy survival. Wide excision is appropriate for localized disease with regional node dissection in patients with suspicious or definite lymph node involvement. Radiotherapy and chemotherapy may be of benefit to some patients.

References

1. Matsusaka T, Watanabe H, Enjoji M: Anaplastic carcinoma of the esophagus: Report of three cases and their histogenetic consideration. Cancer 37:1352–1358, 1976

2. Fisher ER, Palekar A, Paulson JD: Comparative histopathologic, histochemical, electron microscopic and tissue culture studies of bronchial carcinoids and oat cell carcinomas of the lung. Am J Clin Pathol 69:165–172, 1978

3. Gyorkey F, Min KW, Krisko I, et al: The usefulness of electron microscopy in the diagnosis of human tumors. Hum Pathol 6:421–441, 1975

4. McKeown T: Oat-cell carcinoma of the eosophagus. J Pathol Bacteriol 64:889–891, 1952

5. Fer MF, Levenson RM, Cohen MH, et al: Extrapulmonary small cell carcinoma, in Greco FA, Oldham RK, Bunn PA (eds): Small Cell Lung Cancer. New York, Grune and Stratton, 1981, pp 301–325

6. Richardson RL, Weiland LH: Extrapulmonary small cell carcinomas. Semin Oncol 9:484–496, 1982

7. Turnbull AD, Rosen P, Goodner JT, et al: Primary malignant tumors of the esophagus other than typical epidermoid carcinoma. Ann Thorac Surg 15:463–473, 1973

8. Briggs JC, Ibrahim NBN: Oat cell carcinoma of the eosophagus: A clinico-pathological study of 23 cases. Histopathol 7:261–277, 1983

9. Reyes CV, Chejfec G, Jao W, et al: Neuroendocrine carcinomas of the esophagus. Ultrastruc Pathol 1:367–376, 1980

10. Reid HAS, Richardson WW, Corrin B: Oat cell carcinoma of the esophagus. Cancer 45:2342–2347, 1980

11. Scarani P, Betts CM, Fedeli FR, et al: Oat cell carcinoma of the esophagus. Report of a case. Tumori 67:599–603, 1981

12. Rosenthal SN, Lemkin JA: Multiple small cell carcinomas of the esophagus. Cancer 51:1944–1946, 1983

13. Matsusaka T, Watanabe H, Enjoji M: Oat cell carcinoma of the stomach. Fukuoka Acta Medica 67:65–73, 1976

14. Eimoto F, Hayakawa H: Oat cell carcinoma of the stomach. Path Res Pract 168:229–236, 1980

15. Chejfec G, Gould VE: Malignant gastric neuroendocarcinomas: Ultrastructural and biochemical characterization of their secretory activity. Hum Pathol 8:433–440, 1977

16. Bernatz PE: Small cell neoplasms of the stomach. A clinicopathologic study. Master of Science thesis. Graduate School of the University of Minnesota, 1950

17. Toker C: Oat cell tumor of the small bowel. Am J Gastroenterol 61:481–483, 1974

18. Clery AP, Dockerty MB, Waugh JM: Small cell carcinoma of the colon and rectum; a clinicopathologic study. Arch Surg 83:164–171, 1961

19. Gould VE, Chejfec G: Neuroendocrine carcinomas of the colon. Am J Surg Pathol 2:31–38, 1978

20. Mills SE, Allen MS, Cohen AR: Small-cell undifferentiated carcinoma of the colon: a clinicopathological study of five cases and their association with colonic adenomas. Am J Surg Pathol 7:643–651, 1983

21. Petrelli M, Tetangco E, Reid JD: Carcinoma of the colon with undifferentiated, carcinoid, and squamous cell features. Am J Clin Pathol 75:581–584, 1981

22. Damjanov I, Amenta PS, Bosman FT: Undifferentiated carcinoma of the colon containing exocrine, neuroendocrine and squamous cells. Virchows Arch (Pathol Anat) 401:57–66, 1983

23. Schroeder PJ, Snow P: Cloacogenic small cell carcinoma associated with villous adenoma of the rectum. Md State Med J 32:452–453, 1983

24. Albores-Saavedra J, Soriano J, Larraza-Hernandez O, et al: Oat cell carcinoma of the gallbladder. Hum Pathol 15:639–646, 1984

25. Reyes CV, Wang T: Undifferentiated small cell carcinoma of the pancreas: a report of five cases. Cancer 47:2500–2502, 1981

26. Cubilla AL, Fitzgerald PJ: Classification of pancreatic cancer (nonendocrine). Mayo Clin Proc 54:449–458, 1979

27. Corrin B, Gilby ED, Jones JF, et al: Oat cell carcinoma of the pancreas with ectopic ACTH secretion. Cancer 31:1523–1527, 1973

28. Raychowdhuri RN: Oat cell carcinoma and paranasal sinuses. J Laryngol Otol 47:253–255, 1965

29. Koss LG, Spiro RH, Hajdu S: Small cell (oat cell) carcinoma of minor salivary gland origin. Cancer 30:737–741, 1972

30. Weiss MD, de Fries HO, Taxy JB, et al: Primary small cell carcinoma of the paranasal sinuses. Arch Otolaryngol 109:341–343, 1983

31. Leipzig B, Gonzales-Vitale JC: Small cell epidermoid carcinoma of salivary glands: "pseudo"-oat cell carcinoma. Arch Otolaryngol 108:511–514, 1982

32. Kraemer BB, Mackay B, Batsakis JG: Small cell carcinoma of the parotid gland: a clinicopathologic study of three cases. Cancer 52:2115–2121, 1983

33. Ferlito A, Polidoro T: Simultaneous primary oat cell carcinoma (apudoma) and squamous cell carcinoma of the hypopharynx. Otorhinolaryngol 42:146–157, 1980

34. Nagao K, Matsuzaki O, Saija H, et al: Histopathologic studies of undifferentiated carcinoma of the parotid gland. Cancer 50:1572–1579, 1982

35. Olofsson J, Van Nostrand AWP: Anaplastic small cell carcinoma of larynx. Case report. Ann Otol Rhinol Laryngol 81:284–287, 1972

36. Gnepp DR, Ferlito A, Hyams V: Primary anaplastic small cell (oat cell) carcinoma of the larynx: Review of the literature and report of 18 cases. Cancer 51:1731–1745, 1983

37. Posner MR, Weichselbaum RR, Carrol E, et al: Small cell carcinomas of the larynx: Results of combined modality treatments. Laryngoscope 93:946–948, 1983

38. Medina JE, Moran M, Goepfert H: Oat cell carcinoma of the larynx and Eaton-Lambert syndrome. Arch Otolaryngol 110:123–126, 1984

39. Thompson DH, Kao YH, Klos J, et al: Primary small cell (oat cell) carcinoma of the larynx associated with an IgD multiple myeloma. Laryngoscope 92:1239–1244, 1982

40. Culp OS: Primary carcinoma of the trachea. J Thorac Surg 7:471–487, 1938

41. Stenn F: Carcinoma of the trachea: Review of recent literature and report of a case. Arch Otolaryngol 21:190–198, 1935

42. Sweeney EC, Hughes F: Primary carcinoma of the trachea. Histopathol 1:289–299, 1977

43. Pantridge JF: Primary carcinoma of the trachea. Br J Surg 37:48–49, 1949

44. Zarywitz H, Hoffman JB: Primary carcinoma of the trachea. Arch Intern Med 89:454–463, 1952

45. Darch GH: Tracheal neoplasms presenting with mediastinal emphysema. Br J Dis Chest 56:212–213, 1962

46. Wengraf C: Oat cell carcinoma of the trachea. J Laryngol Otol 84:257–274, 1970

47. Jash DK: Oat cell carcinoma of the trachea. J Laryngol Otol 87:681–684, 1973

48. Deckert RE, Burgher LW: Serial flow-volume loops as an aid to management of primary oat cell carcinoma of the trachea. Chest 73:560, 1978

49. Soorae AS, Gibbons JRP: Primary oat cell carcinoma of the trachea. Thorax 34:130–131, 1979

50. Rosai J, Levine G, Weber WR, et al: Carcinoid tumors and oat cell carcinomas of the thymus, in Somers SC (ed): Pathol Annual, vol 11. New York, Appleton-Century-Crofts, 1976, pp 201–226

51. Cohle SD, Tashen JA, Smith FE, et al: ACTH secreting carcinoma of the breast. Cancer 43:2370–2376, 1979

52. Woodard BH, Eisenbarth G, Wallace NR, et al: Adrenocorticotropin production by a mammary carcinoma. Cancer 47:1823–1827, 1981

53. Newmark SR, Dluhy RG, Bennett AH: Ectopic adenocorticotropin syndrome with prostatic carcinoma. Urology 2:666–668, 1973

54. Lovern WJ, Fariss BL, Wettlaufer JN, et al: Ectopic ACTH production in disseminated prostatic adenocarcinoma. Urology 5:817–820, 1975

55. Wenk RE, Bhagavan BS, Levy R, et al: Ectopic ACTH, prostatic oat cell carcinoma, and marked hypernatremia. Cancer 40:773–778, 1977

56. Cramer SF, Aikawa M, Cebelin M: Neurosecretory granules in small cell invasive carcinoma of the urinary bladder. Cancer 47:724–730, 1981

57. Davis BH, Ludwig ME, Cole SR, et al: Small cell neuroendocrine carcinoma of the urinary bladder: report of three cases with ultrastructural analysis. Ultrastruc Pathol 4:197–204, 1983

58. Van Nagell Jr, Donaldson ES, Wood EG, et al: Small cell cancer of the uterine cervix. Cancer 40:2243–2249, 1977

59. Field CA, Dockerty M, Symmonds RE: Small cell cancer of the cervix. Am J Obstet Gynecol 88:447–451, 1964

60. Pazdur R, Bonomi P, Slayton R, et al: Neuroendocrine carcinoma of the cervix. Proc Am Soc Clin Oncol 22:378, 1981

61. Jacobs AJ, Marchevsky A, Gordon RE, et al: Oat cell carcinoma of the uterine cervix in a pregnant woman treated with cis-diammine dichloroplatinum. Gynecol Oncol 9:405–410, 1980

62. Olson N, Twiggs L, Sibley R: Small-cell carcinoma of the endometrium: light microscopic and ultrastructural study of a case. Cancer 50:760–765, 1982

63. Kumar NB: Small cell carcinoma of the endometrium in a 23-year-old woman: light microscopic and ultrastructural study. Am J Clin Pathol 81:98–101, 1984

64. Bannatyne P, Russell P, Wills EJ: Argyrophilia and endometrial carcinoma. Int J Gynecol Pathol 2:235–254, 1983

65. Toker C: Trabecular carcinoma of the skin. Arch Dermatol 105:107–110, 1972

66. Tang CK, Toker C: Trabecular carcinoma of the skin: Further clinicopathologic and ultrastructural study. Mt Sinai J Med 46:516–523, 1979

67. Sibley RK, Rosai J, Foucar E, et al: Neuroendocrine (Merkel cell) carcinoma of the skin. Am J Surg Pathol 4:211–221, 1980

68. Tang CK, Nedwich A, Toker C, et al: Unusual cutaneous carcinoma with features of small cell (oat cell-like) and squamous cell carcinomas. Am J Dermatopath 4:537–548, 1982

69. Silva EG, Mackay B: Small cell neuroepithelial tumor of the skin. Lab Invest 42:151, 1980

70. Taxy JB, Ettinger DS, Wharam MD: Primary small cell carcinoma of the skin. Cancer 46:2308–2311, 1980

14

POORLY DIFFERENTIATED SMALL ROUND CELL MALIGNANCIES OF CHILDHOOD

Richard P. Kadota
Gerald S. Gilchrist
Lester E. Wold

Accurate diagnosis and appropriate management of the small round cell malignancies of childhood is one of the most difficult problems faced by pediatric oncologists and pathologists. Diseases that are usually included under this designation are Ewing's sarcoma, neuroblastoma, non-Hodgkin's lymphoma, and rhabdomyosarcoma. Although the light microscopic appearance of these tumors may be similar, their treatment and prognoses differ considerably. The purpose of this chapter is to review the clinical and pathologic features of the major small round cell malignancies found in children. This review will be organized in a problem-oriented manner approximating situations encountered by the practicing physician. We will address tumors involving bone, tumors in a soft tissue location, and tumors presenting as lymphadenopathy.

POORLY DIFFERENTIATED NEOPLASMS AND TUMORS OF UNKNOWN ORIGIN   ISBN 0-8089-1755-2
© 1986 by Grune & Stratton.

Small Round Cell Malignancies of Bone

General Aspects

The most common primary bone malignancies in children are osteogenic sarcoma and Ewing's sarcoma. Ewing's sarcoma is one of the classic small round cell tumors of childhood while osteogenic sarcoma is excluded by the presence of osteoid. Occasionally, small cell osteosarcoma or large cell Ewing's sarcoma may cause diagnostic confusion, if the existence of these variants is not appreciated.[1,2] Neuroblastoma, non-Hodgkin's lymphoma, and rhabdomyosarcoma may present with skeletal involvement. Neuroblastoma is a neoplasm of early childhood and should be suspected in any patient who is five years old or less. Fifty to 60 percent of neuroblastomas are stage IV tumors at initial diagnosis.[3-5] Bone is a frequent site of metastasis and often produces the symptoms for which medical attention is first sought (Fig. 14-1). Non-Hodgkin's lymphoma occurs uncommonly as a primary bone lesion in the pediatric age group, in contrast to adults.[6] In a recent analysis of 234 patients by the Children's Cancer Study Group, only four percent had bone as the principal site of disease.[7] In a series of 868 malignant bone tumors in the first two decades of life seen at the Mayo Clinic, there were 47 cases of malignant lymphoma in contrast to 230 cases of Ewing's sarcoma and 528 cases of classic osteosarcoma.[8] In rhabdomyosarcoma, bone may be involved by local extension from a soft tissue primary or by hematogenous metastases. Rhabdomyosarcomas originating in the trunk or head and neck region (except orbit) have the greatest likelihood of metastasizing to bone.[9]

Clinical Features

The most frequent presenting complaints of an osseous malignancy are localized pain and swelling. Gait disturbance may occur if a weight-bearing limb is involved. Children present a special challenge because of confusion with nonmalignant disorders such as injury, infection, and arthritis. Often, patients will not seek medical attention until several months after the onset of symptoms. An association with previous trauma may be prominent in the medical history, but in the usual case, the traumatic event has served merely to draw attention to the patient's more serious problem. Depending on the size and spread of the malignancy, there may be systemic complaints such as fever, weight loss, fatigue, and anorexia. Neuroblastoma should be considered in any young child who has an atypical presentation of "failure to thrive" with or without skeletal

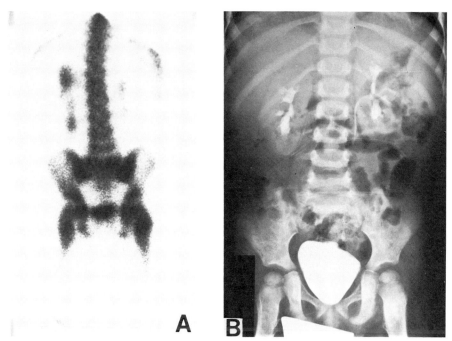

Figure 14-1. *This two-year-old boy presented with bilateral hip pain which was diagnosed initially as toxic synovitis. (A) Bone scan revealed increased uptake in the proximal femurs and pelvis as well as in the area of the right kidney. (B) Note the slight caudal displacement of the right kidney with preservation of the intrarenal architecture and periosteal elevation in the proximal femurs bilaterally. Diagnosis of a right adrenal neuroblastoma with bony metastases was surgically confirmed.*

symptoms. In addition, it should be recalled that acute lymphoblastic leukemia not uncommonly presents with joint swelling and/or bone pain due to leukemic cell infiltration.

On physical exam, a tender mass may be palpable, particularly if the tumor has extended into the surrounding soft tissues. With small bony lesions, only point tenderness may be present. Occasionally, joint findings will predominate if the tumor involves bone at or near the joint space. Most children with Ewing's sarcoma present with a primary lesion in the pelvis or proximal to midfemur, in contrast to osteogenic sarcoma which most often originates in the distal femur or proximal tibia.[8] The patient should be examined thoroughly for local and distant lymphadenopathy as node enlargement occurs with lymphomatous, sarcomatous, and neuroblastoma infiltration. Hepatosplenomegaly suggests lymphoma. An abdominal mass in a young child suggests neuroblastoma. Uncommon but unique physical signs of neuroblastoma include heterochromia iridis and Horner's syndrome secondary to a cervical sympathetic ganglion tumor, bluish or blanching metastatic subcutaneous nodules, opsoclonus/myoclonus, watery diarrhea secondary to vasoactive intestinal peptide secretion, and periorbital ecchymoses and proptosis due to retrobulbar infiltration.[10] Invasion or compression of the spinal cord by neuroblastoma frequently results in significant neurologic deficits.

Diagnostic Evaluation

Radiologic visualization is the customary initial step in the laboratory evaluation of a child with new skeletal complaints. Good quality radiographs can quickly identify patients who need further investigation. As discussed below, certain characteristics are more apt to be associated with malignant lesions rather than with benign ones. However, "classic" x-rays should never be a substitute for tissue diagnosis when a malignancy is being considered. A surprising number of presumptive bone tumors turn out to be skeletal infections at surgery and vice versa.

As recently reviewed by Osborne, certain radiologic features favor a malignant tumor over a benign one.[11] Multiple destructive foci, poorly defined margins between tumor and normal bone, cortical breakthrough with soft tissue extension, and a multilayered periosteal reaction are indicative of rapid, aggressive malignant growth. In contrast, a small lesion with coarse trabeculation and well defined margins is suggestive of a benign disease process. The site of origin and the age of the patient may provide further clues regarding the probability of various bone tumors.[11] In addition, recent use of CT scans and magnetic resonance imaging (Fig. 14-2) has been helpful in defining the extent of skeletal and soft tissue involvement of the primary lesion.

The laboratory evaluation of a child with a suspected bone malignancy should include complete staging studies prior to any attempts at surgical resection. The most common sites of metastases for both rhabdomyosarcoma and Ewing's sarcoma are the lungs, bone marrow, bones, and regional lymph nodes. Non-Hodgkin's lymphoma may involve, in addition to bone, the liver, spleen, bone marrow, lymph nodes, and central nervous system. Neuroblastoma metastasizes most frequently to the liver, subcutaneous tissue, regional lymph nodes, and bone marrow, as well as bone. Skeletal metastases are seen in approximately 50 percent of patients at diagnosis, but lung involvement is unusual. In contrast, Wilm's tumor

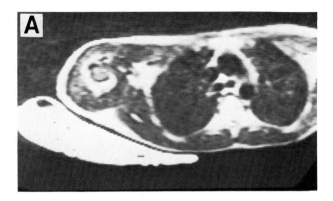

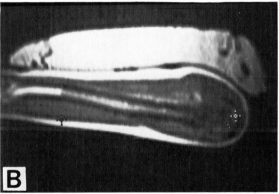

Figure 14-2. *(A,B) Magnetic resonance imaging is a new diagnostic technique which may be helpful to delineate the extent of tumor involvement. The differential diagnosis of this middle and proximal humeral lesion with extension into the surrounding soft tissue is between Ewing's sarcoma and osteogenic sarcoma.*

characteristically metastasizes to the lungs while bony involvement is infrequent.[12] Normal radiographs do not always rule out cancerous skeletal involvement; bone scans may identify lesions which are more extensive or are not readily apparent on plain films.[13–15] Conversely, false-negative bone scans have been reported, particularly involving lesions at the ends of long bones which may be masked by the normally increased uptake of radionuclide at osseous growth centers in children.[16]

Neuroblastoma is unique within the group of small round cell malignancies in that a tumor marker is usually present. Up to 95 percent of patients will have an increased urinary excretion of HVA and/or VMA.[17,18]

Elevated urinary cystothionine may be present in occasional patients with normal levels of VMA.[19,20] Recently, serum neuron-specific enolase has been reported to be elevated in 96 percent of 122 children with metastatic neuroblastoma.[21] In cases with elevated catecholamine levels and characteristic clusters of malignant cells on bone marrow examination, a diagnosis of metastatic neuroblastoma may be made without an invasive surgical procedure.

Pathologic Features

Processing of biopsy tissue should be individualized to meet all potential pathologic needs. A sterile fresh specimen may be collected for tissue culture while fresh cell suspensions may be made for cell surface marker studies. Frozen sections are prepared routinely for intra-operative analysis. Frozen tissue may also be utilized for monoclonal antibody typing of lymphomas and other solid tumors. Tissue fixed in formaldehyde is used for definitive light microscopy review, including special stains. Glutaraldehyde fixation is required for electron microscopic examination. Touch preparations may be particularly helpful if the amount of biopsy material is small. Touch preparations may be used for special stains, alleviating the need for special fixatives. In addition, touch preparations are useful for enzyme histochemical and immunohistochemical techniques.

Ewing's sarcoma is the prototypic osseous malignancy with an undifferentiated histologic appearance. Pathologic features of this tumor have been reviewed recently by Kissane and colleagues from the experience of the Intergroup Ewing's Sarcoma Study.[22] The characteristic morphology is a structureless arrangement of a dimorphic cell population with a paucity of intercellular stroma. Although designated as a small round cell tumor, the predominant cell size is usually two to three times that of a small lymphocyte. Intermingled with such large tumor cells are aggregates of smaller cells with pyknotic, clumpy nuclei. Nuclear morphology is conspicuously bland; generally it consists of oval or round nuclei with finely granular chromatin and small nucleoli. Mitotic figures are uncommon (Figs. 14-3 and 14-4).

The histogenesis of Ewing's sarcoma is not yet resolved. Pathologic examination suggests that the tumor originates in the marrow cavity.[22] There is no consistent relationship, however, to the hematologic malignancies. Thus, it is commonly assumed that Ewing's tumor is of primitive mesenchymal cell origin, although there is an unexplained predominance of osseous lesions.

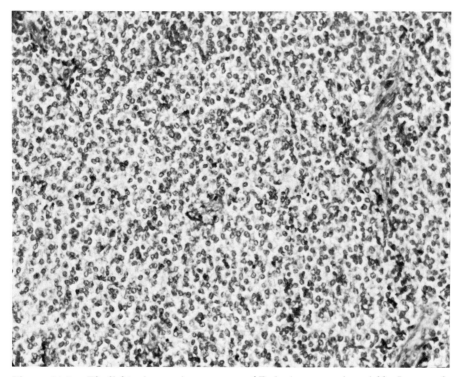

Figure 14-3. *The light microscopic appearance of Ewing's sarcoma is variable. In general, this neoplasm is composed of sheets of small polygonal cells with pale staining cytoplasm. The number of cells with small, dark staining nuclei differs from area to area within a single tumor. There is no significant intercellular stroma (hematoxylin and eosin, X 250).*

Glycogen in Ewing's sarcoma cells is one of the classic findings, but up to one-third of tumors are PAS-negative (Fig. 14-5).[22] In addition, lymphoma, neuroblastoma, and rhabdomyosarcoma may be PAS-positive.[23] Thus, neither the absence nor presence of glycogen supports or negates the diagnosis of Ewing's sarcoma. As mentioned previously, one also should be aware of the occasional histologic variations, small cell osteogenic sarcoma and large cell (atypical) Ewing's sarcoma.[1,2] At this institution, if osteoid formation is equivocal, we tend to diagnose such lesions as Ewing's sarcoma (in contrast to osteogenic sarcoma) and expect it to be radiosensitive.[2]

Childhood non-Hodgkin's lymphoma occurs almost exclusively in 4 histologic patterns, i.e. lymphoblastic, large cell immunoblastic, undiffer-

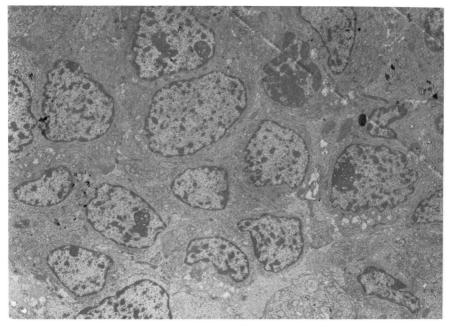

Figure 14-4.   *The ultrastructural appearance of Ewing's sarcoma demonstrates primitive cells which lack cell processes, intracellular filaments, and contain only sparse organelles.*

entiated Burkitt's, and undifferentiated non-Burkitt's subtypes.[24] The latter two lymphoma groups infrequently involve bone, except the jaw in African Burkitt's tumor. Lymphoblastic and large cell immunoblastic lymphomas may occasionally present as primary bony disease, but often can be distinguished by characteristic cellular pleomorphism. Only large cell immunoblastic lymphomas with uniform, noncleaved nuclei may cause diagnostic confusion with the other small round cell malignancies of childhood.[23] Pathologic features of non-Hodgkin's lymphoma are discussed more thoroughly in a subsequent section.

Neuroblastomas present a spectrum of cellular differentiation patterns on light microscopic examination. Features of maturation include neural rosette formation, presence of neural fibrils, enlarged nuclei, and a prominent rim of cytoplasm (Fig. 14-6).[25] Neurosecretory granules at times may be demonstrable by silver staining. PAS-positivity may lead occasionally to confusion with Ewing's sarcoma. The most primitive tumors are very cellular with typical small round cells and scanty cytoplasm. When metastatic to bone, features of differentiation are often not present.

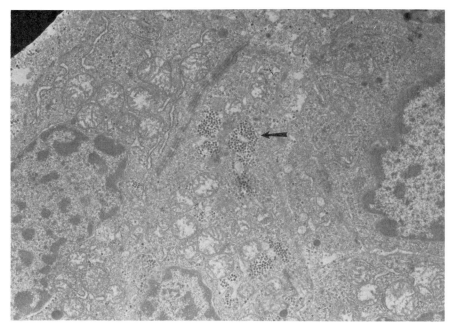

Figure 14-5. *Glycogen is classically present in Ewing's sarcoma and may be appreciated ultrastructurally (arrows) in cases which are PAS-negative at the light microscopic level.*

Electron microscopy may be diagnostic for structures indicative of early neural differentiation such as dense core granules (neurosecretory granules) and abortive neural processes (Fig. 14-7). Recently, monoclonal antibodies have been synthesized which react against neuron-specific esterase and other neuroblastoma antigens.[26-28] Catecholamine fluorescence and neurite growth in tissue culture have also been reported to be highly sensitive and specific techniques.[29]

Bony metastases of rhabdomyosarcoma are not routinely biopsied to make an initial diagnosis and can be presumptively identified by examination of the primary lesion. An additional primitive neoplasm, the polyhistioma, resembles Ewing's sarcoma in microscopic appearance.[30,31] This tumor occurs most frequently in bone of individuals less than 20 years old, usually metastasizing to lungs and other bones within two years from diagnosis. Histologically, the polyhistioma contains a differentiated mesenchymal component, e.g. bone, cartilage or vascular structures, but no muscle. There seems to be a direct conversion of primitive round cells into differentiated tissue without formation of an intermediate mesenchy-

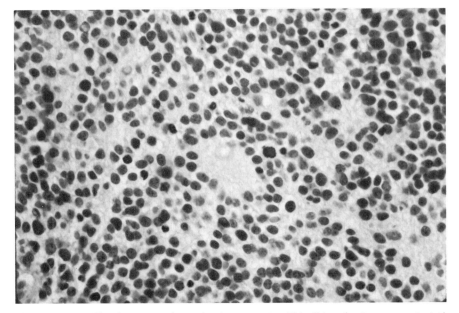

Figure 14-6. *Abortive rosette formation is apparent within this subcutaneous metastatic neuroblastoma. The stromal background shows a "neurofibrillary" quality (hematoxylin and eosin, X 400).*

mal spindle cell.[30] This is the key diagnostic point, as well as being of great conceptual interest.

Small Round Cell Malignancies Involving Soft Tissues

General Aspects

There are several small round cell tumors of childhood which present as a primary lesion in soft tissue. Rhabdomyosarcoma is the classic malignancy of this type. Multiple large series have tabulated that its most common primary locations are the head and neck (30–40 percent), genitourinary system (20–40 percent), and the extremities and trunk wall (15–25 percent).[32-34] Other primary sites (intrathoracic, retroperitoneal, gastrointestinal, hepatobiliary, and the central nervous system) are much less frequent.

Included in rhabdomyosarcoma treatment programs at some institu-

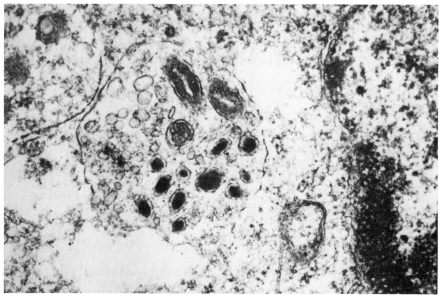

Figure 14-7. *Although optimal preparation for electron microscopy requires special fixation, at times, ultrastructural examination of formalin-fixed tissue may also be helpful. Preservation of the ultrastructural features was sufficient in this case to identify dense core granules within cytoplasmic processes and microtubules to confirm a diagnosis of neuroblastoma.*

tions have been patients whose extraskeletal primitive tumors resembled Ewing's sarcoma.[32] This subset of malignancy has been called extraskeletal Ewing's, extra-osseous Ewing's or soft tissue Ewing's sarcoma.[35] Of 40 cases from an Intergroup Rhabdomyosarcoma Study analysis, extremity, truncal, and retroperitoneal lesions accounted for 18, seven, and seven cases, respectively.[32]

Another small cell malignancy of the soft tissue has been described recently by Askin and colleagues.[36] The typical patient has been an adolescent with a primary lesion in the chest wall or peripheral lung. Thus far, the tumor carries the descriptive name of "malignant small cell tumor of the thoracopulmonary region in childhood". Approximately 25 percent of polyhistiomas (see section on small round cell tumors of bone) have a soft tissue primary location.[30] Neuroblastomas metastasize occasionally to the subcutaneous tissue, but usually do not present a diagnostic problem due the presence of tumor markers and a typically located primary lesion. Non-Hodgkin's lymphoma occurring in an extralymphatic soft tissue location is uncommon in childhood.[7] Similarly, esthesioneuroblastoma and primitive neuroectodermal malignancies rarely cause a diagnostic problem in children.

Clinical Features

The history and findings on physical exam vary with the duration, primary location, and extent of the tumor. In longstanding, aggressive lesions, the patient may display features of a systemic illness with fever, anorexia, and weight loss. More commonly, a soft tissue mass has been present for several days to months which may or may not be painful. In all soft tissue malignancies, it is important to examine regional lymph nodes for evidence of tumor infiltration. Rhabdomyosarcomas metastasize most frequently to the lungs, central nervous system, bone, liver, soft tissue, and bone marrow.[9]

Diagnostic Evaluation

Radiologic evaluation of the primary tumor is key to defining the extent of local infiltration and, hence, operability. Computerized tomography has been especially useful for this purpose, including visualization of enlarged regional lymph nodes. Plain x-rays are useful to screen for bony invasion. Occasionally, angiography assists with delineation of the vascular supply. Search for distant metastases should also be routinely undertaken. Commonly performed procedures are bone marrow (aspirate and biopsy), skeletal survey, bone scan, chest radiograph, chest and abdominal computerized tomography, and, sometimes, nuclear magnetic imaging.

Pathologic Features

The histologic appearance of rhabdomyosarcomas is a spectrum ranging from very primitive mesenchymal cells to those containing mature skeletal muscle elements (Fig. 14-8). The variation within a single tumor specimen may be striking. This spectrum of differentiation has been likened to fetal muscle cell development, i.e. primitive rhabdomyosarcoma cells representing the seven week stage of fetal development while cells with cross striations corresponding to the 10 week stage of normal muscle differentiation.[37] Demonstration of myoblasts is diagnostic, but visualization of typical muscle fiber cross striations under light microscopy by hematoxylin and eosin or PTAH staining has been noted in less than one-half of cases.[38,39]

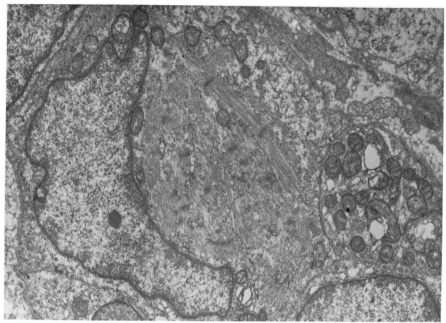

Figure 14-8. *Electron microscopic examination of tumors thought to be consistent with rhabdomyosarcoma on the light microscopic level may show bundles of thick and thin filaments with cross banding, as in this case. Cells in earlier stages of development may show only scattered filaments.*

In poorly differentiated tumors, electron microscopy may be helpful in supporting the diagnosis of rhabdomyosarcoma. Characteristic cytoplasmic filaments, actin (thin filaments: 7 nm diameter) and myosin (thick filaments: 14 nm diameter) may be noted in a hexagonal configuration on cross section. Longitudinally, well-differentiated filaments may form A, I, and Z-bands typical of mature muscle tissue.[23] Another recent advance has been the development of immunohistochemical staining for myoglobin, myosin, and other skeletal muscle proteins. Using an immunoperoxidase technique, improved diagnostic accuracy over conventional methods has been claimed.[40-45] Experience at our institution has shown that approximately 50 percent of rhabdomyosarcomas defined by light microscopy contain myoglobin by immunoperoxidase techniques.

Rhabdomyosarcomas have been divided traditionally into several histopathologic groups by light microscopy. Complications from several large series have revealed that 60–80 percent of tumors were classified as embryonal.[32,38,46] The majority of malignant cells are typically not well-differentiated, sometimes mimicking fibroblasts.[23] Rhabdomyoblasts are interspersed amongst the predominant cell type having oval or round nuclei and prominent eosinophilic cytoplasm with or without cross striations. A subset of embryonal rhabdomyosarcoma has been called "sarcoma botryoides". This variant has been so named by its polypoid appearance attributed to freedom of growth within a hollow body cavity, e.g. the vagina, bladder, ear, etc. Microscopically, there is usually a paucity of cellularity with an abundance of mucoid stroma and scattered rhabdomyoblasts. The tumor typically arises from the submucosa with a basal zone of cells called the "cambium layer" analagous to the zone of maximum growth in a tree.[39] Overall, the embryonal histology has been noted most commonly in genitourinary and head and neck primaries.

Fifteen to 20 percent of rhabdomyosarcomas in childhood have been classified as the alveolar subtype (Fig. 14-9).[32,38,46] As the name implies, the cells of this rhabdomyosarcoma variant are arranged in a configuration reminiscent of pulmonary alveoli. This pattern is formed by loss of tumor cell cohesion resulting in irregular "holes" or "alveolar spaces". Another characteristic feature is the presence of multinucleated giant cells. It has been postulated that these are fused cells based on the observation of transitional forms between rhabdomyoblasts and giant cells.[39] Alveolar lesions have occurred most commonly in the extremities of children who were at least 10 years of age.[9]

Approximately one percent of pediatric rhabdomyosarcomas have been classified as the "pleomorphic" subtype. Loosely arranged large bizarre tumor cells in a fibrous stroma are characteristic.[9,32] Finally, there have been some tumors (less than 10 percent) which were so undifferentiated that they defied further classification. Such primitive malignancies have been termed "small cell undifferentiated mesenchymal sarcoma, type indeterminant" and have been treated on Intergroup Rhabdomyosarcoma Study protocols.[9,32]

Five to 10 percent of patients registered in the Intergroup Rhabdomyosarcoma Study have had tumors identical in appearance to Ewing's sarcoma, although the primary lesion did not originate in a skeletal location. As reviewed by Soule and colleagues, these extraskeletal Ewing's tumors have been divided into two histologic subtypes.[35] Subtype I corresponds to classic Ewing's sarcoma while subtype II is analagous to the "large cell Ewing's variant".

A neoplasm similar in histologic appearance to extraskeletal Ewing's sarcoma is the malignant small cell tumor of the thoracopulmonary region (Askin's tumor).[36] Although the histogenesis of this lesion is unclear,

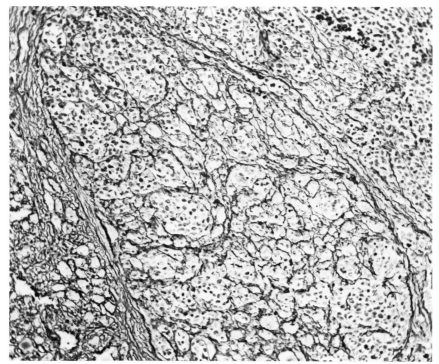

Figure 14-9. *This gluteal lesion shows clustering of neoplastic cells in an alveolar arrangement. Some tumors will show a loss of cell cohesion within the clusters making the alveolar pattern even more prominent (reticulin stain, X 160).*

electron microscopic examination of several cases has suggested neuroepithelial derivation. Recently, positive immunostaining for neuron-specific esterase was noted in eight out of eight cases which also has been useful to confirm the diagnosis of neuroblastoma.[47] Whether some of the thoracic primaries in the Intergroup Rhabdomyosarcoma Study represent examples of Askin's entity is unclear.[48]

Recent pathologic analysis of the Intergroup Rhabdomyosarcoma experience has redefined the tumors into two groups which have prognostic implications (unfavorable and favorable histology).[49,50] The unfavorable histology category is composed of the standard alveolar pattern plus two new classes, anaplastic and monomorphous round cell. Anaplastic rhabdomyosarcoma has been characterized by the focal or diffuse occurrence of

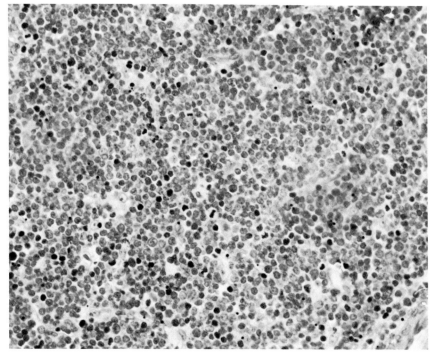

Figure 14-10. *Alveolar, monomorphous round cell, and anaplastic rhabdomyosarcomas have a relatively poor prognosis. This tumor is an example of the monomorphous round cell type described by Palmer (hematoxylin and eosin, X 400).*[49]

enlarged or bizarre mitotic figures and nuclear hyperchromatism with pleomorphism. Monomorphous round cell rhabdomyosarcoma has been descriptively named (Fig. 14-10). The remaining rhabdomyosarcomas have been combined into the "mixed" histology designation with more favorable prognostic implications. This new cytologic classification will be analyzed further in future Intergroup studies.

The Intergroup Rhabdomyosarcoma Study has divided patients into four clinical groups based on the initial extent of disease and surgical resectability:[32]

Group I—localized disease, completely resected
Group II—localized disease, microscopic residual or regional disease, grossly or completely resected

Group III—incomplete resection or biopsy with gross residual disease
Group IV—distant metastases at diagnosis

Overall, these clinical groups have correlated with treatment outcome. However, several notable exceptions have been produced artificially in an effort to preserve organ function.[51] For example, some orbital and genitourinary lesions have been approached with limited surgery or biopsy only, followed by primary chemotherapy with or without irradiation. Since resection was incomplete, these tumors automatically qualified for clinical group III, despite being group I or II disease, if located in a more accessible anatomic area.

Small Round Cell Malignancies Involving Lymph Nodes

General Aspects

It is uncommon for lymphadenopathy to represent malignant disease in childhood. Children characteristically manifest more rapid and exaggerated lymphoid hyperplastic responses to benign inflammatory stimuli compared to adults and have relatively more lymphoid tissue.[52] In a recent series of 239 pediatric patients who underwent peripheral lymph node biopsy at a major children's hospital, four cases of non-Hodgkin's lymphoma, three cases of rhabdomyosarcoma, and three cases of neuroblastoma were discovered.[53] Biopsies performed in 75 children at another center revealed three cases of non-Hodgkin's lymphoma.[54] Unlike solid neoplasms in adults, the presence of an enlarged lymph node with an inapparent primary lesion is relatively rare in pediatrics.

The majority of childhood non-Hodgkin's lymphomas have disseminated beyond the original site of involvement by the time of presentation to a physician. In a recent Children's Cancer Study Group analysis, only 73 of 234 (30 percent) patients had localized disease.[7,55] Twenty-two of these 73 children (30 percent) had peripheral lymph nodes as the primary site of involvement while only three of 161 (two percent) patients with disseminated disease presented with primary peripheral adenopathy. The most common primary locations for childhood non-Hodgkin's lymphomas are abdominal and mediastinal which are most frequently undifferentiated (Burkitt's and non-Burkitt's) and lymphoblastic histologies, respectively.[56–58]

Clinical Features

The history is helpful in distinguishing benign from malignant adenopathy. Nontender lymph node enlargement lasting beyond six to eight weeks warrants biopsy.[53] If the lymph node is growing rapidly, earlier biopsy may be indicated. Many children with disseminated non-Hodgkin's lymphoma or metastatic solid tumors may appear surprisingly well with minimal systemic complaints.

Lymph nodes up to one centimeter in diameter may be palpable in the cervical and inguinal regions in normal children up to 12 years of age.[53] Classic characteristics of malignant adenopathy are large size, lack of tenderness, fixation to deep tissues and to one another (matting). The site of lymph node enlargement is also important. For instance, it has been noted that supraclavicular adenopathy has been associated with malignancy in 14/23 pediatric cases, mainly Hodgkin's disease.[53] Other sites of non-Hodgkin's lymphoma, metastatic rhabdomyosarcoma, and metastatic neuroblastoma, involvement in this series were the cervical and axillary regions which accounted for 4/139 (three percent) and 4/31 (13 percent) of biopsies, respectively.

Diagnostic Evaluation

The diagnostic evaluation of a small round cell tumor presenting as lymphadenopathy varies according to the clinical situation. If non-Hodgkin's lymphoma is suspected or proven, the evaluation includes a chest radiograph (PA and lateral views), chest CT scan, bone scan and/or skeletal survey, bilateral bone marrow aspirations and biopsies, abdominal CT scan or ultrasound, and lumbar puncture. Staging studies for other pediatric solid malignancies are determined by the location of the primary tumor. It should be noted that CT scans accurately delineate mass lesions in children, but may not detect infiltrated abdominal nodes due to the lack of abdominal and retroperitoneal fat in the pediatric age group. Thus, abdominal ultrasonography, liver–spleen scans, gallium scans or lymphangiography may be useful. The recently described technique of bone marrow culture has detected otherwise inapparent malignant spread of non-Hodgkin's lymphoma in selected instances.[59]

The timing of lymph node biopsy also is variable according to the clinical situation. As early biopsy, i.e. prior to completion of staging studies is useful to differentiate between benign and malignant disease processes. Metastatic evaluation is guided then by the tissue diagnosis. The staging laparotomy used routinely in the evaluation of Hodgkin's lymphoma is not indicated in childhood non-Hodgkin's lymphoma due to the characteristic noncontiguous spread of disease in the later. If there is extensive marrow infiltration (greater than 25 percent) by lymphoblastic or Burkitt's lymphoma, surgical biopsy is not necessary because most centers employ treatment regimens similar to those used for acute lymphoblastic leukemia.

Pathologic Features

Non-Hodgkin's lymphoma is the small round cell tumor of childhood most commonly presenting as lymphadenopathy. In children, non-Hodgkin's lymphomas are usually histologically diffuse rather than nodular, have a rapid rate of growth, and tend to disseminate early. They nearly always fall into one of four histologic categories: lymphoblastic (30–40 percent), undifferentiated Burkitt's or undifferentiated non-Burkitt's (30–50 percent) or large cell immunoblastic (15–40 percent).[24,58] In the working formulation proposed by the National Cancer Institute for classification of non-Hodgkin's lymphomas, the childhood tumors are usually high grade.[60] However, small numbers of children were included in this analysis so that correlations with response to therapy and ultimate prognosis remain to be clarified.[24,58] In addition, the concordance rate between pathologist in a recent national cooperative pediatric study (Children's Cancer Study Group) was as low as 50 percent using the aforementioned four histologic categories.[58] The cases entered into this program, therefore, were operationally classified as either lymphoblastic or nonlymphoblastic lymphoma with a much improved rate of concurrence.

Lymphoblastic lymphoma cells are characterized by pleomorphic, convoluted nuclei which are generally smaller than surrounding macrophage nuclei (Fig. 14-11). Key features include a very fine chromatin pattern, indistinct nucleoli, and scanty cytoplasm. Virtually all lymphoblastic lymphomas are of T cell origin as evidenced by E rosette formation, positive staining for terminal deoxynucleotidyl-transferase, and reactions with monoclonal T cell markers. In partially effaced nodes, the lymphoblasts involve the T-dependent paracortical zones. The immunopathologic relationship of lymphoblastic lymphoma to childhood acute lymphoblastic leukemia has not been well defined as there have been heterogenous results using panels of monoclonal antibodies in overlap cases.[61,62]

Undifferentiated lymphomas of the Burkitt's and non-Burkitt's types appear similar morphologically, with a nuclear size that approximates that of a macrophage. Burkitt's cell nuclei tend to have uniform round to oval shape while non-Burkitt's lymphoma nuclei are more pleomorphic in appearance with some binucleate and trinuleate forms. Both lesions feature

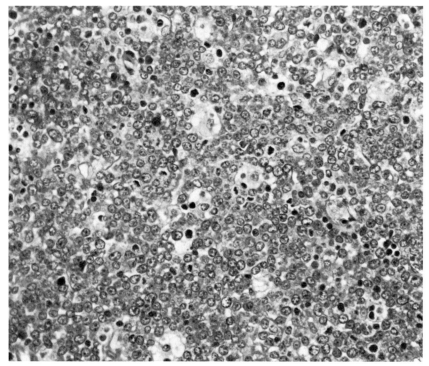

Figure 14-11. *Lymphoblastic lymphoma is the most common subtype of non-Hodgkin's lymphoma occurring in childhood. At low power, the tumor has a "starry sky" appearance due to interspersed macrophages (hematoxylin and eosin, X 400).*

a high mitotic rate and reactive "starry sky" macrophages. Two to five prominent nucleoli per cell are characteristic of Burkitt's lymphoma while the non-Burkitt's cells have three or less, often single, nucleoli (Fig. 14-12). Both types of undifferentiated lymphomas have deeply basophilic cytoplasm which may be markedly vacuolated. Immunologically, both types of undifferentiated lymphomas are routinely of B cell origin with immunoglobulin and, occasionally, Fc and/or C3 receptors demonstrable on the surface of neoplastic cells. In partially involved nodes, the B cell associated germinal centers are primarily affected.

The large cell immunoblastic lymphomas represent a common morphologic endpoint for transformed cells of diverse origin. In children, most tumors have B cell markers with occasional T cell and null cell subtypes.[24] True histiocytic lymphomas are rare.[63,64] As the name implies, the average

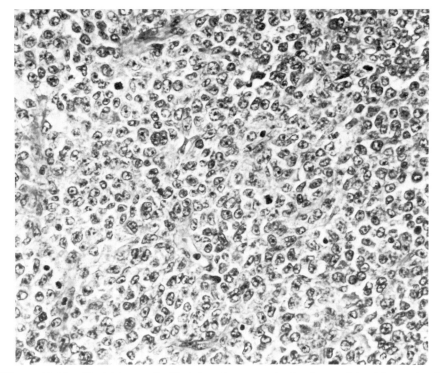

Figure 14-12. *Nuclei in non-Burkitt's lymphomas tend to be pleomorphic with occasional multinucleated forms. Nucleoli are prominent in both Burkitt's non-Burkitt's lymphoma, the latter illustrated in this photomicrograph (hematoxylin and eosin, X 400).*

large cell immunoblastic lymphoma nuclei are larger than the interspersed macrophages. The T cell immunoblasts often have convoluted nuclei reminiscent of lymphoblastic lymphoma cells. B cell immunoblasts have plasmacytoid features with basophilic cytoplasm and juxtanuclear clear zones.[24] True histiocytic lymphomas may be identified by using markers including α-1-anti-trypsin, α-1-anti-chymotrypsin, lysozyme, and Fc and/or C3 receptors without surface immunoglobulin.[63,64]

In the differential diagnosis of small round cell tumors of childhood, lymphoblastic and large cell immunoblastic lymphomas with regular, nonconvoluted nuclei may be confused morphologically with other malignancies, especially if bone is the involved tissue. In nodal disease, the clinical pattern and the use of immunohistochemical stains readily differentiates cases of non-Hodgkin's lymphoma, including those of the null cell type.[65] Recently, the use of the histocompatibility marker, HLA-DR, and a monoclonal antibody specific for a common leukocyte antigen (T200), reliably distinguished 21 small round cell tumors (seven neuroblastomas, seven rhabdomyosarcomas, five Ewing's sarcomas, and two unclassified) from lymphoid malignancies.[66] As noted previously, morphologic subcategorization of non-Hodgkin's lymphomas may be adequate in classic appearing tissue, but is variable between examiners in other situations.

Electron microscopy is not useful for subclassification of non-Hodgkin's lymphomas, but can be helpful in differentiating lymphomas from other small round cell malignancies of childhood. The presence of any ultrastructural cell to cell attachments or basal lamina formation eliminates non-Hodgkin's lymphoma from the differential diagnosis.[25] Pathologic examination of metastatic rhabdomyosarcoma, neuroblastoma, or Ewing's sarcoma involving lymph nodes is usually performed for disease staging purposes rather than to make an initial diagnosis. The most valuable distinguishing point of these solid malignancies is that they do not have lymphocytic, histiocytic or other blood cell markers. Pertinent histopathologic features of the other small round cell tumors of childhood have been discussed elsewhere in this review.

Differential Diagnosis of Difficult Cases

Most cases of small round cell malignancies of childhood may be diagnosed correctly without great difficulty based on clinical features and a classic histological pattern. Problems most frequently arise in the evaluation of bone lesions where the differentiation between Ewing's sarcoma, non-Hodgkin's lymphoma, and metastatic neuroblastoma becomes a challenge. The incidence of small round cell tumors has been estimated to be approximately two cases per 100,000 children per year.[67] Thus, experience with newer diagnostic techniques has been limited to a small number of research facilities. However, pathologic material may be transported between institutions without compromising cytochemical or immunologic investigations, as is often the case with national cooperative group studies. The precise classification of primitive neoplasms is of both biologic and therapeutic importance.

Electron microscopy may be particularly helpful in identifying ultrastructural features characteristic of primitive rhabdomyosarcomas. Prior to the appearance of actin (7 nm) and myosin (14 nm) filaments in embryonic muscle and rhabdomyosarcomas, a feltwork of intermediate (10 nm) filaments is present, often in association with organizing Z-band material. When these two features are observed, they provide presumptive evidence of rhabdomyosarcoma.[25] Another useful feature to identify primitive soft tissue sarcomas are intracytoplasmic, phagocytosed collagen fibers. Such fibers are indicative of matrix degradation and have never been reported in non-Hodgkin's lymphoma, Ewing's sarcoma, or neuroblastoma.[25]

Electron microscopy is also useful to demonstrate several features of primitive neuroblastomas. Dense core granules (catecholamine granules, neurosecretory granules) are 50–200 nm cytoplasmic structures, uniform in size and distribution, frequently peripherally located and found in cell processes mimicking abortive neural processes. These granules should be distinguished from pleomorphic lysosomal granules usually located in the perinuclear Golgi region. Akin to neural rosettes seen under light miscroscopy, the presence of tumor cell clusters with central masses of neuritic processes are pathognomonic of neuroblastoma with or without identifiable dense core granules.[25] Ultrastructural features of neuroblastoma cells also may be identified in colonies growing in a human tumor cloning system.[68]

Recently, antibodies against neuron-specific enolase have been reported to accurately identify neuroblastoma (N = 15) and the malignant small round cell tumor of the thoracopulmonary region (N = 12).[69] Conversely, no reactivity was noted with tissue from Ewing's sarcomas, lymphomas, and soft tissue sarcomas. Some investigators have synthesized a panel of monoclonal antibodies which bind to neuroblastoma cell lines.[27,28] When perfected, antibody analysis would appear preferable to electron microscopy on the basis of cost and time.[27] Catecholamine fluorescence and neurite growth in tissue culture also have been reported to be highly sensitive and specific techniques for confirming the diagnosis of neuroblastoma.[29]

As noted previously, a variety of lymphocytic histiocytic, and other white blood cell markers have been used to diagnose and delineate lineage in cases of non-Hodgkin's lymphoma. Monoclonal antibodies reactive against muscle-specific proteins, i.e. myoglobin,[40] myosin,[41] CPK-MM,[42] CPK-BB,[43] desmin,[44] and Z-protein,[45] also have been useful to identify rhabdomyosarcoma. Panels of monoclonal antibodies against muscle proteins analagous to those reactive with lymphoid antigens may enhance diagnostic accuracy in the future. There are no immunologic markers currently known specific for Ewing's sarcoma. The key pathologic features for the four major small round cell tumors of childhood are summarized in Table 4-1.

Table 14-1
Pathologic Features of the Small Round Cell Malignancies of Childhood

	Ewing's Sarcoma	Neuroblastoma	Non-Hodgkin's Lymphoma	Rhabdomyosarcoma
Light Microscopy	dimorphic, bland cell population often with glycogen	neural rosettes, cell processes	lymphoblastic, Burkitt's, non-Burkitt's, immunoblastic histologies	rhabdomyoblasts with cross striations
Electron Microscopy	scant stroma, abundant glycogen, few organelles	dense core granules, microtubules and neurofilaments within dendritic processes	no cell to cell attachments, cell processes, or dense core granules	actin, myosin, or intermediate filaments, phagocytosed collagen fibers
Immunodiagnosis	no specific markers	neuron-specific enolase; catecholamine fluorescence and neurite growth in cell culture	lymphoid, histiocytic, and other white blood cell markers	muscle protein markers e.g. myoglobin, myosin, CPK, desmin, and Z-protein

Treatment of the Small Round Cell Malignancies of Childhood

Many effective treatment programs for the small round cell tumors of childhood have been developed by cooperative groups and pediatric cancer centers around the world. An extensive review is beyond the scope of this chapter. Results from recent national cooperative groups of which this institution is a member will be summarized for each of the four major small round cell malignancies. Therapeutic regimens for the polyhistioma and malignant small cell tumor of the thoracopulmonary region have not been clearly defined due to the rarity of these lesions.[30,36]

Ewing's Sarcoma

Several approaches have been used in the treatment of patients with Ewing's sarcoma based on the location of the primary tumor and the extent of disease. The Intergroup Ewing's Sarcoma Study has reported a three-year survival rate of 56 percent for nonmetastatic tumors using combination chemotherapy and local irradiation.[70] The most effective regimen, consisting of vincristine, actinomycin D, cyclophosphamide, and Adriamycin (VAC + ADR), resulted in 74 percent of patients free of disease at two years. Children with advanced regional or metastatic tumors fared less favorably, despite four-drug chemotherapy (VAC + ADR) and irradiation to all sites of overt involvement. Eighteen of 33 patients, 12 with metastases and six with advanced regional spread at diagnosis, were disease-free with a median follow-up of 34 months.[71] The long term prognosis is guarded for these individuals as late relapses are a characteristic feature of Ewing's tumor.[72] Survival curves continue to decline for all stages of this malignancy up to six years after diagnosis.[73] Recent, more aggressive treatment programs including autologous bone marrow infusion are hoped to improve future success rates.[74,75] It may be noted that soft tissue Ewing's sarcoma has been successfully managed with treatment programs designed for either rhabdomyosarcoma or Ewing's sarcoma of bone.[35,76]

The role of surgical resection as the primary treatment of Ewing's sarcoma has been resurrected after many years when radiation therapy was considered to be the treatment standard. Complications of radiotherapy including severe fibrosis and contractures, radiation necrosis, pathologic fractures, leg length discrepancy, and secondary malignancies have led to reassessment of the role of surgery.[6,77] Surgery has been advocated for tumors with extensive soft tissue involvement, a pathologic fracture that cannot be managed by other reasonable means, and lesions in the leg of a young, growing child.[6,77] Other investigators have observed acceptable leg function following radiotherapy, concluding that primary amputation for Ewing's sarcoma of the lower extremity is not justified.[78] In a related issue, when an expendable bone is involve with malignancy, e.g. fibula, clavicle, or rib, surgical resection is probably preferable to radiotherapy since there will be no subsequent functional deficit.[6] In conclusion, considerable judgment is necessary to select the proper therapeutic approach for each patient.

Rhabdomyosarcoma

The Intergroup Rhabdomyosarcoma Study has accrued over 1300 cases since 1972. Most patients have been treated with combined modality programs including primary surgery, postoperative radiation, and chemotherapy. The most commonly used drugs have been vincristine, actinomycin D, and cyclophosphamide (VAC).[79] Therapeutic results have been based on the clinical groups outlined in the rhabdomyosarcoma pathology section of this review.

The three-year disease-free survival rate for children with clinical group I disease was 84 percent with and 82 percent without radiotherapy.[79] Recent preliminary data suggests that it may be possible to delete cyclophosphmide from the treatment regimen without jeopardizing survival in this group of patients with resectable disease.[79] For clinical group II lesions, the combination of vincristine and actinomycin D has been equivalent to the standard VAC program with all children receiving postoperative radiotherapy to the tumor bed. The percentage of patients recurrence-free at three years was 70 percent without cyclophosphamide and 62 percent with the drug.[79] In children with clinical group III and IV rhabdomyosarcoma, the addition of Adriamycin to the VAC chemotherapy regimen has not been beneficial. Fifty-seven percent of group III and 29 percent of group IV patients are disease-free survivors at 3 years.[79] Further modifications including the addition of other drugs for treatment of advanced disease are currently being evaluated. As mentioned previously, children with unfavorable histological features are being approached more aggressively in current therapeutic trials.[49,50]

In an effort to minimize long term morbidity by preservation of normal organ function, some children with rhabdomyosarcomas have not undergone immediate surgical resection of their tumors. The value of a primary chemotherapy/radiotherapy approach has been exemplified by cases of rhabdomyosarcoma in the genitourinary region. Twenty-six of 37 patients (70 percent) were recurrence-free at a median of 83 weeks, including 17 who retained functioning bladders. It appears that primary chemotherapy and radiation has improved the bladder salvage rate without diminishing survival.[79] Similarly, rhabdomyosarcomas confined to the orbit have been treated successfully without enucleation.[80]

Neuroblastoma

Treatment and prognosis of neuroblastoma is dependent on the clinical stage of disease at diagnosis. In a classic analysis of 234 children by D'Angio in 1971, the two-year survival rates were: stage I—84 percent, stage II—66 percent, stage III—33 percent, stage IV—5 percent, and stage IVS—84 percent.[3] Patients less than one year of age fared the most favorably in all stages.

In the differential diagnosis of small round cell tumors of childhood, the major concern is to differentiate stage IV neuroblastoma from other malignancies. Unfortunately, when such advanced disease is confirmed, the prognosis is extremely poor (less than 10 percent long term disease-free survival). In the past two decades, minimal improvement has been made, despite multiple combinations of chemotherapy (including vincristine, cyclophosphamide, doxorubicin, dacarbazine, cis-platinum, and VM-26), radiation therapy, and surgery.[28] Similarly, multiagent chemotherapy has had little impact on the survival of nonmetastatic neuroblastoma patients treated with surgical excision and radiotherapy to any residua. The three-year survival rates were 96 percent, 89 percent, and 50 percent for stage I, II, and III disease in the latest Children's Cancer Study Group report.[81]

Clearly, new therapeutic approaches are necessary to combat disseminated neuroblastoma. Modest early success from several centers has been reported utilizing melphalan and other drugs +/–total body irradiation in conjunction with autologous or allogeneic bone marrow transplantation,[75,82,83] Monoclonal antibodies alone or conjugated to toxins or magnetic microspheres may contribute to effective removal of neuroblastoma cells from marrow specimens, or, in the future, in vivo.[28,84] In addition, maturational therapy with retinoic acid has attracted attention recently based on its ability in cultured neuroblastoma cell systems to promote morphologic differentiation and inhibit proliferation.[28]

Non-Hodgkin's Lymphoma

The largest recent series of children treated for non-Hodgkin's lymphoma (N=234) was reported by the Children's Cancer Study Group.[7,55] The patients were divided into two groups of disease involvement, localized and nonlocalized, as well as into two histologic categories, lymphoblastic and nonlymphoblastic. Two therapy programs were compared, the 10-drug LSA2L2 regimen modified from the experience of Wollner,[85] and a four-drug program consisting of cyclophosphamide, vincristine (Oncovin), methotrexate, and prednisone (COMP). The three-year disease-free survival (DFS) for the 73 localized lymphoma patients was 84 percent for both regimens, irrespective of the histologic category. For the children with nonlocalized disease, the LSA2L2 program was more effective compared to COMP when the lymphoblastic histology was present (76 percent versus 26 percent two-year DFS) while the COMP regimen gave better results when nonlymphoblastic disease was being treated (57 percent versus 28 percent two-year DFS) (Fig. 14-13). Central nervous system or bone marrow involvement at diagnosis portended a poor prognosis with a 37 percent two-year DFS rate. However, the LSA2L2 regimen was relatively successful in this situation when the diagnosis was lymphoblastic lymphoma (71 percent two-year DFS) as has been noted by others.[86]

Issues to be resolved in current trials include the efficacy of less intensive treatment for low risk localized disease and an improvement in therapy for patients with disseminated Burkitt's and non-Burkitt's undifferentiated lymphomas. Recent experience would suggest that less treatment for good prognosis patients is feasible, but that improved approaches for diffuse undifferentiated lymphomas are needed.[87-89] A pilot study of 10 patients with disseminated Burkitt's or poor prognosis lymphoblastic lymphoma who underwent allogeneic bone marrow transplantation has resulted in five long term survivors with unmaintained remissions after 18 to 73 months follow-up.[90] Another possibility for treatment of high risk patients includes the usage of monoclonal antibodies for (1) serotherapy and (2) allogeneic or autologous bone marrow transplantation.[10,91]

Conclusion

Diagnosis and management of the small round cell malignancies of childhood has evolved steadily over the past two decades. Improved histopathologic techniques such as electron microscopy and the development of monoclonal antibodies have made the identification of these tumors possible in most cases. Combined modality therapy and the treatment of patients in cooperative groups have advanced our ability to cure these malignancies. Challenges for the future include further understanding of the biology of these cancers and the enhancement of survival, particularly those with metastatic disease.

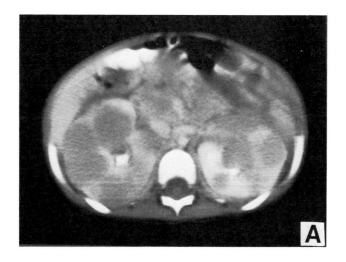

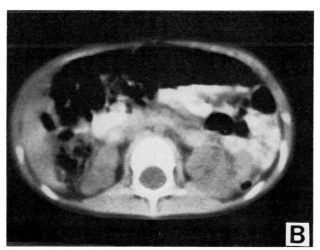

Figure 14-13. *This two-year-old girl presented with widespread Burkitt's lymphoma. Computerized tomography revealed (A) massively infiltrated kidneys and abdominal lymphadenopathy, both of which cleared remarkably with (B) primary chemotherapy.*

371

References

1. Sim FH, Unni KK, Beabout JW, et al: Osteosarcoma with small cells simulating Ewing's tumor. J Bone Joint Surg (Am) 61:207–215, 1979
2. Nascimento AG, Cooper KL, Unni KK, et al: A clinicopathologic study of 20 cases of large-cell (atypical) Ewing's sarcoma of bone. Am J Surg Pathol 4:29–36, 1980
3. D'Angio GJ, Evans AE, Koop CE: Special pattern of widespread neuroblastoma with a favourable prognosis. Lancet 1:1046–1049, 1971
4. Holland T, Donohue JP, Baehner RL, et al: Current management of neuroblastoma. J Urol 124:579–582, 1980
5. Thomas PRM, Lee JY, Fineberg BB, et al: An analysis of neuroblastoma at a single institution. Cancer 53:2079–2082, 1984
6. Pritchard DJ, Unni KK, Gilchrist GS: Small round-cell malignancies of bone, in Sim FH (ed): Diagnosis and Treatment of Bone Tumors: A Team Approach. Thorofare, NJ, Slack, 1983, pp 247–258
7. Anderson JR, Wilson JF, Jenkin DT, et al: Childhood non-Hodgkin's lymphoma: Results of a randomized therapeutic trial comparing a 4-drug regimen (COMP) with a 10-drug regimen (LSA2L2). N Engl J Med 308:559–565, 1983
8. Dahlin DC: Bone Tumors: General Aspects and Data on 6221 Cases (ed 3). Springfield, IL, Charles C Thomas Publisher, 1978
9. Maurer HM: Intergroup Rhabdomyosarcoma Study: Update, November 1978. Natl Cancer Inst Monogr 56:61–68, 1981
10. Altman AJ, Schwartz AD: Tumors of the sympathetic nervous system, in Altman AJ, Schwartz AD (eds): Malignant Diseases of Infancy, Childhood and Adolescence (ed 2). Philadelphia, WB Saunders Company, 1983, pp 368–388
11. Osborne RL: Differential radiologic diagnosis of bone tumors. CA 24:194–211, 1974
12. Gilchrist GS, Telander RL: Tumors of the adrenal medulla and sympathetic chain, in Kelalis PP, King LR, Belman AB (eds): Clinical Pediatric Urology. Second edition. Philadelphia, WB Saunders Company, 1984
13. Howman-Giles RB, Gilday DL, Ash JM: Radionuclide skeletal survey in neuroblastoma. Radiology 131:497–502, 1979
14. Ruymann FB, Newton WA, Ragab AH, et al: Bone marrow metastases at diagnosis in children and adolescents with rhabdomyosarcoma. Cancer 53:368–373, 1984
15. Wolff JA: Diagnostic procedures for evaluation of sarcomas of soft tissue and bone in childhood. Natl Cancer Inst Monogr 56:3–7, 1981

16. Kaufman RA, Thrall JH, Keyes JW, et al: False negative bone scans in neuroblastoma metastatic to the ends of long bones. Am J Roentgenol 130:131–135, 1978

17. Williams CM, Greer M: Homovanillic acid and vanilmandelic acid in diagnosis of neuroblastoma. JAMA 183:134–138, 1963

18. Laug WE, Siegel SE, Shaw KNF, et al: Initial urinary catecholamine metabolite concentrations and prognosis in neuroblastoma. Pediatr 62:77–83, 1978

19. Helson L, Fleisher M, Bethune V, et al: Urinary cystathionine, catecholamine, and metabolites in patients with neuroblastoma. Clin Chem 18:613–615, 1972

20. Rajnherc JR, van Gennip AH, Abeling NGGM, et al: Cystothionuria in patients with neuroblastoma. Med Pediatr Oncol 12:81–84, 1984

21. Zeltzer PM, Marangos PJ, Parma AM, et al: Raised neuron-specific enolase in serum of children with metastatic neuroblastoma. Lancet 2:361–363, 1983

22. Kissane JM, Askin FB, Nesbit ME, et al: Sarcomas of bone in childhood: Pathologic aspects. Natl Cancer Inst Monogr 56:29–41, 1981

23. Triche TJ: Round cell tumors in childhood: Application of newer techniques to the differential diagnosis, in Rosenberg HS, Bernstein J (eds): Perspectives in Pediatric Pathology, vol. 7. New York, Masson Publishing USA, 1982, pp 279–322

24. Callihan TR, Berard CW: Childhood non-Hodgkin's lymphomas in current histologic perspective, in Rosenberg HS, Bernstein J (eds): Perspectives in Pediatric Pathology, vol. 7. New York, Masson Publishing USA, 1982, pp 259–277

25. Triche TJ, Askin FB: Neuroblastoma and the differential diagnosis of small-, round-, blue-cell tumors. Hum Pathol 14:569–595, 1983

26. Tsokos M, Linnoila RI, Chandra RS, et al: Neuron-specific enolase in the diagnosis of neuroblastoma and other small, round-cell tumors in children. Hum Pathol 15:575–584, 1984

27. Kemshead JT, Coakman HB: Use of monoclonal antibodies for the diagnosis of intracranial malignancies and the small round cell tumours of childhood. J Pathol 141:249–257, 1983

28. Seeger RC, Siegel SE, Sidell N: Neuroblastoma: Clinical perspectives, monoclonal antibodies, and retinoic acid. Ann Intern Med 97:873–884, 1982

29. Reynolds CP, German DC, Weinberg AG, et al: Catecholamine fluorescence and tissue culture morphology. Am J Clin Pathol 75:275–282, 1981

30. Jacobson SA: Polyhistioma. Cancer 40:2116–2130, 1977
31. Dehner LP: Soft tissue sarcomas of childhood: Differential diagnostic dilemma of the small blue cell. Natl Cancer Inst Monogr 56:43–59, 1981
32. Gaiger AM, Soule EH, Newton WA: Pathology of rhabdomyosarcoma: Experience of the Intergroup Rhabdomyosarcoma Study, 1972–78. Natl Cancer Inst Monogr 56:19–27, 1981
33. Grosfeld JL, Weber TR, Weetman RM, et al: Rhabdomyosarcoma in childhood: Analysis of survival in 98 cases. J Pediatr Surg 18:141–146, 1983
34. Bale PM, Reye RDK: Rhabdomyosarcoma in childhood. Pathology 7:101–111, 1975
35. Soule EH, Newton W, Moon TE, et al: Extraskeletal Ewing's sarcoma. Cancer 42:259–264, 1978
36. Askin FB, Rosal J, Sibley RK, et al: Malignant small cell tumor of the thoracopulmonary region in childhood. Cancer 43:2438–2451, 1979
37. Patton RB, Horn RC: Rhabdomyosarcoma: Clinical and pathological features and comparison with human fetal and embryonal skeletal muscle. Surgery 52:572–584, 1962
38. Bale PM, Parsons RE, Stevens MM: Diagnosis and behavior of juvenile rhabdomyosarcoma. Hum Pathol 14:596–611, 1983
39. Enzinger FM, Weiss SW: Soft Tissue Tumors. St. Louis, CV Mosby Company, 1983
40. Brooks JJ: Immunohistochemistry of soft tissue tumors. Cancer 50:1757–1763, 1982
41. Koh S-J, Johnson WW: Antimyosin and antirhabdomyoblast sera. Arch Pathol Lab Med 104:118–122, 1980
42. Kahn HJ, Yeger H, Kassim O, et al: Immunohistochemical and electron microscopic assessment of childhood rhabdomyosarcoma. Cancer 51:1897–1903, 1983
43. Tsokos M, Howard R, Costa J: Immunohistochemical study of alveolar and embryonal rhabdomyosarcoma. Lab Invest 48:148–155, 1983
44. Altmannsberger M, Osborn M, Treuner J, et al: Diagnosis of human childhood rhabdomyosarcoma by antibodies to desmin, the structural protein of muscle specific intermediate filaments. Virchows Arch (Cell Pathol) 39:203–215, 1982
45. Mukai M, Iri H, Torikata C, et al: Immunoperoxidase demonstration of a new muscle protein (Z-protein) in myogenic tumors as a diagnostic aid. Am J Pathol 114:164–170, 1984
46. Kingston JE, McElwain TJ, Malpas JS: Childhood rhabdomyosarcoma:

Experience of the Children's Solid Tumour Group. Br J Cancer 48:195–207, 1983

47. Linnoila RI, Tsokos M, Triche TJ, et al: Evidence for neural origin and periodic acid–Schiff–positive variants of the malignant small cell tumor of the thoracopulmonary region ("Askin tumor") (abstract). Lab Invest 48:51A, 1983

48. Raney HB, Ragab AH, Ruymann FB, et al: Soft-tissue sarcoma of the trunk in childhood. Cancer 49:2612–2616, 1982

49. Palmer NF, Foulkes M: Histopathology and prognosis in the second Intergroup Rhabdomyosarcoma Study (IRS-II) (abstract). Proc Annu Mtg Am Soc Clin Oncol 2:229, 1983

50. Ruymann F, Heyn R, Ragab A, et al: Completely resected rhabdo- myosarcoma: Effect of unfavorable histology on recurrence. A report from the Intergroup Rhabdomyosarcoma Study (IRS) (abstract). Proc Annu Mtg Am Soc Clin Oncol 3:86, 1984

51. Donaldson SS, Belli JA: A rational clinical staging system for child- hood rhabdomyosarcoma. J Clin Oncol 2:135–139, 1984

52. Zuelzer WW, Kaplan J: The child with lymphadenopathy. Semin Hematol 12:323–334, 1975

53. Knight PJ, Mulne AF, Vassy LE: When is lymph node biopsy indicated in children with enlarged peripheral nodes? Pediatr 69:391–396, 1982

54. Lake AM, Oski FA: Peripheral lymphadenopathy in childhood. Am J Dis Child 132:357–359, 1978

55. Jenkin RDT, Anderson JR, Chilcote RR, et al: Treatment of localized non-Hodgkin's lymphoma in children: A report from the Children's Cancer Study Group. J Clin Oncol 2:88–97, 1984

56. Murphy SB: Classification, staging and end results of treatment of childhood non-Hodgkin's lymphomas: Dissimilarities from lympho- mas in adults. Semin Oncol 7:332–339, 1980

57. Kjeldsberg CR, Wilson JF, Berard CW: Non-Hodgkin's lymphoma in children. Hum Pathol 14:612–627, 1983

58. Wilson JF, Jenkin RDT, Anderson JR, et al: Studies on the pathology of non-Hodgkin's lymphoma of childhood: I. Role of routine histopathology as a prognostic factor, a report from the Children's Cancer Study Group. Cancer 53:1695–1704, 1984

59. Smith SD, Kisker S, Bush L, et al: Utilization of a human tumor cloning system to monitor for bone marrow involvement in children with non-Hodgkin's lymphoma. Cancer 53:1724–1729, 1984

60. National Cancer Institute sponsored study of classification of non- Hodgkin's lymphomas: summary and description of a working for-

mulation for clinical usage. The non-Hodgkin's lymphoma pathologic classification project. Cancer 49:2112–2135, 1982

61. Bernard A, Boumsell L, Reinherz EL, et al: Cell surface characterization of malignant T cells from lymphoblastic lymphoma using monoclonal antibodies: Evidence for phenotypic differences between malignant T cells from patients with acute lymphoblastic leukemia and lymphoblastic lymphoma. Blood 57:1105–1110, 1981

62. Morgan E: Cell markers in lymphoma syndrome leukemia in children: A pilot study. Med Pediatr Oncol 12:4–8, 1984

63. Isaacson P, Wright DH, Jones DB: Malignant lymphoma of true histiocytic (monocyte/macrophage) origin. Cancer 51:80–91, 1983

64. Koh S-J, Vargas GF, Caces JN, et al: Malignant "histiocytic" lymphoma in childhood. Am J Clin Pathol 74:417–426, 1980

65. Kadin ME: Ia-like (HLA-DR) antigens in the diagnosis of lymphoma and undifferentiated tumors. Arch Pathol Lab Med 104:503–508, 1980

66. Andres TL, Kadin ME: Immunologic markers in the differential diagnosis of small round cell tumors from lymphocytic lymphoma and leukemia. Am J Clin Pathol 79:546–552, 1983

67. Altman AJ, Schwartz AD: The cancer problem in pediatrics: Epidemiologic aspects, in Altman AJ, Schwartz AD (eds): Malignant Diseases of Infancy, Childhood, and Adolescence (ed 2). Philadelphia, WB Saunders Company, 1983, pp 1–21

68. Harris GJ, Zeagler J, Hodach A, et al: Ultrastructural analysis of colonies growing in a human tumor cloning system. Cancer 50:722–726, 1982

69. Tsokos M, Linnoila RI, Triche T, et al: Neuron-specific enolase as an aid to the diagnosis of primitive small round cell tumors of neural origin (abstract). Lab Invest 48:87A, 1983

70. Nesbit ME, Perez CA, Tefft M, et al: Multimodal therapy for the management of primary, nonmetastatic Ewing's sarcoma of bone: An Intergroup Study. Natl Cancer Inst Monogr 56:255–262, 1981

71. Pilepich MV, Vietti TJ, Nesbit ME, et al: Radiotherapy and combination chemotherapy in advanced Ewing's sarcoma—Intergroup Study. Cancer 47:1930–1936, 1981

72. Vietti TJ, Gehan EA, Nesbit ME, et al: Multimodal therapy in metastatic Ewing's sarcoma: An Intergroup Study. Natl Cancer Inst Monogr 56:279–284, 1981

73. Kissane JM, Askin FB, Foulkes M, et al: Ewing's sarcoma of bone: Clinicopathologic aspects of 303 cases from the Intergroup Ewing's Sarcoma Study. Hum Pathol 14:773–779, 1983

74. Cornbleet MA, Corringham RET, Prentice HG, et al: Treatment of

Ewing's sarcoma with high-dose melphalan and autologous bone marrow transplantation. Cancer Treat Rep 65:241–244, 1981

75. Graham-Pole J, Coccia P, Lazarus HM, et al: High-dose melphalan therapy for the treatment of children with refractory neuroblastoma and Ewing's sarcoma. Am J Pediatr Hematol Oncol 6:17–26, 1984

76. Kinsella TJ, Triche TJ, Dickman PS, et al: Extraskeletal Ewing's sarcoma: Results of combined modality treatment. J Clin Oncol 1:489–495, 1983

77. Lewis RJ, Marcove RC, Rosen G: Ewing's sarcoma—functional effects of radiation therapy. J Bone Joint Surg (Am) 59:325–331, 1977

78. Jentzsch K, Binder H, Cramer H: Leg function after radiotherapy for Ewing's sarcoma. Cancer 47:1267–1278, 1981

79. Maurer HM: The Intergroup Rhabdomyosarcoma Study. Cancer Bull 34:108–110, 1982

80. Kadota RP, Evans RG, Gilchrist GS, et al: Morbidity and mortality of pediatric orbital rhabdomyosarcoma (abstract). Proc Am Soc Clin Oncol 2:76, 1983

81. Evans AR, Sather H, Brand W, et al: Results in children with local and regional neuroblastoma managed with and without vincristine, cyclophosphamide, and imidazolecarboxamide: A report from the Children's Cancer Study Group. Am J Clin Oncol 6:3–8, 1984

82. Pritchard J, McElwain TJ, Graham-Pole J: High-dose melphalan with autologous marrow for treatment of advanced neuroblastoma. Br J Cancer 45:86–94, 1982

83. August CS, Serota FT, Koch PA, et al: Treatment of advanced neuroblastoma with supralethal chemotherapy, radiation, and allogeneic or autologous marrow reconstitution. J Clin Oncol 2:609–616, 1984

84. Treleaven JG, Gibson FM, Ugelstad J, et al: Removal of neuroblastoma cells from bone marrow with monoclonal antibodies conjugated to magnetic microspheres. Lancet 1:70–73, 1984

85. Wollner N, Exelby PR, Lieberman PH: Non-Hodgkin's lymphoma in children. Cancer 44:1990–1999, 1979

86. Duque-Hammershaimb L, Wollner N, Miller DR: LSA2L2 protocol treatment of stage IV non-Hodgkin's lymphoma in children with partial and extensive bone marrow involvement. Cancer 52:39–43, 1983

87. Murphy SB, Hustu HO, Rivera G, et al: End results of treating children with localized non-Hodgkin's lymphomas with a combined modality approach of lessened intensity. J Clin Oncol 1:326–330, 1983

88. Magrath IT, Janus C, Edwards BK, et al: An effective therapy for both

undifferentiated (including Burkitt's) lymphomas and lymphoblastic lymphomas in children and young adults. Blood 63:1102–1111, 1984

89. Link M, Donaldson S, Berard C, et al: Effective therapy with reduced toxicity for children with localized non-Hodgkin's lymphoma (NHL) (abstract). Proc Annu Mtg Am Soc Clin Oncol 3:251, 1984

90. O'Leary M, Ramsay NKC, Nesbit ME, et al: Bone marrow transplantation for non-Hodgkin's lymphoma in children and young adults: A pilot study. Am J Med 74:497–501, 1983

91. Appelbaum FR, Thomas ED: Review of the use of marrow transplantation in the treatment of non-Hodgkin's lymphoma. J Clin Oncol 1:440–447, 1983

15

TIME-DEPENDENT CHANGES IN HUMAN TUMORS: IMPLICATIONS FOR DIAGNOSIS AND CLINICAL BEHAVIOR

Geoffrey Mendelsohn
Stephen B. Baylin

The histologic classification of a tumor is based upon morphologic characteristics evident at the particular point in time at which the tumor is sampled and the degree to which the neoplasm resembles the parent tissue in or from which it derives. Pathologists have long recognized that many human tumors contain morphologically heterogeneous populations of cells; tumor classifications such as "adenosquamous carcinoma" reflect this cellular heterogeneity. During recent years, it has become apparent that tumor differentiation is not a static phenomenon. Dynamic relationships exist between a tumor's constituent cell populations involving both reversible and irreversible changes that alter the composition of the tumor as disease progresses. These changes can affect the morphological, biochemical, and functional characteristics of a tumor and obviously play a critical role in determining the features present in a given neoplasm at the time of diagnosis. The ease with which the pathologist is able to recognize features

POORLY DIFFERENTIATED NEOPLASMS AND TUMORS OF UNKNOWN ORIGIN   ISBN 0-8089-1755-2

of the parent tissue and thereby establish an appropriate diagnosis may obviously depend upon the degree to which the neoplasm has altered its cellular characteristics since inception.

The concept of time-dependent change in tumors is important when considering poorly differentiated neoplasms and tumors of unknown origin. Although an appreciation of this aspect of tumor biology may not immediately contribute to the practical problems involved in diagnosing such tumors and in establishing the site of origin, recognition and improved understanding of this phenomenon will surely contribute to enhanced diagnostic capacity.

In this chapter, we will first consider certain basic aspects of the concept of time-dependent changes in tumors and will then use four selected human tumor models to illustrate the pathological and clinical consequences of such changes. Particular attention will be paid to the relationships between morphologic and biochemical changes and clinical course, and an attempt will be made to speculate on how a better understanding of time-dependent changes in selected human tumors may facilitate our ability to identify the tissues of origin of undifferentiated neoplasms.

Time-dependent Changes: The Concept of Tumor Progression

Most of our knowledge of time-dependent changes in tumors has come from nonhuman models; the description of such events has been incorporated in the concept of "tumor progression".[1,2] During the past thirty years, many investigators have monitored the natural course of certain animal tumors as well as changes induced by various therapeutic modalities, and have carefully described the changes that occur with time in these tumors. Foulds,[1] in reviewing experimental studies and in articulating the concept of tumor progression, stressed that innumerable "unit characters", such as morphologic characteristics, biochemical properties, response to hormonal manipulation, and response to various therapeutic modalities, can change with time. A review of salient principles of the concept of tumor progression is given in Table 15-1. Several of these principles warrant special mention.

First, although the concept of tumor progression intimates a time-dependent drift in all cancers, the rate of drift and degree to which it occurs varies considerably not only between different types of tumors, but also for

Table 15-1
Principles of the Concept of Tumor Progression

1. Tumor progression implies time-dependent changes in all neoplasms.
2. Progression occurs independently, and involves independent changes, in individual properties ("unit characters") of a given tumor.
3. The rate and degree of progression vary between different types of tumors, as well as between different lesions of the same tumor type, in the same host.
4. Progression occurs independently of clinically evident tumor growth.
5. Progression may be continuous or discontinuous and may occur gradually or abruptly.
6. Progression is not predictable and may proceed along several alternative pathways of development.

Modified from Foulds L: The experimental study of tumor progression: A review. Cancer Res 14:327–339, 1954, with permission.

tumors within the same diagnostic classification. Differences may even occur between different lesions in the same animal host. Second, the changes which occur in tumors are unpredictable and different unit characters in an individual tumor are involved independently. Finally, the concept of tumor progression as it has evolved from experimental animal studies implies considerable randomness to the series of changes that occur. If this randomness and lack of pattern were to apply to human tumors, it would certainly limit attempts to define changes in cell populations that might have clinical implications.

Since the basis of our medical practice is therapeutic intervention, it is only under exceptional circumstances that we are able to observe the natural course of progression of human neoplasms. As a consequence, while we are accumulating a significant volume of data concerning the effects of various modes of antitumor therapy, we have not yet gathered a sophisticated body of knowledge concerning tumor progression events for the majority of human tumors. In the sections to follow, we will present selected human tumor models which exhibit definable changes in cell populations with time. Using these models, we will attempt to illustrate that the inexorable drift which occurs in these tumors involves recognizable patterns of change in morphology, biochemistry, and functional properties; the drift in these given tumors is not entirely random or unpredictable. Furthermore, we will consider the clinical and therapeutic implications of the time-dependent changes which can occur.

Tumor Progression in Selected Human Neoplasms

Medullary Thyroid Carcinoma

During the past several years, human medullary thyroid carcinoma (MTC) has provided us with a rather unique opportunity to examine the different stages of tumor evolution, to study constituent cell populations in a given tumor, and to follow the changes which occur in these subpopulations of tumor cells during the course of progression of disease. The findings to date have implications and impact on tumor diagnosis and patient management. The specific characteristics of human MTC which permit investigation of constituent cell populations at various developmental stages of the tumor have been detailed previously.[3,4] In brief, the parent cell for the tumor, the thyroid C cell, has been definitively identified[5] and the key morphologic and biochemical features which characterize the C cell have been defined; these include the synthesis and secretion of the polypeptide hormone calcitonin[6,7] and the ability to synthesize biogenic amines via the decarboxylating enzyme L-dopa decarboxylase (APUD properties).[8,9] From a clinical standpoint, familial MTC presents all stages of tumor development from preneoplastic C cell hyperplasia (CCH) to advanced tumor;[4,9–11] hence, a wide spectrum of tumor behavior is available for evaluation. Typically, MTC is characterized by a rather indolent course and patients may survive for 15 to 20 years or even longer with limited or extensive disease. A small cadre of patients, however, develop virulent disease with death resulting from widespread tumor dissemination. This has allowed for the study of biologically different tumors.

During the course of ongoing clinical, biochemical, and morphologic studies of human MTC, we have noted a pattern of loss of differentiated features of tumor C cells during the course of tumor progression in some cases. Two principal patterns of change have emerged. The least common pattern involves a shift in tumor morphology wherein the usual histologic characteristics of MTC are lost and only the persistence of parent cell biochemistry permits identification of the C cell nature of the tumor, allowing the diagnosis of MTC to be confirmed. In two such cases we have seen,[12] the shift has been from histologically well differentiated MTC to diffusely infiltrating small cell carcinoma without amyloid stroma, sclerosis, or other features typical of MTC. In both cases, this change has involved areas of the primary tumors as well as all sampled metastatic tumor nodules. In a third patient who died with widely disseminated MTC, much of the metastatic tumor had the histological features of an anaplastic giant cell carcinoma.[12] In all three cases, positive immunohisto-

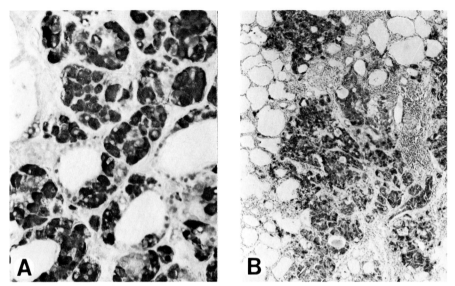

Figure 15-1. *Immunoperoxidase staining for calcitonin in (A) C-cell hyperplasia and (B) early MTC. Note the intense positive staining reaction (dark grey to black in photograph) in the majority of proliferating C cells (uniform calcitonin distribution).*

chemical staining for calcitonin confirmed the true nature of the tumors.[12] The second and more usual form of tumor progression in MTC involves a consistent alteration in the biochemical phenotype of the tumor cells without any concomitant histological alterations. The biochemical change in this cadre of cases is accompanied by significant deterioration in the clinical behavior of the tumors.

The earliest morphologically evident lesion in patients at familial risk for the development of MTC is the preneoplastic stage of C cell hyperplasia (CCH).[9–11] This phase of disease is characterized by a proliferation of C cells whose ability to synthesize and secrete calcitonin is evidenced by elevated circulating calcitonin levels and intense immunostaining for calcitonin within the proliferating C cells (Fig. 15-1). Several studies have shown that the capacity for calcitonin synthesis is retained to a high degree in MTC and, in most cases, changes in C cell mass in patients with MTC can be clinically estimated by monitoring circulating levels of calcitonin.[13–15] In this regard, recent studies from our laboratory[9,16] have shown that microscopic MTC and small, gross tumors localized to the thyroid region are characterized by high concentrations of calcitonin relative to the activity of

L-dopa decarboxylase. In these early stages of disease, immunohistochemical staining for calcitonin is characterized by a homogeneous (uniform) and relatively intense distribution of the hormone throughout the lesions[16] (Fig. 15-1). It would appear from these studies that the morphologic and biochemical phenotype of these early developmental stages of MTC reflect the phenotype of the parent thyroid C cell.

During the course of our studies of patients with MTC, we have encountered a small group of patients in whom the disease has displayed an aggressive, virulent course leading to death from widely disseminated tumor.[16,17] In some of these patients, a discordance between serum calcitonin levels and tumor mass was evident and we have noted a remarkable difference in the biochemical phenotype of systemic metastases in these patients. Sampled lesions from these patients have displayed a deviation from the normal parent C cell phenotype characterized by a complete reversal of the ratios of calcitonin concentration to those of L-dopa decarboxylase and diamine oxidase activity.[16] The marked reduction, and in some cases almost complete loss, of calcitonin correlates with absent, extremely weak, or heterogeneous cellular distribution of calcitonin within the tumors, as evidenced by immunohistochemical staining[16] (Fig. 15-2). Of pivotal importance in regard to the change in phenotype, the primary thyroid tumors, surgically resected as many as five years prior to death, have revealed a similar pattern of cellular heterogeneity for calcitonin.[16] In contrast to the rare situation, in which tumor progression was associated with a loss of the usual histologic characteristics of MTC, in all cases in which the biochemical phenotype has changed with tumor progression, no identifiable changes in tumor histology have been appreciated.

The precise mechanism underlying the loss of parent cell phenotype during the course of tumor progression in human MTC remains unknown at this stage. From the above observations and from our ongoing laboratory studies, however, we would like to postulate that a progressive maturation block occurs during the course of tumor progression resulting in reduced expression of mature phenotypic characteristics, such as the synthesis of calcitonin. There are several features which lend support to such a hypothesis. As we have noted above, the loss of calcitonin reactivity is associated with a relative increase in L-dopa decarboxylase activity. Recent experimental studies of the embryogenesis of mouse pancreas[18] have shown that early stages of endocrine cell development are characterized by increased capacity for biogenic amine synthesis via dopa decarboxylase, following which the normal pancreatic hormones such as glucagon appear. Our studies of MTC might therefore suggest that MTC cells which fail to

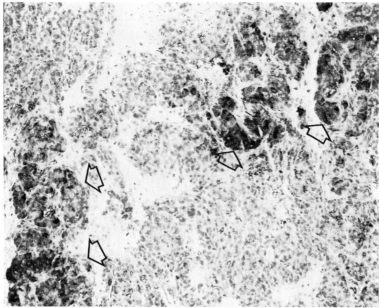

Figure 15-2. *Immunoperoxidase staining for calcitonin in aggressive MTC. Note the heterogeneous distribution of calcitonin positive cells; scattered nests of positive cells (arrows) are present in a region of tumor largely devoid of calcitonin.*

mature retain dopa decarboxylase activity and simultaneously exhibit loss of calcitonin synthesis.

Our recent studies of cultured MTC cells[19] are also consistent with this hypothesis. We have shown that there is an inverse relationship between rate of cell growth and levels of intracellular calcitonin, while L-dopa decarboxylase levels increase during the more rapid growth stages. Individual cell clones were isolated which had low calcitonin levels and gave very high L-dopa decarboxylase to calcitonin ratios during growth. These findings suggest that rapid proliferation of MTC cells, as would be expected in patients with virulent disease, may occur at the expense of cellular differentiation. Some clones of cells may then be particularly unable to differentiate towards the parent cell phenotype. In patients with virulent MTC, therefore, a high rate of cell proliferation plus the evolution of clones with poor maturation potential could well explain the biochemical phenotype we have associated with aggressive disease.

Also of interest to the concept of maturation block associated with tumor progression, recent studies from our laboratory have demonstrated an inverse relationship between CEA, a marker of early cellular differentiation, and calcitonin, a marker for terminal C cell differentiation.[20] In studying the tumors from patients with virulent MTC, we noted that CEA staining was retained, and frequently was most intense, in tumors or regions of tumors from which calcitonin was lost.[20] In our ongoing studies of cultured MTC cells,[19,21] we have also shown reduced calcitonin and most intense immunostaining for CEA during phases of rapid cell replication.

In considering the clinical implications of the above biologic aspects of MTC, certain crucial factors have emerged from the studies. First, the biologic events underlying the loss of parent C cell phenotype in MTC are reflected in a clinically aggressive course of disease and in a poor patient prognosis.[16,17] Second, loss of a specific marker, such as calcitonin, might lead to a significant discrepancy between tumor mass and circulating marker levels. As epitomized by cases which we have previously reported in detail,[16,17] this aspect can make monitoring of clinical course unreliable. Finally, it is obvious that loss of normal parent cell differentiation characteristics in a tumor may render certain diagnoses difficult or even impossible.

Bronchogenic Carcinoma

Lung carcinomas have been a major target of recent investigations. Not only do lung carcinomas account for the largest category of human cancers, but at least four clinically and histologically distinctive subtypes are available for study. The three major differentiated forms of lung carcinoma that arise in the bronchial epithelium are squamous carcinoma, adenocarcinoma, and small cell carcinoma (SCC).[22] The fourth major subtype, large cell undifferentiated carcinoma, encompasses a broad group of carcinomas that lack those specific morphologic differentiating features which characterize the other three subtypes.[22]

During the course of recent clinical, morphologic, and biochemical studies of lung cancer, it has become apparent that there is a considerable overlap between the different histologic subtypes of bronchogenic carcinoma; it has also been observed that small cell carcinoma (SCC) may change with time into other forms of lung carcinoma. In this section, we will examine the interrelationships between the different histologic subtypes of bronchogenic carcinoma, in particular the relationship between SCC and non-small cell carcinomas; we will also address the biologic and clinical implications of time-dependent changes which might occur in SCC.

Precise histologic classification of lung carcinomas is obviously pivotal in instituting correct patient management and therapy. In particular, differentiation of SCC from non-SCC remains crucial from a therapeutic standpoint. Although it has been recognized for many years that mixtures of SCC and non-SCC can occur in lung cancer lesions, it is only in recent years that this very important aspect of lung cancer has been stressed.[23–25] Recent biochemical studies have also shown that the neuroendocrine (APUD) properties which characterize SCC can be found in non-SCC of the lung as well.[26] An analysis of endocrine biochemical parameters has shown that non-SCC of the lung have the capacity for peptide hormone and biogenic amine synthesis, although usually to a lesser degree than SCC; this has led to the postulate that all the major subtypes of bronchogenic carcinoma may be linked along a differentiation continuum.[26,27]

In support of this concept, changes from SCC to non-SCC have been observed both in vivo and in vitro. There are several well-documented cases in which patients with a biopsy-proven initial diagnosis of SCC have, after therapy, shown only non-SCC at autopsy.[25] Currently, all reported cases of such a change in tumor type have involved a drift away from SCC.

The in vivo transition from SCC to non-SCC is supported by recent in vitro studies of human SCC culture lines, which have consistently exhibited a time-dependent change from SCC towards a form of large cell undifferentiated carcinoma.[28–30] Gazdar and associates[29] observed that several established lines of SCC lost their characteristic endocrine (APUD) biochemical parameters when maintained in culture for up to two years. Furthermore, they noted that the loss of APUD biochemistry was accompanied by the acquisition of growth characteristics of non-SCC. Most importantly, sequential studies of tumor cell heterotransplants in the athymic nude mouse revealed a morphologic change from typical SCC to large cell undifferentiated carcinoma.

When considering the cell culture changes observed by Gazdar and others, the key question arises as to whether (1) the large undifferentiated carcinoma cells which evolve in the SCC cultures are linked directly to the SCC cells through a differentiation (or dysdifferentiation) process; or (2) the large cells are selected for with time and have no lineage relationship with respect to SCC.

Recent studies by our group[30,31] provide evidence that SCC and some large cell undifferentiated carcinomas share a common lineage. Initial studies of cell surface proteins in lung cancers showed that SCC cells possess specific cell surface proteins which distinguish them from the cells of non-SCC.[31] Subsequent studies have shown that cloned cell cultures of human large cell undifferentiated carcinoma, established from the pleural fluid of a patient with SCC who was later shown to have mixed SCC–non-SCC at autopsy, simultaneously expressed surface proteins characteristic of both SCC and non-SCC carcioma cells.[30] These data provide convincing evidence in support of the postulate that SCC and some cases of large cell carcinoma do, in fact, share a common lineage and are linked through a continuum of differentiation events.

In studying the evolution of bronchial cancers induced experimentally in the Syrian golden hamster, Reznik-Schuller[32] has provided further evidence linking endocrine (APUD) cells and the cells of squamous carcinoma and adenocarcinoma along a common differentiation pathway. The proliferating cells in the earliest neoplastic lesions induced by N-nitrosomorpholine exhibit characteristic APUD ultrastructural features; with further evolution of the tumors, the neoplastic cells progressively lose their APUD properties and assume first the features of squamous cells, and ultimately, the features of adenocarcinoma cells.[32]

It is important to consider some of the clinical and therapeutic ramifications of such changes in tumor morphology and biochemistry. Recent studies by Goodwin and Baylin[33] have shown that in one SCC culture line, the OH-1 line, subtle losses in endocrine phenotype, which are accompanied by only minimal histologic changes within the SCC category, result in the emergence of profound radiation resistance. This loss of radiation sensitivity accompanying the drift away from SCC parallels the general tendency toward therapeutic resistance that typically characterizes the course of disease in patients with SCC. Certainly, this is a most intriguing possibility and further studies in this area might be most rewarding. In this light, Carney and colleagues[34] have recently shown that this relative radiation resistance is characteristic of all lines of SCC examined which exhibit a drift towards large cell histology.

In a previous review of time-dependent alterations in neoplasms, we proposed a model which we hoped would provide a working construct for considering the dynamic interrelationship between SCC and a form of large cell undifferentiated carcinoma (see Fig. 15-3). In the model, we depicted SCC and a form of large cell carcinoma as forming part of a spectrum of differentiation. It was speculated that the large cell carcinoma might provide a stem cell from which SCC could develop by assuming neuroendocrine differentiation characteristics. The bulk of experimental evidence from tumors indicates that tumor cell differentiation is a dynamic,

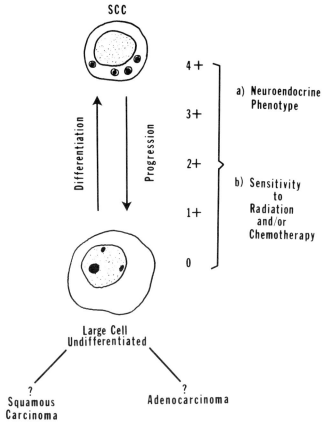

Figure 15-3. *Possible lineage interrelationships between small cell carcinoma (SCC) and large cell undifferentiated carcinoma of the lung. This model depicts how tumor progression might underly a change from SCC to large cell carcinoma. Different degrees of progression would result in tumors with varying admixtures of small and large undifferentiated cells, as is seen in some patients. The 0 to 4+ scale denotes degrees of neuroendocrine differentiation and sensitivity to therapeutic modalities used in patients with SCC. The question marks refer to the possibility that SCC is linked to other types of lung carcinoma as well, through a stem cell with multiple differentiation potentialities. [From Baylin SB and Mendelsohn G: Time-dependent changes in human tumors: Implications for diagnosis and clinical behavior. Semin Oncol 9:504–512, 1982, with permission]*

389

forward-moving process; there is no sound evidence that "retrograde differentiation" or "dedifferentiation" can occur.[3] In our model, we placed large cell carcinoma in the stem cell portion because of its lack of any specific differentiated features. As discussed by Yesner[23] and by ourselves more recently,[27] however, the possibility exists that SCC cells with neuroendocrine features could represent the early stage from which the large cell phenotype emerges. The large cell might then represent a stem cell capable of developing towards the other types of differentiated lung cancer. The work of Reznik-Schuller[32] is intriguing with regard to this possibility.

A critical aspect of this model is that it assumes that transformation events leading to SCC can occur anywhere along the differentiation spectrum in any given patient; the resultant tumors might then contain predominantly small, neuroendocrine cells ("pure" SCC), admixtures of neuroendocrine and stem cells, or predominantly stem cell elements (perhaps representing one form of large cell undifferentiated carcinoma). Such an hypothesis would predict that among patients with SCC of the lung, a heterogeneous spectrum of morphologic types, biochemical phenotypes, and therapeutic sensitivities would be encountered; as we have already discussed, this is in fact the case.

Although the in vitro and in vivo evidence which we have presented might suggest that the drift from SCC to large cell carcinoma which occurs with tumor progression involves differentiation from SCC towards large cell carcinoma, it is possible that the changes reflect a maturation block, i.e. a progressive inability of the tumor cells to differentiate toward SCC.

The clinical implications of a SCC–large cell undifferentiated carcinoma link are considerable. First, the experimental studies showing the emergence of radiation resistance with only a very subtle shift away from SCC in culture[33,34] bring into focus one of the pivotal clinical aspects of tumor progression in SCC. Studies at the National Cancer Institute[35] have indicated that patients with mixed SCC–non-SCC may not respond as well to initial therapy as patients with pure SCC. Second, a significant shift from SCC towards non-SCC during the course of disease progression might result in clinically appreciable losses of endocrine parameters used to monitor tumor burden. Our previous biochemical studies[36] have revealed a loss of neuroendocrine biochemistry in metastatic tumors from some patients with SCC. Such a change might lead to a progressive discrepancy between tumor burden and endocrine (or other) markers with resultant erroneous assessment of clinical course. Finally, in selecting appropriate therapy for patients with both SCC and non-SCC, precise evaluation of cell lineage may prove to be important.

Malignant Melanoma

Malignant melanoma frequently provides an extremely difficult diagnostic problem for the pathologist, particularly in metastatic sites. Diagnostic pathologists need not be reminded of the multitude of histologic appearances that malignant melanoma may assume; clinical oncologists are well aware of the frequency with which a diagnosis of metastatic malignant melanoma is provided or suggested by the pathologist faced with an undifferentiated malignant tumor. Of pivotal importance in this regard is the frequent loss of melanin synthesis which accompanies progression of disease and dissemination of tumor (Fig. 15-4). The current chapter does not provide the appropriate setting in which to review the considerable body of knowledge accrued from experimental studies of malignant melanoma. Rather, we will focus on the clinical situation involving loss of melanin, the traditional diagnostic hallmark of malignant melanoma.

Recently, S-100 protein, an acidic protein present in a variety of neural and neurectodermally derived cells including melanocytes, has been found to be a valuable immunohistochemical marker for malignant melanoma.[37,38] S-100 protein immunocytochemistry in malignant melanomas highlights one of the principles of tumor progression as expounded by Foulds.[1] Immunoreactivity for S-100 protein generally remains intact in malignant melanomas despite loss of melanin with tumor progression; it provides a valuable marker even in completely amelanotic melanomas, a phenomenon not infrequently encountered in metastatic sites (see Fig. 15-4). This fact serves to emphasize Foulds' concept that in any given tumor, progression involves independent changes in different unit characters. In the case of melanoma, dyssynchronous changes in melanin and S-100 provides the clinician or pathologist with a valuable marker to identify melanoma in those cases where melanin is completely lost.

Prostate Carcinoma

Medullary thyroid carcinoma, Lung carcinoma, and malignant melanoma have provided models in which observable tumor progression has involved loss of certain phenotypic features which characterize the parent cell. In contrast, through observation of certain prostate carcinomas, we have been provided with an important, albeit unusual, model in which tumor progression has involved a time-dependent loss of a specific parent cell marker (prostatic acid phosphatase) concomitant with the acquisition of typical neuroendocrine characteristics.[39,40]

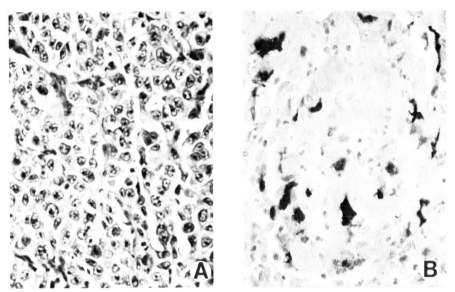

Figure 15-4. *(A) Metastatic amelanotic melanoma presenting clinically as metastatic undifferentiated carcinoma. (B) Despite complete absence of melanin pigment in the tumor, immunoperoxidase staining for S-100 protein demonstrates an intensely positive reaction (black in photograph) in many tumor cells, thereby facilitating the diagnosis of malignant melanoma.*

We have studied three patients who presented with biopsy-proven "regular" adenocarcinoma of the prostate but who, during the course of progression of disease, all developed histologically-proven small cell carcinoma of the prostate.[40] In each case, small cell and adenocarcinomatous components were admixed in primary and/or metastatic sites; in each case, emergence of the small cell component was associated with a loss of prostatic acid phosphatase activity as evidenced by immunocytochemical studies.[40] Of particular interest was the development in one of the patients of clinically florid Cushing syndrome with evidence of ectopic ACTH production concomitant with the change in tumor morphology. The change in morphology from adenocarcinoma to small cell carcinoma included ultrastructural evidence of neuroendocrine dense core granules, as well as immunocytochemical localization of ACTH within the small cell component of the tumor.[39]

While such cases of prostate carcinoma are admittedly rare, they serve to highlight the very important biological phenomenon in which tumor progression may involve not only loss of specific properties, but also acquisition of new properties. These cases also emphasize the caution that must be exercised when utilizing specific tumor products as diagnostic tools or as markers for monitoring course of disease. Loss of specific markers may render correct recognition of a metastatic tumor difficult or even impossible; loss of markers may also result in a discordance between tumor burden and circulating marker levels.

Summary

We have stressed in this chapter that time-dependent events in human tumors may progressively alter their composition (in cell populations, biochemistry, etc.). This process is critical to the diagnosis of a given neoplasm at a set point in time. The time-dependent changes in human tumors probably reflect the classic concept of tumor progression which has been articulated primarily for nonhuman tumor models. We have attempted to provide evidence from selected human tumors that support the basic concept of tumor progression. We have examined shifts in populations of neoplastic cells that have resulted in modifications of the morphologic, biochemical, and ultrastructural characteristics of a series of tumors.

Although individual features of tumors often change independently over time, there are certain patterns of change which, when recognized, may prove invaluable for our understanding of the biology of tumor progression and for enhancing our diagnostic approaches and accuracy.

We have attempted to stress the clinical ramifications of the changes which can occur. Loss of specific differentiating phenotypic features may render correct diagnosis of a carcinoma extremely difficult, especially in metastatic sites. The loss of certain markers during the course of tumor progression may also result in a discordance between tumor burden and assayable circulating marker levels, thereby jeopardizing accurate monitoring of course of disease. In medullary thyroid carcinoma, we have discussed in detail the prognostic implications of deviation of the tumor away from the parent cell phenotype and have shown a correlation between loss of calcitonin content and increasing tumor virulence. In the clinical context, we have considered the possible effects of tumor drift on sensitivity to therapeutic modalities. In this regard, we have focused on the possible relationship between loss of neuroendocrine phenotype in SCC of the lung and the simultaneous emergence of radiation resistance in the cells.

In considering the interrelationships between SCC and non-SCC of the lung, we have examined a model which might explain the time-dependent changes which have been observed in vivo and in vitro, and which might serve as a working construct for further studies in this sphere.

References

1. Foulds L: The experimental study of tumor progression: A review. Cancer Res 14:327–339, 1954
2. Prehn RT: Tumor progression and homeostasis. Adv Cancer Res 23:203–236, 1976
3. Baylin SB, Mendelsohn G: Ectopic (inappropriate) hormone production by tumors: Mechanisms involved and the biological and clinical implications. Endocrinol Rev 1:45–77, 1980
4. Baylin SB, Mendelsohn G: Medullary thyroid carcinoma: A model for the study of human tumor progression and cell heterogeneity, in Owens AH, Coffey D, Baylin SB (eds): Tumor Cell Heterogeneity—Origins and Implications. New York, Academic Press, 1982, pp 9–27
5. Williams ED. Histogenesis of medullary carcinoma of the thyroid. J Clin Pathol 19:114–118, 1966
6. Foster GV, MacIntyre I, Pearse AGE: Calcitonin production and the mitochondrion-rich cells of the dog thyroid. Nature 203:1029, 1964
7. Pearse AGE: Common cytochemical properties of cells producing polypeptide-hormone secretion with particular reference to calcitonin and thyroid C cells. Vet Rec 79:587–590, 1966
8. Hakanson R, Owman C, Sundler F: Aromatic l-amino acid decarboxylase in calcitonin-producing cells. Biochem Pharmacol 20:2187–2192, 1971
9. Baylin SB, Mendelsohn G, Weisburger WR, et al: Levels of histaminase and l-dopa decarboxylase activity in the transition from C-cell hyperplasia to familial medullary thyroid carcinoma. Cancer 44:1315–1321, 1979
10. Wolfe HJ, Melvin KEW, Cervi-Skinner SJ, et al: C-cell hyperplasia preceding medullary thyroid carcinoma. N Engl J Med 289:437–441, 1973
11. Mendelsohn G, Eggleston JC, Weisburger WR, et al: Calcitonin and histaminase in C-cell hyperplasia and medullary thyroid carcinoma. Am J Pathol 92:35–52, 1978
12. Mendelsohn G, Bigner SH, Eggleston JC, et al: Anaplastic variants of medullary thyroid carcinoma. Am J Surg Pathol 4:333–341, 1980

13. Tashjian AH Jr, Howland BG, Melvin KEW, et al: Immunoassay of human calcitonin: Clinical measurement, relation to serum calcium and studies in patients with medullary carcinoma. N Engl J Med 283:890–894, 1970

14. Melvin KEW, Miller HH, Tashjian AH Jr: Early diagnosis of medullary carcinoma of the thyroid gland by means of calcitonin assay. N Engl J Med 285:1115–1120, 1971

15. Wells SA Jr, Baylin SB, Gann DS, et al: Medullary thyroid carcinoma: Relationship of method of diagnosis to pathologic staging. Ann Surg 188:377–384, 1978

16. Lippman SM, Mendelsohn G, Trump DL, et al: The prognostic and biological significance of cellular heterogeneity in medullary thyroid carcinoma. J Clin Endocrinol Metab 54:233–240, 1982

17. Trump DL, Mendelsohn G, Baylin SB: Discordance between plasma calcitonin and tumor-cell mass in medullary thyroid carcinoma. N Engl J Med 301:253–255, 1979

18. Teitelman G, Joh TH, Reis DJ: Transformation of catecholaminergic precursors in glucagon (A) cells in mouse embryonic pancreas. Proc Natl Acad Sci USA 78:5225–5229, 1981

19. Berger CL, de Bustros A, Roos BA, et al: Human medullary thyroid carcinoma in culture provides a model relating growth dynamics, endocrine cell differentiation, and tumor progression. J Clin Endocrinol Metab 59:338–343, 1984

20. Mendelsohn G, Wells SA Jr, Baylin SB: Relationship of tissue carcinoembryonic antigen and calcitonin to tumor virulence in medullary thyroid carcinoma: An immunohistochemical study in early, localized and virulent disseminated stages of disease. Cancer (in press)

21. Mendelsohn G, Gessell M, Berger CL, et al: Relationship of carcinoembryonic antigen and calcitonin immunoreactivity to tumor virulence in medullary thyroid carcinoma. Lab Invest 50:39A, 1984

22. Carter D, Eggleston JC: Tumors of the lower respiratory tract, in Hartmann WH, Cowan WR (eds): Atlas of Tumor Pathology, Second Series. Fasc 17. Washington, DC, Armed Forces Institute of Pathology, 1980

23. Yesner R: Spectrum of lung cancer and ectopic hormones, in Sommers SC, Rosen PP (eds): Pathology Annual, Part I. New York, Appleton-Century-Crofts, 1978, pp 217–240

24. Brereton HD, Matthews MM, Costa J, et al: Mixed anaplastic small-cell and squamous-cell carcinoma of the lung. Ann Intern Med 88:805–811, 1978

25. Abeloff MD, Eggleston JC, Mendelsohn G, et al: Changes in morphological and biochemical characteristics of small cell carcinoma of the lung—a clinicopathologic study. Am J Med 66:757–764, 1979

26. Berger CL, Goodwin G, Mendelsohn G, et al: Endocrine-related biochemistry in the spectrum of human lung carcinoma. J Clin Endocrinal Metab 53:422–429, 1981

27. Baylin SB, Mendelsohn G: Time-dependent changes in human tumors: Implications for diagnosis and clinical behavior. Semin Oncol 9:504–512, 1982

28. Gazdar AF, Carney DN, Russell EK, et al: Establishment of continuous, clonable cultures of small-cell carcinoma of the lung which have amine precursor uptake and decarboxylation cell properties. Cancer Res 40:3502–3507, 1980

29. Gazdar AF, Carney DN, Guccion JG, et al: Small cell carcinoma of the lung: Cellular origin and relationship to other pulmonary tumors, in Greco FA, Oldham RK, Bunn PA Jr (eds): Small Cell Lung Cancer. New York, Grune & Stratton, 1981, pp 145–175

30. Goodwin G, Shaper JH, Abeloff MD, et al: Analysis of cell surface proteins delineates a differentiation pathway linking endocrine and non-endocrine human lung cancers. Proc Natl Acad Sci USA 80:3807–3811, 1983

31. Baylin SB, Gazdar AF, Minna JD, et al: A unique cell-surface protein phenotype distinguishes human small cell from non-small-cell lung cancer. Proc Natl Acad Sci USA 79:4650–4654, 1982

32. Reznik-Schuller H: Sequential morphologic alterations in the bronchial epithelium of Syrian golden hamsters during N-nitorsomorpholine-induced pulmonary tumorigenesis. Am J Pathol 89:59–66, 1977

33. Goodwin G, Baylin SB: Relationships between neuroendocrine differentiation and sensitivity to γ-radiation in culture line OH-1 of human small cell lung carcinoma. Cancer Res 42:1361–1367, 1982

34. Carney DN, Mitchell JB, Kinsella TJ: In vitro radiation and chemotherapy sensitivity of established cell lines of human small-cell lung cancer and its large-cell morphologic variants. Cancer Res 43:2806–2811, 1983

35. Matthews MJ: Effects of therapy on the morphology and behavior of small cell carcinoma of the lung—a clinicopathologic study, in Muggia F, Rozencweig M (eds): Lung Cancer: Progress in Therapeutic Research. New York, Raven Press, 1979, pp 155–165

36. Baylin SB, Weisburger WR, Eggleston JC, et al: Variable content of histaminase, L-dopa decarboxylase and calcitonin in small-cell carci-

noma of the lung. Biologic and clinical implications. N Engl J Med 299:105–110, 1978

37. Clark HB, Cruz DS, Hartman BK, et al: S-100 protein, an immuno-histochemical marker for malignant melanoma and other melanocytic lesions. Lab Invest 46:13A, 1982

38. Warner TFCS, Lloyd RV, Hafez GR, et al: Immunocytochemistry of neurotropic melanoma. Cancer 53:254–257, 1984

39. Vuitch MF, Mendelsohn G: Relationship of ectopic ACTH production to tumor differentiation: A morphologic and immunohistochemical study of prostatic carcinoma with Cushing's syndrome. Cancer 47:296–299, 1981

40. Schron DS, Gipson T, Mendelsohn G: The histogenesis of small cell carcinoma of the prostate: An immunohistochemical study. Cancer 53:2478–2480, 1984

16

THE USE OF MONOCLONAL
ANTIBODIES IN THE
HISTOPATHOLOGIC DIAGNOSIS
OF HUMAN MALIGNANCY

Kevin C. Gatter
David Y. Mason

On the 22nd of March 1887 at the celebration dinner for the 90th birthday of the Kaiser Wilhelm I, the Crown Prince Frederick, heir to the throne, rose to propose the toast. His normally clear voice was noticeably hoarse, making his words difficult to hear. In the succeeding months his throat was examined by several eminent German doctors, who found a swelling on the left vocal cord but were unable to reach any clear diagnosis. On the 20th of May 1887, and again on the 7th of June, the celebrated English laryngologist Dr. (later Sir) Morell MacKenzie took biopsies from the Crown Prince's larynx. Both biopsies were sent to Rudolf Virchow, the best known pathologist of his day, for histologic examination.

This story, dating back almost a century, serves as a reminder of the antiquity of surgical pathology as a diagnostic technique. It also provides an early example of a major weakness inherent in histological examination, namely that the pathologist bases his diagnosis on subjective visual assessment of cell and tissue morphology. In the case of the Crown Prince,

POORLY DIFFERENTIATED NEOPLASMS AND TUMORS OF UNKNOWN ORIGIN   ISBN 0-8089-1755-2
© 1986 by Grune & Stratton.   All rights of reproduction in any form reserved.

Virchow was unable to decide from the two fragments he received whether the Crown Prince's lesion was malignant. He issued lengthy and inconclusive reports indicating to us how early pathologists became adept at prevarication. Nor was Virchow more successful when MacKenzie sent larger pieces some months later.

In the years which have elapsed since this episode, many pathologists have explored ways in which diagnostic accuracy may be enhanced. Few of these procedures, however, have proved to be of practical use in the routine laboratory, and the pathologist of today bases his reports on material which has been processed and stained by methods which are essentially identical to those used in Virchow's day.

In the present chapter we review whether the latest of these diagnostic aids, immunocytochemical labeling with monoclonal antibodies, can succeed where other, ostensibly equally promising and innovative, techniques have failed. This topic will be reviewed under the following four headings.

1. Distinction between benign and malignant states
2. Identification of the cell type of the neoplasm
3. Assessment of the grade of a malignancy
4. Detection of tumor metastases

Although monoclonal antibodies have only recently been introduced into diagnostic pathology, their number makes it impossible to review all of the literature. This chapter will therefore be based on our own experience in Oxford and will refer to other studies which compliment them or fill in some of the numerous gaps which we have been unable to touch.

Monoclonal Antibodies and the Technical Aspects of Immunohistology

Techniques for the production of monoclonal antibodies and the selection of reagents specifically for immunohistological use are now well established.[1-4] Many histologists remain unconvinced, however, as to the advantages of using monoclonal antibodies, rather than polyclonal antisera, for immunocytochemistry. The comparative properties of these two types of antibody are set out in Table 16-1, which summarizes the strong arguments for preferring monoclonal antibodies in most instances in view of their specificity, purity, and wide availability.[2-5] A more succinct expression of the ideas behind this table, however, is to be found in a story told by Cesar Milstein. He describes a restaurant in which a diner orders a mouth watering list of dishes only to find that they had all been mixed together (for reasons obscure) by the chef before reaching the table. Milstein suggests that this inedible mixture of avocado, orange sorbet, chablis and saddle of lamb resembles the mixture of antibodies to be found in a polyclonal antiserum. In contrast, monoclonal antibodies represent the individual dishes presented alone. The value of this story lies in the fact that it neatly replies to a question sometimes raised about monoclonal antibodies: "Why should they be so much better than polyclonal antibodies when, after all, they are only antibodies and not fundamentally different types of reagents?"

The major technical aspects of monoclonal antibody immunohistology concern antibody labeling methods and the preparation of tissue sections.

Labeling Methods

There are several immunoenzymatic techniques in current use, all of which are both sensitive and reliable. Details of those presently used in our laboratory are given in the Appendix although there are several technical sources to which the interested reader may be referred.[6-8] We continue to use a simple two stage immunoperoxidase method for the immunohistological screening of new monoclonal antibodies. In this technique the antigenic sites, to which the primary mouse monoclonal antibody binds, are revealed using a commercial peroxidase conjugated rabbit antibody against mouse immunoglobulin (Ig) (Fig. 16-1). Although this technique is perfectly satisfactory not only for screening new monoclonal antibodies but also for most diagnostic cases it does have the limitation that occasionally the labeling reactions obtained are weak. For immunological diagnosis we use one or other of two more sensitive techniques (see Appendix for details). The first is a three stage immunoperoxidase procedure (Fig. 16-1) in which the monoclonal antibody and the peroxidase conjugated second stage antibody are followed by a third peroxidase conjugate (directed against Ig from the species in which the second antibody has been raised). The alternative technique is the alkaline-phosphatase anti-alkaline-phosphatase (APAAP) technique (Fig. 16-1).[9] In this procedure the primary mouse monoclonal antibody is linked to a monoclonal anti-alkaline phosphatase antibody (previously complexed with alkaline phosphatase) by a sheep anti-mouse antiserum (see Appendix). The principle is the same as that of the well-known peroxidase:anti-peroxidase (PAP) technique.[10] The alkaline phosphatase label is revealed using a substrate containing naphthol AS-MX and Fast Red. The APAAP technique circumvents the

Table 16-1

Comparative Features of Monoclonal and Polyclonal Antibodies
as Immunocytochemical Reagents

Characteristic	Monoclonal Antibodies	Polyclonal Antibodies
Range of antigens detectable	Potentially very large	Limited to those antigenic constituents which can be purified to homogeneity.
Purity of antibody preparations	Most, if not all, of the antibody produced by a hybridoma cell line is specific for a single antigen.	Only a minor proportion (rarely more than 20 percent) of the antibody present in an immune serum is specific for the immunizing antigen. The remainder consists mainly of antibodies produced by the animal in the past in response to previous antigenic stimuli, or of antibody against contaminating antigens present in the immunizing preparation. These nonspecific antibodies are a common cause of unwanted immunocytochemical staining reactions.
Homogeneity of antibody	Each hybridoma cell line produces multiple copies of a single immunoglobulin molecule, all of which possess the same antigen-binding site. In consequence they usually react not only with one molecule, but with a single antigenic determinant (epitope) on the molecule.	The antibodies in a polyclonal antiserum which are specific for the immunizing antigen are usually highly heterogenous (in terms of antigen-binding affinity) and are normally directed against a number of different epitopes on the immunizing antigen. Consequently they are usually not as effective in discriminating between related molecules as are monoclonal antibodies.

Table 16-1, *continued*
Comparative Features of Monoclonal and Polyclonal Antibodies
as Immunocytochemical Reagents

Characteristic	Monoclonal Antibodies	Polyclonal Antibodies
Availability of antibodies	Monoclonal antibodies can be produced in unlimited amounts and in consequence laboratories throughout the world can perform immunocytochemical investigations using identical reagents.	The preparation of satisfactory polyclonal reagents involves considerable expenditure of time and effort (in purification of the immunizing antigen, in specificity testing and in elimination of unwanted antibodies) and at the end of these procedures the amount of available antiserum is often small. This consideration severely restricts the distribution of polyclonal antibodies of valuable specificity on a side scale.

problems which may be encountered in immunoperoxidase procedures because of endogenous peroxidase in tissues, and is thus particularly useful in hematopathology. Furthermore it is possible to enhance the sensitivity of the APAAP technique if required by repeating the second and third antibodies in the sequence (Fig. 16-1, details in Appendix).

Tissue Preparation

Fresh unfixed tissue remains the material of choice for immunostaining since a large number of antigens cannot be reliably revealed in fixed tissue. In addition, freshly received material also allows the pathologist to handle it optimally in order to achieve the very best quality of conventional sections, which is necessary for comparison with, and the interpretation of, immunohistology.

In view of the practical difficulties inherent in obtaining and storing fresh material two developments may be of interest to the surgical pathologist. One is the availability of monoclonal antibodies, albeit in limited amounts at present, which give good immunoenzymatic staining reactions on conventionally fixed, paraffin-embedded sections. The use of some of these in diagnosis will be referred to in the following text, and no doubt other antibodies of this type will become available in the future.

Recent experiments in our laboratory have shown that it is possible

IMMUNOENZYMATIC LABELLING TECHNIQUES

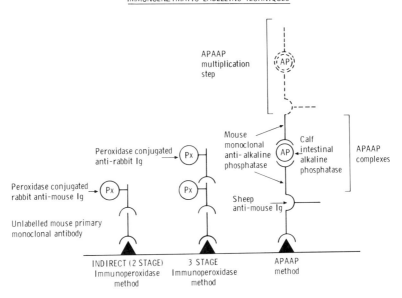

Figure 16-1. *Schematic illustration of the immunoenzymatic labeling techniques in use in our laboratory. The three-stage immunoperoxidase method only differs from the indirect (two-stage) in that after the first peroxidase conjugated antibody has bound to the primary monoclonal antibody a second peroxidase conjugated antibody is added which binds to the first. The alkaline phosphatase:anti-alkaline phosphatase (APAAP) method is essentially identical to the well known peroxidase:anti-peroxidase (PAP) method except that alkaline phosphatase is used as the enzymatic label rather than peroxidase. This technique depends on the ability of the anti-mouse Ig antiserum (second stage) to bind via one antigen combining site to the primary monoclonal antibody and via the other to alkaline phosphatase. The sensitivity of the technique may be considerably enhanced by repeating the second and third stages (shown in the diagram by dotted lines) up to two times.*

to avoid antigenic denaturation in paraffin-embedded samples if the tissue is freeze-dried, rather than fixed, before embedding. These experiments were undertaken after it became apparent that all currently recognized histological fixatives, including the mixture of periodate, lysine, and paraformaldehyde (PLP), cause an unacceptable degree of antigenic denaturation. Unfixed biopsies are rapidly frozen in liquid nitrogen and freeze-dried on an Edwards-Pearce tissue drier before vacuum-embedding in paraffin wax.[11,12] To date we have tested more than 40 monoclonal antibodies on this material and all have worked as well, if not better, than on cryostat sections. In addition, the blocks have been kept at room temperature for more than one year without loss of reactivity.

The Immunohistological Analysis of Malignancy with Monoclonal Antibodies

Distinction Between Benign and Malignant States

The distinction of benign from malignant tumors is one of the most important and frequent tasks of the surgical pathologist. Although the distinction can be made in most instances on clinical or conventional morphologic grounds, it is impossible to diagnose a minority of biopsies in this way.

Many pathologists have turned to monoclonal antibodies as a means to solve such problems. The simplest solution would be an antibody specifically recognizing malignant cells. Much effort has been expended in the search for such a reagent but until now no reliable antibody of this sort has been found. As we have discussed elsewhere[3] the problems inherent in discovering such an antibody, at least by the "blunderbus" approach of raising antibodies against whole malignant cells or crude cell extracts, are more complex than may appear at first sight. Further studies along these lines may only, if ever, be successful if molecular entities specifically associated with neoplastic transformation are found by other means and antibodies are then raised to them as a secondary step.

It may be added, however, that although malignancy-specific monoclonal antibodies remain elusive, one area in which immunocytochemistry may aid in recognizing malignancy is by identifying cell types in a location to which they do not belong. Examples include the recognition of epithelial cells in lymph nodes, bone marrow, and brain which are likely to be metastatic deposits.

Immunocytochemical studies of lymphoid disease have also been successful in recognizing certain patterns of staining indicative of malignancy. Findings such as the expression of a single light chain, a single T cell subset, aberrant combinations or a completely "new" antigen such as Leu-1 in CLL have proved reliable indicators of malignant lymphoma.[3,13,14] The pattern of staining seen with selected panels of monoclonal antibodies has also been helpful in distinguishing benign lymphoid reactions from malignant lymphoma. One example is the distinction between reactive hyperplasia and follicular lymphoma where malignancy is indicated by light chain monoclonality, absence of immune complexes in germinal centers, and breakdown of mantle zone regularity.

Identification of the Cell Type of the Neoplasm

Although the search for an antibody or antibodies able to distinguish benign from malignant lesions has been disappointing, significant advances have been made using them to distinguish between different types of malignancy. Advances in clinical oncology are making increasing demands on the surgical pathologist for a reliable identification of tumor type. Conventional morphologic study may only allow a diagnosis of "anaplastic malignant tumor" a term which is often of little practical value to the clinician. The diagnosis of such cases is often complicated by poor tissue morphology, distortion, or crushing artifact due to biopsy by an endoscopic procedure.

Monoclonal antibodies can now make an important contribution in this field in distinguishing between different large cell undifferentiated tumors (usually in adults), in classifying lymphomas, in deciding on the origin of epithelial tumors, and in the differential diagnosis of the "small round blue cell tumor" of childhood.

Large Cell Undifferentiated Tumors

This group of tumors comprises anaplastic carcinoma, malignant lymphoma, malignant melanoma, and sarcoma. In our initial studies of such cases we applied a panel of monoclonal antibodies directed against epithelial and nonepithelial antigens to fresh biopsies and were able to classify the great majority as either lymphoma or carcinoma.[15] In routine laboratories, however, such diagnostic problems are usually only recognized after the tissue has been fixed and paraffin-embedded. We have thus sought monoclonal antibodies which will react with routinely processed material and have been able in the past two years to find a small number of such reagents.[16] The antibodies comprising this panel and typical results achieved with them on anaplastic tumors are shown in Table 16-2.

At the time of writing (August 1984) we have studied 90 anaplastic tumors which have been referred either by other pathologists (due to diagnostic difficulty) or by oncologists (due to an unexpected clinical response of the patient). It is clear from the results of this study (summarized in Table 16-3) that in most of these cases the differential diagnosis rested between lymphoma and carcinoma. Although the latter diagnosis was favored by the referring pathologist, in the majority of instances, immunohistological labeling revealed, contrary to this expectation, that the majority of the tumors were lymphomas (Table 16-3). This revision of diagnosis, provided it was made in time, often led to a major change in the

Table 16-2
Typing of Large Cell Undifferentiated Tumors

	Leukocyte Common Antigen (Dako-LC)	Epithelial Membrane Antigen (Dako-EMA)	Cytokeratins (KL1, 5.2)[53,54]	S-100 Protein (S1.61)[55]	"Melanoma Associated Antigen" (NK1/C3)[22,23]
Carcinoma	−	±	+	∓	∓
Lymphoma	+	∓	−	∓	∓
Sarcoma	−	−	∓	∓	−
Melanoma	−	−	−	+	+

± = majority of cases positive, though some negative
∓ = majority of cases negative, though some positive

clinical management of the patient. Examples of such cases are illustrated in Figures 16-2 and 16-3.

It may be surprising that of 90 anaplastic tumors only one turned out to be an amelanotic melanoma, which is frequently considered in the differential diagnosis in this type of tumor. It is unlikely that we have missed any melanomas since all melanomas studied to date have been negative for lymphoid and epithelial markers. Most melanomas express, even if only focally, either the S-100 protein[17-21] or the antigen recognized by antibody NK1/C3[22,23] (Fig. 16-4). These latter antibodies cannot be relied

Table 16-3
Results of Staining 90 Routinely Fixed and Processed Anaplastic Tumors

Number of Cases	Leukocyte Common Antigen	Epithelial Membrane Antigen	Cytokeratins	S-100 Protein	Melanoma Associated Antigen	cIg	Diagnostic Conclusion
64	+	−*	−	∓	∓	−	Lymphoma
2	−	+	−	−	−	+	Lymphoma
1	−	−	−	−	−	+	Lymphoma
14	−	+	+	∓	∓	−	Carcinoma
3	−	−	+	∓	∓	−	Carcinoma
4	−	+	−	−	−	−	Carcinoma
1	−	−	−	+	+	−	Melanoma
1	−	−	−	−	−	−	Sarcoma

* = 5 cases showed dot-like positivity in many tumor cells
∓ = majority of cases negative, though some were positive

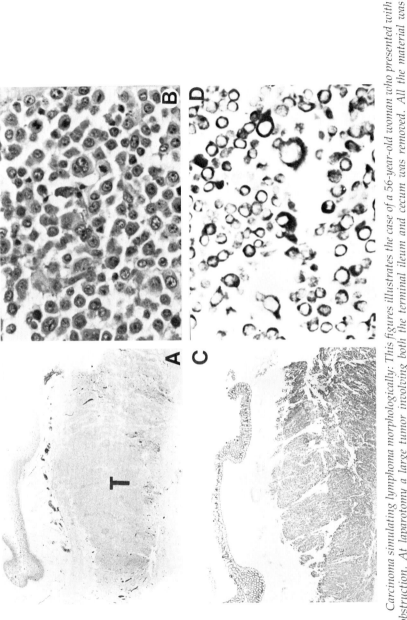

Figure 16-2. Carcinoma simulating lymphoma morphologically: This figures illustrates the case of a 56-year-old woman who presented with small bowel obstruction. At laparotomy a large tumor involving both the terminal ileum and cecum was removed. All the material was routinely fixed and embedded. In (A) it can be seen that the tumor (T) is mainly located in the muscular layer of the bowel and although multiple sections were taken no connection with the overlying epithelium could be found. In view of the lack of cellular adhesiveness and the regular cytological features (shown at higher power in B) a diagnosis of large cell lymphoma was favored by the referring pathologists. However, in (C) and at higher power in (D) the tumor, and its overlying epithelium, can be seen to be strongly labeled by the anticytokeratin antibody KL1 which works reliably in routinely fixed paraffin-embedded sections. The tumor cells were completely negative for the leukocyte common antigen indicating that the most likely diagnosis is an anaplastic carcinoma of the bowel histologically simulating a large cell lymphoma.

408

upon alone, however, since they also stain, although usually more weakly, a considerable number of carcinomas and lymphomas.

A practical point emerging from these studies is the value of using a panel of monoclonal antibodies to distinguish anaplastic tumors. Many previous studies relied on only one or two antibodies, leaving many tumors unstained, thus precluding a firm diagnosis. As the number of tissues and tumors examined has increased, rare cross reactions of individual antibodies have come to light, which by themselves, could lead to a misleading diagnosis. The most striking example at present concerns monoclonal antibodies against the epithelial membrane antigen (EMA). Original studies suggested that these antibodies were specific for epithelial cells and could be used to distinguish carcinomas from lymphomas[24] and to recognize micrometastases in either bone marrow or lymph nodes.[25,26] It had been noted in passing that anti-EMA antibodies usually labeled occasional plasma cells weakly, although this was considered of little importance since plasma cells could be easily distinguished morphologically from tumor cells.[27] On investigating this phenomenon in detail, however, it became clear that most cases of myeloma and a small number of pleomorphic lymphomas also express EMA.[28] Myeloma cells are usually easily recognized morphologically and serologically, and cytoplasmic Ig can generally be detected. However, EMA-positivity in more anaplastic myelomas in which the leukocyte common antigen is usually absent, or in pleomorphic lymphomas could be misleading since many of these tumors resemble anaplastic carcinomas. The use of a panel of monoclonal antibodies helps to circumvent this problem since the leukocyte common antigen has been present (except in anaplastic myeloma) and cytokeratin intermediate filaments absent in such cases studied to date.

Lymphoma Classification

Immunocytochemistry has had the greatest influence on tumor classification in the field of lymphoma pathology. It may seem strange that a group of tumors which look so similar should be easily subclassifiable by immunocytochemistry whereas epithelial tumors, in which morphologic differences are often striking, show considerable antigenic similarity. Detailed studies of non-Hodgkin's lymphomas have attempted to correlate morphologic classifications with immunologic features.[29] It is evident that the majority of non-Hodgkin's lymphoma have either a B or T cell phenotype and that in many cases the immunophenotype cannot be predicted from the morphology.[30] The recent international comparative classification system for non-Hodgkin's lymphoma[31] takes no account of

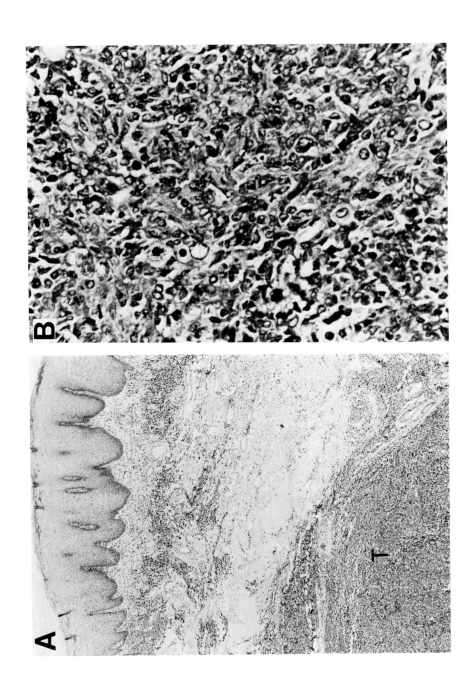

410

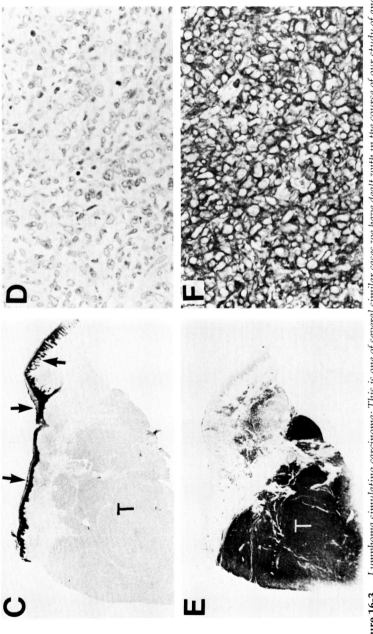

Figure 16-3. *Lymphoma simulating carcinoma: This is one of several similar cases we have dealt with in the course of our study of anaplastic tumors. An oral biopsy was removed from a woman in her forties which was thought on clinical grounds to be a carcinoma. In (A) the tumor (T) can be seen beneath the oral epithelium and is composed of a pleomorphic neoplastic infiltration showing (B) marked cellular cohesiveness. Morphologic opinion favored the diagnosis of poorly differentiated squamous cell carcinoma with a differential diagnosis of malignant fibrous histiocytoma. However, immunocytochemical staining with the panel of monoclonal antibodies which reacts with routinely processed tissue showed the tumor (T) to be negative for epithelial markers (C and D). Note that in (C) the oral mucosa is positively labeled by the anticytokeratin KL1 (arrows). Positive staining for the antileukocyte antigen recognized by PD7/26 (E and F) indicated that the tumor was likely to be a pleomorphic lymphoma rather than a carcinoma or sarcoma. Fresh tissue was not available in this case to subclassify the lymphoma. In view of distant lymphadenopathy the patient was treated with lymphoma chemotherapy and remains alive and well one year later.*

411

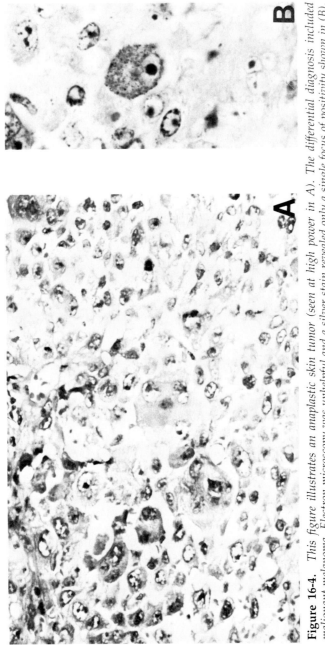

Figure 16-4. This figure illustrates an anaplastic skin tumor (seen at high power in A). The differential diagnosis included malignant melanoma. Electron microscopy was unhelpful and a silver stain revealed only a single focus of positivity shown in (B). Immunocytochemically the tumor was negative for epithelial (C) and leukocyte markers (not shown) but strongly positive for the melanoma associated antigen recognized by NK1/C3 (D) and for the S-100 protein (not shown). In our experience in this particular context this phenotype is characteristic of malignant melanoma.

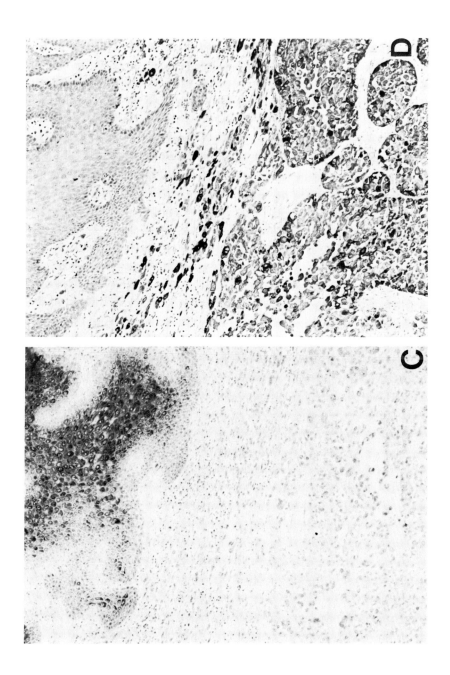

413

immunophenotype. It may therefore need progressive modification if the increasing use of monoclonal antibodies reveal patterns of relevance to clinical management. The Kiel lymphoma group has recently published a detailed review of its data on this subject.[32]

Immunological studies of the cellular constituents of Hodgkin's disease have revealed characteristic patterns in the different histological subtypes. This can be useful in the classification of Hodgkin's disease and in its differentiation from non-Hodgkin's lymphomas.[33,34] The nature and origin of the Reed-Sternberg cell has long eluded pathologists. There have been many attempts to raise specific antibodies against Hodgkin's cell. A recent antibody, Ki-1, raised against a Hodgkin's disease derived cell line (L428), stained Hodgkin's cells in all subtypes of Hodgkin's disease and a subpopulation of large cells in normal lymphoid tissue.[35] Initial hopes that these normal cells were the counterparts of Reed-Sternberg cells and that the antibody would help in the diagnosis of Hodgkin's disease received a setback from the finding of Ki-1-positive cells in other malignant lymphoid conditions, principally pleomorphic large cell lymphomas, previously often classified as "malignant histiocytosis". Study of these conditions has shed considerable light on the relationship between Hodgkin's disease and these non-Hodgkin's lymphomas and provided strong evidence that both are derived from either activated T or B cells.[36] Clearly immunocytochemistry has placed lymphoma diagnosis in a state of flux which detailed clinicopathological studies should begin to elucidate in the next few years.

The Origin of Epithelial Tumors

There have been many immunocytochemical studies aimed at detecting the origin of epithelial tumors though none has been entirely reliable or accurate. The most promising approach to the recognition of different epithelial tumors comes from studies of the intermediate filament cytoskeletal structures of epithelial cells. Moll et al.[37] have shown that epithelial intermediate filaments are made up of a family of at least 19 different cytokeratins and that these appear to have unique patterns of distribution in individual tissues. Whether this distribution pattern can be utilized to determine the origin of human tumors awaits the development of monoclonal antibodies specific for each cytokeratin. Biochemical studies of these cytokeratin filaments in a variety of human tumors have shown, however, that the picture is more complex than that seen in normal tissues: many tumors, such as carcinoma of the lung, possess cytokeratins which are not present in the organ from which they originate.[38]

In our own studies of human lung cancer we have analyzed 54 surgical resection specimens with a large panel of monoclonal antibodies, including

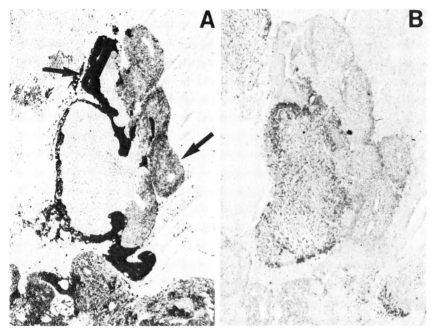

Figure 16-5. *Two consecutive sections from a carcinoma of the lung shows (A), the overlap of antigenic profiles which can be seen in many lung tumors. Areas of squamous cell differentiation (arrows) are positively stained by the anticytokeratin antibody LP34 surrounding a negative area of small cell differentiation. (B), in contrast, illustrates that the central area of small cell differentiation is positively labeled by the antineural antibody UJ13A whereas the surrounding squamous area is negative. In this example the antigenic patterns are based on a clearly different morphology. Similar overlapping staining patterns may be seen, however, in many lung tumors in the absence of obvious morphologic differentiation.*

those against a variety of cytokeratins, and prekeratins.[39] Although immunophenotypes characteristic of the different histological categories of lung tumor could be identified, we were struck by the considerable overlap of antigenic profiles (Fig. 16-5). This suggests that there may be a greater similarity between the different histological categories of lung tumor than has hitherto been assumed.

The Small Round Blue Cell Tumors of Childhood

These form a group of tumors which include lymphoma, Wilms' tumor, Ewing's tumor, rhabdomyosarcoma, neuroblastoma, and myeloid sarcoma, in which individual cases may be impossible to classify morphologically. Monoclonal antibodies are currently available which may be useful in their differential diagnosis (Figs. 16-6 and 16-7). Those studies performed to date, however, have concerned themselves with tumors which were readily distinguishable clinically and morphologically. These and our own unpublished observations are summarized in Table 16-4. The important study remaining to be completed is to collect a series of truly indistinguishable small cell pediatric tumors to ascertain whether they can be distinguished immunologically. These cases should then be followed clinically to determine whether the immunocytochemical differentiation has been of benefit to the patients' therapeutic or prognostic course.

Assessment of the Grade of a Malignancy

The first indication that immunocytochemistry might be helpful in distinguishing tumors of high grade malignancy, i.e. those rapidly prolif- erating, from those of low grade, came from studies of the distribution of transferrin receptors in lymphomas.[40] Transferrin receptor is required for iron transport into cells and its expression can be shown to occur in vitro in dividing but not in resting cells. However, some normal tissues (testis, basal layer of skin, macrophages) possess numbers of transferrin receptors as high, if not higher, than many malignant tissues.[41] In addition, although a series of high grade malignancies will possess higher concentrations of transferrin receptors than low grade malignancies, this cannot be predicted for individual cases, i.e. some high grade malignancies have low numbers as determined by immunostaining.

In view of the unreliability of antitransferrin receptor antibodies as a marker for grade of malignancy, our attention has recently turned to a new monoclonal antibody (designated Ki67) which appears to stain a nuclear antigen expressed by cells in cycle.[42] Studies of normal and malignant tissues have shown that the number of cells expressing Ki67 bears a direct relationship to known proliferation rates. Studies comparing Ki67 expres- sion with autoradiography have shown that the two methods give good comparability.[43] Studies of Ki67 expression in malignant lymphomas, lung tumors, and inflammatory bowel disease[44] suggest that this antibody may provide a more reliable and accurate guide to the rate of cellular prolifer- ation and hence, in the case of tumors, to the grade of malignancy, than transferrin receptor or any other currently available marker.

Detection of Tumor Metastases

It is known that in many human malignancies, especially carcinoma of the lung and breast, a large number of patients must have metastatic disease at presentation, since many die not of locally recurrent tumor, but

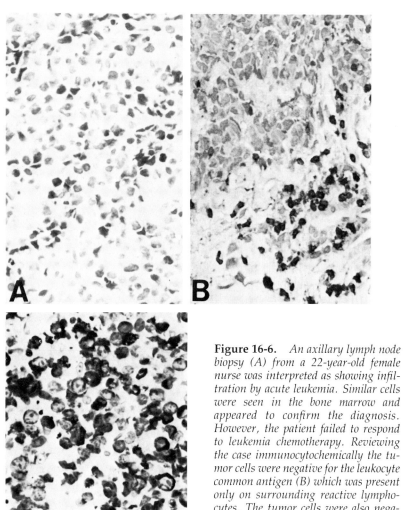

Figure 16-6. *An axillary lymph node biopsy (A) from a 22-year-old female nurse was interpreted as showing infiltration by acute leukemia. Similar cells were seen in the bone marrow and appeared to confirm the diagnosis. However, the patient failed to respond to leukemia chemotherapy. Reviewing the case immunocytochemically the tumor cells were negative for the leukocyte common antigen (B) which was present only on surrounding reactive lymphocytes. The tumor cells were also negative for all other leukemia markers. Staining for desmin intermediate filaments (C) showed strong positivity suggesting the diagnosis of rhabdomyosarcoma. This was confirmed by a later nasal biopsy in which typical muscle cell striations were seen in infiltrating tumor cells.*

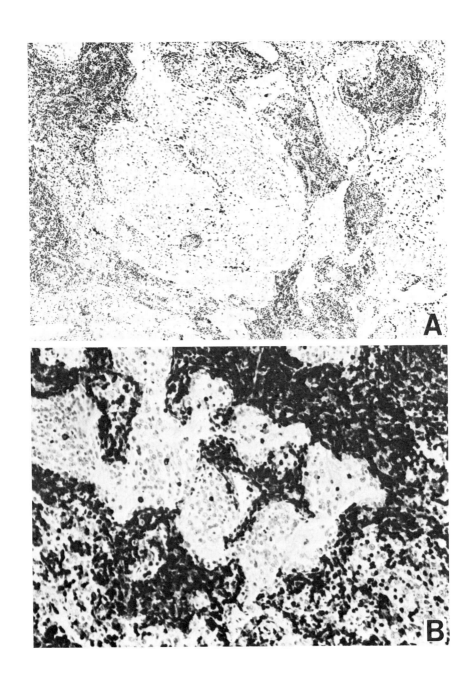

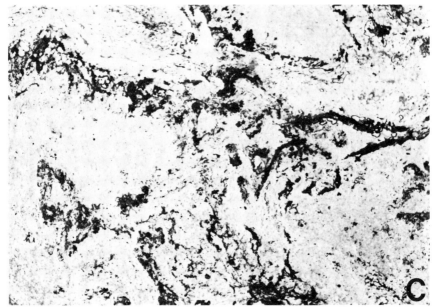

Figure 16-7. *Fig. illustrating the typical staining pattern seen on a neuroblastoma. (A) is a conventional H and E section showing pale areas of neuroblastoma surrounded by more darkly staining lymphocytes. In (B) these lymphocytes are strongly labeled by the antileukocyte antibody 2B11 whereas the tumor cells are negative. Staining for neural intermediate filaments (C) shows positivity with the tumor particularly in those areas where there is neuropil-like differentiation.*

Table 16-4

Typing of Typical Small Blue Cell Tumors of Childhood by Means of Monoclonal Antibody Immunohistology and Enzyme Histochemistry

Tumor type	Leukocyte Common Antigen	Neuro-filaments	Desmin	Granulocytic Antigen	Chloroacetate Esterase
Lymphoma/leukemia	+	−	−	−	−
Neuroblastoma	−	+	−	−	−
Rhabdomyosarcoma	−	−	+	−	−
Ewing's sarcoma	−	−	−	−	−
Myelosarcoma	∓	−	−	+	+

419

of distant spread. In spite of sophisticated improvements in radiological investigation, the detection rate of early metastatic disease remains low. Monoclonal antibodies have recently been introduced into in vivo radiolocalization experiments[45,46] and into pathological staging procedures in an effort to improve this detection rate. In vivo diagnostic imaging, although of immense potential importance, is beyond the scope and experience of the authors and will not be further discussed here.

The bone marrow is known to be one of the commonest sites of metastatic spread in common human malignancies such as carcinoma of breast and lung. Investigations of bone marrow samples have shown that immunoenzymatic labeling with antiepithelial monoclonal antibodies provides a reliable means of detecting small metastatic deposits even when these constitute only a few scattered individual cells.[47,48] Investigations are currently in progress to detect micrometastases in the bone marrow of patients at presentation with carcinoma of the breast and lung. In the case of breast carcinoma it has been shown that antiepithelial antibodies are able to detect micrometastatic deposits in 2 percent of patients which were unsuspected by conventional examination.[47]

In a similar immunocytochemical study of breast cancer, micrometastases were detected, post mastectomy, in axillary lymph nodes which had been reported as uninvolved both clinically and histologically.[49] Similarly early metastatic disease can be detected immunocytochemically in serious effusions[27,50,51] and in cerebrospinal fluid[52] at a time when conventional examination is unable to locate such cells.

The ability of immunohistologic techniques to detect single metastatic cells in lymphoid tissue and bone marrow is well-established. An important question, however, concerns the reliability and relevance of this investigation. It must be established whether the percentage of patients developing late metastatic disease without local recurrence equals the number in whom micrometastases are detectable by immunocytochemical testing. This will at least ensure that the correct patients are treated if these techniques are used to select candidates for early chemotherapy, or other treatment, trials.

Conclusion

In conclusion we should like to return to the story of the German Crown Prince with which this chapter opened. This episode took place when surgical pathology was in its infancy. Virchow's reports were scholarly descriptions but consisted of negative observations. The clinical management was possibly complicated rather than aided by his reports; the ripples of controversy surrounding the case extended far beyond the immediate circle of court physicians, occupying much space in ensuing years in both the medical and popular press. Correspondents to leading medical journals even questioned the ethicality of taking biopsies for microscopic diagnosis. Those of us interested in seeing that diagnostic immunocytochemistry thrives at this early stage in its development hope that similar setbacks will not threaten its development, and that this chapter will be of some value in pointing out that although these techniques have as yet failed to fulfill the claims made by their most optimistic supporters, this should not distract attention from the very real advances which have already been made.

Appendix

Preparation and Storage of Tissue Samples

Tissue for Cryostat Sections

Fresh tissue biopsies (no larger than 1 cm^3 may be kept satisfactorily for many years in a $-70°C$ freezer when placed in a soft plastic capsule, surrounded by normal saline or tissue-mounting medium and snap-frozen in liquid nitrogen. Simply wrapping frozen tissue samples in foil has not proved a reliable means of preservation especially if stored in a conventional $-20°C$ freezer.

Freeze-Drying Specimens for Immunocytochemistry

Fresh tissue specimens should be sliced to a thickness of 2–4 mms (the thinner the better), snap-frozen in liquid nitrogen, and placed, without any prefixation, on the freezing plate of a tissue freeze-drier, e.g. Edwards-Pearce ETD4. Tissue is dried under vacuum for approximately 24 hours. Individual laboratories should establish their own drying times which may vary depending on the nature of the tissue and its pathological condition. When dry, the tissue is allowed to reach room temperature before being vacuum-embedded in clean paraffin wax at approximately 60°C. These paraffin blocks may be stored at room temperature with no apparent loss of antigenicity.

Practical Details of Staining Procedures

Preparation of Cryostat Tissue Sections

1. Cut cryostat sections (approximately 5 to 8 μ) from snap-frozen tissue samples.
2. Air dry slides for between two and 24 hours. Optimal drying (and hence good preservation of tissue morphology and antigenic reactivity) is achieved by placing slides in the vacuum chamber of a freeze-drying apparatus. However, this is not essential and sections dried in the atmosphere usually give fully satisfactory results.
3. If slides are not to be stained immediately, they should be stored at −20°C. It is convenient to put slides back to back in pairs and then to wrap them in aluminum foil before freezing.
4. Shortly before staining, slides should be removed from the freezer and allowed to reach room temperature before removing the foil.
5. Sections are fixed in acetone at room temperature for 10 minutes and then allowed to air dry.

Preparation of Routinely Fixed Paraffin Sections

These are prepared as for routine histological examination. Tissues should preferably have been fixed in Bouin's fixative or in formol sublimate (B5) before paraffin-embedding. Sections are prepared for staining by dewaxing, hydrating, and washing in Tris buffered saline. If required endogenous peroxidase activity may be blocked by exposing sections (either before or after hydration) to methanol containing one percent H_2O_2 for 15 to 30 minutes.

Preparation of Freeze-dried Paraffin Sections

Freeze-dried tissues are more brittle than conventionally prepared blocks so that sections are easier to cut if a disposable microtome blade is used. Sections are dewaxed with xylene, post-fixed in acetone for 5–10 minutes, and may be stained by any of the procedures below preferably without drying at any stage. Brief post-fixation (less than 15 minutes) in fixatives other than acetone appears to have no deleterious effects and may enhance morphologic preservation in some cases. If the slides are not to be stained immediately they should be stored at $-20°C$ since antigenic deterioration occurs after several days at room temperature.

Two-stage Immunoperoxidase Staining Procedure

1. Apply the primary monoclonal antibody to the slide. When staining *cryostat sections* the antibody is added directly to dry acetone-fixed sections; if sections are hydrated before addition of the antibody the intensity of specific staining will be reduced. When staining *paraffin sections* or *cell smears*, excess buffer is removed from around the area to be stained before applying the antibody. Supernatants can be used undiluted. Some antibodies, however, give equally good results when diluted by up to one in 20 in Tris buffered saline (TBS) so that, in the interests of economy, individual laboratories should check the optimal dilution for their own use. Ascitic fluid containing monoclonal antibodies should always be diluted with many samples working well at dilutions above one in 10,000.
2. Wash briefly in TBS. Several brief immersions in the washing buffer will be sufficient to remove unbound monoclonal antibody, and longer than one minute is not necessary.
3. Incubate with peroxidase-conjugated rabbit anti-mouse Ig (Dakopatts a/s). This reagent should be diluted between one in 10 and one in 50 in TBS (the optimal dilution to be determined in individual laboratories). Normal human serum is added to this reagent at a final concentration of one in 20 in order to block cross reactivity against human Ig. Incubation is continued for 30 minutes.
4. Wash in TBS (as above).
5. Add diaminobenzidine/H_2O_2 substrate to slides (see below) and incubate for approximately eight minutes.
6. Wash in tap water and counterstain with hematoxylin.
7. Mount directly in aqueous mountant or dehydrate and mount in a medium such as DPX.

Three-stage Immunoperoxidase Staining Technique

1. Apply the primary monoclonal antibody to the slide. When staining *cryostat sections* the antibody is added directly to dry acetone-fixed sections; if sections are hydrated before addition of the antibody the intensity of specific staining will be reduced. When staining *paraffin sections* or *cell smears* excess buffer is removed from around the area to be stained before applying the antibody. Supernatants may be diluted

more than in the two-stage procedure, i.e. up to one in 50 in TBS. The antibody should be left on the slide for 30 minutes to one hour.

2. Wash briefly in TBS. Several brief immersions in the washing buffer will be sufficient to remove unbound monoclonal antibody, and longer than one minute is not necessary.

3. Incubate with peroxidase-conjugated rabbit anti-mouse Ig (Dakopatts a/s). This reagent should be diluted between one in 10 and one in 50 in TBS (the optimal dilution to be determined in individual laboratories). Normal human serum is added to this reagent at a final concentration of one in 20 in order to block cross reactivity against human Ig. Incubation is continued for 30 minutes.

4. Wash in TBS (as above).

5. Incubate with peroxidase-conjugated swine anti-rabbit Ig (Dakopatts a/s). This reagent should be diluted between one in 10 and one in 50 in TBS. Normal human serum is added to this reagent at a final concentration of one in 20 in order to block cross reactivity against human Ig. Incubation is continued for 30 minutes.

6. Wash in TBS (as above).

7. Add diaminobenzidine/H_2O_2 substrate to slides (see below) and incubate for approximately eight minutes.

8. Wash in tap water and counterstain with hematoxylin.

9. Mount directly in aqueous mountant or dehydrate and mount in a medium such as DPX.

Immunoperoxidase Substrate

Dissolve 6 mgs 3,3 Diaminobenzidine (Sigma Catalogue No. D5637) in 10 mls 0.1M TBS in a glass vessel. Immediately before use add 30 μls of 3% H_2O_2 and pipette directly onto sections.

Immunoalkaline Phosphatase Staining Technique
(APAAP Method)

1. Apply the primary monoclonal antibody to the slide and incubate for 30 minutes to 1 hour.

2. Wash in TBS.

3. Add anti-mouse Ig antiserum. Numerous suitable reagents are available commercially, e.g., Dako rabbit anti-mouse Ig. The optimal working concentration varies but in practice it is impossible to use this reagent at too high a concentration and consequently one should err on the generous side. The concentration used in this laboratory is 1 in 25

(in TBS). It may be necessary to add normal human serum (1 in 20) to block cross-reactivity against human immunoglobulin. Incubation is carried out for 30 minutes.

4. Wash in TBS.
5. Add APAAP complexes (see below) and incubate for 1 hour.
6. Wash in TBS.
7. Add alkaline phosphatase substrate (see below) and incubate for 15 minutes.
8. Wash in tap water and counterstain with haematoxylin.
9. Wash in tap water, transfer to distilled water and mount in an aqueous mounting medium (e.g. Apathy's). N.B. Do not dehydrate and mount in nonaqueous mountant since the reaction product will be dissolved.

Preparation of APAAP Complexes

Alkaline phosphatase (Type 1 bovine intestinal enzyme from Sigma, Catalogue No. P3877) is added at a concentration of 5 mg/ml to monoclonal anti-alkaline phosphatase. The optimal dilution of this reagent should be determined by titration. When the antibody is in the form of tissue culture supernatant optimal results are usually obtained if the reagent is used undiluted or when diluted by only a few fold. Antibody in the form of ascitic fluid on the other hand can be used after dilution by a factor of at least 1 in 500.

It is recommended that the APAAP complexes be prepared at least 18 hours before staining. This reagent is then stable for at least 2 weeks at 4°C. On occasions, it may be preferable to prepare the complexes using bovine intestinal alkaline phosphatase of high purity (e.g. Sigma Type 7, Catalogue No. P4502), since on occasion enzymes present in the crude Type 1 preparation appear to damage cryostat sections. If the higher purity enzyme is used it should be added to the anti-alkaline phosphatase at a correspondingly lower concentration.

Alkaline Phosphatase Substrate

Dissolve 2 mg naphthol-AS-MX phosphate (Sigma Catalogue No. N4875) in 0.2 mLs of dimethyl formamide in a glass tube. Add 9.8 mls of 0.1 M tris buffer, pH 8.2. This solution is made up fresh each time. Immediately before staining dissolve Fast Red TR salt (Sigma Catalogue No. F1500) at a concentration of 1 mg/ml and filter directly onto slide. If it is required to block endogenous alkaline phosphatase activity levamisole should be added to the substrate solution at a concentration of 1 mM.

References

1. Bastin JM, Kirkley J, McMichael AJ: Production of Monoclonal Antibodies: A practical guide, in McMichael AJ, Fabre JW (eds): Monoclonal Antibodies in Clinical Medicine. London, Academic Press, 1982, pp 503–517
2. Mason DY, Cordell JL, Pulford KAF: Production of Monoclonal Antibodies for Immunocytochemical Use, in: Bullock GR, Petrusz P (eds): Immunocytochemistry 2. London, Academic Press, 1982, pp 175–216
3. Gatter KC, Falini B, Mason DY: The use of monoclonal antibodies in histopathological diagnosis. Recent Advances in Histopathology 12:35–67, 1984
4. Sikora K, Smedley HM: Monoclonal Antibodies. London, Blackwell Scientific Publications, 1984
5. Warnke RA, Gatter KC, Mason DY: Monoclonal antibodies as diagnostic reagents. Recent Advances in Clinical Immunology 3:163–186, 1983
6. Bullock GR, Petrusz P (eds): Techniques in Immunocytochemistry 1, London, Academic Press, 1982
7. Polak M, Van Noorden S (eds): Immunocytochemistry: Practical Applications in Pathology and Biology. London, Wright PSG, 1983
8. Cuello AC (ed): Immunohistochemistry. London, John Wiley and Sons, 1984
9. Cordell JL, Falini B, Erber WN, et al: Immunoenzymatic labeling of monoclonal antibodies using immune complexes of alkaline phosphatase and monoclonal anti-alkaline phosphatase (APAAP Complexes). J Histochem Cytochem 32:219–229, 1984
10. Sternberger LA, Hardy PH, Cuculis JJ, et al: The unlabelled antibody method of immunohistochemistry. J Histochem Cytochem 18:315–321, 1970
11. Stein H, Gatter KC, Heryet A, et al: Freeze-dried paraffin-embedded human tissue for antigen labelling with monoclonal antibodies. Lancet 1:71–73, 1984
12. Stein H, Gatter KC, Asbahr H, et al: The use of freeze-dried paraffin embedded sections for immunohistological staining with monoclonal antibodies. Lab Invest (in press)
13. Gatter KC, Cordell JL, Falini B, et al: Monoclonal antibodies in diagnostic pathology: Techniques and applications. J Biol Res 2:369–395, 1983
14. Burns BF, Warnke RA, Doggett RS, et al: Expression of a T-cell antigen (Leu-1) by B-cell lymphomas. Am J Pathol 113:165–171, 1983

15. Gatter KC, Abdulaziz Z, Beverley P, et al: Use of monoclonal antibodies for the histopathological diagnosis of human malignancy. J Clin Pathol 35:1253–1267, 1982

16. Gatter KC, Alcock C, Heryet A, et al: The differential diagnosis of routinely processed anaplastic tumors using monoclonal antibodies. Am J Clin Pathol 82:33–43, 1984

17. Cochran AJ, Wen DR, Herschmann HR, et al: Detection of S100 protein as an aid to the identification of melanocytic tumours. Int J Cancer 30:295–297, 1982

18. Stefansson K, Wollmann R, Jerkovic M: S100 protein in soft tissue tumours derived from Schwann cells and melanocytes. Am J Pathol 106:261–268, 1982

19. Nakajima T, Watanbe S, Sayo Y, et al: Immunohistochemical demonstration of S100 protein in malignant melanoma and pigmented naevus and its diagnostic application. Cancer 50:912–918, 1982

20. Springall DR, Gu J, Cocchia D, et al: The value of S100 immunostaining as a diagnostic tool in human malignant melanomas. Virchows Arch (Pathol Anat) 400:331–343, 1983

21. Gatter KC, Pulford KAF, Vanstapel MJ, et al: An immunohistological study of benign and malignant skin tumours: epithelial aspects. Histopathology 8:209–227, 1984

22. Mackie RM, Campbell I, Turbitt ML: Use of NK1 C3 monoclonal antibody in the assessment of benign and malignant melanocytic lesions. J Clin Pathol 37:367–372, 1984

23. Van Duinen SG, Ruiter DJ, Hageman P, et al: Immunohistochemical and histochemical tools in the diagnosis of amelanotic melanoma. Cancer 53:1566–1573, 1984

24. Sloane JP, Ormerod MG: Distribution of epithelial membrane antigen in normal and neoplastic tissues and its value in diagnostic tumor pathology. Cancer 47:1786–1795, 1981

25. Sloane JP, Ormerod MG, Imrie SF, et al: The use of antisera to epithelial membrane antigen in detecting micrometastases in histological sections. Br J Cancer 42:392, 1980

26. Dearnaley DP, Ormerod MG, Sloane JP, et al: Detection of isolated mammary carcinoma cells in marrow of patients with primary breast cancer. J Roy Soc Med 76:359–364, 1983

27. To A, Dearnaley DP, Ormerod MG, et al: Epithelial membrane antigen: Its use in the cytodiagnosis of malignancy in serous effusions. Am J Clin Pathol 78:214–219, 1982

28. Delsol G, Gatter KC, Stein H, et al: Human lymphoid cells may

express epithelial membrane antigen: Implications for the diagnosis of human neoplasms. Lancet 2:1124–1129, 1984

29. Lennert K, Mohri N, Stein H, et al: The histopathology of malignant lymphoma. Br J Haematol 31 (Suppl):193–203, 1975

30. Jaffe ES, Strauchen JA, Berard CW: Predictability of immunologic phenotype by morphologic criteria in diffuse aggressive non-Hodgkin's lymphomas. Am J Clin Pathol 77:46–49, 1982

31. National cancer institute sponsored study of classifications of non-Hodgkin's lymphomas. Cancer 49:2112–2135, 1982

32. Stein H, Lennert K, Feller A, et al: Immunohistological analysis of human lymphoma: Correlation of histological and immunological categories. Adv Cancer Res 42:67–147, 1984

33. Poppema S, Bhan AK, Reinherz EL, et al: In situ immunologic characterization of cellular constituents in lymph nodes and spleen involved by Hodgkin's disease. Blood 59:226–232, 1982

34. Abdulaziz Z, Mason DY, Stein H, et al: An immunohistological study of the cellular constituents of Hodgkin's disease using a monoclonal antibody panel. Histopathology 8:1–25, 1984

35. Schwab U, Stein H, Gerdes J, et al: Production of a monoclonal antibody specific for Hodgkin and Sternberg-Reed cells of Hodgkin's disease and a subset of normal lymphoid cells. Nature 299:65–67, 1982

36. Stein H, Gerdes J, Wainscoat J, et al: The expression of the Hodgkin's disease associated antigen Ki-1 in reactive and neoplastic lymphoid tissue. Blood (in press)

37. Moll R, Franke WW, Schiller DL, et al: The catalog of human cytokeratins: Patterns of expression in normal epithelia, tumors and cultured cells. Cell 31:11–24, 1982

38. Moll R, Krepler R, Franke WW: Complex cytokeratin polypeptide patterns observed in certain human carcinomas. Differentiation 23:256–269, 1983

39. Gatter KC, Dunnill MS, Pulford KAF, et al: Human lung tumours: A correlation of antigenic profile with histological type. Histopathology (in press)

40. Habeshaw JA, Lister TA, Stansfeld AG, et al: Correlation of transferrin receptor expression with histological class and outcome in non-Hodgkin lymphoma. Lancet 1:498–501, 1983

41. Gatter KC, Brown G, Strowbridge I, et al: Transferrin receptors in human tissues: their distribution and possible clinical relevance. J Clin Pathol 36:539–545, 1983

42. Gerdes J, Schwab U, Lemke H, et al: Production of a mouse mono-

clonal antibody reactive with a human nuclear antigen associated with cell proliferation. Int J Cancer 31:13–20, 1983

43. Gerdes J, Lemke H, Baisch H, et al: Cell cycle analysis of cell proliferation associated human nuclear antigen defined by the monoclonal antibody Ki-67. J Immunol 133:1710–1715, 1984

44. Franklin WA, McDonald GB, Stein HO, et al: Immunohistological demonstration of abnormal colon crypt cell kinetics in ulcerative colitis. Hum Pathol (in press)

45. Farrands PA, Pimm MV, Embleton MJ, et al: Radioimmunodetection of human colorectal cancers by an anti-tumour monoclonal antibody. Lancet 2:397–400, 1982

46. Epenetos AA, Mather S, Granowska M, et al: Targeting of iodine-123-labelled tumour-associated monoclonal antibodies to ovarian, breast and gastrointestinal tumours. Lancet 2:999–1004, 1982

47. Redding WH, Monaghan P, Imrie SF, et al: Detection of micrometastases in patients with primary breast cancer. Lancet 2:1271–1274, 1983

48. Ghosh AK, Hatton C, O'Connor N, et al: Detection of metastatic tumour cells in routine bone marrow smears by immuno-alkaline phosphatase labelling with monoclonal antibodies. Br J Haematol (in press)

49. Wells CA, Heryet A, Brochier J, et al: The immunocytochemical detection of axillary micrometastases in breast cancer. Br J Cancer 50:193–197, 1984

50. Ghosh AK, Spriggs AI, Taylor-Papadimitriou J, et al: Immunocytochemical staining of cells in pleural and peritoneal effusions with a panel of monoclonal antibodies. J Clin Pathol 36:1154–1164, 1983

51. Ghosh AK, Mason DY, Spriggs AI: Immunocytochemical staining with monoclonal antibodies in cytologically "negative" serous effusions from patients with malignant disease. J Clin Pathol 36:1150–1153, 1983

52. Coakham HB, Garson JA, Brownell B, et al: Use of monoclonal antibodies to identify malignant cells in cerebrospinal fluid. Lancet 1:1095–1098, 1984

53. Viac J, Reano A, Brochier J, et al: Reactivity pattern of a monoclonal antikeratin antibody (KL1). J Invest Dermatol 81:351–354, 1983

54. Makin CA, Bobrow LG, Bodmer WF: Monoclonal antibody to cytokeratin for use in routine histopathology. J Clin Pathol 37:975–983, 1984

55. Vanstapel MJ, Peeters B, Cordell J, et al: Production and identification of monoclonal antibodies directed against an antigenic determinant common to the alpha and beta chain of S100. Lab Invest 52:232–238, 1985

17

CHROMOSOME ABNORMALITIES IN SOLID TUMORS: POTENTIAL APPLICATIONS TO TUMOR RECOGNITION

Michael A. Cornbleet
Harvey M. Golomb

The observation in 1960 by Nowell and Hungerford of a specific chromosomal abnormality seen only in patients with chronic myeloid leukemia (CML)[1] led to considerable optimism that similar changes would be found in other malignancies that would help in understanding the origins of the malignant state. Subsequent progress, however, was delayed until the technical methods for examining chromosomes were improved and refined with the development of various banding techniques.[2] With each new methodological advance, the proportion of patients with acute leukemia who could be shown to have clonal chromosomal abnormalities has increased, so that a recent report described such changes in 46 of 49 patients for whom adequate material was available.[3] Furthermore, careful re-evaluation of a group of 21 patients with "Philadelphia-negative CML" has shown that in each case except one, the morphologic diagnosis met the criteria etablished by the French–American–British (FAB) group for other myelodysplastic syndromes.[4] In the hematological malignancies, karyotypic information has thus had increasing significance in establishing both the diagnosis and prognosis of patients. In the "solid" tumors, however, progress has been slower, with relatively few specific nonrandom changes identified. This is largely a consequence of the complexity of the karyotypic abnormalities commonly found in solid tumors, compounded with the difficulty of obtaining sufficient metaphases of adequate morphology for the accurate characterization of very subtle changes in banding pattern. Since the only material available for study from patients who present with cancers of unknown origin is by definition obtained from sites of metastatic disease, the changes observed tend to be extremely complex, representing the endpoint of karyotypic evolution. Material for cytogenetic analysis is commonly obtained from bone marrow, malignant effusions, or tumor deposits in lymph nodes or skin. In addition, a significant number of observations have been made as a result of cytogenetic analysis of continuous cell lines growing in culture.

In this chapter, we propose to review some of the problems involved in studying solid tumor karyotypes and to discuss those abnormalites that have been described as having diagnostic significance. Specific chromosome changes in hematological malignancies have recently been the subject of several reviews[5,6] and will not be discussed in detail here. Chromosome morphology will be described using the Paris Nomenclature.[7] Gain of a whole chromosome is indicated by a plus sign before the number, and a minus sign indicates a loss. A plus or minus sign after a number indicates gain or loss of a part of a chromosome. The letters "p" and "q" refer to the short and long arms of the chromosome, respectively; "i" and "r" stand for "isochromosome" and "ring chromosome." Mar is marker, del is deletion, ins is insertion and inv is inversion. Translocations are identified by a "t" followed by the chromosomes involved in the first set of brackets; the chromosome bands in which the breaks occurred are indicated in the second brackets.

Cytogenetic Methods for Solid Tumors

The objective of all cytogenetic methods is to obtain a representative sample of dividing tumor cells as quickly as possible after their removal from the patient. Accomplishing this ensures that any chromosomal abnormalities have the greatest chance of being those present in stem cells residual in the patient. The technical problems involved in achieving this objective have been recently reviewed[8] (Table 17-1). If the tumor is not already in the form of a single cell suspension, as from a malignant effusion

Table 17-1
Cytogenetic Techniques for Solid Tumors

Reference	Duration of Culture	Overall Success (%)	Enzymatic or Mechanical Disaggregation	Permits Normal Cell Growth
Short-term liquid:				
11	2–3 days	80	Both	Yes
10	16–48 hours	n.d.	Both	Yes
16	2–14 days	80	Mech	Yes
Tissue explant:				
17	4–6 weeks	50	Mech	Yes
Soft agar:				
9	2–7 days	50	Mech	No

n.d. = not determined

Derived from Yunis JJ: New chromosome techniques in the study of human neoplasia. Hum Pathol 12:540–549, 1981.

or bone marrow, a necessary first step is the disaggregation of a solid tumor sample, either by mechanical means or as a result of enzyme action. The former, however, has the disadvantage of a relatively low yield of viable cells. In most studies, a period of culture has also been necessary as direct preparations of cells from solid tumors rarely yield mitotic figures of adequate morphology for Giemsa-banding.[9] The most frequently employed methods of disaggregation employ collagenase, alone or with another enzyme (often deoxyribonuclease), to produce single cell suspensions. In one study, 14 of 19 tumors dissociated with collagenase, and cultured for 16–48 hours, showed sufficient numbers of metaphases to permit chromosome analysis.[10] When compared to mechanical methods, enzymatic disaggregation produced significantly more analyzable metaphases in each slide (5.2 versus 0.8), permitting adequate karyotypic analysis in 85 percent of the enzymatically treated samples. There were no significant differences between the karyotypes observed in cells obtained by mechanical disaggregation compared with those obtained enzymatically, suggesting that the latter technique does not modify the karyotype of the tumor. In this study, it was not clear that the addition of DNAse I added appreciably to the yield or morphology of the metaphase cells.[11]

An alternative method of obtaining a single cell suspension has been to use fine needle aspiration (FNA), a method widely used to obtain material for cytological diagnosis. Out of 21 lymph node biopsies in patients with malignant lymphoma, analyzable chromosomes were obtained from 14 biopsies representing 11 cases.[12] In this series, aspiration of subcutaneous deposits was less successful, and the authors comment that the technique may be less suitable for tumors with an infiltrative growth pattern. There are two proposed advantages of this method. First, it provides for the immediate suspension of cells with no mechanical or enzymatic step necessary. Second, it is a simple procedure from the patient's point of view which permits repeated study during the course of the illness. The authors also mention that the same method has been tried with promising results in other solid tumors, including breast and bronchial carcinomas, though further experience was needed before any conclusions about more widespread applicability could be drawn.

Cells already in suspension are frequently found in malignant effusions; these cells have been used in cytogenetic studies which have also helped to identify the malignant etiology of the effusions. Cytogenetic and cytologic analyses have been found to be complementary in the diagnosis of such effusions.[13,14] In the study of Dewald et al., direct examination of the effusion was found to be superior to culture methods for malignant effusions, whereas only 12 percent of studies on uncultured cells yielded metaphases suitable for analysis in the later study. These authors comment, however, that very few of their specimens were received fresh.

The clonogenic tumor stem cell assay has also been utilized to enhance the mitotic index of cells in culture. Using a soft agar cloning technique, Trent and Salmon were able to successfully analyze by banding 13/16 tumors (including 8/9 ovarian cancers) and to assess the modal chromosome number in 37/62 tumors (80 percent).[9] The enhancement in the number of analyzable mitoses seen with this technique was attributed to the selective circumstances of growth in agar culture, which resulted in the proliferation of only 50–200 tumor stem cells out of some 500,000 cells plated in each Petri dish. In a subsequent report, the use of uncultured single cell suspensions of either solid ovarian tumors or their effusions has been compared with cells grown in soft agar culture for 24–96 hours. Cells so cultured were shown to have similar modal number, structural variants, and marker chromosomes as direct cultures, but also have numeric enhancement of tumor mitoses and improved banding morphology.[15]

Clonal Chromosome Abnormalities in Solid Tumors

Small Cell Lung Cancer

Small cell lung cancer accounts for approximately 25 percent of all cases of lung cancer and is associated with a rapidly fatal clinical course in the absence of treatment. In 1982, Whang-Peng et al. reported from the

National Cancer Institute that a specific, acquired chromosomal abnormality was found in 100 percent of the metaphases of 12 of 12 cell lines cultured from human small cell lung cancer, and also in two-day tumor cultures of fresh specimens from three patients.[16,17] A deletion in the short arm of chromosome 3 (3p−) was identified in at least one chromosome 3, and analysis of the shortest region of overlap localized the deletion to the region 3p14–23. In addition, abnormalities of chromosomes 1, 2, and 10 were noted in 13 of 16 lines, though specific bands were not consistently involved. Five of five cell lines derived from lung cancers other than small cell, and two lymphoblastoid lines, failed to show the same abnormality. Of the cell lines, five were derived from previously untreated patients, and all had been in culture for between four and 96 months (retaining enzymatic and electron microscopy characteristics of small cell tumors). The same deletion was identified in short-term (two-day) cultures from three patients, one of whom also showed it in direct preparations of bone marrow. The modal chromosome numbers in these preparations were 78, 68, and 80.

However, in a study of bone marrow preparations from patients with small cell lung cancer and known bone marrow infiltration at the University of Chicago, the deletion of 3p could not be identified in any of five patients, and four appeared to have normal karyotypes (P Hoffman, personal communication).

Ovarian Cancer

Ovarian cancer, the leading cause of death from gynecological cancer, was responsible for 11,200 deaths in the United States in 1980. A wide variety of structural changes had been described in studies of the chromosomes from ovarian cancer cells, but no specific changes were reported until 1979,[18] when Trent and Salmon reported a nonrandom abnormality of chromosome 6 (6q−). Using single cell suspensions derived from either solid tumors or effusions, six ovarian malignancies were studied after 24–96 hours in soft agar culture. Only one patient had received prior chemotherapy and a variety of different histological subtypes were represented. The modal chromosome number in these tumors varied from 37–72, with a range of 26–250. The loss of a single sex chromosome was the most common numeric change, being noted in all six samples. Abnormalities of chromosome 1 (including deletions, duplications, translocations, inversions, and isochromosome formation) were also common (occurring in four of six patients), but the most consistent structural alteration was a simple deletion of a portion of the long arm of chromosome 6 (6q−)(q15−

21:) also in four of six patients. The deleted segment was not observed to be translocated within the genome, and could not be identified in the marker chromosomes found in these cells.

A deletion of chromosome 6 was also observed in a study of twelve patients with papillary serous adenocarcinoma of the ovary reported by Wake et al.[19] In this study, which included five primary and seven metastatic tumors grown in tissue culture medium for two days, 19 clonal chromosomal abnormalities were identified, of which 6q− and 14q+ were the most frequent. Although all twelve tumors had complex karyotypes with many rearranged chromosomes, analysis by banding showed the preferential involvement of 1 as a gain and the X chromosome as a loss. The 6q− and 14q+ chromosomes were each identified in 10 cases, and both markers were found in 8 cases. In six of the tumors, the additional segment of chromosome 14 appeared similar in size and banding pattern to the segment missing from chromosome 6, suggesting that the markers had arisen as a result of a reciprocal translocation. However, this could not be confirmed in the remaining six cases, as the breakpoints were not identical and the added material did not match the deleted portion. The translocation t(6;14)(q21:q24) was suggested to be specifically associated with papillary serous adenocarcinoma.

A recent report from the National Cancer Institute, however, failed to confirm the specificity of the 6q− abnormality.[20] Forty-four patients were successfully analyzed by banding of cells derived either from direct preparations or short-term culture of cells obtained mostly from ascitic fluid. All patients showed aneuploidy with numerical abnormalities; 39 patients had structural chromosomal abnormalities. There was considerable variation in cell chromosome number including wide ranges within single samples. All chromosome pairs were involved in structural abnormalities, the most frequently involved being 1 followed by 3, 2, 9 and 10. Chromosome 6 abnormalities were present in 17 patients; in 9 patients they were clonal. Of the three patients showing 6q21−, none had this abnormality in 50 percent or more of their cells, and of 13 patients with serous papillary cystadenocarcinoma, only 2 had clonal deletions of 6q (6q23− and 6q24−) while 3 patients had deletions in 6q in only one cell each. Six of 15 patients with abnormalities of 14 had 14q+ and in no case could the additional material be identified as coming from 6. These authors comment that the t(6;14) marker might be an artifact produced by the culture in agar, since it has also been seen in melanoma cells grown in the same system.[21] Alternatively, the discrepancy might be a result of differences in the source of cultured material, since their report described the karyotypes of cells from metastatic tumor deposits present in malignant effusions, rather than primary tumor samples. This seemed to them an unlikely explanation, as they felt that markers of this type were more likely to remain than to disappear as the karyotype becomes increasingly complex in metastatic tissue. At present, the utility of this marker in the diagnosis of ovarian cancer must be regarded as provisional.

Carcinoma of the Colon

Cytogenetic studies employing banding have been performed in only a small number of patients with large bowel cancer, and a complex range of abnormalities have been described. In a report of 31 patients successfully studied by banding (out of a total of 56 patients) at the University of Chicago, Reichmann et al. found three to have apparently normal karyotypes. Fifty-two percent of patients had between 44 and 52 chromosomes and the remainder had between 56 and 91 chromosomes, a distribution similar to that observed in a large series reported prior to the use of banding.[22] Of the nonrandom changes observed, 8 was the chromosome most frequently gained (six cases), and 17 was the chromosome most frequently lost. Chromosome 1 was the most frequently involved in rearrangements, which involved either arm and translocations to other chromosomes. No specific region of the chromosome appeared selectively involved in these rearrangements, but in many cases only an approximate karyotype could be obtained.

A later report of the cytogenetic analysis of primary tumors from 10 patients with adenocarcinoma of the large bowel showed all except one to have numerical and/or structural abnormalities, and all but two with abnormal clones were hyperdiploid, including one triploid and another near-triploid. In this study structural and numeric changes most commonly involved chromosomes 7 (six patients) and 12 (six patients).[23]

Testis Cancer

Testicular cancer is at present regarded as the solid tumor with the greatest potential for cure with currently available therapy. Little information, however, has been available about possible consistent karyotypic changes in these tumors. In 1980, Wang et al. reported the results of trypsin–Giemsa banding studies on 14 cell lines derived from 11 patients with testicular cancer.[24] Five were derived from teratocarcinomas, three from embryonal carcinomas, one from a teratoma, and five from tumors containing mixed histologic components. All had been in culture for between 3 and 96 months, undergoing between 7 and 56 passages in culture. Nine of the lines were derived from patients who had received no therapy at the time tissue was obtained, five from primary tumors, and the rest from a variety of metastatic sites. All of the lines had a hyperdiploid chromosome number, with modal chromosome numbers between 51 and 115. Chromosome 1 was found to be involved in numeric and structural changes in every line, with trisomy for the q arm found as the common chromosomal aberration for all cell lines studied. The breakpoints in chromosome 1 in the different structural changes were nonrandom and were most frequently at the regions p36, p22, p12, and q36. These structural changes produced morphologically identical marker chromosomes in different cases.

A specific chromosomal marker in seminoma and malignant teratoma of the testis has recently been described by Atkin and Baker. Twelve primary tumors (nine seminoma, one spermatocytic seminoma, one anaplastic teratoma, and one combined tumor) were studied either directly or after short-term culture.[25] A small metacentric marker, identified in all the tumors, was found to be an isochromosome (12p) in preparations from the four tumors with the most favorable morphology, but in the other tumors a different origin could not be excluded. The tumors were all hyperdiploid, and abnormalities of chromosome 1 were present in most. This marker has also been identified in two of four cell lines derived from metastatic embryonal carcinoma of the testis (N Vogelzang, personal communication).

Malignant Melanoma

Few studies of chromosome abnormalities in malignant melanomas utilizing modern banding techniques have been described; the reports that do exist have largely concerned long-term cultures. A recent report described the results of analyzing a variety of premalignant, malignant, and metastatic melanocytic lesions, including sequential analysis of a primary melanoma and five metastatic deposits removed over an 18-month period.[26] Five nevi had normal karyotypes, while each of the tumors had a predominantly abnormal karyotype. Ten of the 11 advanced melanomas had one or more aberrations involving chromosome 1, with nine having deletions or translocations of 1p that involved the proximal segment (1p12→1p22). Six advanced tumors had additional material involving 7q (including an extra chromosome 7 in four cases and 7q+ in two cases). Nine melanomas, including the early tumor, had alterations in chromosome 6. In the tumor studied sequentially, nearly identical karyotypes were observed over an 18-month period. Considering their results in conjunction with previous studies, the authors suggest that the proximal portion of 1p carries a gene importantly involved in the development of malignant melanoma. The observation of polysomy for chromosome 7 is also unusual; abnormalities of this chromosome are most commonly a loss of part, or all, of the chromosome seen in various hematological malignancies.

Renal Cell Cancer

Rarely, renal cell cancer is found to afflict several members of one family over several generations. In one such family, a heritable balanced translocation t(3;8) has been reported.[27] In an individual from a second family, a translocation involving 3p and the entire chromosome 11 was identified in 22 of 30 cells from the primary tumor studied by banding,[28] although the breakpoint differed in this tumor, being identified in band 3p13 or 14 in the t(3;11) and in band 3p21 in the t(3;8).

In a single case report, the karyotype of a sporadic renal cell carcinoma (in a woman of 76) analyzed by trypsin–Giemsa banding of uncultured tumor tissue showed normal karyotypes in only four of 40 metaphases analyzed. Thirty-six cells had between 51 and 76 chromosomes, and several marker chromosomes were consistently identified. All metaphases contained two normal chromosomes 3, together with a marker chromosome characterized as a t(3;17)(3qter→3q21::17q25→17pter). A normal chromosome 17 was present in only a few metaphases.[29] Thus, although chromosome 3 has been consistently implicated in abnormalities associated with renal cell cancer in reported cases, no concordance exists as to the regions of the chromosome involved, and the significance of the observations remains to be clarified.

Sarcomas

Employing a disaggregation method utilizing collagenase and short-term culture, Becher et al. were able to study the karyotypes of 15 of 29 cases of soft tissue sarcoma.[30] Four had a normal karyotype; a variety of histological subtypes were represented among the remainder. All but one were metastatic tumors, and eight had received prior radiation or chemotherapy. The majority of cases were found to have modal chromosome numbers in the hypodiploid or near diploid range. Chromosomes 1 and 2 were most frequently involved in structural abnormalities.

One of the patients with Ewing's sarcoma studied by Becher et al. was noted to have a complex translocation involving chromosomes 2, 12, and

22. The band in number 22 at which the break occurred (q11−12) was also involved in translocations identified in all of four further cases of Ewing's sarcoma, although the other chromosomes involved varied, chromosomes 2 and 11 in one case, 9 and 20 in the second, 11 in the third, and two separate translocations involving chromosomes 1 and 11 in the fourth.[31] An identical translocation involving t(11;22) has been reported in four cell lines derived from Ewing's tumor.[32]

Childhood Tumors

Although individually rare, cancers in children have been relatively intensively studied in the hope that clues derived from the study of tumors with an inherited origin may be more widely applicable. In two such tumors, retinoblastoma and Wilms' tumor with aniridia, observed chromosome changes differ in at least some cases from those described previously, in that the abnormalities are constitutional, i.e. seen in all somatic cells and not only tumor cells.

Retinoblastoma

Retinoblastoma is the most common eye tumor of children, and a tendency to recur within families has long been identified. Most patients (60 percent), however, have no family history of eye tumors, and in these it is usually unilateral. Bilateral retinoblastoma is always hereditary and is associated with a very high incidence of second tumors. Two forms of the heritable type occur, the majority (nearly 40 percent of all cases) in which no constitutional karyotype change is detectable, and a small group in which a deletion or translocation of a portion of the long arm of chromosome 13 (always involving band 13q14) is observed in all cells. These two groups have clinical similarities in early age of onset and frequency of bilaterality; a gene believed responsible for the former has been mapped to the same band that is missing in the latter type.[33] The more general significance of a gene (or genes) at this site is suggested by the observation of deletions or rearrangements involving 13q14 in the tumor cell karyotypes of five of six cases with normal constitutional karyotypes[34] in which fresh tumors were studied after short-term (72 hours) culture, although a study in which retinoblastoma cells were studied in tissue culture or after passage in nude mice found no particular relationship between retinoblastoma and chromosome 13.[35] In the largest study reported so far, Benedict et al. have described three nonrandom changes identified in 15 retinoblastoma tumors, a loss of chromosome 13, an iso (6p), or a trisomy 1q.[36] In addition, one tumor showed a deletion of 13q14, with no deletion present in a fibroblast cell line established from the same patient. As a result of their study, and those of others, Benedict et al. suggest that either a total loss of one 13 or a deletion that includes one 13q14 may play an important role in the development of retinoblastoma. They further suggested that the *normal* chromosome 13 is the one that is lost and that the remaining 13 contains the "first hit" proposed in the Knudson hypothesis.[37] Loss of the normal gene locus would then result in the complete loss of the "retinoblastoma susceptibility gene" located at 13q14. In this model, the retinoblastoma gene is a recessive gene at the tumor level. Because of the close linkage between the esterase-D locus and the retinoblastoma gene, it has been possible to study the apparently normal chromosomes in several tumors; several pieces of evidence favor the conclusion that homozygosity for a recessive gene at the retinoblastoma locus is an important step in the development of the tumor. For example, patients in whom the esterase-D polymorphism (i.e. patients with the 2–1 esterase-D pattern in nontumor cells) and in whom two structurally normal chromosomes 13 were present in their tumors, have been shown to have only one esterase-D allele present in the tumor. This has been interpreted as suggesting that one 13 had been lost, with reduplication of a 13 carrying a submicroscopic deletion at the retinoblastoma locus.[38] Further clarification of the significance of this gene and its mechanism of action may have far-reaching implications.

Wilms' Tumor With Aniridia

The association of Wilms' tumor in children with aniridia (and other anomalies) was first reported in 1964.[39] In 1978, Riccardi et al. demonstrated that deletions of chromosome 11 (specifically band p13) could account for at least some cases of this association.[40] Two subsequent reports have identified interstitial deletions involving band 11p13 in three Wilms' tumors in patients without aniridia or other congenital abnormalities and who had normal constitutional karyotypes,[41,42] suggesting a situation analogous to that in retinoblastoma.

Neuroblastoma

A third childhood tumor with both a hereditary and nonhereditary pattern, but with no identified constitutional changes, is neuroblastoma, a tumor of infancy with a peak incidence at birth. In 1977, Brodeur et al. reported deletions of 1p in three of six neuroblastomas,[43] and several reports since then have described similar changes in approximately half the tumors and cell lines studied.[44] In 11 of 14 cell lines with structural

rearrangements of 1p, the abnormality included deletions of bands
1p32→1pter, rendering the cells monosomic for this genetic material.[45]
Two reported patients, one with familial neuroblastoma, have had balanced translocations involving a common breakpoint at 11q23.[46,47]

Discussion

In the 70 years since Boveri first proposed that abnormalities in the
chromosomal constitution of cells could result in malignancy,[48] a number
of chromosome changes have been identified as specific for certain malignancies, most consistently in the case of the Philadelphia chromosome in
chronic myeloid leukemia. Studies in this field were severely hampered
until the development of banding techniques in the early 1970s permitted
not only the identification of individual chromosomes but also delineation
of the specific region of a chromosome that was involved in a deletion or
translocation. Since then, several more specific changes have been identified, particularly those associated with the different subtypes of acute
nonlymphocytic leukemia.[5] In the case of the solid cancers, however,
technical difficulties have continued to slow progress towards identifying
similarly specific changes. Coupled with the considerable complexity of the
karyotypes commonly encountered are difficulties in obtaining sufficient
metaphases likely to represent the true karyotype of the malignant cell in
vivo. These difficulties have led to the consideration of alternative strategies for selectively studying the malignant cell population, such as the soft
agar cloning assay or the use of cell lines, which have, in recent years,
substantially increased the number of reports of chromosome changes in
solid tumors. A recurring caveat in such reports, however, is the concern
that the identified changes might represent selection artifacts of the culture
system, rather than changes significant in the evolution of the malignant
state.

It has been increasingly evident that changes in the organization or
structure of genetic material are of fundamental importance in this evolution, and that the rapidly unfolding "oncogene story" has led to a
confluence of several lines of research in molecular genetics and cytogenetics that has already been very productive. Several oncogenes have now
been localized to the sites of chromosome breaks in the better delineated
translocations. For example, the abl oncogene has been shown to move
from 9q to 22q in chronic myeloid leukemia,[49] and the myc gene from 8q to
a site on 14q adjacent to the heavy chain gene complex.[50] The exchange of
segments between chromosomes in this way might lead to the activation of

these genes by any of several mechanisms, for example by altering the relationship between a gene and either its own or a more active promoter. The site of the deletion observed in the Wilms-aniridia syndrome (11p13) is also the site of the Harvey-ras 1 gene,[51] but it is not clear whether the deletion actually involves any or all of the gene, or of a suppressor of its activity. The different types of chromosome abnormalities seen in cancer cells have been classified by Gilbert into three groups;[52] (1) reciprocal translocations in which there is no significant loss of structural material, e.g. t(8;14) and t(9;22), (2) deletions or nonreciprocal rearrangements resulting in the loss of structural material at specific sites, e.g. del (11p) in the Wilms-aniridia syndrome, and (3) duplication of whole chromosomes or chromosome segments. While these different rearrangements have clearly differing implications for gene function (either quantitative or qualitative) that are only beginning to be understood, the functions of some oncogene products have recently become clearer. The product of the simian sarcoma virus (sis) gene, a protein of molecular weight 28,000, has been found to show striking homology with parts of the large domain of platelet-derived growth factor (PDGF), which is released from alpha granules of platelets during clotting and is a powerful mitogen.[53] Those human tumors found to express the cellular homologue of the sis gene (sarcomas and gliomas) are derived from cell types sensitive to PDGF and which express receptors for it.[54] Activation of an oncogene thus might lead to the production by a cell of a powerful growth factor for which it itself expresses a receptor, offering an attractive hypothesis to explain the growth of tumors unhindered by external regulation.

As exciting as these developments are, they do indicate a major obstacle for the cytogeneticist at the light microscope. In one of the most intensively studied of the oncogenes, the EJ oncogene in human bladder carcinoma, the difference between the transforming gene and its cellular homologue has been shown to reside in a single base pair.[55,56] Since the average metaphase band observed in a light microscope preparation contains 5×10^6 base pairs, a deletion or duplication of one-third of a band (or 2×10^6 base pairs) would be difficult to detect with conventional methods.[57] It is thus highly probable that many important changes will be beyond the resolution of the most careful cytogenetic analysis.

Although few specific chromosomal changes have been identified in human solid tumors, some chromosomes do appear to be more frequently involved in rearrangements than do others. Thus, chromosome 1 has been implicated in malignant melanoma, neuroblastoma, and testicular cancer (Table 17-2), as well as in cervical cancer[58] and ovarian cancer.[59] Chromosome 1 abnormalities are not, however, confined to solid tumors, having

Table 17-2
Clonal Chromosome Abnormalities in Solid Tumors

Tumor	Chromosome Abnormality	Reference
Small cell lung cancer	del 3p(p14;p23)	16, 17
Ovarian cancer	t(6;14) or 6q −	18, 19
Colon cancer	+8, − 17, others	22
Testis cancer	1p −, i(12p)	24, 25
Malignant melanoma	1p −	26
Renal cell cancer	t(3,8),	27
	t(3,11)(p23or24;p15)	28
Ewing's sarcoma	t(22,?)(q12;?)	31, 32
Retinoblastoma	13q −	33, 34
Wilms' tumor	11p −	39, 40, 41
Neuroblastoma	1p −	43, 44, 45

been observed also in a variety of hematologic malignancies[60] and in malignant lymphomas.[61] The diversity of the malignancies in which changes in chromosome 1 are found, prompted Rowley to speculate that structural rearrangements affecting genes localized to this chromosome provide one mechanism associated with an increased malignant potential. Among the genes so far localized to 1q are those for UDP glucose pyrophosphorylase, guanylate kinase 1 and 2, and 5s ribosomal RNA, while among those on the short arm are the N-ras oncogene, the gene for nerve growth factor, and the U1 small nuclear RNA genes believed to have important functions in gene splicing.[62] Alterations in the structure, function, or dose of any of these genes might be expected to significantly affect the proliferative potential of a cell.

Despite the established diagnostic and prognostic utility of cytogenetic analysis in hematologic[63] and lymphoid malignancies,[61] it is apparent from the foregoing review that few changes of direct clinical significance have so far been identified in solid cancers. While cytogenetic analysis may assist in identifying a poorly differentiated lymphoma if a characteristic abnormality such as the t(8;14) of Burkitt's lymphoma[64] is observed, similarly specific changes that would differentiate among carcinomas have proved elusive. With the increasing sophistication of molecular genetic technology, the availability of oncogene and other cellular DNA probes may substantially alter the diagnostic approach to these patients in the not too distant future. It is already apparent that the relationship between the nature of the oncogene activated and the type of malignancy is not simple, since in a study of the expression of 15 cellular oncogenes in fresh tumors of twenty different types, more than one oncogene was transcriptionally active in all tumors. In many of the 14 patients from whom normal tissue was also available, the ratio of differential expression between normal and malignant tissue varied widely.[65] The hope exists that specific patterns of oncogene expression may be found to have diagnostic as well as etiologic implications. The results of these studies will certainly provide new insights into the biology of malignant transformation.

Acknowledgment

Dr. Cornbleet was a recipient of the Hamilton-Fairley Travelling Fellowship of the Cancer Research Campaign of Great Britain.

References

1. Nowell P, Hungerford DA: A minute chromosome in human chronic granulocytic leukemia. Science 132:1497, 1960
2. Caspersson T, Farber S, Foley GE, et al: Chemical differentiation along the metaphase chromosomes. Exp Cell Res 49:219–222, 1968
3. Yunis JJ: Recurrent chromosomal defects are found in most patients with acute non-lymphocytic leukemia. Cancer Genet Cytogenet 11:125–137, 1984
4. Pugh WC, Pearson MG, Rowley JD, et al: Ph[1]-negative CML: A morphologic reassessment (abstr). Proc ASCP 1983
5. Pearson MG, Larson RA, Golomb HM: Clinical significance of chromosome patterns in malignant disease, in Rowley JD, Ultmann JE (eds): Chromosomes and Cancer: From Molecules to Man. New York, Academic Press, 1983, pp 311–333
6. Hart JS: Chromosome abnormalities in human cancer. Cancer Treat Rev 10:173–183, 1983
7. Paris Conference on Standardization in human cytogenetics, in: Birth Defects, Orig. Artic Series, Vol 8. No. 7. New York, Natl Foundation-March of Dimes, 1971
8. Yunis JJ: New chromosome techniques in the study of human neoplasia. Hum Pathol 12:540–549, 1981
9. Trent JM, Salmon S: Human tumour karyology: marked analytic improvement by short-term agar culture. Br J Cancer 41:867–874, 1980

10. Kusyk CJ, Edwards CL, Arrighi FE, et al. Improved methods for cytogenetic studies of solid tumours. JNCI 63:1199–1203, 1979

11. Wake N, Slocum HK, Rustum YM, et al: Chromosomes and causation of human cancer and leukemia: XLIV A method for chromosome analysis of solid tumours. Cancer Genet Cytogenet 3:1–10, 1981

12. Kristofferson U, Olsson H, Mark-Vendel E, et al: Fine-needle aspiration biopsy: A useful tool in tumour cytogenetics with special reference to malignant lymphomas. Cancer Genet Cytogenet 4:53–60, 1981

13. DeWald GW, Hicks GA, Dines DE, et al: Cytogenetic diagnosis of malignant pleural effusions. Mayo Clinic Proc 57:488–494, 1982

14. Watts KC, Boyo-Ekwueme H, To A, et al: Chromosome studies on cells cultured from serous effusions. Acta Cytol (Baltimore) 27:38–44, 1983

15. Trent JM, Salmon SE: Karyotypic analysis of human ovarian carcinoma cells cloned in short-term agar culture. Cancer Genet Cytogenet 3:279–291, 1981

16. Whang-Peng J, Kao-Shan CS, Lee EC, et al: Specific defect associated with small cell lung cancer: deletion 3p(14–23). Science 215:181–182, 1982

17. Whang-Peng J, Bunn PA, Kao-Shan CS, et al: A non-random chromosomal abnormality del 3p(14–23) in human small cell lung cancer (SCLC). Cancer Genet Cytogenet 6:119–134, 1982

18. Trent JM, Salmon SE: Karyotypic analysis of human ovarian cancer cells cloned in agar (abstr). Am J Human Genet 31:379, 1979

19. Wake N, Hreshchyshyn MM, Piver SM, et al: Specific cytogenetic changes in ovarian cancer involving chromosomes 6 and 14. Cancer Res 40:4512–4518, 1980

20. Whang-Peng J, Knutsen T, Douglas EC, et al: Cytogenetic studies in ovarian cancer. Cancer Genet Cytogenet 11:91–106, 1984

21. Trent JM, Rosenfeld SB, Meyskens FL: Chromosome 6q involvement in human malignant melanoma. Cancer Genet Cytogenet 9:177–180, 1983

22. Reichmann A, Martin P, Levin B: Chromosomal banding patterns in human large bowel cancer. Int J Cancer 28:431–440, 1981

23. Ochi H, Takeuchi J, Holyoke D, et al: Possible specific chromosome changes in large bowel cancer. Cancer Genet Cytogenet 10:121–122, 1983

24. Wang N, Trend B, Bronson DL, et al: Nonrandom chromosome abnormalities in chromosome #1 in human testicular cancers. Cancer Res 40:796–802, 1980

25. Atkin NB, Baker MC: i(12p): Specific chromosomal marker in semi-

noma and malignant teratoma of the testis? Cancer Genet Cytogenet 10:199–204, 1983

26. Balaban G, Herlyn M, DuPont G IV, et al: Cytogenetics of human malignant melanoma and premalignant lesions. Cancer Genet Cytogenet 11:429–439, 1984

27. Cohen AJ, Li FP, Berg S, et al: Hereditary renal cell carcinoma associated with a chromosomal translocation. N Engl J Med 301:592–595, 1979

28. Pathak S, Strong LC, Ferrell RE, et al: Familial renal cell carcinoma with a 3:11 chromosome translocation limited to tumour cells. Science 217:939–941, 1982

29. Ferti-Passantonopoulou A, Panani A, Raptis S: G-banded karyotype of a primary renal-cell carcinoma. Cancer Genet Cytogenet 11:227–232, 1984

30. Becher R, Wake N, Gibas H, et al: Chromosome changes in soft tissue sarcoma. JNCI 72:823–831, 1984

31. Aurias A, Rimbaut C, Buffe D, et al: Chromosome translocations in Ewings sarcoma (letter). N Engl J Med 309:496–497, 1983

32. Turc-Carel C, Philip I, Berger M-P, et al: Chromosome translocations in Ewings sarcoma (letter). N Engl J Med 309:497–498, 1983

33. Sparkes RS, Murphree AL, Lingua RW, et al: Gene for hereditary retinoblastoma assigned to human chromosome 13 by linkage to esterase-D. Science 219:971–973, 1983

34. Balaban G, Gilbert F, Nichols W, et al: Abnormalities of chromosome #13 in retinoblastomas from individuals with normal constitutional karyotypes. Cancer Genet Cytogenet 6:213–221, 1982

35. Gardner HA, Gallie BL, Knight LA, et al: Multiple karyotypic changes in retinoblastoma tumour cells: Presence of normal chromosome 13 in most tumours. Cancer Genet Cytogenet 6:201–211, 1982

36. Benedict WF, Banerjee A, Coret M, et al: Nonrandom chromosomal changes in untreated retinoblastomas. Cancer Genet Cytogenet 10:311–333, 1983

37. Knudson AG: Mutation and cancer: A statistical study of retinoblastoma. Proc Natl Acad Sci 68:820–823, 1971

38. Godbout R, Gallie BL, Dryja TP: Lack of expression of one esterase-D isoenzyme in retinoblastoma tumour cells. Invest Opth Vis Sci 24 (suppl):294, 1983

39. Miller RW, Fraumeni JF, Manning MD: Association of Wilms tumour with aniridia, hemihypertrophy and other congenital malformations. N Engl J Med 270:922–927, 1964

40. Riccardi VM, Sujansky E, Smith AC, et al: Chromosomal imbalance in

the Aniridia-Wilms tumour association: 11p interstitial deletion. Paediatrics 61:604–610, 1978

41. Kaneko Y, Egues MC, Rowley JD: Interstitial deletion of short arm of chromosome 11 limited to Wilms tumour cells in a patient without aniridia. Cancer Res 41:4577–4578, 1981

42. Slater RM, de Kraker J: Chromosome number 11 and Wilms tumour. Cancer Genet Cytogenet 5:237–245, 1982

43. Brodeur GM, Sekhon GS, Goldstein MN: Chromosomal aberrations in human neuroblastoma. Cancer 40:2256–2263, 1977

44. Gilbert F, Balaban G, Moorhead P, et al: Abnormalities of chromosome 1p in human neuroblastoma tumours and cell lines. Cancer Genet Cytogenet 7:33–42, 1982

45. Brodeur GM, Green AA, Hayes FA, et al: Cytogenetic features of human neuroblastomas and cell lines. Cancer Res 41:4678–4686, 1981

46. Hecht F, Kaiser-McCaw B: Chromosomes in familial neuroblastoma. J Paediatrics 98:334, 1981

47. Moorhead PS, Evans AE: Chromosomal findings in patients with neuroblastoma, in Evans AE (ed): Advances in Neuroblastoma Research. Raven Press, New York, 1980 pp 109–118

48. Boveri T: Zur Frage der Enstehung Maligner Tumoren. Gustav Fischer Verlag, Jena, 1914

49. De Klein A, van Kessel AG, Grosveid G, et al: A cellular oncogene is translocated to the Philadelphia chromosome in chronic myeloid leukaemia. Nature 300:765–767, 1982

50. Neel BG, Jhanwhar SC, Chaganti RS, et al: Two human c-onc genes are located on the long arm of chromosome 8. Proc Natl Acad Sci 79:7842–7846, 1982

51. De Martinville B, Giacalone J, Shih C, et al: Oncogene from human EJ bladder carcinoma is located on the short arm of chromosome 11. Science 219:498–501, 1983

52. Gilbert F: Chromosomes, Genes and Cancer: A classification of chromosome abnormalities in cancer. JNCI 71:1107–1114, 1983

53. Waterfield MD, Scrace GT, Whittle N, et al: Platelet-derived growth factor is structurally related to the putative transforming protein p28[sis] of simian sarcoma virus. Nature 304:35–39, 1983

54. Weiss R: Oncogenes and growth factors. Nature 304:12, 1983

55. Tabin CJ, Bradley SM, Bargamann CI, et al: Mechanism of action of a human oncogene. Nature 300:143–149, 1982

56. Reddy EP, Reynolds RK, Santos E, et al: A point mutation is responsible for the acquisition of transforming properties by the T24 bladder carcinoma oncogene. Nature 300:149–152, 1982

57. Rowley JD: Mapping of human chromosomal regions related to neoplasia: Evidence from chromosome 1 and 17. Proc Natl Acad Science 12:5729–5729, 1977

58. Atkin NB, Baker MC: Chromosome 1 in cervical carcinoma. Lancet 2:984 (letter) 1977

59. Atkin NB, Pickhall VJ: Chromosome 1 in 14 ovarian cancers. Human Genet 38:25–33, 1977

60. Rowley JD: Abnormalities of chromosome 1: Significance in malignant transformation. Virchows Arch B Cell Pathol 29:139–144, 1978

61. Kaneko Y, Rowley JD, Variakojis D, et al: Prognostic implications of karyotype and morphology in patients with non-Hodgkins lymphoma. Int J Cancer 32:683–692, 1983

62. McKusick VA: Human Gene Map. Johns Hopkins Hospital, November, 1983

63. Larson RA, Le Beau MM, Vardiman JW, et al: The predictive value of initial cytogenetic studies in 148 adults with acute non-lymphocytic leukaemia: a 12-year study (1970–1982). Cancer Genet Cytogenet 10:219–234, 1983

64. Zech L, Haglund U, Nilsson K, et al: Characteristic chromosomal abnormalities in biopsies and lymphoid cell-lines from patients with Burkitt and non-Burkitt lymphomas. Int J Cancer 17:47–56, 1976

65. Salmon DJ, deKernion JB, Verma IM, et al: Expression of cellular oncogenes in human malignancies. Science 224:256–262, 1984

18

THE HUMAN TUMOR CLONOGENIC ASSAY AND OTHER CELL CULTURE TECHNIQUES: POTENTIAL APPLICATIONS TO THE STUDY OF UNDIFFERENTIATED NEOPLASMS OR CANCERS OF UNKNOWN ORIGIN

William W. Grosh
Daniel D. Von Hoff

Contemporary concepts of the cellular kinetics of normal self-renewing tissues and neoplasms are based upon the existence of a stem cell population. These stem cells are believed to retain the ability to reproduce themselves and to parent a differentiating line of mature cells with different functions and reduced capacity for self-renewal.[1,2] The stem cell concept is well-established in a number of normal tissues including the mucosa of the gastrointestinal tract and cell lineages of the hematopoietic system.[3-6] Since neoplasms frequently retain many of the morphologic and physiologic features of normal tissues, it intuitively seems reasonable that stem cells would also be present in neoplasms. Recent evidence supports this supposition.[1,7-10] Similarly, since marrow stem cells comprise a very small

POORLY DIFFERENTIATED NEOPLASMS AND TUMORS OF UNKNOWN ORIGIN   ISBN 0-8089-1755-2
© 1986 by Grune & Stratton.   All rights of reproduction in any form reserved.

percentage (one percent) of the marrow indigenes, tumor stem cells are hypothesized to comprise only a small percentage of the tumor cells. This view is also supported by recent data.[1,7,8] The human tumor stem cell assay (HTSCA) is based on the concept that certain cells within a malignancy, stem cells, can renew themselves and the other tumor cell populations. The cell populations that lack this self-renewing capacity (nonstem cells) are therefore of less import in a therapeutic sense, since they would eventually die out. The HTSCA is an in vitro cell culture system that purports to identify stem cell activity. Since the cells to be tested are plated as single cell suspensions and their capacity for growth is deduced by the subsequent formation of clones or colonies, the term clonogenic assay (CA) appears more appropriate. There is no conclusive proof that these clonogenic cells correspond to the putative stem cells of the parent malignancy. This contention can, however, be supported by data derived from the use of the CA in culturing spontaneous human tumors and from an analysis of the cellular composition of the colonies that develop. First, comparison of the cells that comprise the colonies and the parent tumor suggests a high degree of histologic and cytogenetic similarity.[11,12] Second, cells derived from colonies plucked from the CA can form tumors in nude mice or parent long-term cell culture lineages in liquid media.[13–15] Third, a relatively high degree of correlation between the chemoresponsiveness identified in the CA and actual in vivo results has been demonstrated,[11,12,16,17] suggesting that if the kinetic cellular models described for malignancies are valid, the CA must be assessing stem cells or another population of tumor cells with similar chemoresponsiveness.

The CA is still in its infancy as a technique. This chapter describes potential uses of the CA and other cell culture techniques as research and clinical tools for evaluating certain poorly differentiated neoplasms and carcinomas that arise from unknown primary sites.

Poorly Differentiated Neoplasms and Carcinomas of Unknown Primary Site

Patients with unclassifiable malignancies, poorly differentiated or undifferentiated neoplasms classifiable as lymphoma, carcinoma, or sarcoma, and those with better differentiated metastatic carcinomas with unknown sites of origin present the clinical oncologist with knotty problems regarding their evaluation, prognosis, and therapy. Unraveling this Gordian knot is clinically relevant because the administration of appropriate therapy may be curative or palliative for patients with many different

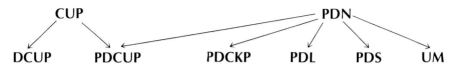

Figure 18-1. *Summary of the inter-relationships of poorly differentiated neoplasms (PDN), carcinomas of unknown primary (CUP), and their subtypes.*

CUP:	*carcinoma with an unknown primary site*
DCUP:	*well- or moderately well-differentiated CUP*
PDCUP:	*poorly differentiated CUP*
PDN:	*poorly differentiated neoplasm*
PDKP:	*poorly differentiated neoplasm with a known primary site*
PDL:	*poorly differentiated lymphoma/leukemia*
PDS:	*poorly differentiated sarcoma*
UM:	*unclassifiable malignancy*

malignancies even if advanced disease is present. Poorly differentiated neoplasms can usually be categorized as hematologic, sarcomatous, or carcinomatous by utilizing the powers of light microscopy, electron microscopy and immunocytochemistry, although their exact morphologic position within these general categories may remain unclear.[18–22] Neoplasms that cannot be placed within this nomenclature should be described as unclassifiable malignancies (UM) (Fig. 18-1). The pathologic diagnosis of UM may vary considerably in its incidence among different institutions, but in the experience of the authors it is rare. In one study, however, 56 cases of undifferentiated large cell malignancy drawn from a six-year review of biopsy results were evaluated pathologically by light microscopy, electron microscopy, and histochemical methods. Despite these methods, six of these cases (10.8 percent) could not be classified as a lymphoma, carcinoma, or sarcoma.[18] More common than the diagnosis of UM is the classification of a neoplasm as a poorly differentiated or undifferentiated carcinoma (PDC), lymphoma (PDL), or sarcoma (PDS). Among these entities the diagnosis of PDC is encountered most frequently. Poorly differentiated carcinomas may occur with occult or identifiable primary sites. The term PDCUP will refer to those PDC with an unknown primary and PDCKP to those with a known primary site. Metastatic carcinomas have been accepted as having an unknown primary site, in this chapter, if a search for a primary site directed by clinical or laboratory abnormalities was unrewarding. A negative exhaustive search for a primary lesion was not required. This chapter will review the current applicability of the CA for selecting chemotherapy prospectively in other malignancies, data regarding its potential use in poorly differentiated neoplasms and CUP, and potential investigational avenues for the future use of cell culture techniques including the CA to clarify the sites of origin and therapy of these malignancies.

The Clonogenic Assay

Methodology and Problems

The CA is a complicated laboratory procedure; it is outlined in Figure 18-2. Tumors arrive in the laboratory as a solid (i.e., a portion of a colonic carcinoma) or liquid (i.e., malignant effusion) specimen. These specimens are converted into clean single cell suspensions by mechanical and enzymatic disaggregation and by washing several times in media to remove debris. These cells are cytologically evaluated for viability and malignancy, brought to the appropriate concentration, exposed to a panel of drugs (each generally at several concentrations to establish a dose response curve) for one hour, rewashed, and plated in a layer of media and agar overlying a similar feeder layer in a Petri dish (double layer culture system). The plates are then examined within 24 hours in an inverted microscope to ensure that a good single cell suspension was plated and that clumps of cells that could be confused with colonies are not present. If the plates are acceptable, colony counts are performed at seven-day intervals comparing growth in control plates to that in drug-treated plates.

Many technical problems are encountered in the use and interpretation of the CA due to its complexity. Many tumor specimens are hard to make into adequate, viable single cell suspensions and some never provide sufficient cell yield or colony growth (more than 30 colonies/500,000 cells plated) for drug activity testing or other manipulations. To improve these results it may be necessary to individualize growth conditions and interpretive criteria (i.e., defining a colony as consisting of 30 to 50 cells) for specific tumor types. It is impossible to mimic in vivo drug kinetics and exposures accurately in the CA even for single antineoplastic agents. The dose response curves obtained with single agents are often unusual in shape with illogical plateaus and higher degrees of colony growth as drug concentrations are escalated. Many investigators therefore perform dose response curves (at least 3 drug doses) when testing an antineoplastic agent in the CA. Drug combinations and drugs requiring metabolism (cyclophosphamide) are difficult to assess given contemporary techniques. Finally, the in vitro responses of the subset of cells that grow in the CA may

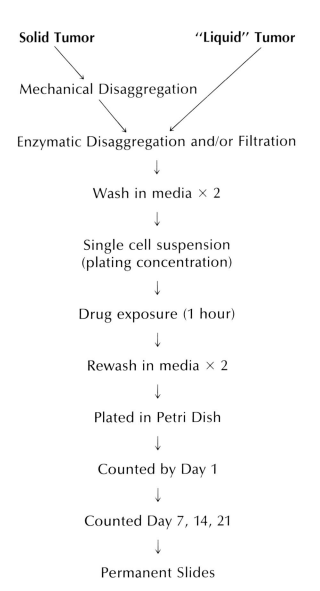

Solid Tumor   **"Liquid" Tumor**

Mechanical Disaggregation

Enzymatic Disaggregation and/or Filtration

↓

Wash in media × 2

↓

Single cell suspension
(plating concentration)

↓

Drug exposure (1 hour)

↓

Rewash in media × 2

↓

Plated in Petri Dish

↓

Counted by Day 1

↓

Counted Day 7, 14, 21

↓

Permanent Slides

Figure 18-2. *Methodology of the Clonogenic Assay (CA)*

or may not be representative of the responses in vivo of the stem cells of the malignancy. Clearly this is an artificial in vitro system involving many manipulations that are brutal to a cell. There are many potential methodologic sources for discordance between in vitro and in vivo chemosensitivity. The system, by exerting selective growth pressures (i.e., media, disaggregation), may examine only a subset of the clonogenic cells present in the tumor in vivo. Despite these problems the test of this assay as a clinical tool is whether or not it can reproducibly predict chemoresponsiveness in vivo and whether or not that data can be prospectively employed to improve the response rates and survival of patients with cancer.

Contemporary Clinical Utility in Diverse Malignancies

The test of the CA as a predictor of chemotherapeutic responsiveness lies in its comparison with the responses seen to the same agents in the patient from which the tumor specimen was obtained. The published data describing the use of the CA specifically in poorly differentiated neoplasms and CUP consists of 19 cases.[23] Clearly this is a very limited experience. These malignancies and their more differentiated counterparts with known primary sites clearly share many similarities despite their incongruities. It intuitively seems reasonable to consider the correlation of in vitro drug activity predicted by the CA and the actual in vivo response seen in large groups of unselected tumors as potentially reflective of the results that will be seen in poorly differentiated neoplasms and CUP. The results and clinical impact of the CA in more common malignancies can be used as models to sketch its potential impact in the poorly differentiated neoplasms and CUP. The correlations noted from an initial large retrospective study evaluating the predictive capacity of the CA in a diversity of malignancies are delineated in Table 18-1.[24] These data suggest a true positive (sensitive in vivo and in vitro) rate of 60 percent and a true negative rate (resistant in vivo and in vitro) of 97 percent, and have been supported by the results of other researchers.[11,25,26] More recent trials utilizing the CA modified by some technical improvements have suggested improved true positive predictive rates (71 percent to 85 percent) and slightly lower true negative rates (85 percent to 91 percent).[16,27]

The highly accurate prediction of resistance and less accurate prediction of sensitivity could be anticipated. There is no reason to believe that these problems would be any less when studying poorly differentiated neoplasms or CUP. Clinically it is quite evident that while a malignancy

Table 18-1

Composite Update of Correlations of In Vitro–In Vivo Sensitivity to Anticancer Drugs (January 1980)

Investigative Group	No. Pts	No. Clinical Trials for Correlations	Tumor Sensitive Both In Vitro and In Vivo	Tumor Sensitive In Vitro Resistant In Vivo	Tumor Resistant In Vitro Sensitive In Vivo	Tumor Resistant Both In Vitro and In Vivo
Tucson	96	193	34	20	5	134
San Antonio	105	151	7	8	3	133
Total	201	344	41	28	8	267
			(60% true positive)			(97% true negative)

From Salmon SE and Von Hoff DD: In vitro evaluation of anti-cancer drugs with the human tumor stem cell assay. Semin Oncol 8:377–385, 1981.

With the χ^2 test the association of in vitro and in vivo results was highly significant ($p < 10^{-9}$)

457

may respond to a chemotherapeutic regimen in one site it may fail to respond in another. Tumor heterogeneity and problems with adequate drug delivery to the tumor may explain this phenomenon in part. Resistance (progression) defined at any tumor site would theoretically predict that an objective response (complete or partial) could not occur; whereas sensitivity demonstrated at one site would not necessarily predict that all other sites will respond. These considerations alone imply that the CA would more accurately predict resistance than sensitivity. A definable discordance rate between the chemosensitivity of different sites of malignant involvement and between the chemosensitivity of different areas within the same malignant site supports these considerations.[28]

Despite the described predictive accuracy of the assay, its impact on the selection of chemotherapy is further diluted by technical problems inherent in the assay technique. These problems, obtaining adequate single cell suspensions and evaluable degrees of growth given contemporary methods, are likely to remain when studying poorly differentiated neoplasms or CUP and to minimize the impact of the CA in clinical situations. A flow diagram demonstrating this point in patients with resistant ovarian carcinoma is displayed in Figure 18-3. In order to effectively screen a series of chemotherapeutic agents for one that is active in a malignancy, five to eight or more drugs must usually be tested.[29,30] Only 50 percent of the specimens obtained provide sufficient cell yields to test five or more drugs and produce sufficient growth to analyze their chemosensitivity. The use of five to eight drugs allows the identification of an active agent 75 percent of the time, or in 38 percent of all specimens in this case. If we accept a true positive predictive rate of 70 percent for the CA, a drug will be identified in about 25 percent of specimens that will produce an in vivo response which is commensurate with the results of empirically selected therapy in patients with resistant ovarian carcinoma.[31,32] An active drug will be identified in less than 25 percent of specimens if any of these estimates are unrealistically optimistic. Similar results were noted in a nonrandomized prospective study where in vivo responses occurred in 25 percent of 246 single agent clinical trials performed with drugs identified as active in vitro in the CA whereas 14 percent of 358 empirically directed single agent trials developed responses.[16]

Two studies provide intriguing information regarding the use of the CA for the prospective choice of chemotherapy in patients with ovarian carcinoma.[25,31] In one nonrandomized study the CA was performed on tumor specimens from patients in relapse after primary combination chemotherapy. Twenty-four patients received drugs delineated as active

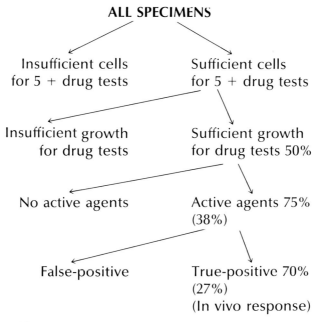

Figure. 18-3. *Clinical impact of the CA in ovarian carcinoma*

by the CA; twenty-eight, who had active drugs delineated by the CA, received empiric therapy. Objective response rates and survival were statistically significantly better in those patients whose therapy was directed by the CA than in either of the empirically treated groups (Table 18-2).[31] In a second study, patients were randomized to receive either cyclophosphamide, doxorubicin and platinum, or a three drug combination chosen by the CA as being the three most active agents. All patients had untreated stage III or IV ovarian carcinoma. Eligibility criteria for entry into the protocol included sufficient growth of the tumor in the CA to allow screening with a 10 drug chemotherapeutic agent panel (Table 18-3). Objective response rates were 85 percent using CA directed therapy and 64 percent using empiric CAP therapy.[25] Both of these studies suggest that the CA may indeed be a means of selecting active therapy for patients with ovarian carcinoma.

The results of the CA may, however, predict an inactive agent in nearly all specimens that grow sufficiently for evaluation (50 percent of all specimens). Although this negative information is less appealing than the

Table 18-2
CA Directed Therapy of Ovarian Carcinoma in Relapse after
Primary Combination Chemotherapy

Therapy*	HTSCA Best Drug(s) (1 drug—59%) (2 drugs—32%) (3 drugs—9%)	Empiric Drug(s) (Sensitive to one or more drugs in HTSCA)	Empiric Drug(s) (Sensitive to no drugs in HTSCA)
No. of Patients	24	28	31
Objective Responses (%)	55	19	16 (p < 0.01)
Survival (mo) (mean)	14 ± 3	6 ± 1	6 ± 1 (p < 0.02)
Response Duration (mo)	5.1	1.1	1.4

Adapted from Alberts DS, Leigh SA, Moon TE, et al: Improved survival for relapsing ovarian cancer (OV CA) patients (pts) using the human tumor clonogenic assay (HTCA) to select chemotherapy (CRx): An update. Abstracts IV conf on Hum Tumor Clon, abstr. 31, 1984.
* Not randomized, Clinical Measurable Disease.

identification of an active chemotherapeutic agent, the reliable prediction of failure to respond could significantly reduce toxicity and help in the selection of potentially active therapeutic agents by excluding inactive agents from clinical trials.

Although these data in diverse tumor types are encouraging and may hold similar promise for poorly differentiated neoplasms and CUP, proof that the results of drug screens performed with the CA are clinically relevant, have a salutary therapeutic impact, and are cost-effective can best be developed in prospective randomized studies. Such studies are in

Table 18-3
Ovarian Carcinoma: Primary Chemotherapy—Randomized
Prospective Comparison of Combination Chemotherapy
Chosen by CA vs CAP

Therapy	Best 3 Drugs HTSCA	Empiric CAP
Objective Response	17 (85%)	16 (64%)
Stable + Progressive Disease	3 (15%)	9 (36%)

Adapted from Welander Homesly HD, Jobson VW: Multiple factors predicting responses to combination chemotherapy in patients with ovarian cancers. Abstracts of the Fourth Human Tumor Cloning Conference, Tuscon, Arizona, 1984, abstract 29.
Eligibility: Stage III or IV Epithelial Ovarian Carcinoma. Successful HTSCA growth + 10 drug panel.

progress. Given the multiple problems inherent in the CA, it cannot be presently supported as a means for determining therapy. This caveat is supported in the case of PDCUP by the potentially dramatic and durable responses seen in patients that meet the criteria for "extragonadal germ cell cancer".[20,21] It is the belief of the authors that their therapy should consist of the Einhorn regimen, irrespective of in vitro results of the CA, since the value of CA in selecting or narrowing therapy for those patients or other patients with CUP is as yet unproven.

Results with Poorly Differentiated Neoplasms

The results of studies describing the predictive validity of drug activity testing in the CA in diverse tumor types[25,31] are promising but clearly hampered by technical features. Some data suggest that low plating efficiency may be less of a problem among PDCKP. Several tumor types, including head and neck carcinoma and lung cancer, appear to demonstrate higher plating efficiencies (PE) (more colonies formed for each 500,000 cells plated) for their poorly differentiated subtypes than for their well-differentiated ones.[33-35] This suggests that PDC and poorly differentiated CUP might have higher PEs than more differentiated tumors. One might anticipate that malignancies like PDC, which tend to grow rapidly in vivo, would have high relative clonogenicity and rapid growth rates in vitro which could facilitate their evaluability in the CA. This may not be the case, however, or may only occur if the appropriate in vitro environment (i.e., media, growth factors, cell to cell interactions) can be provided.

In an effort to evaluate this question and to assess the predictive accuracy of the CA in PDCUP, the 11,000 CA performed at the San Antonio Health Sciences Center and recorded in the computerized data bank were reviewed. Specimens obtained from patients with poorly differentiated neoplasms with no known primary disease sites were identified. Twenty-five specimens were identified in this manner, obtained from 20 individual patients. Specimens from 10 of these patients (50 percent) demonstrated growth (more than five colonies/500,000 cells plated) but only five of these specimens (25 percent) when cultured in the CA, produced sufficient colonies for drug assays (more than 30 colonies/500,000 cells plated). None of the patients whose drug activity could be assessed in vitro received any of the same antineoplastic agents in vivo subsequently. There are, therefore, no available correlations between in vivo and in vitro drug activities.

A literature review identified one report of 19 patients with CUP studied in the CA.[23] Four patients had undifferentiated carcinomas and many of the remaining 15 were poorly differentiated adenocarcinomas. All

19 cases reported had grown sufficiently in the CA to test drug activity, but the number of cases of CUP that did not grow was not delineated and the results of the group were analyzed as a whole allowing no separate evaluation of PDCUP. Overall chemoresponsiveness of the group was very low.

These data are very limited because of the small number of CA involved. While they cannot support any definitive conclusions they do spotlight specific problems and potentials. First of all, PDCUP may not demonstrate any dramatically greater PE in the CA, as currently performed, than other malignancies, despite their in vivo virulence. This may in part be the result of their biologic heterogeneity. It has become evident that different malignancies may require individualized approaches in the CA with reference to the media and techniques used and the criteria for interpreting growth. Examples of the individualization of techniques and media include the enhancement of clonogenicity of myeloma cells by vigorous T cell depletion and the addition of nonproliferating human fetal lung fibroblasts,[32,36] of lung cancer cells by utilizing the Courtney-Mills assay system,[37] and of small cell lung cancer (as opposed to large cell and adenocarcinoma) by the addition of red blood cells in the Courtney-Mills system.[37] Conditioned medium from a variety of sources and other media additives are being studied in a diversity of tumors to assess their ability to enhance clonogenicity.[38] Specific media may be developed that significantly enhance or unleash the in vitro clonogenicity of a particular malignancy, bridle the clonogenicity of another, and lead to selective culture systems. The methods used to interpret the growth that does occur may need to be individualized for specific malignancies. Such technical advances may improve the predictive accuracy of the assay and alter the percentage of studies with evaluable degrees of growth. Ovarian carcinoma colonies that grow in the CA, for example, seem to demonstrate a hierarchy of size that may relate to the clonogenic capacity of the cells that originate them, and therefore to their stem cell nature.[39] Large colonies may be more representative of the stem cell population than small ones. Counting large colonies alone (greater than 124 cells), for example, may provide more predictive assessments of chemosensitivity. Melanoma colonies in the CA, on the other hand, do not appear to have any such hierarchy and may require different interpretive techniques.[40]

Specific culture conditions and interpretive methods may need to be developed for different malignancies to maximize their clonogenicity and obtain the highest predictive accuracy of chemoresponsiveness. Since the malignancies encompassed by the terms PDC and CUP probably include tumors of diverse origins, these features may make consistent high levels of clonogenic activity difficult to achieve and thereby lessen the overall potential impact of CA results obtained. If media with significant specificity for a particular tumor type are developed the growth of an unknown tumor in a panel of these might provide evidence of the nature of the tumor. Further discriminating features may arise from other avenues of research.

The incidence of PDCUP described in the series (20 cases in 11,000) contrasts sharply with a higher incidence seen in another institution.[41] There are many variables that may produce marked differences in the incidence of a specific tumor type between two referral institutions, including different environs, referral patterns, and areas of research interest. In the case of poorly differentiated neoplasms the criteria for tumor classification are complex and interpretive and may vary among different institutions. These variations could produce cohorts of patients in several institutions composed of biologically different malignancies that carry the same diagnosis.

Results with Carcinomas of Unknown Primary Site

Our literature review identified one report detailing the use of the CA in CUP.[23] In this report the results of 19 patients whose CUP grew in the CA were reviewed. The total number of CUP placed in culture was not described. Four patients had undifferentiated carcinomas and many of the remaining 15 had poorly differentiated adenocarcinomas. Sensitivity was observed in only 6 (3.4 percent) of 178 drug assays (less than 30 percent survival colonies) although intermediate chemoresponsiveness (30 to 50 percent survival) was noted in 14 percent. The number of in vitro–in vivo comparisons were too small to comment on the predictive accuracy of the CA for clinical response but a high degree of in vitro drug resistance was noted. Among drugs studied in six or more tumors, only interferon (50–800 units of leukocyte, lymphoblastoid, and fibroblast) suggested sensitivity (equal or less than 30 percent colony survival) and only in 3.2 percent of cases, while intermediate activity (30–50 percent colony survival) was noted in greater than 25 percent of tumors studied with Bisantrene (26.6 percent), Vinblastine (28.5 percent), Mitomycin C (33.3 percent) and Melphalan (42.8 percent). Cisplatin produced only intermediate activity in 14.2 percent of tumors studied.

In an effort to further evaluate the impact of the CA on the selection of chemotherapy for patients with PDC and CUP, we reviewed the San Antonio data base of over 11,000 patients' malignancies studied in the CA. We identified 297 carcinomas of unknown primary site within this data base. Further classification was made on 167 malignancies: 144 as

Table 18-4

Growth of 297 Carcinomas of Unknown Primary Site (CUP) in
Soft Agar

Type of CUP	No. with $\geq$ 30 colonies/ Total Attempted	Percent Evaluable
Adenocarcinoma	67/144	47
Squamous cell	4/21	19
Small cell	0/2	0
CUP (could not be further classified)	43/130	33
Totals	114/297	38

adenocarcinomas, 21 as squamous cell carcinomas, and 2 as small cell
carcinomas, all with unknown primary sites. One hundred thirty malignancies could not be classified more definitively than as carcinomas of
unknown primary site (this does not mean that they are necessarily
PDCUP). Table 18-4 details the percent of tumors in each category with
adequate (more than 30 colonies) growth in soft agar. Thirty-eight percent
of the CUP plated (114 of 297) produced more than 30 colonies and were
evaluable for in vitro drug sensitivity. As noted in Table 18-4, CUP with
histological features of adenocarcinoma developed evaluable degrees of
growth most frequently (47 percent). Single agent treatment, based on the
results of the CA, was administered to 23 of the 114 patients whose tumors
were evaluable in the CA. Table 18-5 details the in vitro–in vivo correlations
in those 23 patients. As depicted in Table 18-5 the true positive rate for the
assay was 9/11 (82 percent) and the true negative rate 10/12 (83 percent).
These parameters of predictive validity are comparable with the in vitro–in
vivo correlations noted with other tumor types.[16]

Table 18-5

In Vitro and In Vivo Single Agent Comparisons for 23 Patients
with CUP

Total Correlations	Sensitive* In Vitro and In Vivo	Sensitive In Vitro, Resistant In Vivo	Resistant In Vitro, Sensitive In Vivo	Resistant In Vitro and In Vivo
23	9	2	2	10

* Sensitive in vitro is defined as $\leq$ 50 percent survival of tumor colony forming units while
in vivo responses are defined as partial or complete responses only.

Table 18-6
In Vitro Activity of Standard and Investigational Agents
Against Adenocarcinoma of Unknown Primary

Agent	Concentration (μg/ml)	No. $\leq$ 50% Survival/ No. Tested	% In Vitro Response
5 Flourouracil	6.0	7/39	15%
Adriamycin	0.04	4/41	9%
BCNU	0.30	2/9	22%
Bleomycin	0.10	0/5	0%
Chlorambucil	0.10	1/5	20%
DTIC	0.10	1/5	20%
Melphalan	0.10	4/38	10%
Mitomycin C	0.10	2/12	16%
Methotrexate	0.30	3/13	23%
Cisplatin	0.02	4/33	12%
Vincristine	0.05	1/10	10%
Vinblastine	0.05	14/40	35%
VP-16	0.30	1/5	20%
Fludarabine	1.0	3/10	30%
Bisantrene	0.5	6/22	27%
Mitoxantrone	0.05	1/8	12%
MGBG	0.10	3/8	37%
Echinomycin	0.001	4/11	36%
Tiazofurin	10.0	2/15	13%
Vinzolidine	0.05	6/6	100%

The CA, in addition to its potential use in identifying active antineoplastic agents for use in an individual patient, may also prove useful as a screening test evaluating the antineoplastic activity of new agents in specific tumor types. Table 18-6 details the in vitro responses noted with adenocarcinomas of unknown primary site in the CA to both standard and investigational antineoplastic agents (one hour exposure time). As noted in that table, the in vitro response rate to the conventional agents at clinically achievable concentrations are generally 20 percent or less. Vinblastine is a notable exception with an in vitro response rate of 35 percent. It is of interest that vinblastine is not commonly employed in adenocarcinoma of unknown primary site treatment regimens. Among the investigational drugs tested it is encouraging to note several with substantial in vitro activity against tumors in this category. Most notable are 30 percent or better response rates with the new nucleoside analog fludarabine (2-fluoro-ara-AMP), the new bifunctional intercalator echino-

Table 18-7
In Vitro Activity of Standard and Investigational Agents
Against Carcinoma of Unknown Primary which could not be
classified further

Agent	Concentration (μg/ml)	No. $\leq$ 50% Survival/ No. Tested	% In Vitro Response
5 Flourouracil	6.0	3/28	10%
Adriamycin	0.04	5/32	15%
BCNU	0.30	1/8	12%
Bleomycin	0.10	0/6	0%
Chlorambucil	0.10	2/6	33%
DTIC	0.10	1/3	33%
Melphalan	0.10	2/17	11%
Mitomycin C	0.10	1/14	7%
Methotrexate	0.30	0/5	0%
Cisplatin	0.02	1/17	5%
Vincristine	0.05	2/8	25%
Vinblastine	0.05	3/19	15%
Fludarabine	1.0	1/2	50%
Bisantrene	0.5	2/11	18%
Mitoxantrone	0.05	1/5	20%
MGBG	0.10	1/4	25%
Echinomycin	0.001	0/4	0%
Tiazofurin	10.0	0/8	0%
Vinzolidine	0.05	2/3	66%

mycin, the older agent MGBG (methylglyoxalbisguanylhydrazone), and the new vinca alkaloid, vinzolidine. All of these new agents should have a phase II trial in patients with adenocarcinoma with unknown primary sites. Table 18-7 details the in vitro responses to both standard and investigational agents noted for the CUP which could not be further classified.

Perspectives for Future Impact of the Clonogenic Assay and Tissue Culture Techniques on Poorly Differentiated Carcinoma

Much of the current enthusiasm surrounding the CA centers on its potential utility as an in vitro test to predict the chemoresponsiveness of a spontaneous human tumor in vivo. Although there are numerous problems surrounding the use of the CA as a clinical tool, the use of the CA and liquid media culture techniques as a research tool to study poorly differentiated neoplasms and CUP could produce many rewards. These techniques could clarify the pathobiology, genetics, growth rates, and nutritional requirements of these tumors. They could also allow investigation of the impact of growth factors on maintenance, evaluation of phase II agents, and evaluation of the mechanisms of drug resistance in these tumors. These data might allow subdivision of these heterogeneous tumor categories into groups with biologic, therapeutic, and prognostic relevance as well as provide insight into new avenues for therapy.

The CA may also provide a mechanism for assessing new or discarded antineoplastic agents for activity in these classes of malignancies (drug screening function).[42] This general concept is the basis of an National Cancer Institute Contract Study evaluating the CA as a means of rapidly developing Phase II data for new antineoplastic agents.[43-46] Data developed in the CA with new investigational and old agents has already been presented in CUP. These screening studies can be performed in the CA using a bank of human tumors cryopreserved as single cell suspensions or maintained in long-term cultures in liquid media.

The research applications of the CA are not limited to drug testing, however. It can provide basic biologic data characterizing the malignant cells involved. The CA provides a tumor-enriched cell population that divides actively. These populations can be used to perform cytogenetics without the confusion of normal fibroblasts common in liquid cultures, and without the frustrating inability to find a mitotic figure, a problem in direct samples from tumors.[47] The genetic features of small cell lines may be an important criterion for dividing them into clinically and biologically relevant subsets.[48] Specific genetic abnormalities are being described for increasing numbers of malignancies,[49] and the availability of methods to determine the presence or absence of oncogenes are increasingly more relevant.[49,50] As suggested in SCCL cell lines, these kinds of data may ultimately provide important information relevant to PDC and CUP.

The PE in the CA of SCCL[33,51] and several other tumors including breast cancer,[52,53] and head and neck cancer[54,55] appears to be of prognostic import. Higher plating efficiencies among these tumors are associated with clinically more aggressive disease. Among SCCL cell lines the PE in the CA can be used to aid in subsetting the lines into prognostically relevant categories with biologic differences.[48] Similar considerations may apply to CUP and PDC.

Growth requirements can be assessed utilizing the CA. These include hormonal agents, nutritional factors, and growth factors.[38,56] These approaches might lead to the development of new therapeutic options.

Perspectives: Liquid Media Culture

The CA is a cell culture system that visualizes a cell population with clonogenic capabilities; it has the advantage of prohibiting fibroblastic overgrowth. The constituent cells of a fresh specimen intuitively seem more representative of the natural tumor, despite the brutal manipulations and artificial environment of the CA, than a liquid media cell line that has suffered these pressures and separation from its native site for many passages. The CA has the disadvantage, however, of being a short-term (28-day) cell culture system. Initiating liquid media cultures from spontaneous tumors, on the other hand, is hampered by the overgrowth of fibroblasts which develop anchorage dependent growth on the culture flask floor. This fibroblast growth is prohibited by the underlayer in the double agar layer system of the CA. While long-term liquid media cell cultures have been initiated from colonies plucked from CA plates, these attempts are not consistently successful (10 percent),[57] and higher success rates have been achieved by some investigators, by directly plating prepared tumor specimens in liquid media.[58]

Small Cell Carcinoma of the Lung

The results and implications of research with SCCL in liquid media cell culture are relevant to PDN and CUP. This relevance is enhanced by certain clinical similarities between SCCL and PDCUP that satisfy criteria for the "extragonadal germ cell cancer syndrome." Both are undifferentiated histologically, clinically rapidly progressive, and usually fatal (median survival three to four months from diagnosis) if untreated, but have dramatic objective response rates (95 percent and 55 percent respectively) with appropriate therapy. The durable complete response rates in both malignancies, however, appears to be similar and low (10–15 percent).[59,60]

A serum-free medium (HITES) that selectively supports the growth of SCLC cells and not stromal cells has been developed.[61] Seventy-five percent of histologically positive SCCL specimens plated in this medium have demonstrated growth, compared to 44 percent of those plated in serum supplemented media.[57] Only one (a non-SCCL) of 20 other human tumors (including nine non-SCCL) grew in this medium.[57,59] The fact that only 10 percent of non-SCCL (NSCCL) grow in a media system that supports continued growth of SCCL 75 percent of the time demonstrates the selectivity of this media system. This research along with others has provided more than 50 SCCL cell lines for study.[62–64] Study of these cell lines disclosed several biologic subsets. The criteria for subsetting these cell lines include their growth characteristics (i.e., loose floating, tight floating, or adherent cell clusters), doubling times, presence and levels of c-myc oncogene and heavy staining regions, production of biomarkers (creatinine kinase-BB (CK-BB) neuron-specific enolase (NSE), bombesin (BN), and dopa decarboxylase (DDC), colony-forming efficiency in agarose, and tumorigenicity in nude mice. Differences between SCCL and NSCCL cell lines were also noted for epidermal growth factor (EGF) receptors, BN receptors, and gastrin releasing peptide (GRP) receptors. SCCL cells expressed high affinity receptors for BN/GRP[65] and may require BN/GRP as an autocrine growth factor.[66] On the basis of these criteria, SCCL cell culture lines could be divided into classical, variant and, multipotent groups[51] and distinguished from NSCCL malignancies.[48] These data are intriguing from several points of view and suggest many areas of research to evaluate poorly differentiated neoplasms and CUP. First, HITES medium (serum-free) appears to provide a culture system that is fairly selective for SCCL. Similar serum-free selective media are being devised for other malignancies.[67] Serum-free media remove the "indispensible" but undefinable and nonspecific "black box" from the culture system; their selectivity might thus provide a means of distinguishing between tumor types. Perhaps, for example, UM could be segregated using their growth in selective media and other probes into PDL, PDC, PDS. Second, other biologic features of the SCCL cell lines, biomarkers, growth patterns, and genetic features were found to be useful to categorize them into subsets that appear clinically and therapeutically relevant. Third, the ability to grow SCCL in serum-free media provides a model in which substances can be evaluated for activity as growth factors. Different serum lots may contain a diverse assortment and varying concentrations of growth inhibitors or stimulators that complicate these assays. Fourth, this research has provided insight into the genesis and interrelationships of SCCL and NSCCL. Multipotent cell lines demonstrated in vitro "differentiation" and developed morphologies consistent with adenocarcinoma and squamous cell carcinoma. This in vitro data is an intriguing parallel to clinically observed morphologic alterations in SCCL which include the appearance of large cell carcinoma, squamous cell carcinoma (keratin-positive), and adenocarcinoma (mucin-positive) in biopsy specimens of some patients with SCCL and recurrent malignant disease.[68] The NSCCL cells of the multipotent lineages, however, displayed (or retained) certain features suggestive of SCCL ancestry which included presence of the del (3) (pl4-23) chromosomal marker, higher PE in the CA, high specific activities of CK-BB and intermediate levels of NSE.[69] These data have suggested that SCCL and NSCCL might all arise from a common precursor in the bronchial epithelium.[48] Fifth, cellular alterations associated with disease progression and drug resistance have been described using these cell lines. Variant SCCL lines were more resistant to chemotherapy and radiotherapy in vivo than classical SCCL lines. Many of these variant SCCL lines exhibited double minute chromosomes or homogeneous staining regions representative of gene amplification, 20 to 50 fold amplifications of c-myc DNA and high levels of m-RNA.[48] These same lines had a higher plating efficiency in the CA and enhanced tumorigenicity in nude mice. These alterations may represent biologic adaptations that translate clinically into progressive and resistant disease. Finally, new areas for antineoplastic therapy are suggested by these studies. These currently include monoclonal antibodies directed against BN/GRP receptors, approaches to reverse c-myc oncogene amplification, and the use of established cell lines in the CA to identify appropriate therapy for the patient from whom the specimen came. Biomarkers identified by these studies are being evaluated in prospective clinical trials in patients with lung cancer to study their prognostic value.[48]

Since poorly differentiated neoplasms and CUP are heterogeneous categories of malignancies, they are likely to demonstrate a diversity of biologic features if evaluated in similar systems. These diverse biologic features may allow clinically relevant subsets to be identified. These techniques could also provide insight into the mechanisms of drug resistance and the genesis of these malignancies.

Ovarian Carcinoma

A series of long-term cell lines has been developed from patients with untreated ovarian carcinoma (OC).[70] Biologic features of these cell lines have been investigated including their responsiveness to antineoplastic agents, patterns of cross resistance, karyotype, capacity for substrate independent growth, tumorigenicity in athymic mice, and steroid hormone receptor status.[70] These cell lines are of special interest because they can now function as probes in well-characterized in vivo animal model systems (i.e., subcutaneous xenografts and intraperitoneal implantation in nude mice) to further clarify the biologic characteristics of OC and methods of drug resistance in OC.[70] If the mechanisms by which a malignant cell becomes drug resistant can be identified, methods to overcome that resistance may be devised. The investigation of melphalan resistance in OC, analyzed using these cell lines, is one example. Gluthathione levels have been noted to be elevated in resistant cell lines. In vitro resistance can be reversed by growing the cells in cysteine-free media or by a specific inhibitor of glutathione synthesis.[71] These results are potentially clinically relevant.

Summary

Contemporary oncologic therapy can produce curative or useful palliative results for patients with many types of malignancy. The selection of appropriate therapy is essential and is predicated upon identifying the site of origin of the malignancy and its morphology. This image of the malignancy, focused by other features including stage and clinical performance status, coarsely describes its natural history and pattern of response to antineoplastic agents. Poorly differentiated neoplasms and CUP, by depriving the oncologist of more specific data on morphology and site of origin, limit the ability to select appropriate treatment and can cripple therapeutic efforts. Certain clinical features of these malignancies can be used to guide therapy. For example, PDCUP that fit the "extragonadal germ cell cancer syndrome" (as discussed by Hainsworth and Greco elsewhere in this book), should, in the opinion of the authors, be treated with Einhorn's regimen, since dramatic objective responses may occur. Durable objective responses occur in 10–15 percent of patients whose prognosis otherwise would be dismal.[59,60] Among other patients with CUP, clinical and pathological features can be used to narrow therapeutic options, but objective response rates are low. Patients with other PDN provide similar difficulties in selecting therapy.

Cell culture methods, including the CA and liquid media culture systems could potentially assist the clinician either by determining in vitro the responsiveness of the malignancy (whether or not its type were known) to antineoplastic therapy, or by identifying the nature of the malignancy more clearly. The CA, as evaluated in diverse tumor types, is reasonably accurate at predicting in vivo chemoresponsiveness, but its impact is diluted by technical problems.[11,16,24-26] Data supporting the use of the CA as a means of selecting therapy for patients with ovarian carcinoma is developing, but these studies contain only small numbers of patients and may or may not be relevant to other tumor types such as poorly differentiated neoplasms or CUP.[25,31] Individualized methods may be required for studying different types of malignancy in the CA. Insufficient data is available to characterize the growth patterns of PDCUP in the CA using contemporary methodology. In a small series of 20 cases, reported herein, the PE of PDCUP appeared to be low in the CA. Sufficient colony formation to test drug activity (greater than 30 colonies/500,000 cells plated) occurred in only 25 percent of the cases. If these low PEs are verified, initial research efforts should be directed at improving the PE. No in vivo–in vitro comparisons of drug activity could be made. There is no available data regarding the use of the CA in evaluating PDL or PDS. Thirty-eight percent of 297 CUP developed evaluable degrees of growth in the CA, as reported herein, and the predictive accuracy of the CA was comparable to that reported in larger studies including diverse tumor types, however, the same problems remain.[16,24] Although recent data generated in patients with ovarian carcinoma is suggestive, there is no conclusive proof that the CA directed therapy offers any advantage over empirically selected therapy in any malignancy.

The CA may also provide a system in which to test the activity of old and new investigational agents. Such a screen performed in small numbers of patients with CUP demonstrated that more than 30 percent of cases were sensitive in vitro to several new agents including fludarabine, echinomycin, and vinzolidine as well as the older agents, MGBG and vinblastine. These screening studies may be utilized to identify agents that warrant clinical trials.

Cell culture methods, including the CA and long-term liquid media cultures ultimately may have greater impact on the therapy of malignancies by providing basic biologic data. Contemporary cell culture research in SCCL demonstrates this point. SCCL lineages, grown in liquid culture, can be segregated into biologically, prognostically, and therapeutically relevant subsets on the basis of in vitro biologic parameters.[48,51] SCCL, which appear morphologically indistinguishable at present when biopsied may be further distinguished with regard to biology, natural history, prognosis, and responsiveness using these subsets.[48,51] These methods offer the hope that tumor categories which are clearly heterogeneous but cannot currently be further classified morphologically (i.e., PDN and CUP) might be segregated into relevant subsets using biologic criteria. Features that can be evaluated utilizing the CA and liquid culture methods are multiple and include clonogenicity, drug activity, patterns of drug cross resistance, radiation responsiveness, karyotypes, biomarker (i.e., NSE, DDC and BN) elaboration, tumorigenicity in nude mice, media requirements (i.e., hormonal and mineral), and growth factors. Simple and useful tests, perhaps centering on genetic abnormalities, biomarkers, or selective growth media, may emerge allowing these tumors to be segregated into clinically relevant subgroups enhancing the specificity and sensitivity of current morphologic categorization.

References

1. Steel GG: Cell kinetics and cell survival, in Bagshawe KD (ed): Medical Oncology—Medical Aspects of Malignant Disease. Oxford, Blackwell Scientific Publications, 1975, p 49

2. Laftha LG: Stem cell concepts, in Potten CS (ed): Stem Cells, Their Identification and Characterisation. New York, Churchill Livingstone, 1983, p 1

3. Lord BI: Haemopoietic stem cells, in Potten CS (ed): Stem Cells, Their Identification and Characterisation. New York, Churchill Livingstone, 1983, p 118

4. Potten CS, Hendry JH: Stem cells in murine small intestine, in Potten CS (ed): Stem Cells, Their Identification and Characterisation. New York, Churchill Livingstone, 1983, p 155

5. Pike BS, Robinson WA: Human bone marrow colony growth in agar-gel. J Cell Pysiol 76:77, 1970

6. Metcalf D: In vitro cloning techniques for hematopoietic cells: clinical applications. Am Int Med 7:483, 1977

7. Hill RP, Bush RS: A lung colony assay to determine the radiosensitivity of the cells of a solid tumor. Int J Rad Biol 15:435, 1969

8. Brown CH, Carbone PP: In vitro growth of normal and leukemic human bone marrow. J Natl Can Inst 46:989, 1971

9. Buick RN, MacKillop WJ: Measurement of self-renewal in culture of clonogenic cells from human ovarian carcinoma. Brit J Can 44:349–355, 1981

10. Thomson SP, Meyskens FL: Method for measurement of self-renewal capacity of clonogenic cells from biopsies of metastatic human malignant melanoma. Cancer Res 42:4606–4613, 1982

11. Salmon SE, Hamburger AW, Soehnlen B, et al: Quantitation of differential sensitivity of human tumor stem cells to anti-cancer drugs. N Engl J Med 298:1321–1327, 1978

12. Von Hoff DD, Casper J, Bradley E, et al: Association between human tumor colony-forming assay results and response of an individual patient's tumor to chemotherapy. Am J Med 70:1027–1032, 1981

13. Carney DN, Gazdar AF, Bunn PA, et al: Demonstration of the stem cell nature of clonogenic cells from lung cancer patients. Stem Cells 1:149–164, 1981

14. Sandbach J, Von Hoff DD, Clark G, et al: Direct cloning of human breast cancer in soft agar culture. Cancer 50:1315–1321, 1982

15. Von Hoff DD, Forseth B, Metelmann HR, et al: Direct cloning of human malignant melanoma in soft agar. Cancer 50:696–701, 1982

16. Von Hoff DD, Clark GM, Stogdill BJ, et al: Prospective clinical trial of human tumor cloning system. Cancer Res 43:1926–1931, 1983

17. Alberts DS, Salmon SE, Chen HS, et al: In vitro clonogenic assay for predicting response of ovarian cancer to chemotherapy. Lancet 2:340–342, 1980

18. Azar HA, Espinoza CG, Richman AV, et al: "Undifferentiated" large cell malignancies; an ultra-structural and immunocytochemical study. Hum Pathol 13:323–333, 1982

19. Gyorkey F, Min KW, Krisko I: The usefulness of electron microscopy in the diagnosis of human tumors. Hum Pathol 6:421, 1975

20. Greco FA, Oldham RK, Fer M: The extragonadal germ cell cancer syndrome. Sem Oncol 9:448–456, 1982

21. Richardson RL, Schoumacher RA, Fer M, et al: The unrecognized germ cell cancer syndrome. Ann Int Med 94:181–186, 1981

22. Silverman C, Marks JE: Metastatic cancer of unknown origin: epidermoid and undifferentiated carcinomas. Sem Oncol 9:435–441, 1982

23. Greenberg BR, Salmon SE: Human tumor clonogenic assay in patients with unknown primary carcinomas. J Clin Oncol 2:46–50, 1984

24. Salmon SE, Von Hoff DD: In vitro evaluation of anti-cancer drugs with the human tumor stem cell assay. Sem Oncol 8:377–385, 1981

25. Welander CE, Holmesley HD, Jobson VW: In vitro chemotherapy testing of gynecologic tumors: basis for planning therapy? Am J Ob Gyn 147:188–195, 1983

26. Grosh WW: unpublished data

27. Salmon SE: Preclinical and clinical application of chemosensitivity testing. Abstracts IV Conf on Hum Tumor Clon, abstr. 28, 1984

28. Kern DH, Bertelsen CA, Tanigawa N, et al: Heterogeneity of chemosensitivity response of human tumors. Abstracts IV Conf on Hum Tumor Clon, abstr. 8, 1984

29. Ajani JA, Sahu SK, Spitzer G, et al: Prospective study of human tumor stem cell assay with correlation between in vitro sensitivity and number of drugs tested. Abstracts IV Conf on Hum Tumor Clon, abstr. 41, 1984

30. Moon TE, Salmon SE, White CS, et al: Quantitative association between the invitro human tumor stem cell assay and clinical response to cancer chemotherapy. Cancer Chemother Pharmacol 6:211–218, 1981

31. Alberts DS, Leigh SA, Moon TE, et al: Improved survival for relapsing ovarian cancer (OV CA) patients (pts) using the human tumor

clonogenic assay (HTCA) to select chemotherapy (CRx): An update. Abstracts IV Conf on Hum Tumor Clon, abstr. 31, 1984

32. Selby P, Buick RN, Tannock I: A critical appraisal of the "Human tumor stem-cell assay". New Engl J Med 298:1321–1327, 1978

33. Callahan SK, Coltman CA, Kitten C, et al: Tumor cloning assay: application and potential usefulness in lung cancer management, in Greco FA (ed): Biology and Management of Lung Cancer, New York, Martinas Nijhoff Publishers, 1983, pp 51–72

34. Kish JA, Crissman JD, Haas C, et al: Parameters for predicting growth of squamous head and neck tumors in the human tumor stem cell assay. Proc AACR 24:10, 1983

35. Mattox DE, Von Hoff DD: Culture of human head and neck cancer stem cells using soft agar. Arch Otolaryngol 106:672–674, 1980

36. Durie BGM, Christiansen JA, Vela EE: Recent observations on enhanced cloning of multiple myeloma in vitro. Abstracts IV Conf on Hum Tumor Cloning, abstr. 15, 1984

37. Twentyman PR, Walls GA: Factors influencing the clonogenicity of human lung cancer cells. Abstracts IV Conf on Hum Tumor Clon, abstr. 50, 1984

38. Spitzer G, Umbach G, Tomasovic B, et al: Conditioned media (CM) and tissue culture supplements (TCS) for in vitro growth of human tumors. Abstracts IV Conf on Hum Tumor Clon, abstr. 57, 1984

39. Buick RN: Aspects of the cell renewal hierarchy in human ovarian carcinoma. Abstracts IV Conf on Hum Tumor Clon, abstract 1, 1984

40. Meyskens FL Jr, Thomson SP, Moon TE: Self-renewal of melanoma colonies in agar: similar colony formation from replating primary colonies of different sizes. Abstracts IV Conf on Hum Tumor Clon, abstr. 2, 1984

41. Greco FA: personal communication

42. Carney DN, Gazdar AF, Minna JD: In vitro chemosensitivity of clinical specimens and cell lines of small cell lung cancer. Proc ASCO abstr. C-37, 1982

43. Shoemaker R, Wolpert-DeFilippes M, Kern D, et al: Recent results of new drug screening trials with a human tumor colony forming assay (HTCFA). Abstracts IV Conf on Hum Tumor Clon, abstr. 32, 1984

44. Lathan B, Von Hoff DD, Clark GM: Comparison of in vitro prediction and clinical outcome for two anthracene derivatives: mitoxantrone and bisantrene. Abstracts IV Conf on Hum Tumor Clon, abstr. 33, 1984

45. Salmon SE: Preclinical and clinical application of chemosensitivity testing. Abstracts IV Conf on Hum Tumor Clon, abstr. 28, 1984

46. Lathan B, Von Hoff DD, Melink TJ, et al: Screening of Phase I drugs in the human tumor cloning system (HTCS) to pinpoint areas of emphasis in Phase II studies. Abstracts IV Conf on Hum Tumor Clon, abstr. P27, 1984

47. Trent JM, Crossen PE: Cytogenetic and cytokinetic analysis of human tumor colony forming cells (TCFUs). Abstracts IV Conf on Hum Tumor Clon, abstr. 11, 1984

48. Minna JD: The Richard and Hinda Rosenthal Foundation Award Lecture: Recent advances of potential clinical importance in the biology of lung cancer. Proc AACR 25:393–394, 1984

49. Bloomfield CD, (Chairperson) Trent JM, Chapelle A (Panelists): Recent Advances in Cytogenetics: Educational Symposium and Workshops. ASCO Educational Symposium and Workshop Booklet, 1984, pp 57–65

50. Schimke RT: Gene amplification, drug resistance and cancer. Cancer Res 44:1735–1742, 1984

51. Carney DN, Dazdar AF, Nau M, et al: Prognostic implications of the biological heterogeneity of cultured cell lines (CL) from patients with small cell lung cancer (SCLC). Abstracts IV Conf on Hum Tumor Clon, abstr. 7, 1984

52. Aapro MS, Schafer P, Cillo C: Colony growth and patient survival in primary or metastatic breast cancer. Abstracts IV Conf on Hum Tumor Clon, abstr. 30, 1984

53. Rashid R, Hug V, Spitzer F, et al: Correlation of in vitro growth characteristics of human breast carcinoma with their histological grading. Abstracts IV Conf on Hum Tumor Clon, abstr. P8, 1984

54. Kish JA, Crissman J, Haas C, et al: Growth predictive parameters in the HTSCA for squamous cell carcinoma of the head and neck. Abstracts IV Conf on Hum Tumor Clon, abstr. 59, 1984

55. Johns ME, Mills SE: Cloning efficiency: A possible prognostic indicator in squamous cell carcinoma of the head and neck. Cancer 52:1401–1404, 1983

56. Todaro GJ, Fryling CM, DeLavco JE: Transforming growth factors produced by certain human tumor cells: Polypeptides that interact with epidermal growth factor receptors. Proc Natl Acad Sci 77:5258–5262, 1980

57. Carney DN, Broder L, Edelstein M, et al: Experimental studies of the biology of human small cell lung cancer. Cancer Treat Rep 67:27–35, 1983

58. Matern J, Volm M: Clinical relevance of predictive tests for cancer chemotherapy. Cancer Treat Rev 9:267–298, 1982

59. Carney DS, Gazdar AF, Oie HK, et al: The invitro growth and characterization of small cell lung cancer, in Greco FA (ed): Biology and Management of Lung Cancer. Boston, Martinus Nijhoff, 1983, p 1–24

60. Greco FA, Oldham RK: Clinical management of patients with small cell lung cancer, in Greco FA, Oldham RK, Bunn PA (eds): Small Cell Lung Cancer. New York, Grune & Stratton, 1981, p 353–379

61. Carney DN, Bunn PA, Gazdar AF, et al: Selective growth in serum-free hormone supplemented medium of tumor cells obtained by biopsy from patients with small cell carcinoma of the lung. Proc Natl Acad Sci USA 78:3185–3189, 1981

62. Hayashi I, Sato G: Replacement of serum by hormones permits the growth of cells in a defined medium. Nature 259:132–134, 1976

63. Ham RG, McKeehan WL: in Jacoby WB, Pastan IH (eds): Methods in Enzymology, vol. 43. New York, Academic Press, 1979, pp 44–93

64. Barnes D, Sato G: Methods for growth of cultured cells in serum-free medium. Ann Biochem 102:255–270, 1980

65. Moody TM, Pert CB, Gazdar AF, et al: High levels of intracellular bombesin characterize human small cell lung cancer. Science 214; 1246–1248, 1981

66. Cuttita F, Carney DN, Mulshine J, et al: Anti-idiotypic antibodies (AIA) which block bombesin receptor interaction of human small cell lung cancer. Proc AACR 25:864, 1984

67. Murakami H, Masui H: Hormonal control of human colon carcinoma cell growth in serum-free medium. Proc Natl Acad Sci, USA 77:3464–3468, 1980

68. Fer M, Grosh WW, Greco FA: Morphologic changes in small cell lung cancer, in Greco FA (ed): Biology and Management of Lung Cancer. Boston: Martinus Nijhoff, 1983, p 109

69. Minna JD, Carney DN, Alvarez R, et al: Heterogeneity and homogeneity of human small cell lung cancer, in Owens AH Jr, Coffey DS, Baylin SB (ed): Tumor Cell Heterogeneity—Origins and Implications. New York, Academic Press, 1982, p 51

70. Hamilton TC, Young RC, Ozols RF: Novel in vivo and in vitro models for the study of ovarian cancer (OC). Abstracts IV Conf on Hum Tumor Clon, abstr. 44, 1984

71. Ozols RF, Green JA, Vistica DT, et al: Reversal of melphalan (E) resistance (R) in human (GSH) levels. Abstracts IV Conf on Hum Tumor Clon, abstr. 38, 1984

19

HORMONE RECEPTORS IN HUMAN MALIGNANCY OF UNKNOWN ORIGIN: POTENTIAL UTILITY IN CLINICAL MANAGEMENT

John S. Meyer

Identification of receptors for hormones has had a great impact on the understanding of endocrine physiology and has been translated into advances in the management of breast carcinoma. After Jensen and coworkers described estrogen receptors in breast carcinomas in 1967,[47] evidence that presence of estrogen receptor (ER) predicted hormonal responsiveness accumulated rapidly.[76] Shortly thereafter, Knight and coworkers showed that ER was predictive of the short-term course of primary breast carcinoma, and that patients with ER-negative carcinomas were at relatively high risk for early relapse.[57] Subsequently, a number of studies have confirmed that ER is predictive of the short-term course of breast carcinoma, although chiefly for axillary node-positive rather than node-negative patients. The same relationships also apply to progesterone receptor,[17,105] which has prognostic significance chiefly in the node-positive group of patients. Not all studies have shown, however, that progesterone receptor assay results are prognostic.[5,43]

Other receptors that have been detected on breast carcinoma include

POORLY DIFFERENTIATED NEOPLASMS AND TUMORS OF UNKNOWN ORIGIN ISBN 0-8089-1755-2
© 1986 by Grune & Stratton.

androgen (dihydrotestosterone) receptors (AR)[111,123] in approximately 20 percent of carcinomas, and glucocorticoid receptors in 33–50 percent of carcinomas.[3,107] Prolactin receptors (PlR) are present in many experimental mammary gland carcinomas,[20] and prolactin is necessary for in vitro development of mouse mammary gland and mammary gland carcinomas.[84,89,112] Insulin also is necessary for in vitro growth of mammary tissues.[50,89,112] Oka and Topper presented evidence that insulin, not prolactin, may be a direct mitogen for mammary gland epithelium, with prolactin acting to sensitize the epithelium to insulin.[88] By use of a dehydrogenase assay as a measure of stimulation of breast carcinoma explants in vitro, 32 percent were shown to be prolactin-dependent,[97] and growth hormone was required for the prolactin effect.[26]

PlR, located within the cell membranes, has been detected in approximately 50 percent of breast carcinomas.[13,90] A weak correlation between presence of PlR and ER and PgR exists.[13] PlR has not found a role in management of breast carcinoma because it has not correlated well with clinical or pathologic features.[13] Prolactin failed to stimulate DNA synthesis of human breast carcinomas in vitro,[119] although it is necesary for induction and maintenance of many mammary carcinomas of rats and mice. Plasma prolactin levels have not consistently been different between breast carcinoma patients and controls,[14,87] although some studies have shown increased levels in breast carcinoma patients.[95]

Receptor Analysis and Interpretation of Results

The Nature of Receptors

Receptors have three distinguishing characteristics: (1) Specificity for a particular class of ligands as defined by physiologic effect. Examples of different classes are estrogens, progestins, glucocorticoids, mineralocorticoids, and androgens. (2) High affinity for the specific ligands. (3) Saturability, which results from the presence of only a limited number of high affinity binding sites. Saturability can be demonstrated by prevention of radioligand binding by a relatively small excess of unlabeled ligand.

The position of receptors within the cell depends on the diffusability of its specific ligands. Lipid-soluble steroid hormones can diffuse through cell membranes, and their receptors are found within the cell sap. Polypeptides lack diffusability into the cell, and their receptors are found attached to the cell membranes. For a review of physiology of steroid hormonal receptors, see Chan and O'Malley[15] and Baxter and Funder.[7] In brief, steroid hormones are thought to stimulate cells through the following series of events. The steroid diffuses through the cell membrane and binds to receptor within the cytoplasm or nucleus. If bound in the cytoplasm, the receptor-hormone complex translocates to the nucleus where it binds to chromatin. The result is stimulation of messenger RNA synthesis with subsequent protein synthesis within the cytoplasm. In certain tissues such as mammary epithelium and endometrium, this may lead to cell division. The sequence is different for polypeptide hormone receptor interaction. The complex remains in the cell membrane, and the effect on intracellular constituents is mediated by second messengers, for example, cyclic adenosine monophosphate.

Methods of Analysis and Interpretation

Virtually all steroid hormonal receptor assays now are being done by use of radiolabeled ligands. Most steroid receptor assays have been performed on the soluble cytoplasmic component (cytosol) obtained by ultracentrifugation of the homogenized tumor. Fewer studies have utilized nuclei.[59,121] Results of the nuclear assay usually agree with those of the cytosol assay, but nuclear binding may predict hormonal response better than cytoplasmic binding.[59,64]

The assays depend on some method of separating receptor-bound ligand from unbound ligand prior to determination of bound radioactivity (Table 19-1). The methods commonly used are dextran-charcoal, hydroxylapatite, and ultracentrifugation in a sucrose gradient. Dextran-charcoal absorbs unbound and weakly bound ligand, and it is removed by centrifugation prior to counting bound radioactivity. Hydroxylapatite binds the receptor-ligand complex, allowing the unbound radioactivity to pass through the column. Different assay methods have their own particular advantages or disadvantages. For example, oxidation products of estradiol may not be absorbed by dextran-charcoal, and the tyrosinase oxidation products of tritiated estradiol have been misinterpreted as ER in the dextran-charcoal assay.[74,122] This problem is circumvented by hydroxylapatite, to which the oxidation products of estrogen do not bind, and by sucrose gradient ultracentrifugation which leaves the oxidation products in the supernatant. The nonresponsiveness of melanoma to antiestrogenic therapy underscores the impression that the supposed ER is artefact.[22]

Another potential problem is misinterpretation of the serum sex steroid binding globulin (SSBG) as ER. The dextran-charcoal assay will not reliably distinguish between these two binding proteins. In sucrose gradients, ER sediments at 4S and 8S, whereas SSBG sediments at 4S, and SSBG

Table 19-1
Methods of Assay of Steroidal Receptors

Method	Advantages	Disadvantages
Dextran-charcoal, single point	Simplicity	Does not distinguish high from low affinity
Dextran-charcoal, Scatchard plot	Quantitative, measures affinity	Does not distinguish 8S and 4S moieties, or ER from SSBG
Hydroxylapatite, Scatchard plot	Quantitative, measures affinity. Eliminates interference from ligand metabolites.	
Gel electrophoresis	Separates ER from other binders such as SSBG. Distinguishes 8S from 4S.	Expensive, time-consuming
Gradient centrifugation	Distinguishes 8S and 4S binders. Eliminates interference from ligand metabolites.	Expensive, time-consuming
Immunoassay	High sensitivity, specificity, can be done on frozen microsections	Still under development. Must be validated against standard binding assays and hormonal therapy response rates.
Fluoresceinated estradiol histochemical assay	Can be done on microsections	Requires supersaturating concentrations of fluoresceinated ligand. Never proven to be specific for receptor proteins.

482

and ER can also be separated by electrophoresis. SSBG often contaminates breast carcinoma cytosols,[86] but the contamination does not appear to be sufficient to produce false-positive assays in breast carcinoma cytosols.[83]

A great deal of effort has been expended on development of histochemical methods to reveal steroid hormonal receptors which would permit assay of small amounts of material such as needle biopsies or cytologic preparations. Unfortunately, the histochemical methods have foundered because attachment of marker molecules such as fluorescein to the steroid ligands has invariably reduced their affinity for the receptors. This, together with the low content of the receptors within cells, has necessitated use of supersaturating concentrations of the labeled ligands. The result has been nonspecific binding and poor correlation with standard biochemical assays.[6,61,73,91,110] Further evidence of the invalidity of these methods comes from their inability to identify breast carcinomas that will respond to hormonal therapy.[72] When adapted to flow cytometry, histochemical assays may give more reliable results. The high intensity laser beam available in the flow cytometer enables the concentration of ligand to be reduced below saturating levels, rendering the conditions of the assay more like those of the biochemical assay.[113] Further investigation will show whether this approach is clinically useful.

The recent availability of antibodies to ER offers the prospect of a valid immunohistochemical assay.[35,93] Preliminary studies with a monoclonal antibody have shown excellent correlation between visualization of receptor binding by frozen section immunofluorescence or immunoperoxidase and the biochemical assay.[25] Results thus far have been poor with paraffin-embedded, formalin-fixed sections.

Besides the SSBG, other nonreceptor proteins capable of binding steroid hormones may be present in tumors. Kesterson reported a 4S nonsaturable estrogen and progesterone binder in cystosarcoma phyllodes.[54] Whether a progesterone binding protein commonly present in meningiomas is truly a progesterone receptor is controversial, with results of one study indicating that it is specific for progestins,[9] whereas another study found that the protein also bound estradiol-17β, diethylstilbestrol, dihydrotestosterone, and dexamethasone.[99] This wide range of binding clearly would place it outside the definition of a progesterone receptor. These experiences warrant careful evaluation of reports of steroid hormonal receptors in tumors, particularly tumors of organs that do not display obvious endocrine responsiveness. Before a steroid binding protein can be considered to qualify as a receptor it should demonstrate, as a minimum, saturability, specificity, and high affinity for the ligand. The case would be further strengthened by demonstration of nuclear binding of

the receptor-ligand complex, and by evidence of a biochemical or morphologic response to the ligand. These conditions are met by but few reports
of receptors discovered in human tumors, and until they are met such
"receptors" should be accepted as receptor-candidates only.

Problems with Sampling

Heterogeneity within tumors can complicate the interpretation of
results of receptor assays. Allegra noted concordance of results of ER
assays from multiple metastatic sites of breast carcinoma in 85 percent of 27
patients.[2] Results of assay of the primary breast carcinoma agreed with
later results on recurrent or metastatic carcinoma in 83 percent of 23
patients.[10] A similar rate of agreement is achieved when results of assays
on paired samples of primary breast carcinomas and primary versus
axillary metastases are compared. Receptor-negative primary lesions followed by receptor-positive metastases can be accounted for by sampling
error or relatively low cellularity of some forms of primary breast carcinoma
in comparison to their metastases.[82] Davis noted agreement between
central and peripheral samples of breast carcinomas assayed for ER and
PgR in 87 percent of 30 cases.[23] Harland noted agreement in 89 percent of
synchronous multiple ER assays on 38 patients, 87 percent of synchronous
multiple PgR assays in 38 patients, 77 percent of asynchronous ER assays
in 88 patients, and 70 percent of asynchronous PgR assays in 87 patients.[40]
When therapy has intervened between sampling of the primary tumor and
sampling of a metastasis, a lesser degree of concordance can be expected.[41]
One cause of disconcordance may be selection of receptor-negative variants during hormonal therapy. Both receptor-positive and receptor-
negative stemlines may exist in tumors even before therapy. Prey noted
clonal heterogeneity in two of eight primary breast carcinomas by flow
cytometric DNA measurements.[92] These observations indicate a risk that
receptor assays on any one sample from a tumor may not be representative
of other areas of the tumor or of other metastatic sites.

Effects of Prior Therapy on Receptors

High levels of specific circulating steroids can be expected to reduce
the amounts of assayable receptors by competition with the ligand.
Possibly for this reason, breast carcinomas assayed during pregnancy
seldom are positive for ER or PgR,[117] and high circulating estrogen levels
are associated with low levels of ER in tumors of premenopausal women.[83]
Similar decreases in ER and PgR occur in the normal endometrium and

endometrial carcinoma during treatment with progestins.[46] In the normal endometrium, both ER and PgR decline during the progestational phase.[8] Tamoxifen therapy for one to four weeks usually resulted in a decrease in cytosol in ER within breast carcinomas, and had variable effects on cytosol PgR.[118] Progestational therapy of endometrial carcinomas resulted in nuclear translocation of PgR and disappearance of PgR from the cytosol within one week.[68] Cytotoxic chemotherapy did not appear to affect ER content in breast carcinoma.[56] In evaluating receptor assay results on metastatic tumors, these effects of physiologic hormonal variation and therapeutic use of hormones need to be considered.

Steroid Hormonal Receptor Assay Results in Specific Tumors

Breast Carcinomas

Approximately 60 percent of breast carcinomas contain appreciable amounts of ER, and approximately 50 percent contain PgR (Tables 19-2 and 19-3). ER and PgR are less likely to be present in tumors with anaplastic nuclei and with rapid proliferative rates than in more slowly proliferative carcinomas with lesser nuclear anaplasia.[80] For example, medullary carcinomas are seldom receptor-positive. Infiltrating lobular carcinomas, although they are poorly differentiated in that they form no glandular structure and infiltrate in a single cell pattern, are commonly receptor-positive. Given a metastatic adenocarcinoma or poorly differentiated carcinoma with minimal nuclear anaplasia that is receptor-negative, breast carcinoma could be ruled out with some security provided hormonal therapy had not recently been given that might affect the receptor status. If the nuclei were highly anaplastic, negative receptor values would not be evidence against origin in the breast.

Glucocorticoid receptor (GCR) is present in many breast carcinomas, and two types of glucocorticoid binders have been detected. One binder resembles the plasma binding protein, transcortin, in its 4S sedimentation coefficient and relatively low affinity ($Kd = 10^{-8}$ mole/liter). This high capacity binder binds cortisol but not fluorinated glucocorticoids and appears to act as an intracellular reservoir for cortisol. A low capacity, 8S binding protein with a $Kd = 10^{-9}$ mole/liter is less often present and is considered to be a true glucocorticoid receptor. It binds both cortisol and fluorinated glucocorticoids such as dexamethasone.[31] Presence of GCR in breast carcinoma is highly correlated with presence of ER.[4,31]

Table 19-2
Estrogen Receptor Assay Results in Various Tumors

Tumor	Reference	Assay method	No. cases	Positive No.	Positive %
Breast carcinoma primary	59	1, 5, 6, 8	1000	521	52
Breast carcinoma primary	56	3, 6	171	85	50
Breast carcinoma met	56	3, 6	79	39	49
Breast carcinoma met	47	3, 6, 9	133	46[†]	35[†]
Breast carcinoma met	76	Various, 9	580	298	51
Breast carcinoma primary	115	1, 5, 6	605	481	80
Breast carcinoma met	115	1, 5, 6	150	180	72
Breast carcinoma met	11	1, 5, 6	55	44	80
Breast carcinoma primary	83	1, 5, 6	349	198	57
Breast carcinoma axillary met	83	1, 5, 6	34	13	38
Breast carcinoma recurrent-met	83	1, 5, 6	40	17	43
Breast carcinoma	98	1, 3, 5, 6, 9	500	225	45
Breast carcinoma	63	4, 9	270	148	55
Breast carcinoma	4	1, 5, 6	328	174	54
Colorectal carcinoma	1	1, 5, 6	33	10	30
Colorectal carcinoma	79	3, 6	19	5	26
Colorectal carcinoma	55	3, 6	6	0	0
Endometrium carcinoma primary	71	1, 3, 5, 6	44	36	82
Endometrium carcinoma met	71	1, 3, 5, 6	13	6	46
Endometrium carcinoma	52	1, 5, 6	113	94	83
Endometrium carcinoma	68	1, 5, 6	58	58	100
Endometrium carcinoma	37	1, 5, 6	35	23	66
Head and neck squamous carcinoma	85	3, 6	9	0	0
Malignant melanoma	16	1, 5, 6	27	10	37
Malignant melanoma	32	1, 5, 6	35	16	46
Malignant melanoma	74	3, 6	20	0	0

		Assay methods			
Malignant melanoma	36	1, 3, 6	15	13	87
Meningioma	102	1, 5, 6	6	1	25
Meningioma	9	1, 5, 6, 7	20	0	0
Meningioma	99	1, 3, 5, 6, 7	26	8[‡]	31[‡]
Meningioma	67	1, 5, 6	34	6	18
Meningioma	114	1, 5, 6	8	0	0
Ovary benign	120	1, 5, 6	25	5	20
Ovary malignant	120	1, 5, 6	49	35	72
Ovary malignant	48	1, 5, 6	13	5	38
Ovary germ cell carcinoma	100	1, 5, 6	9	2	22
Ovary granulosa cell	100	1, 5, 6	3	1	33
Ovary carcinoma	102	1, 5, 6	68	40	58
Pleomorphic adenoma	85	3, 6	5	2	40
Renal parenchymal carcinoma	19	4	23	14	61
Renal parenchymal carcinoma	75	1, 6	8	7	87
Renal parenchymal carcinoma	51	1, 3, 5, 6	7	0[#]	0[#]
Sarcoma	16	1, 3, 4, 6	66	13	20
Thyroid papillary carcinoma	85	3, 6	4	1	25
Uterine cervix carcinoma, mostly squamous	38	1, 5, 6	49	15	62
Uterine cervix adenoca	34	1, 6	18	10	56
Uterine cervix squamous carcinoma	34	1, 6	8	6	75
Uterine cervix squamous carcinoma	33	1, 5, 6	24	7	29
Uterine cervix adenoca	33	1, 5, 6	6	4	67
Vulva and vagina squamous carcinoma	33	1, 5, 6	12	0	0

[*] Assay methods: 1. Dextran-charcoal, 2. Hydroxylapatite, 3. Sucrose gradient, 4. Electrophoresis, 5. High affinity proven, 6. Saturable, 7. Specificity proven, 8. Nuclear binding, 9. Therapeutic response to hormonal therapy correlates with presence of receptor.

[†] Borderline patients grouped with negatives.

[‡] Competitive studies with other classes of steroids suggested nonspecificity of binding.

[#] Negative by dextran-charcoal assay. Minimal amounts of 4S binding detected by sucrose gradient ultracentrifugation in four tumors.

Table 19-3
Progesterone Receptor Assay Results in Various Tumors

Tumor	Reference	Assay method[*]	No. cases	Positive No.	Positive %
Breast carcinoma primary	106	1, 5, 6, 7	23	7	30
Breast carcinoma primary	115	1, 5, 6	605	386	64
Breast carcinoma met	115	1, 5, 6	150	71	47
Breast carcinoma met	11	1, 5, 6, 9	55	31	56
Breast carcinoma	4	1, 5, 6	176	67	38
Colorectal carcinoma	1	1, 5, 6	30	13	43
Endometrium carcinoma primary	71	1, 3, 5, 6	44	31	77
Endometrium carcinoma met	71	1, 3, 5, 6	13	5	38
Endometrium carcinoma	52	1, 5, 6	113	92	82
Endometrium carcinoma	68	1, 5, 6	58	36	62
Malignant melanoma	36	1, 6	15	11	74
Meningioma	109	1, 5, 6	6	4	67
Meningioma	9	1, 5, 6, 7	20	18	90
Meningioma	99	1, 3, 5, 6, 7	26	18[†]	69[†]

488

Meningioma	67	1, 5, 6	34	26	76
Meningioma	114	1, 5, 6	8	7	87
Ovary benign	120	1, 5, 6	25	5	20
Ovary malignant	120	1, 5, 6	49	14	29
Ovary malignant	48	1, 5, 6	13	6	46
Ovary germ cell carcinoma	100	1, 5, 6	9	2	22
Ovary granulosa cell	100	1, 5, 6	3	3	100
Ovary carcinoma	102	1, 5, 6	68	27	39
Prostate carcinoma	29	2, 6	8	3	37
Renal parenchymal carcinoma	19	4	23	14	61
Renal parenchymal carcinoma	51	1, 3, 5, 6	12	0‡	0‡
Sarcoma	16	1, 3, 5, 6	66	1	2
Uterine cervix adenocarcinoma	34	1, 6	19	12	63
Uterine cervix squamous carcinoma	34	1, 6	9	5	56

* Assay methods: refer to Table 19-2.
† Competitive studies with other classes of steroids suggested nonspecificity of binding.
‡ Very small amounts of 8S receptor detected in two tumors, small amounts of 4S in five by sucrose gradient centrifugation. Binding by dextran-charcoal assay was beneath levels considered positive for breast carcinoma in all cases.

Androgen receptors are present in 30 percent of breast carcinomas. As is the case for the other steroidal receptors, androgen receptors are more likely to be present if one or more of the other receptors are present.[4]

Estrogen and progesterone receptors may have different significance in predicting hormonal responsiveness of breast carcinoma. Theoretically ER may be present in the absence of an intact hormonal stimulatory pathway. This may occur if the ER is defective and unable to bind within the nucleus.[101] PgR is inducible in mammary carcinomas by administration of estrogen.[58,78] Following this line of reasoning, presence of progesterone receptor should be more predictive of hormonal responsiveness than presence of ER alone. This has, in fact, been borne out by clinical experience in some[11,77] but not in all[42] evaluations.

Endometrial Carcinomas

The relationship in endometrial carcinomas between nuclear anaplasia and receptor status parallels that of breast carcinomas. The majority of endometrial carcinomas with low levels of nuclear anaplasia and high levels of histologic differentiation have high levels of both ER and PgR. Less well-differentiated carcinomas with high grade nuclear anaplasia are likely to be negative for receptors,[52,62,71] or may have high levels of ER but lack PgR.[68] The 8S forms of both ER and PgR are commonly present.[71] The quantitative measurement of PgR content is predictive for response to progestin therapy.[68]

Carcinomas of the Uterine Cervix

Both ER and PgR are detectable in the majority of uterine cervical adenocarcinomas and also in many squamous cell carcinomas (Tables 19-2 and 19-3). The quantitative levels of saturable binding reported have been less for cervical carcinomas than endometrial carcinomas, in accord with the general lack of hormonal responsiveness of the cervical carcinomas.

Ovarian Tumors

Both estrogen and progesterone receptors have been reported in ovarian carcinomas of a variety of types. One would expect endometrioid carcinomas to have receptors, but receptors have also been noted in high proportions of papillary serous and mucinous carcinomas and even in granulosa cell tumors.[81] Presence of the receptors in ovarian tumors can be explained by their presence in the normal ovary,[45,120] or by derivation of some ovarian carcinomas from the surface peritoneal epithelium. The latter is capable of a deciduoid response during pregnancy and therefore presumably contains receptors. In fact, Hamilton demonstrated high affinity estradiol-17β and anti-estrogen binding in cultured rat ovarian surface epithelium.[39] Evolution of carcinomas from endometriosis can also account for presence of receptors.

Carcinoma of the Prostate Gland

Since 80 percent of prostatic carcinomas respond to hormonal therapy (estrogen supplementation or androgen deprivation), the great majority presumptively contain androgen receptors (AR). Assays for AR have been hampered by the need to separate AR from SSBG which binds testosterone and 5α-dihydrotestosterone with affinity comparable to that of AR. This problem has been overcome by use of a ligand, methyltrienolone (R1881), that binds to AR but not to SSBG.[30] R1881 also binds to PgR, but this binding can be blocked with triamcinolone acetonide. Using R1881, AR was found in 20 of 25 metastatic prostatic carcinomas. The observation that 15 of the 18 AR-positive tumors responded to castration and only one of the five AR-negative tumors responded supports the validity of the assay. AR assay is not likely to be employed widely for discrimination between prostatic carcinoma and other tumors because of its complexity and the diagnostic utility of more readily available acid phosphatase assays.

Carcinoma of the Renal Parenchyma

Low levels of ER and PgR have been reported in many renal paren-chymal carcinomas. The significance of these findings is questionable because of the low response rates to progestin therapy (approximately 2 percent).[44] Furthermore, the careful study of Karr and coworkers[51] failed to reveal specific binding of estrogen or progestin above the levels considered negative for breast carcinomas, although traces of 4S and rarely 8S binding were sometimes found.

Malignant Melanoma

The problem of distinguishing between oxidation products of tritiated estradiol and receptor-bound ligand have been discussed above. Because of this problem the dextran-charcoal assay cannot be used for melanomas, and they should be assayed by some method such as hydroxylapatite, electrophoresis, or sucrose gradient ultracentrifugation that can distinguish between receptor-bound ligand and the oxidation products.[122] Since the oxidizing enzyme tyrosinase is responsible for both pigment formation and the assay artefact, it is not surprising that pseudoreceptor binding is found in pigmented rather than nonpigmented melanomas.[74] However, evidence does exist for presence of ER in some melanomas. A 4-5S diethylstilbestrol-suppressible binder has been detected in human melanoma cell lines, and a study in nude mice of these cell lines demonstrated growth-inhibition by estrogen.[116] Grill found both 4S and 8S binding of estradiol-17β in several malignant melanomas assayed by the sucrose gradient centrifugation method.[36] These findings should stimulate further investigation of estrogen receptor in melanoma.

Colorectal Adenocarcinoma

Although little evidence for steroidal hormonal influences on colorectal adenocarcinoma exists, a minority of colorectal adenocarcinomas do contain estrogen-binding proteins consistent with ER. ER has been identified both by dextran-charcoal[1] and sucrose gradient[79] techniques. No significance of the ER for stage, histologic grade, prognosis, or therapeutic response has yet emerged.

Sarcomas

The only extensive study of soft tissue sarcomas, by Chaudhuri and coworkers,[16] reports the occurrence of ER in 20 percent of 66 tumors, GCR in 33 percent of 63 tumors and AR in 27 percent of 59 tumors. Only one sarcoma, Kaposi's type, was positive for PgR. The significance of these observations is unclear except that sarcomas represent another type of tumor that can yield positive receptor assays. No pattern of receptor positivity by type of sarcoma was discernible in Chaudhuri's data except that none of the 17 fibrosarcomas, ten malignant fibrous histiocytomas, or five synovial sarcomas assayed was positive for ER. ER, AR, and GCR each were found in one or more examples of liposarcoma, angiosarcoma, leiomyosarcoma, and rhabdomyosarcoma. Given the hormonal responsiveness of the myometrium, it is not surprising that its smooth muscle tumors often contain ER.[21]

Meningiomas

Meningiomas only rarely may present in such a way as to be confused with tumors of unknown primary site. They are mentioned here because of their anomalous positivity in PgR assays. Receptor assays were initially undertaken to explain examples of exacerbation of meningioma symptoms during pregnancy, and remission of the symptoms after parturition.[66] ER has been detected in meningiomas less frequently than PgR. The question of whether the steroid-binding is to receptors or to nonreceptor-binding proteins is still being debated.[9,99] Recent evidence indicates that the PgR is present by criteria of affinity, saturability and specificity.[67] The absence of ER in presence of PgR was documented by assays of both cytosol and nuclei for ER.[67] The presence of PgR in meningiomas appears to be independent of induction by action of estrogen in concert with ER. Data pertaining to response to hormonal manipulation are not available.

Malignant non-Hodgkin's Lymphomas

Many of these lymphomas appear to have GCR. High levels of receptors forecasted response to single agent glucocorticoid therapy.[12]

Cystosarcoma Phyllodes and Fibroadenoma

Rao reported PgR in the majority of fibroadenomas and cytosarcoma phyllodes of the breast in absence of ER.[94] Presence of 8S progestin binding, high affinity, saturability, and specificity were demonstrated. Therefore, cystosarcoma and fibroadenoma resemble meningioma in that PgR seems to be present without presence of ER. The discrepancy between Rao's results and those of Kesterson,[54] who failed to find PgR in cystosarcoma, is unexplained, and constitutes another example of controversy concerning the nature of steroid-binding in tumors.

Other Tumors that May Have Steroid Hormonal Receptors

Colburn and Buonassisi reported ER in cultures of endothelial cells,[18] anticipating the discovery of ER in angiosarcomas.[16] Given the relationship between hepatocellular adenomas and use of contraceptive estrogenic and progestogenic steroid hormones,[28,69,70] the finding of steroid hormonal receptors in hepatocellular adenomas and carcinomas would be expected. Low concentrations of ER have been verified in normal human liver which can account for the effect of estrogens on rates of synthesis of certain proteins in the liver.[27,108] ER and PgR have been reported in a case of hepatoblastoma.[24] Saturable estradiol-binding consistent with ER has been reported in carcinoid tumors.[53]

Rosen[96] recently reported ER in chronic lymphocytic leukemia (CLL) cells in eight of 11 patients, a finding that can explain occasional reports of response of otherwise refractory CLL to estrogenic therapy. ER has been detected in rat thymus cells,[65] and in a transformed human B lymphocyte cell line.[96] Stark reported high levels of estrogen receptors in a tumor of nodular sclerosing Hodgkin's disease.[103] The tumor was strongly positive both by dextran-charcoal and Scatchard plot and sucrose gradient ultracentrifugal analyses. Since the small population of Hodgkin's cells usually present in this lesion could hardly account for the high levels of estrogen receptor, the receptor may have been present in the lymphocytic–histiocytic inflammatory component of the tumor.

Other tumors in which presence of steroid hormonal receptors seems anomalous but in which they have been reported include carcinoma of the lung.[49] High levels of estrogen-binding consistent with ER but of unproved specificity or affinity were reported in one gallbladder carcinoma, one pancreatic carcinoma, and one osteosarcoma.[104] Molteni studied a variety of tumors of the head and neck by sucrose gradient ultracentrifugal analysis and found high levels of 4S ER in one of five pleomorphic adenomas of the parotid gland.[85] One of four papillary carcinomas of the thyroid gland and another pleomorphic adenoma had lesser amounts of 4S ER. Nine squamous cell carcinomas and three malignant melanomas were essentially devoid of ER.

AR has been described in juvenile angiofibroma of the nasopharynx in absence of ER and PgR.[60] This observation explains the unique restriction of this tumor to juvenile males, and raises the question of androgen dependence analogous to that of prostatic carcinoma.

Conclusions

Our survey has documented occurrence of positive assays in a wide spectrum of malignancies. Both tumors of endocrine target organs and tumors of organs not generally considered to be under endocrine control can give positive assays. Whether or not all of the positive assays actually represent specific steroidal receptors is not clear, but they cannot be distinguished from true receptors by the assays in common use. For these reasons, receptor assays are not useful for localization of primary site. Tumors of endocrine-responsive organs (for example, breast, endometrium) can be receptor-negative, and tumors of other tissues (liver, kidney, pancreas, large bowel, melanomas, and even malignant lymphomas) can unexpectedly be positive for sex steroid receptors.

The only tumors in which the sex steroidal receptor status is useful in planning therapy are breast and endometrial carcinomas. A carcinoma of unknown primary site presenting in a woman should be screened for ER and PgR if its histologic pattern is not incompatible with either of those primary sites. If the histologic pattern is not compatible with adenocarcinoma, assays for ER and PgR would not be helpful and would constitute a waste of resources unless being done in the context of an investigative protocol. This is true because hormonal responsiveness has not been convincingly documented in a variety of tumors other than those of mammary, prostatic, and endometrial origin in which receptors have been found. Insofar as current information indicates, results of ER and PgR assays would not help in planning therapy of metastatic carcinoma of the uterine cervix, intestine, liver, pancreas, kidney, sarcoma, or malignant melanoma. Any of these malignancies, however, might give positive assay results. Therefore, we do not recommend that receptor assays be done on tumors of unknown primary site unless origin in breast, prostate, or endometrium is suspected. In addition, receptor assays might also be useful if clinical data from a given patient are suggestive of hormonal responsiveness.

The receptor assay cannot now be used either to establish or to refute a primary site, nor does it have established utility at present in planning therapy or establishing the prognosis of the ordinary patient with cancer of unknown primary site. On the other hand, sufficient information is not yet available to determine whether or not receptor assay results will eventually find a place in management of cancers of unknown primary site or of endocrine nontarget organs. Carefully planned studies are needed to answer this question. Such studies should use assay methods capable of distinguishing specific receptor-binding from nonspecific binders and products of ligand catabolism.

References

1. Alford TC, Do HM, Geelhoed GW, et al: Steroid hormone receptors in human colon cancers. Cancer 43:980–984, 1979
2. Allegra JC, Barlock A, Huff KK, et al: Changes in multiple or sequential estrogen receptor determinations in breast cancer. Cancer 45:792–794, 1980
3. Allegra JC, Lippman ME, Thompson EB, et al: Steroid hormone receptors in human breast cancer (abstr). Proc Am Assoc Cancer Res 19:336, 1978
4. Allegra JC, Lippman ME, Thompson EB, et al: Relation between the

progesterone, androgen and glucocorticoid receptors in human breast cancer. Cancer Res 39:1447–1454, 1979

5. Andersen JA, Mattheiem WH: Markers and prognostic factors in breast cancer disease; workshop report. Eur J Cancer Clin Oncol 19:1699–1707, 1983

6. Barrows GH, Stroupe SB, Riehm JD: Nuclear uptake of a 17β-estradiol-fluorescein derivative as a marker of estrogen dependence. Am J Clin Pathol 73:330–339, 1980

7. Baxter JD, Funder JW: Hormone receptors. N Engl J Med 301:1149–1161, 1979

8. Bayard F, Damilano S, Dobel P, et al: Cytoplasmic and nuclear estradiol and progesterone receptors in human endometrium. J Clin Endocrinol Metab 46:635–638, 1978

9. Blankenstein MA, Blaauw G, Lamberts SWJ, et al: Presence of progesterone receptors and absence of estrogen receptors in human intracranial meningioma cytosols. Eur J Cancer Clin Oncol 19:365–370, 1983

10. Block GE, Jensen EV, Polley TL Jr: The prediction of hormonal dependency of mammary cancer. Ann Surg 182:342–352, 1975

11. Bloom ND, Tobin EH, Schreibman B, et al: The role of progesterone receptors in the management of advanced breast cancer. Cancer 45:2992–2997, 1980

12. Bloomfield DC, Smith KA, Hildebrandt L, et al: The therapeutic utility of glucocorticoid receptor studies in non-Hodgkin's malignant lymphoma, in Iacobella S, King RJB, Lindner HR, Lippman ME (eds): Hormones and Cancer. New York, Raven Press, 1979, pp 361–370

13. Bonneterre J, Peyrat JP, Vandewalle B, et al: Prolactin receptors in human breast cancer. Eur J Cancer Clin Oncol 18:1157–1162, 1982

14. Boyns AR, Cole EN, Griffiths K, et al: Plasma prolactin in breast cancer. Eur J Cancer 9:99–102, 1973

15. Chan L, O'Malley BW: Mechanism of action of the sex steroid hormones. New Engl J Med 294:1322–1328, 1372–1381, 1430–1437, 1976

16. Chaudhuri PK, Walker MJ, Beattie CW, et al: Distribution of steriod hormone receptors in human soft tissue sarcomas. Surgery 90:149–90:149–153, 1981

17. Clark GM, McGuire WL, Hubay CA, et al: Progesterone receptors as a prognostic factor in stage II breast cancer. N Engl J Med 309:1343–1347, 1983

18. Colburn P, Buonassisi V: Estrogen-binding sites in endothelial cell cultures. Science 201:817–819, 1978

19. Concolino G, Marocchi A, Conti C, et al: Human renal cell carcinoma as a hormone-dependent tumor. Cancer Res 38:4340–4344, 1978

20. Costlow ME, McGuire WL: Autoradiographic localization of prolactin receptors in 7,12-dimethylbenz[α]anthracene-induced rat mammary carcinoma. J Natl Cancer Inst 58:1173–1175, 1977

21. Cramer SF, Meyer JS, Kraner JR, et al: Metastasizing leiomyoma of the uterus. S-phase fraction, estrogen receptor, and ultrastructure. Cancer 45:932–937, 1980

22. Creagan ET, Ingle JN, Green SJ, et al: Phase II study of tamoxifen in patients with disseminated malignant melanoma. Cancer Treat Rep 64:199–201, 1980

23. Davis BW, Zava DT, Locher GW, et al: Receptor heterogeneity of human breast cancer as measured by multiple intratumoral assays of estrogen and progesterone receptor. Eur J Cancer Clin Oncol 20:375–382, 1984

24. Demanes DJ, Friedman MA, McKerrow JM, et al: Hormone receptors in hepatoblastomas: a demonstration of both estrogen and progesterone receptors. Cancer 50:1828–1832, 1982

25. DeSombre ER: Steroid receptors in breast cancer, in McDivitt RW, Oberman HA, Ozzello L, Kaufman N (eds): The Breast. Baltimore/London, Williams and Wilkins, 1984, pp 149–174

26. De Souza I, Morgan L, Lewis UJ, et al: Growth-hormone dependence among human breast cancers. Lancet 2:182–184, 1974

27. Duffy MJ, Duffy GJ: Estrogen receptors in the human liver. J Steroid Biochem 9:233–235, 1978

28. Edmondson HA, Henderson B, Benton B: Liver-cell adenomas associated with use of oral contraceptives. N Engl J Med 294:470–472, 1976

29. Ekman P: The application of steroid receptor assay in human prostate research and clinical management. Anticancer Res 2:163–172, 1982

30. Ekman P, Snochowski M, Zetterberg A, et al: Steroid receptor content in human prostatic carcinoma and response to endocrine therapy. Cancer 44:1173–1181, 1979

31. Fazekas AG, MacFarland JK: Macromolecular binding of glucocorticoids in human mammary carcinoma. Cancer Res 37:640–645, 1977

32. Fisher RI, Neifeld JP, Lippmann ME: Oestrogen receptors in human malignant melanoma. Lancet 2:337–338, 1976

33. Ford LC, Berek JS, Lagasse LD, et al: Estrogen and progesterone

receptor sites in malignancies of the uterine cervix, vagina and vulva. Gynecol Oncol 15:27–31, 1983

34. Gao YL, Twiggs LB, Leung BS, et al: Cytoplasmic estrogen and progesterone receptors in primary cervical carcinoma: clinical and histopathologic correlates. Am J Obstet Gynecol 146:299–306, 1983

35. Greene GL, Nola C, Engler JP, et al: Monoclonal antibodies to human estrogen receptor. Proc Natl Acad Sci USA 77:5115–5119, 1980

36. Grill HJ, Benes P, Manz B, et al: Steroid hormone receptors in human melanoma. Arch Dermatol Res 272:97–101, 1982

37. Hähnel R, Martin JD, Masters AM, et al: Estrogen receptors and blood hormone levels in endometrial carcinoma. Gynecol Oncol 8:209–225, 1979

38. Hähnel R, Martin JD, Masters AM, et al: Estrogen receptors and blood hormone levels in cervical carcinoma and other gynecological tumors. Gynecol Oncol 8:226–233, 1979

39. Hamilton TC, Davies P, Griffiths K: Estrogen receptor-like binding in the surface epithelium of the rat ovary. J Endocrinol 95:377–385, 1982

40. Harland RN, Barnes DM, Howell A, et al: Variation of receptor status in cancer of the breast. Br J Cancer 47:511–515, 1983

41. Holdaway IM, Bowditch JV: Variation in receptor status between primary and metastatic breast cancer. Cancer 52:479–485, 1983

42. Holdaway IM, Mountjoy KG, Harvey VJ, et al: Clinical applications of receptor measurements in breast cancer. Br J Cancer 41:136–139, 1980

43. Howat JMT, Barnes DM, Harris M, et al: The association of cytosol oestrogen and progesterone receptors with histological features of breast cancer and early recurrence of disease. Br J Cancer 47:629–640, 1983

44. Hrushesky WJ, Murphy GP: Current status of the therapy of advanced renal carcinoma. J Surg Oncol 9:277–288, 1977

45. Jacobs BR, Suchocki S, Smith RG: Evidence for a human ovarian receptor. Am J Obstet Gynecol 138:332–336, 1980

46. Jänne O, Kauppila A, Kontula K, et al: Female sex steroid receptors in human endometrial hyperplasia and carcinoma, in Wittliff JL, Dapunt O (eds): Steroid Receptors and Hormone Dependent Neoplasia. Innsbruck, Austria, Masson, 1980, p 37

47. Jensen EV, DeSombre ER, Jungblut PW: Estrogen receptors in hormone-responsive tissues and tumors, in Wissler RW, Dao LLY, Woods S (eds): Endogenous Factors Influencing Host-tumor Balance. Chicago, University of Chicago Press, 1967, p 15

48. Jolles CJ, Freedman RS, Jones LA: Estrogen and progestogen therapy in advanced ovarian cancer: a preliminary report. Gynecol Oncol 16:352–359, 1983

49. Jones LA, Blocker SH, Rusch VH, et al: Specific estrogen binding protein in human lung cancer. Proc Am Assoc Cancer Res 25:208 (abstract), 1984

50. Juergens WG, Stockdale FE, Topper YJ, et al: Hormone-dependent differentiation of mammary gland in vitro. Proc Natl Acad Sci USA 54:629–634, 1975

51. Karr JP, Pontes JE, Schneider S, et al: Clinical aspects of steroid hormone receptors in human renal cell carcinoma. J Surg Oncol 23:117–124, 1982

52. Kauppila A, Kujansuu E, Vihko R: Cytosol estrogen and progestin receptors in endometrial carcinoma of patients treated with surgery, radiotherapy, and progestin. Clinical correlates. Cancer 50:2157–2162, 1982

53. Keshgegian AA, Wheeler JR: Estrogen receptor protein in malignant carcinoid tumor. Cancer 45:293–296, 1980

54. Kesterson GHD, Georgiade N, Seigler HF, et al: Cystosarcoma phyllodes: a steroid hormone and ultrastructure analysis. Ann Surg 190:640–647, 1979

55. Kiang DT, Kennedy BJ: Estrogen receptor assay in the differential diagnosis of adenocarcinoma. JAMA 238:32–34, 1977

56. Kiang DT, Kennedy BJ: Factors affecting estrogen receptors in breast cancer. Cancer 40:1571–1576, 1977

57. Knight WA, Livingston RB, Gregory EJ, et al: Estrogen receptor as an independent prognostic factor for early recurrence in breast cancer. Cancer Res 37:4669–4671, 1977

58. Koenders AJM, Geurts-Moespot A, Zolingen SJ, et al: Progesterone and estradiol receptors in DMBA-induced mammary tumors before and after ovariectomy and after subsequent estradiol administration, in McGuire WL, Raynaud JP, Baulieu EE (eds): Progesterone Receptors in Normal and Neoplastic Tissues. New York, Raven Press, 1977, pp 71–84

59. Leake RE, Laing L, Calman KC, et al: Oestrogen receptor status and endocrine therapy of breast cancer: response rates and status stability. Br J Cancer 43:59–66, 1981

60. Lee DA, Rao BR, Meyer JS, et al: Hormonal receptor determination in juvenile nasopharyngeal angiofibromas. Cancer 46:547–551, 1980

61. Lee SH: Cancer cell estrogen receptor of human mammary carcinoma. Cancer 44:1–12, 1979

62. Lindahl B, Alm P, Borg A, et al: Correlations between estradiol-17β and progesterone cytosol receptor concentration, histologic differentiation, and ^{3}H-thymidine incorporation in endometrial carcinoma. Anticancer Res 2:203–207, 1982

63. Maass H, Engel B, Trams G: Steroid hormone receptors in human breast cancer and the clinical significance. J Steroid Biochem 6:743–749, 1975

64. MacFarlane JK, Fleiszer D, Fazekas AG: Studies on estrogen receptors and regression in human breast cancer. Cancer 45:1998–2003, 1980

65. Malacarne P, Piffanelli A, Indelli M, et al: Estradiol binding in rat thymus cells. Hormone Res 12:224–232, 1980

66. Manganiello PD, Mentz RC, Andros GJ: Probable parasellar meningioma in a pregnant woman. Obstet Gynecol 53 (suppl): 43s–46s, 1979

67. Markwalder TM, Zava DT, Goldhirsch A, et al: Estrogen and progesterone receptors in meningiomas in relation to clinical and pathological features. Surg Neurol 20:42–47, 1983

68. Martin PM, Rolland PH, Gammerre M, et al: Estradiol and progesterone receptor in normal and neoplastic endometrium: correlations between receptors, histopathological examination and clinical response under progestin therapy. Int J Cancer 23:321–329, 1979

69. Mays ET, Christopherson WM, Mahr MM, et al: Hepatic changes in young women ingesting contraceptive steroids. Hepatic hemorrhage and primary hepatic tumors. JAMA 235:730–732, 1976

70. McAvoy JM, Tompkins RK, Longmire WP Jr: Benign hepatic tumors and their association with oral contraceptives. Case reports and survey of the literature. Arch Surg 111:761–767, 1976

71. McCarty KS Jr, Barton TK, Fetter BF, et al: Correlation of estrogen and progesterone receptors with histologic differentiation in endometrial adenocarcinoma. Am J Pathol 96:171–184, 1979

72. McCarty KS Jr, Hiatt KB, Budwit DA, et al: Clinical response to hormone therapy correlated with estrogen receptor analyses. Biochemical vs. histochemical methods. Arch Pathol Lab Med 108:24–26, 1984

73. McCarty KS Jr, Reintgen DS, Seigler HF, et al: Cytochemistry of sex steroid receptors: a critique. Breast Cancer Res Treat 1:315–325, 1982

74. McCarty KS, Wortman J, Stowers S, et al: Sex steroid receptor analysis in human melanoma. Cancer 46:1463–1470, 1980

75. McDonald MW, Diokno AC, Seski JC, et al: Measurement of

progesterone receptor in human renal cell carcinoma and normal renal tissue. J Surg Oncol 22:164–166, 1983

76. McGuire WL, Carbone PP, Sears ME, et al: Estrogen receptors in human breast cancer: an overview, in McGuire WL, Carbone PP, Vollmer EP (eds): Estrogen Receptors in Human Breast Cancer. New York, Raven Press, 1975, p 1–7

77. McGuire WL, Horwitz KB, Pearson OH, et al: Current status of estrogen and progesterone receptors in breast cancer. Cancer 39:2934–2947, 1977

78. McGuire WL, Raynaud JP, Baulieu EE: Progesterone receptors, introduction and overview, in McGuire WL, Raynaud JP, Baulieu EE (eds): Progesterone Receptors in Normal and Neoplastic Tissues. New York, Raven Press, 1977, pp 1–7

79. McLendon JE, Appleby D, Claudon DB, et al: Colonic neoplasms: tissue estrogen receptor and carcinoembryonic antigen. Arch Surg 112:240–241, 1977

80. Meyer JS, Bauer WC, Rao BR: Subpopulations of breast carcinoma defined by S-phase fraction, morphology, and estrogen receptor content. Lab Invest 39:225–235, 1978

81. Meyer JS, Rao BR, Valdes R Jr, et al: Progesterone receptor in granulosa cell tumor. Gynecol Oncol 13:252–257, 1982

82. Meyer JS, Schechtman K, Valdes R Jr: Estrogen and progesterone receptor assays on breast carcinoma from mastectomy specimens. Cancer 52:2139–2143, 1983

83. Meyer JS, Stevens SC, Vandillen N, et al: Estrogen receptor assay of mammary carcinomas. Effects of testosterone-estradiol-binding globulin (TEBG) and serum estradiol-17β. Am J Clin Pathol 72:564–570, 1979

84. Mills ES, Topper YJ: Some ultrastructural effects of insulin, hydrocortisone, and prolactin on mammary gland explants. J Cell Biol 44:310–328, 1970

85. Molteni A, Warpeha RL, Brizio-Molteni I, et al: Estradiol receptor-binding protein in head and neck neoplastic and normal tissue. Arch Surg 116:207–210, 1981

86. Murayama Y, Sakuma T, Udagawa H, et al: Sex hormone-binding globulin and estrogen receptor in breast cancer: technique and preliminary clinical results. J Clin Endocrinol Metab 46:998–1006, 1978

87. Ohgo S, Kato Y, Chihara K, et al: Plasma prolactin responses to thyrotropin-releasing hormone in patients with breast cancer. Cancer 37:1412–1416, 1976

88. Oka T, Topper YJ: Is prolactin mitogenic for mammary epithelium? Proc Natl Acad Sci USA 69:1693–1696, 1972
89. Pasteels JL, Heuson JC, Heuson-Stiennon J, et al: Effects of insulin, prolactin, progesterone and estradiol on DNA synthesis in organ culture of 7,12dimethylbenz[α]anthracene-induced rat mammary tumors. Cancer Res 36:2162–2170, 1976
90. Pearson OH, Manni A, Chambers M, et al: Role of pituitary hormones in the growth of human breast cancer. Cancer Res 38:4323–4326, 1978
91. Pertschuk LP, Gaetjens E, Carter AC, et al: An improved histochemical method for detection of estrogen receptors in mammary cancer. Comparison with biochemical assay. Am J Clin Pathol 71:504–508, 1979
92. Prey MU, Meyer JS, Stone KR, et al: Heterogeneity of breast carcinomas determined by flow cytometric analysis. J Surg Oncol 29:35–39, 1985
93. Raam S, Richardson GS, Bradley F, et al: Translocation of cytoplasmic estrogen receptors to the nucleus: immunohistochemical demonstration utilizing rabbit antibodies to estrogen receptors of mammary carcinomas. Breast Cancer Res Treat 3:179–199, 1983
94. Rao BR, Meyer JS, Fry CG: Most cystosarcoma phyllodes and fibroadenomas have progesterone receptor but lack estrogen receptor: stromal localization of progesterone receptor. Cancer 47: 2016–2021, 1981
95. Rose DP, Pruitt BT: Plasma prolactin levels in patients with breast cancer. Cancer 48:2687–2691, 1981
96. Rosen ST, Maciorowski Z, Wittlin F, et al: Estrogen receptor analysis in chronic lymphocytic leukemia. Blood 62:996–999, 1983
97. Salih H, Flax H, Brander W, et al: Prolactin dependence in human breast cancers. Lancet 2:1103–1105, 1972
98. Savlov ED, Wittliff JL, Hilf R: Further studies of biochemical predictive tests in breast cancer. Cancer 39:539–541, 1977
99. Scheartz MR, Randolph RL, Cech DA, et al: Steroid hormone binding macromolecules in meningiomas. Failure to meet criteria of specific receptors. Cancer 53:922–927, 1984
100. Schwartz PE, MacLusky N, Sakamoto H, et al: Steroid receptor proteins in nonepithelial malignancies of the ovary. Gynecol Oncol 15:305–315, 1983
101. Shyamala G: Estradiol receptors in mouse mammary tumors: absence of the transfer of bound estradiol from the cytoplasm to the nucleus. Biochem Biophys Res Comm 46:1623–1630, 1972

102. Spona J, Gitsch E, Salzar H, et al: Estrogen- and gestagen-receptors in ovarian carcinoma. Gynecol Obstet Invest 16:189–198, 1983
103. Stark JJ, Lloyd JW, Schellhammer PR: Estrogen receptor activity in a case of Hodgkin's disease. Ann Intern Med 95:186–187, 1981
104. Stedman KE, Moore GE, Morgan RT: Estrogen receptor proteins in diverse human tumors. Arch Surg 115:244–248, 1980
105. Stewart JF, Rubens RD, Millis RR, et al: Steroid receptors and prognosis in operable (stage I and II) breast cancer. Eur J Cancer Clin Oncol 19:1381–1387, 1983
106. Terenius L: Estrogen and progesterone binders in human and rat mammary carcinoma. Eur J Cancer 9:291–294, 1973
107. Teulings FAG, Van Gilse HA: Demonstration of glucocorticoid receptors in human mammary carcinomas. Horm Res (Basel) 8:107–116, 1977
108. Thompson C, Hudson P, Lucier G: Correlation of hepatic estrogen receptor concentrations and estrogen-mediated elevations of very low density lipoproteins. Endocrinology 112:1389–1397, 1983
109. Tilzer LL, Plapp FV, Evans JP, et al: Steroid receptor proteins in human meningiomas. Cancer 49:633–636, 1982
110. Tominaga T, Kitamura M, Saito T, et al: Comparative histochemical and biochemical assays of estrogen receptors in breast cancer patients. Gann 72:60–65, 1981
111. Trams G, Maass H: Specific binding of estradiol and dihydrotestosterone in human mammary cancers. Cancer Res 37:258–261, 1977
112. Turkington RW: Induction of milk protein synthesis by placental lactogen and prolactin in vitro. Endocrinology 82:56–83, 1968
113. Van NT, Raber M, Barrows GH, et al: Estrogen receptor analysis by flow cytometry. Science 224:876–879, 1984
114. Vaquero J, Marcos ML, Martinez R, et al: Estrogen- and progesterone-receptor proteins in intracranial tumors. Surg Neurol 19:11–13, 1983
115. Vihko R, Jänne O, Kontula K, et al: Female sex steroid receptor status in primary and metastatic breast carcinoma and its relationship to serum steroid and peptide hormone levels. Int J Cancer 26:13–21, 1980
116. Walker MJ, Chaudhuri PK, Das Gupta TK, et al: Influence of host sex on the growth of human melanoma. Proc Soc Exper Biol Med 165:96–99, 1980
117. Wallack MK, Wolf JA Jr, Bedwinek J, et al: Gestational carcinoma of the female breast. Current Problems in Cancer 7:1–58, 1983
118. Waseda N, Kato Y, Imura H, et al: Effects of tamoxifen on estrogen

and progesterone receptors in human breast cancer. Cancer Res 41:1984–1988, 1981

119. Welsch CW, de Iturri GC, Brennan MJ: DNA synthesis of human, mouse and rat mammary carcinomas in vitro. Influence of insulin and prolactin. Cancer 38:1272–1281, 1976

120. Willcocks D, Toppila M, Hudson CN, et al: Estrogen and progesterone receptors in human ovarian tumors. Gynecol Oncol 16:246–253, 1983

121. Zava DT, Chamness GC, Horwitz KB, et al: Human breast cancer: biologically active estrogen receptor in the absence of estrogen? Science 196:663–664, 1977

122. Zava DT, Holdhirsch A: Estrogen receptor in malignant melanoma: fact or artefact? Eur J Cancer Clin Oncol 19:1151–1159, 1983

123. Zava DT, McGuire WL: Human breast cancer: androgen action mediated by estrogen receptor. Science 199:787–788, 1978

20

GENE REARRANGEMENTS AS SPECIFIC CLONAL MARKERS IN HUMAN NEOPLASMS

Ajay Bakhshi
Andrew Arnold
John J. Wright
Katherine A. Siminovitch
Thomas A. Waldmann
Stanley J. Korsmeyer

Recent developments in the fields of immunology and cell biology have provided a variety of new tools applicable to the diagnosis of human cancer. Although the diagnosis of a given tumor is generally founded in the correlation of clinical, gross, and light microscopic features, these newer techniques have provided the means of clarifying the cellular lineage and stage of differentiation of tumors. For example, the use of immunologic reagents to identify cell surface determinants has resulted in new schemes for classifying hematologic malignancies and has markedly advanced our understanding of their biology. Moreover, these insights are improving our recognition of good and poor prognostic categories and may enable the development of tailor-made, effective therapies.[1,2] In addition to determination of specific cellular lineage and stage of differentiation, these approaches have been important for the demonstration of clonality within

POORLY DIFFERENTIATED NEOPLASMS AND TUMORS OF UNKNOWN ORIGIN   ISBN 0-8089-1755-2
© 1986 by Grune & Stratton.   All rights of reproduction in any form reserved.

malignant expansions of cells. The demonstration that a population of cells was monoclonal has been a central piece of information distinguishing a malignant from a benign proliferation of cells.[3] Within B lymphoid proliferations the presence of only one light chain class or the secretion of immunoglobulin with restricted electrophoretic mobility has served as a clonal marker.[4] In other cellular lineages, the presence of a specific cytogenetic abnormality or the presence of one of two distinguishable glucose-6-phosphate dehydrogenase isoenzymes in a heterozygous female has also served as a clonal marker.[5,6]

Not infrequently, however, these approaches to demonstrate clonality or lineage may be inapplicable or inconclusive. This is frequently because of the admixture of large numbers of non-neoplastic cells with neoplastic cells. In addition, cells that are genetically committed to a given lineage but are early in differentiation may not yet express surface markers solely restricted to that lineage. Finally, purely technical factors, such as avid Fc receptors or the inability to obtain mitotic cells for karyotypic analysis can result in ambiguous findings.[7,8] To overcome these limitations we turned to a recombinant DNA approach. Specifically, we utilized the DNA rearrangements that assemble the antigen specific receptors in B cells and in T cells. This was first accomplished with the human immunoglobulin (Ig) genes but has been extended to the use of T cell antigen receptor genes. Such an analysis can overcome these limitations because it is sensitive enough to detect a clonal population that comprises but one to five percent of the total cells within a mixed population. Furthermore, it is capable of identifying cells which are lineage-committed at the DNA level but may not express other lineage-restricted surface markers. Finally, interchromosomal rearrangements, that often translocate oncogenes, promise to make a great impact on tumor diagnosis and classification.

Gene Rearrangements Generate Unique Clonal Markers

The immunoglobulin genes, in their embryonic or germline form, are organized as discontinuous, separated DNA segments.[10] Early in its development, a cell committed to B cell differentiation must first rearrange its heavy chain and then its light chain gene subsegments.[11] This DNA rearrangement, as shown for the kappa light chain gene in Figure 20-1, juxtaposes one of many available variable (V_K) regions with one of five joining (J_K) segments.[12] This rearranged allele is then transcribed into mRNA, where the intervening sequence between V_K/J_K and C_K is removed

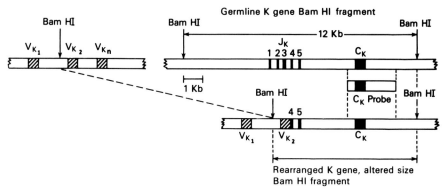

Figure 20-1. *Schematic representation of the germline and a rearranged κ gene allele. In the germline form there are multiple variable (V$_κ$) regions, five fully functional joining (J$_κ$) regions but only one constant (C$_κ$) region. The germline C$_κ$ region is contained within a 12kb BamHI fragment. In B cells a DNA rearrangement juxtaposes a single V$_κ$ and J$_κ$ region. This rearrangement introduces a new 5' BamHI site thereby altering the size of the BamHI fragment recognized by the C$_κ$ probe.*

by RNA splicing. This processed RNA is then translated into the κ light chain protein. The heavy chain variable region peptide contains additional information contributed by diversity (D$_H$) gene subsegments.

The process of V/J (or V/D/J) joining at the DNA level generates a marker unique to an individual cell and its progeny.[13–15] These DNA rearrangements produce a change in the location of restriction sites to the left (5') of the joining gene subsegments. For example, the new sites brought in by a V$_κ$ element are distinct for each different V$_κ$ gene subsegment utilized. Rearranged Ig genes thus are found on different sized DNA restriction fragments when compared to germline DNA. Furthermore, polyclonal B cells would possess numerous different immunoglobulin–gene rearrangements each of which would be below the threshold of sensitivity of a Southern blot. In contrast, a monoclonal expansion of B cells represents the progeny of a single cell and would thus have multiple copies of the same unique DNA rearrangement. When this monoclonal expansion constitutes over one percent of the test sample a distinct band, which serves as a marker for this clonal expansion, is clearly detectable.[9,16]

Rearrangements of heavy and light chain immunoglobulin genes are mandatory in mature B cells which produce immunoglobulin. These rearrangements occur in an ordered sequence with heavy chain gene rearrangements preceding light chain gene rearrangements and κ gene rearrangements occuring before λ. In distinction, most non-B cell lineages retain their immunoglobulin genes in the germline configuration. Thus, all 25 T cell tumors we have examined retain germline light chain genes and most (23/25) retain germline heavy chain genes as well.[13] All nonlymphoid malignancies examined including acute myelogenous leukemia, acute and chronic myeloid phases of chronic myelogenous leukemia, monocytic leukemia, promyelocytic leukemia, and carcinomas retained germline light chain genes and usually germline heavy chain genes.

The genes coding for the β and α chain of the T cell receptor have recently been cloned.[17–20] They are similar to the immunoglobulin gene locus both in terms of their organization and method of assembly. These loci undergo a mandatory rearrangement in any T cell bearing an antigen receptor and only occassionally rearrange in non-T cells. They thus provide a T cell associated clonal marker at the DNA level. This set of genetic markers provides the opportunity to establish the clonality of T cell neoplasms and to determine the developmental hierarchy of T cell receptor gene rearrangements.

Immunoglobulin Gene Rearrangements Establish a Diagnosis of B Cell Lymphoma

The distinction between a lymphoma and an undifferentiated carcinoma could not be made histologically on either the presenting gastric mass or a malignant pleural effusion in the case shown in Figure 20-2.[9] An extensive search for lymphocyte surface markers including the monoclonal antibodies B1, BA-1, BA-2, and Lyt3 was negative. Staining for the T-200 pan-leukocyte antigen and terminal deoxynucleotidyl transferase was also negative. Furthermore, electron microscopy revealed no evidence of epithelial differentiation. When DNA from the malignant cells was examined, however, clonal heavy chain and kappa light chain gene rearrangements were demonstrated. The β chain of the T cell receptor was retained in its germline form. This is strong evidence favoring a diagnosis of malignant lymphoma of B cell origin with accompanying therapeutic implications.

A recent study indicates that among tumors referred to as primitive, anaplastic, or undifferentiated because they lack identifiable gross or light microscopic features, the most likely diagnosis is lymphoma.[21] Lymphocyte receptor gene rearrangement analysis would be appropriate in this group of tumors. If rearrangements are detected, as illustrated by the case presented, the diagnosis of a lymphoma can be made. If this analysis is

Gastric mass, malignant pleural effusion

Histopathology, cytology: large cell lymphoma *vs.* undifferentiated carcinoma

EM: no epithelial differentiation

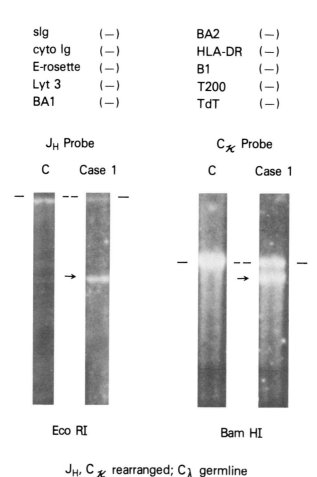

sIg	(−)	BA2	(−)
cyto Ig	(−)	HLA-DR	(−)
E-rosette	(−)	B1	(−)
Lyt 3	(−)	T200	(−)
BA1	(−)	TdT	(−)

J_H Probe $C_\varkappa$ Probe

C   Case 1   C   Case 1

Eco RI   Bam HI

J_H, $C_\varkappa$ rearranged; C_λ germline

Figure 20-2. *Southern blot analysis of Ig gene configuration from a case with undifferentiated carcinoma. When probed with a heavy chain joining (J_H) probe and a constant κ (C_κ) probe in EcoRI and BamHI digests respectively, both heavy and light chain rearrangements were detected (arrows) when compared to the germline configuration (dash marks). Thus while histopathology and surface phenotypic analysis were unable to differentiate large cell lymphoma from undifferentiated carcinoma, the molecular analysis proved the diagnosis of B cell lymphoma.*

extended to include the genes involved in interchromosomal rearrangements the diagnostic potential of this molecular biological approach should be even greater.

Establishment of Monoclonality and Cellular Lineage in Lymphomas with Ambiguous Phenotypes

Three lymphomas we examined had a preponderance of T cells (73 percent to 89 percent) and had only a small number of B cells in their biopsy specimens. Yet all three had heavy chain gene rearrangements. Two cases had light chain gene rearrangements as well, thereby firmly establishing the presence of a monoclonal B cell population. In addition, examination of these two DNA samples with the β chain T cell receptor gene showed no clonal rearrangements thereby insuring that there were no clonal T cells present. Thus, these two lymphomas are B cell malignancies with a large number of infiltrating non-neoplastic T cells. In other lymphomas, immunologic marker analysis may reveal a preponderance of B cells in biopsy tissues, but no single immunoglobulin light chain isotype will be predominant. Such cases are felt to be B cell lymphomas, but clonality cannot be established by such routine analysis. An additional group, though unequivocally lymphomas, have no clear majority of either T or B cells by surface marker analysis. Such cases are ideally suited for analysis of immunoglobluin gene and T cell receptor gene rearrangement. This determination would allow their assignment to a T or B cell lineage lymphoma.

Detection of Clonal B Cells in Lymphoid Proliferations

In an immunocompromised patient, the distinction between benign and malignant lymphoid proliferations is especially difficult on histologic grounds alone. In this setting the demonstration of clonality, often based on the presence of a single light chain (κ or λ) has served as important information favoring a malignancy. Surface marker analysis of a progressively enlarging lymph node in a patient with Wiskott-Aldrich syndrome revealed the presence of both κ and λ bearing B cells and many Lyt 3 positive cells consistent with a diagnosis of atypical follicular hyperplasia. DNA analysis, however, revealed the presence of a minority population of clonal B cells with rearranged heavy and light chain genes. In contrast, another typical follicular hyperplasia and four hyperplastic benign tonsils did not have detectable immunoglobulin gene rearrangments. It is possible that clonal B cell populations in the setting of immunodeficiency might represent truly benign B cell expansions still under some regulatory control. Alternatively they may represent the early detection of malignant cells that will ultimately become the dominant cell in these lymph nodes.

Serial Examination for Clonal Persistence, Clonal Recurrence, or Clonal Evolution

These sensitive and specific DNA level markers of T and B cells can be used to determine (1) clonal persistence (2) clonal recurrence, and (3) clonal evolution. Specimens could be obtained following therapy for lymphoma or leukemia and then analyzed for clonal gene rearrangements to confirm histologic or surface marker evidence that remission has indeed been achieved. Serial examination of bone marrow specimens, for example, from patients in remission may allow the early detection of recurrences before other histologic or tumor-associated markers become detectable. Finally, such a marker would allow the natural history of a clone of cells to be determined by serial examinations of involved cells. A dramatic example of the potency of this approach was provided by a serial study of affected cells from a patient with chronic myelogenous leukemia (CML) (Fig. 20-3).[14] During the chronic phase the granulocytes bearing the t(9;22) Philadelphia chromosome retained germline immunoglobulin heavy and light chain genes. During two separate lymphoid blast crises the lymphoid cells shared a new cytogenetic marker, having lost chromosme 7, 45XY-7 t(9;22). In addition, they possessed identical heavy chain gene rearrangements indicating that both blast crises could be traced to a common progenitor cell with doubly rearranged heavy chain genes. The two lymphoid blast crises did have a distinguishing Ig gene marker, however. The first crisis had a λ light chain gene rearrangement whereas the second crisis had germline light chain genes. The immediate precursor cells which gave rise to the separate lymphoid blast crises were thus different in their genetic maturation. This indicated that clonally affected B cell precursors in CML are capable of sequential rearrangement of first heavy and then light chain genes.

Bakhshi, et al.

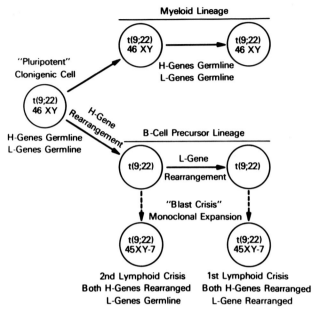

Figure 20-3. *Clonal evolution in chronic myelogenous leukemia (CML). The pleuripotent stem cell of CML bearing the Philadelphia chromosome t(9;22) marker retains germline immunoglobulin genes during myeloid differentiation. When the affected cells pursue B cell differentiation they undergo sequential rearrangements of first heavy chain and then light chain genes. Separate episodes of lymphoid blast crisis can represent discrete genetic steps of B cell maturation. [Reproduced from Bakhshi et al: Lymphoid blast crises of chronic myelogenous leukemia represent stages in the development of B-cell precursors. N Engl J Med 309:826–831, 1983. With permission of the New England Journal of Medicine.]*

Chromosomal Translocations Rearrange Genes at the Breakpoints

Chromosomal translocations are often specifically associated with distinct neoplasms.[22,23] Since the initial discovery of the Philadelphia chromosome in the neoplastic cells of patients with chronic myelogenous leukemia, specific chromosomal rearrangements have been described in several subtypes of human leukemias and lymphoma. The translocation best characterized at the molecular level is the one typically found in

Burkitt's lymphoma.[24-26] This reciprocal chromosomal translocation involves the distal segment (q24–qter) of the long arm of chromosome 8, where the c-myc oncogene is located, and the precise chromosomal segments on chromosome 14, 22, or 2 bearing the heavy chain, λ chain and κ chain immunoglobulin genes respectively. In its most common form the c-myc oncogene translocates to the heavy chain locus on chromosome 14 at band q32. In the variant t(8;22) and t(2;8) translocations, the c-myc oncogene remains on chromosome 8, but the constant regions of the λ and κ chain, respectively, translocate to a region distal (3') to the c-myc oncogene. The consequence of these translocations is an altered regulation of expression of the c-myc gene on the translocated chromosome.[27]

The immunoglobulin heavy chain locus on band 14q32 is also involved in the translocations that occur in other human B cell neoplasms.[28-29] Thus, a translocation between chromosomes 11q13 and 14q32 has been observed in chronic lymphocytic leukemia, small cell lymphocytic, and diffuse large cell lymphomas. In addition, a translocation between 18q21 and 14q32 has been noted within follicular and some diffuse lymphomas. One side of the chromosomal break involves a transcriptionally active gene within the B cell lineage (the immunoglobulin heavy chain locus), while the other side, by analogy with c-myc, may contribute an oncogene. When introduced into its new surroundings its expression may become deregulated (possibly by removing normal negative controls and/or being influenced by the immunoglobulin enhancer) and represent an important step in transformation. In an attempt to identify and characterize a putative new transforming gene, we and Tsujimoto et al. have cloned the t(14;18) chromosomal breakpoint from lymphomas bearing this translocation.[30,31]

The chromosomal translocations not only provide important insights into the pathogenesis of human neoplasia but may also provide molecular probes specific for an individual neoplasm. Furthermore, they may be applied diagnostically where a translocation is suspected but an adequate karyotype cannot be obtained. For example, c-myc rearrangements can be detected in over half of the cases with Burkitt's lymphoma. Those that cannot be detected have breakpoints that may be further away on the 5' or 3' side of the c-myc gene. When flanking region probes are available it should be possible to detect rearrangements more uniformly. In chronic myelogenous leukemia the c-abl oncogene is translocated from chromosome 9 to a limited region of 5.8kb on chromosome 22. Similarly, in the commonly occuring follicular lymphomas, we have demonstrated that the breakpoints are clustered within a 4kb region on chromosome 18 and an 11kb segment of chromosome 14.[30] As more loci (for example, those on chromosomes 17 and 15 involved in the translocation observed in acute promyelocytic leukemia) are defined, this approach would have a broader application in identifying these translocations at a DNA rearrangement level. In addition to refining molecular cytogenetics these rearrangements would be unique for an individual tumor. They could, therefore, be used to address issues such as clonality, clonal evolution, clonal persistence, and clonal recurrence in a wide variety of neoplasms which bear chromosomal translocations.

The study of oncogenes can also have additional impact in predicting susceptibility to cancer and in providing objective information regarding prognosis. For example, it may allow the development of genetic screening assays which identify persons at risk for specific types of malignancy. Restriction fragment length polymorphisms around a given oncogene (genetic variation in the location of restriction endonuclease sites) may prove to be associated with an increased risk of cancer just as polymorphisms around the insulin gene have been linked with non-insulin requiring diabetes mellitus.[32] Similarly, mutations, insertions, or deletions within the oncogene itself may serve as markers of susceptibility.

The prognostic value of this molecular biologic approach is illustrated by the example of neuroblastomas. Neuroblastoma is a neoplasm which at times undergoes spontaneous regression as well as differentiation to a normal tissue counterpart in an unpredictable fashion. It has become apparent that the chromosome 1 abnormalities in neuroblastoma may be due to abnormalities of a specific oncogene n-myc, which shares sequence homology with c-myc.[33] The homogenous staining regions within chromosomes, as well as the extra chromosomal double minutes seen in neuroblastoma are cytogenetic manifestations of n-myc amplification. These findings implicate n-myc in the biologic behavior of neuroblastomas.[34] This contention is strongly supported by several recent observations:

1. There is minimal n-myc expression in stage 1 and stage 2 neuroblastoma tissues where tumor progression and patient death is unlikely; however, half of the cases with the more advanced stages 3 and 4 show a 3–300 fold increase in n-myc expression.[35]

2. It has also been noted that the ability to establish neuroblastoma cell lines in vitro from tumor tissues correlates with poor patient outcome. Conversely, it is difficult to derive cultured lines from patients with a good prognosis.[36] Correspondingly, neuroblastoma lines (8/9) express high levels of n-myc.

3. When the n-myc probe was hybridized in situ to human neuroblastoma tumor material it was observed to hybridize specifically to undifferentiated (small round and/or pleomorphic) tumor cells. It has

long been known that neuroblastoma lacking undifferentiated neuro-blasts blasts has a good prognosis, whereas composite tumors containing both differentiated and undifferentiated cells carry the prognosis of an undifferentiated neoplasm. The results with in situ hybridization substantiate the view that the biologically aggressive cells in neuroblastoma are, in fact, the small undifferentiated neuroblast.[37] It may be possible, therefore, using a combination of conventional and molecular biologic approaches, to predict in advance of treatment those patients with a poor prognosis. Those patients would be candidates for aggressive therapy, while those with more benign tumors require less aggressive or little therapy.

Conclusion

The molecular biologic approaches described in this chapter are already being used or have potential utility in the diagnosis and classification of neoplasms. The apparently random assembly of a single variable and joining Ig segment from multiple germline alternatives generates a unique clonal marker identifying an individual B cell and its progeny. Similarly, assembly of the T cell antigen receptor and the movement of genes at the breakpoints of interchromosomal recombinations generate unique markers for those cells and their progeny. This specificity is complemented by the sensitivity of this methodology which allows clonal cells to be identified when they contribute only one to five percent of the total DNA analyzed. Furthermore, since these rearrangements are DNA level markers, the expression of these genes is not required for their detection. DNA is extractable from fresh or frozen specimens, enhancing the applicability of this method for routinely available clinical material. The application of these molecular genetic approaches should greatly improve our ability to identify, classify, follow, and indeed predict the natural history of human neoplasms.

References

1. Aisenberg AC: Cell surface markers in lymphoproliferative disease. N Engl J Med 304:331–336, 1978
2. Rudders RA, Ahl ET Jr, DeLellis RA: Surface marker and histopathologic correlation with long term survival in advanced large-cell non-Hodgkin's lymphoma. Cancer 47:1329–1335, 1981

3. Fauget GB, Webb HH, Agee JF, et al: Immunologically diagnosed malignancy in Sjogren's pseudolymphoma. Am J Med 65:424–429, 1978

4. Levy R, Warnke R, Dorfman RF, et al: The monoclonality of human B-cell lymphomas. J Exp Med 145:1014–1028, 1977

5. Rowley JD, Fukuhara S: Chromosome studies in non-Hodgkin's lymphomas. Sem Oncol 7:225–266, 1980

6. Fialkow PJ, Jacobson RJ, Papayannopoulou T: Chronic myelocytic leukemia: clonal origin in a stem cell common to the granulocyte erythrocyte platelet and monocyte/macrophage. Am J Med 63:125–130, 1977

7. Stein RS, Cousar J, Flexner JM, et al: Correlations between immunologic markers and histopathologic classifications: clinical implications. Sem Oncol 7:244–254, 1980

8. York JC, Glick AD, Collins RD: Unclassified leukemias and lymphomas. Sem Oncol 9:497–503, 1982

9. Arnold A, Cossman J, Bakhshi A, et al: Immunoglobulin gene rearrangements as unique clonal markers in human lymphoid neoplasms. N Engl J Med 309:1593–1599, 1983

10. Tonewaga S: Somatic generation of antibody diversity. Nature 302:575–581, 1983

11. Korsmeyer SJ, Bakhshi A, Arnold A, et al: Genetic rearrangements of human immunoglobulin genes, in Greene MI, Nisonoff A (eds): The Biology of Idiotypes. Plenum Press, New York, 1984, pp 75–79

12. Hieter PA, Korsmeyer SJ, Waldmann TA, et al: Human immunoglobulin κ light-chain genes are deleted or rearranged in λ-producing B-cell. Nature 290:368–372, 1981

13. Korsmeyer SJ, Arnold A, Bakhshi A, et al: Immunoglobulin gene rearrangement and cell surface antigen expression in acute lymphocytic leukemias of T-cell and B-cell precursor origins. J Clin Invest 71:301–313, 1983

14. Bakhshi A, Minowada J, Arnold A, et al: Lymphoid blast crises of chronic myelogenous leukemia represent stages in the development of B-cell precursors. N Engl J Med 309:826–831, 1983

15. Korsmeyer SJ, Hieter PA, Ravetch JV, et al: Developmental hierarchy of immunoglobulin gene rearrangements in human leukemic pre-B-cells. Proc Natl Acad Sci USA 78:7096–7100, 1981

16. Cleary MI, Warnke R, Sklar J: Monoclonality of lymphoproliferative lesions in cardiac transplant recipients. N Engl J Med 310:477–482, 1984

17. Yanagi Y, Yoshikai Y, Leggett K, et al: A human T-cell specific cDNA

clone encodes a protein having extensive homology to immunoglobulin chains. Nature 308:145–149, 1984

18. Hedrick SM, Cohen DI, Nielson EA, et al: Isolation of cDNA clones encoding T-cell specific membrane-associated proteins. Nature 308: 149–153, 1984
19. Chien Y, Becker DM, Lindsten T, et al: A third type of murine T-cell receptor gene. Nature 312:31–35, 1984
20. Saito H, Kranz DM, Takagaki Y, et al: A third rearranged and expressed gene in a clone of cytotoxic T lymphocytes. Nature 312;36–40, 1984
21. Gatter KC, Alcook C, Heryet A, et al: The differential diagnosis of routinely processed anaplastic tumors using monoclonal antibodies. Am J Clin Pathol 82:33–43, 1984
22. Klein G: The role of gene dosage and genetic transpositions in carcinogenesis. Nature 294:313–318, 1982
23. Yunis JJ: The chromosomal basis of human neoplasia. Science 221:227–236, 1983
24. Taub R, Kirsh I, Morton C, et al: Translocation of the c-myc gene into the immunoglobulin heavy chain locus in human Burkitt's lymphoma and murine plasmacytoma cells. Proc Natl Acad Sci USA 79:7837–79:7837–7841, 1982
25. Dalla-Favera R, Martinotti S, Gallo R, et al: Translocation and rearrangements of the c-myc oncogene locus in human undifferentiated B-cell lymphomas. Science 219:963–967, 1983
26. Leder P, Battey J, Lenoir G, et al: Translocation among antibody genes in human cancer. Science 222:765–771, 1983
27. Erikson J, Ar-Rushdi A, Driwinga HL, et al: Transcriptional activation of the translocated c-myc oncogene in Burkitt lymphoma. Proc Natl Acad Sci USA 80:820–824, 1983
28. Yunis JJ, Oken MT, Kaplan ME, et al: Distinctive chromosomal abnormalities in histologic subtypes of non-Hodgkins lymphoma. N Engl J Med 307:1231–1236, 1982
29. Fukuhara S, Rowley JD, Variakojis D, et al: Chromosome abnormalities in poorly differentiated lymphocytic lymphoma. Cancer Res 39:3119–3131, 1979
30. Bakhshi A, Jensen JP, Goldman P, et al: Cloning the chromosomal breakpoint of t(14;18) bearing human lymphomas: clustering around J_H on chromosome 14 and near a transcriptional unit on chromosome 18. Cell (in press)
31. Tsujimoto Y, Finger LR, Yunis JJ, et al: Cloning of the chromosome

breakpoint of neoplastic B-cells with the t(14;18) chromosome translocation. Science 226:1097–1099, 1984

32. Rotwein PS, Chirgwin J, Provine M, et al: Polymorphism in the 5′ flanking region of the human insulin gene: a genetic marker for non-insulin-dependent diabetes. N Eng J Med 308:65–71, 1983

33. Schwab M, Varmus HE, Bishop JM, et al: Chromosome localization in normal human cells and neuroblastomas of a gene related to c-myc. Nature 308:288–291, 1984

34. Schwab M, Alitalo K, Klempnauer K-H, et al: Amplified DNA with limited homology to myc cellular oncogene is shared by human neuroblastoma cell lines and a neurobastoma tumour. Nature 305:245–248, 1983

35. Broudeur GM, Seeger RC, Schwab M, et al: Amplification of N-myc in untreated human neuroblastomas correlates with advanced disease stage. Science 224:1121–1124, 1984

36. Reynolds CP, Frenkel EP, Smith RG: Growth characteristics of neuroblastoma in vitro correlate with patient survival. Trans Assoc Am Phys 93:203–211, 1980

37. Schwab M, Ellison J, Busch M, et al: Enhanced expression of the human gene N-myc consequent to amplification of DNA may contribute to malignant progression of neuroblastoma. Proc Natl Acad Sci USA 81:4940–4944, 1984

21

POTENTIAL VALUE OF CELL KINETICS IN MANAGEMENT OF CANCERS OF UNKNOWN ORIGIN

John S. Meyer

Cancer of undetermined origin (CUO) has infrequently been a topic of study. No such title is found in the *Index Medicus,* nor in most textbooks. This heterogeneous group of tumors contains subsets with characteristics that differ in accord with their different progenitor tissues, although the metabolic and cell kinetic characteristics of the tissue of origin may be modified during neoplastic transformation. The physician needs methods for classification of the subsets in order to predict prognosis and plan therapy. Cells in different kinetic stages vary in susceptibility to many currently available antineoplastic agents, and kinetic properties of tumor cells could be useful in predicting response to therapy,[66,67] as well as to estimate tumor growth rate and prognosis.[38,73] Since studies of cell kinetics in CUO are virtually nonexistent, we will approach the topic through a review of cell kinetics of cancers of known primary site.

Comparative Cell Kinetics of Tumors

At present, the only body of kinetic data large enough to permit comparison among different anatomic sites and histologic categories is from thymidine labeling, which measures the proportion of cells in the

POORLY DIFFERENTIATED NEOPLASMS AND TUMORS OF UNKNOWN ORIGIN   ISBN 0-8089-1755-2
© 1986 by Grune & Stratton.   All rights of reproduction in any form reserved.

DNA synthetic phase (S phase) of the cell cycle.[32] Since the duration of the S phase does not appear to differ a great deal from one type of tumor to another, the thymidine labeling index (TLI) can be used to compare the rates of cellular proliferation.[32] A summary of the published data indicates that neoplasms can be divided into groups dependent on rates of proliferation. Our data (Table 21-1), which are derived entirely from a standardized in vitro labeling procedure,[34] allow comparison of different neoplasms without interference by variations from one technique to another. They are generally in close agreement with published data (Table 21-2). From analysis of these data, we have made the following seven observations.

First, benign neoplasms tend to have lower TLIs than malignant neoplasms. However, some carcinomas with metastatic capability have low TLIs. Noteworthy examples are adenocarcinomas of the thyroid and prostate glands, well-differentiated lymphocytic lymphomas, some breast carcinomas, and sarcomas.

Second, malignant tumors with low TLIs tend to have prolonged courses and/or low rates of recurrence after primary therapy. Examples that illustrate this principle are carcinoids, papillary and follicular carcinomas of the thyroid, adenocarcinoma of the prostate, some breast carcinomas, and well-differentiated lymphocytic lymphoma.

Third, malignant neoplasms with high TLIs run rapid courses once metastases have appeared. Notable examples supporting this rule are germ cell tumors, alimentary tract adenocarcinomas, Burkitt's and "histiocytic" lymphomas, small cell and most other carcinomas of the lung, and medullary carcinoma of the breast.[56]

Fourth, in various primary sites, high TLI tumors are more aggressive than low TLI tumors. This is true for breast,[19,35,37,73] transitional cell carcinomas of the urinary bladder,[69] and malignant lymphomas (Tables 21-1 and 21-2). This relationship does not appear to hold for colorectal carcinomas,[40] but the unimodal distribution of TLIs of colorectal carcinomas suggests that the great majority of them comprise a single kinetic population. In this population the spread of TLIs might reflect summation of sampling, diurnal, and other variabilities rather than fixed differences between kinetically distinctive subsets of tumors.

Fifth, the relationship between the proliferative rates of neoplasms of a given anatomic site and their degrees of histologic differentiation is variable. For example, the TLIs of well-differentiated tubular carcinomas of the breast fall in the low portion of the broad range for duct-forming carcinomas, whereas medullary carcinomas, which by definition are poorly differentiated, have high TLIs. However, infiltrating lobular (small cell) carcinomas of the breast also are poorly differentiated but usually have low TLIs.[33,37] The proliferative indices of central nervous system gliomas follow a close inverse relationship to the degree of differentiation.[23] Verrucous carcinoma, an unusually well-differentiated, nonmetastasizing variant of squamous cell carcinoma, is distinguished by low TLIs.[53] Presence of estrogen receptors, an expression of biochemical differentiation in breast carcinomas, is associated with low TLIs.[33,63] A weak inverse relationship was found between TLI and histologic differentiation of colorectal adeno-carcinoma.[7,40]

Sixth, a metastatic tumor has the same or sometimes a higher prolif-erative index than the primary lesion. Data indicate that the proliferative index may increase for breast carcinoma,[38] malignant melanoma (Tables 21-1 and 21-2), and prostatic carcinoma.[41]

Seventh, the capacity to metastasize is not closely related to the rate of cell production as measured by the TLI. For example, infiltrating lobular carcinomas of the breast,[33] well-differentiated carcinomas of the thyroid gland, and prostatic adenocarcinomas have low TLIs (Table 21-1) but high propensity to metastasize.

Applications to Cancers of Undetermined Origin

How can the above observations be applied to the problem of metastatic cancers of unknown origin? CUO is usually rapidly progres-sive.[43] The median survival has been one to three months, and only a small minority of patients have lived for a few years after diagnosis. Nonethe-less, some benefit would accrue from identification of patients with expectancy for survival of months or years rather than only weeks. The TLI or other cell kinetic measurements, for example, S phase fraction (SPF) measurements by flow cytometry,[4,39,48] could define such subsets. Cell kinetic information, however, must be interpreted in conjunction with the extent of dissemination of the cancer. We have noted that although the TLI is very useful for prediction of the relapse-free interval in breast carcinoma patients, the relapse-free survival curves for high and low TLI groups differ less for high stage than for low stage disease. For example, in stage 1 breast carcinoma patients treated by radical mastectomy, below median TLI was associated with a probability of relapse within four years of 10 percent, versus 50 percent for TLI above the median. In stage 2, the respective probabilities were 28 percent versus 50 percent and in stage 3, 44 percent versus 72 percent.[35] Tubiana and Silvestrini also noted a strong relation-

Table 21-1
Thymidine Labeling Indices (TLI) of Human Neoplasms

Tumor type	No.	%TLI Mean[*]	%TLI S.D.	Range
Benign				
Pheochromocytoma	5	0.06	0.08	0.00–0.15
Ovary, thecoma-fibroma	2	0.12		0.10–0.15
Kidney, oxyphile adenoma	5[*]	0.17	0.14	0.05–0.40
Parathyroid, adenoma	7	0.19	0.28	0.00–0.80
Thyroid, adenoma	7	0.32	0.45	0.00–1.30
Leiomyoma, nonuterine	6	0.33	0.25	0.00–0.70
Fibroadenoma of breast, stroma	13	0.53	0.48	0.00–1.30
Leiomyoma of myometrium	9	0.64	0.70	0.05–1.90
Granular cell tumor	3	0.65	0.53	0.10–1.15
Angiofibroma of nasopharynx	3	0.68	0.29	0.35–0.85
Eosinophilic granuloma, histiocytes	2	1.15		0.50–1.80
Proliferative myositis, fasciitis	4	1.21	1.19	0.30–2.90
Villous and tubular adenomas of large bowel	16	9.60	6.90	0.45–25.30
Questionable or Low Grade Malignancy				
Carcinoid, ileum	3	0.20	0.01	0.20–0.21
Carcinoid, bronchus	3	0.25	0.15	0.10–0.40
Thyroid, follicular carcinoma	2	0.35		0.10–0.60
Islet cell carcinoma of pancreas	1	0.38		
Desmoid tumor	3	0.43	0.28	0.20–0.75
Carcinoid, thymus	1	0.45		
Dermatofibrosarcoma protuberans	3	0.48	0.25	0.20–0.65
Carcinoid, stomach	1	0.70		
Thyroid, papillary carcinoma	7	0.70	0.68	0.10–2.05
Liposarcoma, well-differentiated (lipoma-like)	2	0.82		0.28–1.35
Ovary, granulosa cell tumor	2	3.38		2.60–4.15
Urothelium, transitional cell carcinoma, Grade I[(69)]	9	3.4	1.68	0.8–5.9
Verrucous carcinoma	4	5.60	1.38	4.30–6.70
Cystosarcoma phyllodes, stroma	8	6.44	6.07	1.00–16.40
Other malignant tumors				
Malignant lymphoma, well-differentiated lymphocytic	4	1.11	0.52	0.60–1.80
Prostate, adenocarcinoma	22	1.29	1.21	0.14–3.90
Kidney, clear cell carcinoma	7	2.14	3.08	0.35–9.00
Malignant melanoma, primary	6	3.09	1.89	0.25–5.80
Leiomyosarcoma, viscero–genital	3	3.77	2.35	1.07–5.30
Sarcomas, miscellaneous soft tissue	13	4.60	3.66	0.20–11.90
Liposarcoma	5	4.66	7.27	0.28–17.60

Table 21-1   *(continued)*

Tumor type	No.	%TLI Mean[*]	S.D.	Range
Malignant fibrous histiocytoma	4	6.59	3.99	0.77–9.80
Breast carcinoma, primary	437	6.78	6.15	0.05–35.60
Malignant melanoma, metastatic	9	6.82	4.72	0.45–13.80
Malignant mesothelioma	5	7.65	3.93	2.60–12.45
Urothelium, transitional cell carcinoma, Grade II[(69)]	8	8.2	8.2	0.7–26.1
Ovary, adenocarcinoma	5	8.22	4.24	2.60–14.40
Lung, adenocarcinoma	4	8.68	6.57	1.25–17.25
Breast carcinoma, metastatic	89	8.83	6.65	0.35–28.80
Gallbladder and bile ductal adenocarcinoma	3	8.87	3.54	6.60–12.95
Carcinoma, undetermined origin	6	11.26	6.40	2.95–16.90
Endometrium, adenocarcinoma	5	12.50	7.87	2.75–24.45
Urothelium, flat carcinoma in situ[(69)]	10	12.90	12.90	1.75–42.80
Squamous cell carcinoma, various sites	14	13.89	6.87	4.70–24.40
Stomach, adenocarcinoma	6	17.00	11.83	4.00–35.90
Lung, large cell carcinoma	4	17.45	10.13	8.06–30.14
Colorectal adenocarcinoma[(40)]	90	17.80	8.70	2.20–40.10
Urothelium, transitional cell carcinoma, Grade III[(69)]	14	18.0	7.9	1.0–32.5
Malignant lymphoma, diffuse large cell ("histiocytic")	16	21.08	10.69	5.45–45.80
Lung, small cell carcinoma	3	22.13	4.99	18.36–27.80
Malignant lymphoma, small transformed cell	3	22.87	3.62	19.00–26.20
Testis, seminoma	5	31.25	19.93	13.65–65.50
Testis, embryonal and teratocarcinoma	4	49.75	5.22	42.25–54.00

[*] Two patients; one patient had 4 adenomas.

ship between the TLI of breast carcinoma and probability of early relapse.[64,72]

At present, the primary determinants of selection of drugs for cytotoxic therapy of tumors are the site of origin and the histologic type. Because the majority of CUO are either adenocarcinomas or poorly differentiated cancers and most such carcinomas have high TLIs, the TLI

Table 21-2
Thymidine Labeling Indices (TLI) of Human Tumors Reported
from Other Laboratories

Tumor type	No.	%TLI, mean
Benign		
Phenochromocytoma[32]	2	0.1
Squamous papilloma of larynx[32]	12	5.8
Questionable or Low Grade Malignancy		
Meningioma[32]	4	1.3
Basal cell carcinoma[32]	22	8.1
Other Malignant Tumors		
Kidney, clear cell carcinoma[32]	9	0.6
Malignant lymphoma, well differentiated lymphocytic[13+32]	13	0.8
Prostate, adenocarcinoma[32]	8	1.4
Astrocytoma, Grade II[32]	2	2.0
Plasma cell myeloma[32]	33+	2.1
Kidney, granular cell carcinoma[32]	9	3.2
Urinary bladder, transitional cell carcinoma, Grade I[32]	15	3.7
Breast carcinoma, primary	623	3.9
Malignant lymphoma, nodular poorly differentiated lymphocytic[13]	6	4.2
Malignant lymphoma, poorly differentiated lymphocytic	27	4.7
Sarcomas of soft tissue[32]	37	4.9
Lung, adenocarcinoma[26]	7	6
Urinary bladder, transitional cell carcinoma, Grade II[32]	9	6.9
Malignant melanoma, primary[32+59]	44	7.9
Astrocytoma, Grades III and IV (gliobalstoma)[32]	17	8.4
Stomach, signet ring carcinoma[7]	4	8.5
Malignant lymphoma, mixed lymphocytic and "Histiocytic"[13+32]	20	8.7
Breast carcioma, metastatic[32]	80	9.3
Neuroblastoma[32]	17	12.6
Malignant melanoma, metastatic[32]	11	12.8
Squamous cell carcinoma, various sites[26+32]	200	14.6
Malignant lymphoma, "histiocytic"	31	15.0
Stomach, adenocarcinoma, tubular[7]	42	15.5
Lung, small cell carcinoma[26+32]	22	16.3
Lung, large cell carcinoma[26]	10	18
Colorectum, adenocarcinoma[7+32]	75	19.4
Stomach, adenocarcinoma, unspectified subtype[32]	5	22.7
Urinary bladder, transitional cell carcinoma, Grades II and IV[32]	14	23.0
Burkitt's lymphoma[32]	39	25.0

will not usually be helpful in determining a primary site. Adenocarcinomas with low TLIs, chiefly originating in the breast, prostate gland, kidney, and thyroid, do not comprise a large proportion of CUO. However, kinetic studies can distinguish this group of slowly progressive tumors from the more common rapidly progressive tumors.

The kinetic status of the carcinoma can be an important consideration for planning cytotoxic therapy. Thymidine labeling studies indicate that among solid tumors in adults, only those with high proliferative indices have shown appreciable rates of long-term complete remissions with cytotoxic therapy. They include germ cell tumors, "histiocytic" lymphomas, Burkitt's lymphoma, and small cell carcinoma of the lung (Table 21-1). Therefore, patients with poorly differentiated tumors with TLI (SPF) in excess of 15 percent to 20 percent might benefit from intensive chemotherapy with intent to eliminate the disease.

Attempts to subdivide small cell lung carcinomas into histologic subtypes that will predict response to chemotherapy have met with inconsistent results.[11,45] Recent flow cytometric analysis of DNA in these tumors has shown not only high S phase fractions, but also varying degrees of aneuploidy and multiple tumor stemlines in some cases.[74] The latter finding indicates a degree of genetic instability that could affect responsiveness to cytotoxic therapy and development of resistant strains. Conclusive studies relating proliferative and ploidy indices of a given type of tumor to responsiveness to therapy would be pertinent, but are not yet available. Scarffe observed a significant association between high SPF and complete remission in malignant lymphomas treated with cytotoxic agents,[60] but Silvestrini noted that complete remissions were more frequent with low rather than high TLI.[65]

Detailed cytokinetic studies in animal tumor models whereby cytotoxic therapy can be optimized to the tumor cell kinetics[66,67] are seldom practical for human neoplasms. S phase labeling, however, can be accomplished in vitro even with small surgical biopsies.[34] By use of this technique, relationships between the proliferative index and therapeutic responsiveness of a variety of tumors could be studied.[22] A newer technology substitutes 5-bromodeoxyuridine (BrdU) for tritiated thymidine as an S phase label. The labeled cells are detected by a monoclonal antibody to BrdU.[21] This method reproduces the results of thymidine labeling and avoids the delay attendant on exposure of autoradiographs. Flow cytometric measurement of the DNA index provides another potentially useful approach, and by using BrdU as an S phase marker, the accuracy of %S measurements by flow cytometry may be improved.[15,42]

Measurement of DNA Content ("Ploidy") and %S by
Flow Cytometry

Flow cytometry can define tumors with normal or nearly normal DNA content (diploid) and clearly abnormal DNA content (aneuploid). As we use *diploid,* it implies DNA content indistinguishable from normal by flow cytometry. Cytogenetic abnormalities may nonetheless be present in these tumors.[5] Aneuploid tumors are usually hyperdiploid, but occasionally are hypodiploid. In a series of 261 patients with a variety of different tumors reported by Barlogie, 81 percent were aneuploid.[4] The frequency of aneuploidy differs according to the type of tumor (Table 21-3). By mathematical analysis of the DNA histogram the percent of cells in the various phases of the cell cycle (G_1, S, G_2+M) can be estimated. Barlogie noted that a high G_1+G_0 fraction, indicative of low proliferative activity, and ploidy level (DNA index) not exceeding 1.5 times diploid were associated with survival, whereas low G_1+G_0 fraction and DNA index over 1.5 were associated with early mortality.[4] High DNA indices in carcinoma of the breast are associated with high TLI[39] and with high %S (percent of cells in DNA synthesis) by flow cytometric analysis.[47,48,55] Diploid tumors tend to proliferate slowly (Fig. 21-1), and tumors with high DNA content tend to proliferate more rapidly (Fig. 21-2).[5] Although a correlation between the DNA index and proliferative indices does exist, it is not sufficiently high to predict proliferative activity in a given tumor. We have observed TLIs under one percent in metastatic islet cell carcinoma (Fig. 21-3) and in a metastasizing carcinoid tumor, each of which had a prominent aneuploidy. Some breast carcinomas have high TLIs despite diploid DNA indices,[39] and large cell malignant lymphomas are not infrequently diploid by flow cytometry,[62] although as a class they are rapidly proliferative by thymidine labeling.[36,49,65] We have also noted diploid malignant lymphomas with high TLIs (Fig. 21-4) and multiple hyperdiploid populations in breast carcinomas with low TLIs (Fig. 21-5).

Experience relating DNA flow cytometric data to survival in patients with cancer is scanty. Braylan reported a significant negative correlation between the %S and survival in 27 patients with malignant lymphoma.[8] Since the TLI correlates significantly with the %S of breast carcinoma measured by flow cytometry,[30,39] we suspect that the %S will also be a stage-independent prognostic factor. The prognostic significance of the DNA index apart from its correlation with the proliferative index is only beginning to emerge. Presence of aneuploid clones has been significantly associated with early relapse after primary treatment in carcinoma of the ovary,[17] malignant lymphomas,[14] and the mycosis fungoides–Sezary syn-

Table 21-3
DNA Indices of Human Solid Tumors

Tumor type	No.	Aneuploid, %	Reference
Brain tumors, collected reports	81	48	5
Breast carcinoma	588	70	6, 12, 16, 28, 30, 39, 47, 55, 70
Colorectal adenocarcinoma	180	76	29, 51, 16, 57
Kidney, parenchymal carcinoma	90	50	3, 16
Leukemia, childhood acute, collected reports	411	24	5
Leukemia, adult acute myelogenous	339	11	5
Leukemia, adult acute lymphocytic	123	46	5
Lung, squamous cell carcinoma	20	100	46, 54
Lung, adenocarcinoma	31	94	46, 54
Lung, small cell carcinoma	38	71	54, 74
Lymphoma, well-differentiated lymphocytic	9	33	13
Lymphoma, non-Hodgkin's intermediate grade[*]	54	59	13, 14
Lympnoma, non-Hodgkin's, high grade[†]	34	79	13, 14
Lymphomas, non-Hodgkin's, various grades, collected reports	360	53	5
Lymphoma, large B cell	10	50	62
Lymphoma, small B cell	16	25	62
Lymphoma, T cell	12	17	62
Melanoma, primary	40	73	16, 68
Melanoma, metastatic	87	80	16, 68
Mycosis fungoides	63	63	13, 14
Ovary, carcinoma	177	62	16, 17, 27
Plasma cell myeloma	177	76	4, 9
Prostatic carcinoma, collected reports	147	62	5
Sarcoma, primary	46	50	16
Sarcoma, metastatic	42	71	16
Squamous cell carcinoma of skin	220	82	61
Testicular cancer	74	93	61
Thyroid, follicular carcinoma	4	25	25
Thyroid, anaplastic carcinoma	2	100	25
Urinary bladder, invasive carcinoma[‡]		67	31
Urinary bladder, papillary carcinoma in situ[‡]		42	31
Urinary bladder, carcinoma, various grades, collected reports	511	83	5
Uterine cervix, carcinoma	91	94	24, 29

[*] According to Rappaport classification: nodular poorly differentiated lymphocytic, nodular mixed, diffuse poorly differentiated lymphocytic.

[†] According to Rappaport classification: nodular histiocytic, diffuse mixed, diffuse histiocytic, diffuse undifferentiated.

[‡] Flow cytometry obtained on bladder washings; aneuploidy rate could be underestimated because of inadequate sampling of some tumors.

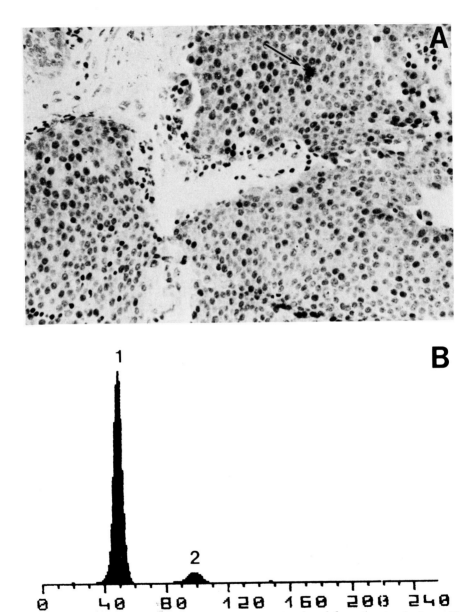

Figure 21-1. *(A) Autoradiograph of diploid carcinoid of ileum after incubation with tritiated thymidine. A single labeled nucleus is covered by dark silver grains (arrow), TLI = 0.2 percent (X 270). (B) Flow cytometric DNA histogram of ileal carcinoid. Note the single G_1/G_0 peak (1), single G_2/M peak (2), and no appreciable number of events in the intervening S phase region.*

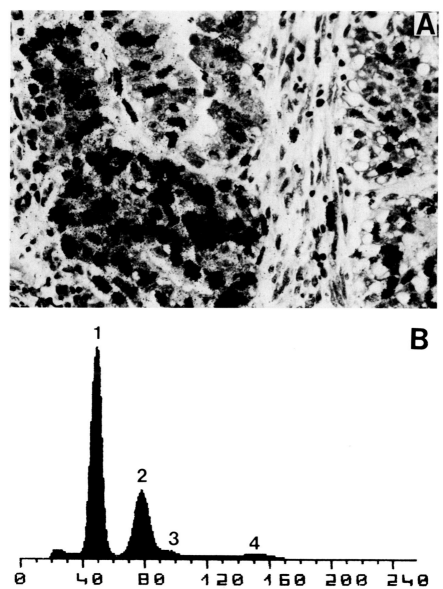

Figure 21-2. *(A) Autoradiograph of aneuploid testicular teratocarcinoma after incubation with tritiated thymidine. Note labeling of approximately half of the malignant epithelial nuclei and of fewer nuclei in the intervening stroma. The TLI of the epithelium varied from 24 percent in better differentiated areas to 50 percent or more in areas like that shown (X 270). The nuclei are large in comparison to those of the diploid carcinoid (See Figure 21-1A). (B) Flow cytometric DNA histogram of testicular teratocarcinoma shows diploid cells (1) and hyperdiploid neoplastic G_1/G_0 population (2) (DNA index = 1.60). Peak 3 represents the diploid G_2/M cells, and peak 4 the hyperdiploid G_2/M cells. A large number of hyperdiploid S phase cells is present between peaks 3 and 4.*

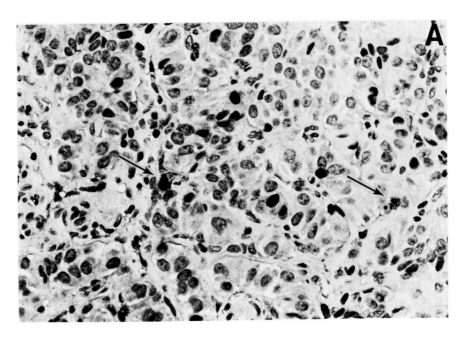

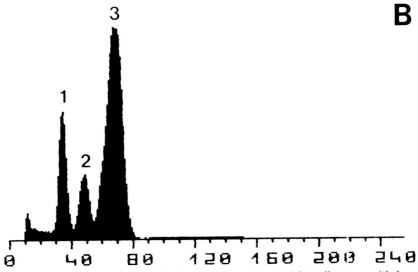

Figure 21-3. (A) Autoradiograph of aneuploid malignant islet cell tumor with hepatic metastases after incubation with tritiated thymidine. Two labeled nuclei are shown (arrows), TLI = 0.4 percent (X 270). (B) Flow cytometric DNA histogram of islet cell carcinoma shows a diploid G_1/G_0 peak (2) flanked by hypodiploid G_1/G_0 peak (1) with DNA index = 0.72 and a hyperdiploid G_1/G_0 peak (3) with DNA index = 1.41. The profile dips to the baseline briefly to the right of peak 3, indicating a paucity of S phase cells, and the merged G_2/M peaks of the diploid and hyperdiploid populations follow.

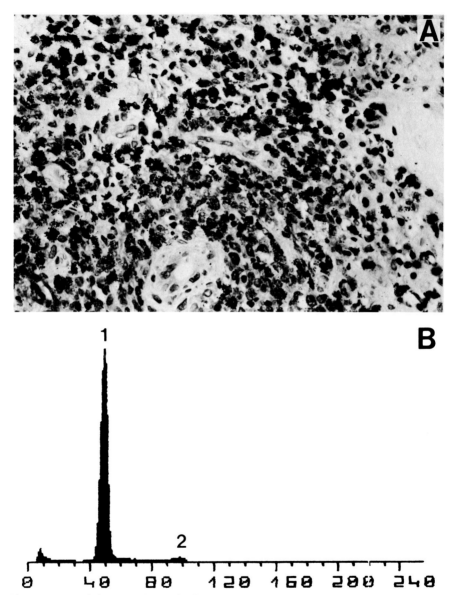

Figure 21-4. *(A) Autoradiograph of diploid diffuse large cell ("histiocytic") malignant lymphoma after incubation with tritiated thymidine. Numerous nuclei are labeled, particularly near the blood vessels (lower center), TLI = 27.4 percent (X 270). (B) Flow cytometric DNA histogram of diffuse large cell lymphoma shows a single G_1/G_0 peak in the diploid position (1) and a single G_2/M peak (2). The elevated plateau between the two peaks indicates the presence of many S phase cells.*

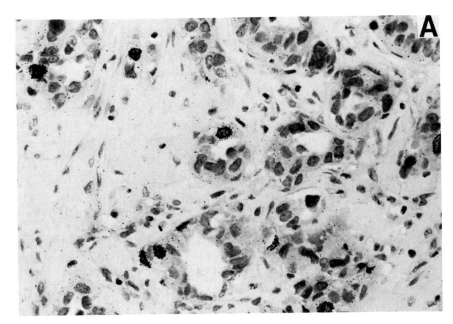

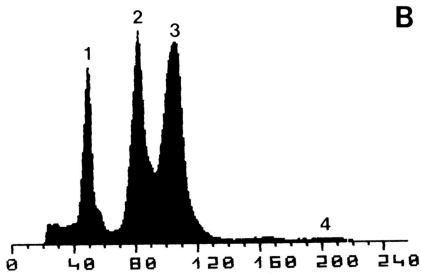

Figure 21-5. *(A) Autoradiograph of aneuploid breast carcinoma after incubation with tritiated thymidine. Note several labeled nuclei (TLI = 1.85 percent). The nuclei are relatively large in comparison to those of the diploid carcinoid (see Fig. 21-1(A)) and histiocytic lymphoma (Fig. 21-4(B)) (X 270). (B) Flow cytometric DNA histogram of breast carcinoma shows diploid G_1/G_0 peak (1) followed by two hyperdiploid peaks (2, 3) with DNA indices = 1.65, 2.11. The shoulder on the right side of the diploid peak is consistent with a minor population of slightly hyperdiploid carcinoma cells. The G_2/M cells belonging to the most hyperdiploid population form a low peak (4). Between peaks 3 and 4 are hyperdiploid S phase cells and the G_2/M cells of the population forming peak 2.*

drome.[10] A similar trend was observed in malignant melanoma.[68] By Feulgen microdensitometry, which gives ploidy results analogous to those from flow cytometry, Atkin and Auer and coworkers have shown that aneuploidy is associated with high mortality in breast carcinoma patients.[1,2]

Presence of multiple stemlines with different DNA indices has been noted frequently in adenocarcinoma of the large intestine,[50] small cell carcinomas of the lung,[74] large cell lymphomas,[13] malignant melanoma,[68] and in breast carcinomas (Fig. 21-5).[52] Teodori has reported that most uterine tumors lack aneuploid populations, some small cell lung carcinomas are quasidiploid, most gastric carcinomas have a single aneuploid population, and most adenocarcinomas of the lung have more than one aneuploid population.[71] Ruta succeeded in culturing three stemlines from a single supraclavicular metastasis of breast carcinoma.[58] The clones, which were carried for more than a year in vitro, had modal chromosome numbers of 72, 80, and 88. This confirms, by cytogenetic analysis, the impression of polyclonality from DNA flow cytometry. The significance of multiple stemlines in terms of other biologic characteristics, for example, growth rate, sensitivity to hormonal and cytotoxic agents, is not known. Histologic characteristics of nuclear anaplasia predict hyperdiploidy.[3]

Very little is known about the cytogenetic stability of human malignancies. Those tumors in which multiplicity of aneuploid clones is most common would appear to be the most unstable. Instability may relate to a combination of rapid proliferation and high rate of cell loss. In this combination of circumstances the number of antecedent cell divisions in a tumor of a given size is greatly increased relative to that of a slowly proliferative, low cell loss tumor of the same size.[20] Given a fixed mutational rate, the probability of a mutation is proportional to the number of cell divisions. We know of one study designed to show changes of the DNA index of tumors with passage of time. In a group of nine patients with ovarian carcinoma studied initially and after relapse, Friedlander noted no significant change in the DNA index.[18]

Conclusions

Both the labeling index, by use of tritiated thymidine or BrdU, and flow cytometry have roles to play in the evaluation of malignant neoplasms, and both should be useful in helping to define cancers of unknown primary site. Since kinetic data cannot always be extracted reliably from complex DNA histograms, the labeling index gives more reliable proliferative indices than does flow cytometry. Flow cytometry contributes a DNA index and can detect polyclonality when multiple DNA indices occur in the same tumor. Presence of more than one aneuploid clone in a tumor may be of particular interest if this type of genetic instability correlates with appearance of drug-resistant mutants. Well-planned prospective studies should contribute useful information.

Acknowledgments

Jeanne Ruperto was technically responsible for the thymidine labeling. Kenneth Stone, Ph.D. operated the flow cytometer. Robert Henry helped prepare the illustrations. Meredith Hammer provided secretarial assistance and typed the manuscript.

References

1. Atkin NB: Modal deoxyribonucleic acid value and survival in carcinoma of the breast. Br Med J 1:271–272, 1972
2. Auer G, Eriksson E, Azavedo E, et al: Prognostic significance of nuclear DNA content in mammary adenocarcinomas in humans. Cancer Res 44:394–396, 1984
3. Baisch H, Otto U, König K, et al: DNA content of human kidney carcinoma cells in relation to histological grading. Br J Cancer 45:878–886, 1982
4. Barlogie B, Johnston DA, Smallwood L, et al: Prognostic implications of ploidy and proliferative activity in human solid tumors. Cancer Genet Cytogenet 6:17–28, 1982
5. Barlogie B, Raber MN, Schumann J, et al: Flow cytometry in clinical cancer research. Cancer Res 43:3982–3997, 1983
6. Bichel P, Poulsen HS, Andersen J: Estrogen receptor content and ploidy of human mammary carcinoma. Cancer 50:1771–1774, 1982
7. Bleiberg H, Buyse M, van den Heule B, et al: Cell cycle parameters and prognosis of colorectal cancer. Eur J Cancer Clin Oncol 20:391–20:391–396, 1984
8. Braylan RD, Diamond LW, Powell ML, et al: Percentage of cells in the S-phase of the cell cycle in human lymphoma determined by flow cytometry. Correlation with labeling index and patient survival. Cytometry 1:171–174, 1980
9. Bunn PA Jr, Krasnow S, Makuch RW, et al: Flow cytometric analysis

of DNA content of bone marrow cells in patients with plasma cell myeloma: clinical implications. Blood 59:528–535, 1982

10. Bunn PA Jr, Whang-Peng J, Carney D, et al: DNA content analysis by flow cytometry in mycosis fungoides and Sezary syndrome. J Clin Invest 65:1440–1448, 1980

11. Burdon JGW, Sinclair RA, Henderson MM: Small cell carcinoma of the lung. Prognosis in relation to histologic subtype. Chest 76:302–304, 1979

12. Chassevent A, Daver A, Bertrand G, et al: Comparative flow DNA analysis of different cell suspensions in breast carcinoma. Cytometry 5:263–267, 1984

13. Costa A, Mazzini G, Delbino G, et al: DNA content and proliferative characteristics of non-Hodgkin's lymphoma: determined by flow cytometry and autoradiography. Cytometry 2:185–191, 1981

14. Diamond LW, Nathwani BN, Rappaport H: Flow cytometry in the diagnosis and classification of malignant lymphoma and leukemia. Cancer 50:1122–1135, 1982

15. Dolbeare F, Gratzner HG, Pallavicini MG, et al: Flow cytometric measurement of total DNA content and incorporated bromodeoxyuridine. Proc Natl Acad Sci USA 80:5573–5577, 1983

16. Frankfurt OS, Slocum HK, Rustum YM, et al: Flow cytometric analysis of DNA aneuploidy in primary and metastatic human solid tumors. Cytometry 5:71–80, 1984

17. Friedlander ML, Hedley DW, Taylor IW, et al: Influence of cellular DNA content on survival in advanced ovarian cancer. Cancer Res 44:397–400, 1984

18. Friedlander ML, Taylor IW, Russell P, et al: Cellular DNA content— a stable feature in epithelial ovarian cancer. Br J Cancer 49:173–179, 1984

19. Gentili C, Sanfilippo O, Silvestrini R: Cell proliferation and its relationship to clinical features and relapse in breast cancers. Cancer 48:974–979, 1981

20. Goldie JH: A model for the relation between tumor growth rates and curability. Eighth Annual Meeting, Cell Kinetics Society, Memphis, Tennessee, 1984

21. Gratzner HG: Monoclonal antibody to 5-bromo- and 5-iododeoxyuridine: a new reagent for detection of DNA replication. Science 218:474–475, 1982

22. Hart JS, Livingston RB, Murphy WK, et al: Neoplasia, kinetics, and chemotherapy. Sem Oncol 3:259–267, 1976

23.   Hoshino T, Wilson CB: Cell kinetic analysis of human malignant brain tumors (gliomas). Cancer 44:956–962, 1979

24.   Jacobsen A, Bichel P, Sell A: DNA distribution in biopsy specimens from human cervical carcinoma investigated by flow cytometry. Virchows Arch (B) Cell Pathol 29:337–342, 1979

25.   Johannessen JV, Sobrinho-Simoes M, Lindmo T, et al: The diagnostic value of flow cytometric DNA measurements in selected disorders of the human thyroid. Am J Clin Pathol 77:10–25, 1982

26.   Kerr KM, Robertson AMG, Lamb D: *In vitro* thymidine labelling of human pulmonary neoplasms. Br J Cancer 47:245–252, 1983

27.   Krug H, Ebeling K: Impulszytophotometrische Charakterisierung von malignen Ovarialtumoren. Arch Geschwulstforsch 46:214–224, 1978

28.   Kute TE, Muss HB, Anderson D, et al: Relationship of steroid receptor, cell kinetics and clinical status in patients with breast cancer. Cancer Res 41:3524–3529, 1981

29.   Linden WA, Beck HP, Baisch H, et al: Flow cytometric analysis of cervical smears and solid tumors. Acta Pathol Microbiol Scand (A) 274(suppl):443–447, 1981

30.   McDivitt RW, Stone KR, Meyer JS: A method for dissociation of viable human breast cancer cells that produces flow cytometric kinetic information similar to that obtained by thymidine labeling. Cancer Res 44:2628–2633, 1984

31.   Melamed MR, Klein FA: Flow cytometry of urinary bladder irrigation specimens. Hum Pathol 15:302–305, 1984

32.   Meyer JS: Growth and cell kinetic measurements in human tumors. Pathol Ann 16:53–81, 1981

33.   Meyer JS, Bauer WC, Rao BR: Subpopulations of breast carcinoma defined by S-phase fraction, morphology, and estrogen receptor content. Lab Invest 39:225–235, 1978

34.   Meyer JS, Connor RE: In vitro labeling of solid tissues with tritiated thymidine for autoradiographic detection of S-phase nuclei. Stain Technol 52:185–105, 1977

35.   Meyer JS, Friedman E, McCrate MM: Prediction of early course of breast carcinoma by thymidine labeling. Cancer 51:1879–1886, 1983

36.   Meyer JS, Higa E: S-phase fractions of cells in lymph nodes and malignant lymphomas. Arch Pathol Lab Med 103:93–97, 1979

37.   Meyer JS, Hixon B: Advanced stage and early relapse of breast carcinomas associated with high thymidine labeling indices. Cancer Res 39:4042–4047, 1979

38.   Meyer JS, Lee JY: Relationships of S-phase fraction of breast carcinoma in relapse to duration of remission, estrogen receptor content,

therapeutic responsiveness, and duration of survival. Cancer Res 40:1890–1896, 1980

39. Meyer JS, Micko S, Craver JL, et al: DNA flow cytometry of breast carcinoma after acetic-acid fixation. Cell Tissue Kinet 17:185–197, 1984

40. Meyer JS, Prioleau PG: S-phase fractions of colorectal carcinomas related to pathologic and clinical features. Cancer 48:1221–1228, 1981

41. Meyer JS, Sufrin G, Martin SA: Proliferative activity of benign human prostate, prostatic adenocarcinoma and seminal vesicle evaluated by thymidine labeling. J Urol 128:1353–1356, 1982

42. Mortsyn G, Hsu SM, Kinsella T, et al: Bromodeoxyuridine in tumors and chromosomes detected with a monoclonal antibody. J Clin Invest 72:1844–1850, 1983

43. Neumann KH, Nystrom JS: Metastatic cancer of unknown origin: nonsquamous cell type. Sem Oncol 9:427–434, 1982

44. Newburger AE, Weinstein G: Cell proliferation patterns in human malignant melanoma, in vivo. Cancer 46:308–313, 1980

45. Nixon DW, Murphy GF, Sewell CW, et al: Relationship between survival and histologic type in small cell anaplastic carcinoma of the lung. Cancer 44:1045–1049, 1979

46. Olszewski W, Darzynkiewicz Z, Claps ML, et al: Flow cytometry of lung carcinoma: a comparison of DNA stemline and cell cycle distribution with histology. Ann Quant Cytol 4:90–94, 1982

47. Olszewski W, Darzynkiewicz Z, Rosen PP, et al: Flow cytometry of breast carcinoma. I. Relation of DNA ploidy level to histology and estrogen receptor. Cancer 48:980–984, 1981

48. Olszewski W, Darzynkiewicz Z, Rosen PP, et al: Flow cytometry of breast carcinoma: II. Relation of tumor cell cycle distribution to histology and estrogen receptor. Cancer 48:985–988, 1981

49. Peckham MJ, Cooper EH: The pattern of cell growth in reticulum cell sarcoma and lymphosarcoma. Eur J Cancer 6:453–463, 1970

50. Petersen SE, Bichel P, Lorentzen M: Flow-cytometric demonstration of tumor-cell subpopulations with different DNA content in human colorectal carcinoma. Eur J Cancer 15:383–386, 1979

51. Petersen SE, Lorentzen M, Bichel P: A mosaic subpopulation structure of human colorectal carcinomas demonstrated by flow cytometry. Acta Pathol Microbiol Scand (A) 274(suppl):412–416, 1981

52. Prey MU, Meyer JS, Stone KR, et al: Heterogeneity of breast carcinomas determined by flow cytometric analysis. J Surg Oncol 29:35–39, 1985

53. Prioleau PG, Santa Cruz DJ, Meyer JS, et al: Verrucous carcinoma. A

light and electron microscopic, autoradiographic, and immunofluorescence study. Cancer 45:2849–2857, 1980

54. Raber MN, Barlogie B, Farquhar D: Determination of ploidy abnor-
     mality and cell cycle distribution in human lung cancer using DNA
     flow cytometry (abstr). Proc Am Assoc Cancer Res 21:40, 1980

55. Raber MN, Barlogie B, Latreille J, et al: Ploidy, proliferative activity
     and estrogen receptor content in human breast cancer. Cytometry
     3:36–41, 1982

56. Ridolfi RL, Rosen PP, Port A, et al: Medullary carcinoma of the breast.
     A clinicopathologic study with 10 year follow-up. Cancer 40:1365–
     1385, 1977

57. Rognum TO, Refsum SB, Thorud E: Cell kinetics of human colonic
     adenocarcinomas. II. Relationship between ploidy pattern, tumour
     spread and cell kinetic parameters (abstr). Cell Tissue Kinet 17:304,
     1984

58. Ruta C, Natale RB, Edwards J: Direct evidence of heterogeneity in the
     stem cell population of a breast cancer metastasis (abstr). Proc Am
     Assoc Cancer Res 25:30, 1984

59. Sasaki K, Takahashi M, Ogino T, et al: An autoradiographic study on
     the labeling index of biopsy specimens from gastric cancers. Cancer
     (in press)

60. Scarffe JH, Crowther D: The pre-treatment proliferative activity of
     non-Hodgkin's lymphoma cells. Eur J Cancer 17:99–108, 1981

61. Schumann: Unpublished observations quoted by Barlogie B, et al:
     Cancer Res 43:3982–3997, 1983

62. Shackney SE, Skramstad KS, Cunningham RE, et al: Dual parameter
     flow cytometry studies in human lymphomas. J Clin Invest 66:1281–
     1294, 1980

63. Silvestrini R, Diadone MG, Di Fronzo G: Relationship between
     proliferative activity and estrogen receptors in breast cancer. Cancer
     44:665–670, 1979

64. Silvestrini R, Diadone MG, Motta R, et al: Predictivity of cell kinetics
     on clinical outcome of human tumors. Cell Tissue Kinet 17:289–290
     (abstract), 1984

65. Silvestrini R, Piazza R, Riccardi A, et al: Correlation of cell kinetic
     findings with morphology of non-Hodgkin's malignant lymphomas.
     J Natl Cancer Inst 58:499–504, 1977

66. Skipper HE: Kinetics of mammary tumor cell growth and implications
     for therapy. Cancer 28:1479–1499, 1971

67. Skipper HE, Schabel FM Jr, Mellett LB, et al: Implications of biochem-
     ical, cytokinetic, pharmacologic, and toxicologic relationships in the

design of optimal therapeutic schedules. Cancer Chemother Rep 54:431–450, 1970

68. Sondergaard JO, Larsen JK, Moller U, et al: DNA ploidy-characteristics of human malignant melanoma analyzed by flow cytometry and compared with histological and clinical course. Virchows Arch (Cell Pathol) 42:43–52, 1983

69. Sufrin G, Meyer JS, Martin SA, et al: Proliferative activity of urothelium and tumors of renal pelvis, ureter, and urinary bladder evaluated by thymidine labeling. Urology 23(suppl):15–22, 1984

70. Taylor IW, Musgrove EA, Friedlander ML, et al: The influence of age on the DNA ploidy levels of breast tumors. Eur J Cancer Clin Oncol 19:623–628, 1983

71. Teodori L, de Vita R, Mauro F: Flow cytometrically determined ploidy level as an indicator of cellular heterogeneity of human solid tumors (abstr). Cell Tissue Kinet 17:303–304, 1984

72. Tubiana M, Pejovic MH, Chavaudra N, et al: The long-term prognostic significance of the thymidine labeling index in breast cancer. Int J Cancer 33:441–445, 1984

73. Tubiana M, Pejovic MJ, Renaud A, et al: Kinetic parameters and the course of the disease in breast cancer. Cancer 47:937–943, 1981

74. Vindelov LL, Hansen HH, Christensen IJ, et al: Clonal heterogeneity of small-cell anaplastic carcinoma of the lung demonstrated by flow-cytometric DNA analysis. Cancer Res 40:4295–4300, 1980

22

UNDIFFERENTIATED NEOPLASMS AND CANCERS OF UNKNOWN PRIMARY: A CLINICOPATHOLOGICAL PERSPECTIVE

Nicholas J. Robert
Marc B. Garnick
Emil Frei, III

The management of patients with undifferentiated neoplasms or cancers of unknown primary site presents a formidable problem. The common denominator in both heterogeneous groups of patients is that the cell of origin is unknown, the natural history or response to therapy cannot be predicted, and treatment plans usually cannot be based on the specific features of the tumor. The approach to the patients harboring a neoplasm that falls into either category requires a team effort with input from both clinical and laboratory disciplines. We will summarize our current approach to the patient with undifferentiated neoplasm or cancer of unknown origin, with an emphasis on the clincopathologic perspective.

The first group of patients present a problem in identifying the type of neoplasm. The bisopsy reveals an undifferentiated neoplasm without further qualifications. It is unclear whether the cell lineage is ectodermal, endodermal, or mesenchymal. In practical terms, the questions are usually

POORLY DIFFERENTIATED NEOPLASMS AND TUMORS OF UNKNOWN ORIGIN   ISBN 0-8089-1755-2

whether the neoplasm is carcinoma vs. lymphoma vs. sarcoma, or adeno-carcinoma vs. squamous cell carcinoma vs. small cell carcinoma. The second group of patients present with a tissue diagnosis usually of specific neoplasm, e.g., adenocarcinoma without a known primary. An anatomic site or origin cannot be determined in approximately 0.5–10 percent of all patients with a diagnosis of cancer.[1-4] These situations pose special problems with respect to diagnosis and therapy. There has been a tendency to order tests in a "shotgun" manner with the hopes of obtaining more information. The yield from performing numerous diagnostic studies however, is often low. These tests becomes time-consuming and expensive; they are inconvenient to the patients and they postpone treatment.[5-6] Another tendency is to oversimplify the diagnostic possibilities. All young men with poorly differentiated carcinomas, for example, would be treated as if they have germ cell cancer, or patients with an undifferentiated neoplasm would be treated as if they have lymphoma. This approach, while useful in certain circumstances, may not fully utilize the recent advances in diagnostic tests that may provide greater specificity in diagnosis and subsequent treatment.

There is obviously a need for a multidisciplinary organized approach to these problems. Today, there are a number of cancers that can be cured or at least effectively palliated even though the cancer is disseminated (Table 22-1). In a recent review it was estimated that there now are fourteen disseminated forms of cancer that are potentially curable.[7] In the next five to ten years, it is hoped that many additional categories of neoplastic disease will be added. Any approach to the patient with an undifferentiated neoplasm or "cancer of unknown origin" must ensure that these treatable tumors are identified.

The Evaluation of Patients with a Tumor of Unknown Origin

The Initial Clinical Evaluation

The initial clinical assessment should be thorough. The patient who is admitted with brain metastases may have metastatic melanoma, which will be appreciated only after a close examination of the skin. A careful history may reveal factors such as exposure to asbestos, a disappearing pigmented skin lesion, a family history of breast cancer, or exposure to unusual toxins. A physical examination should pay particular attention to the skin, lymph nodes, oral cavity, and rectum. In women, deliberate examination of the breasts and pelvic organs should be done. Similarly, in men, examination

Table 22-1
Role of systemic treatment in certain tumors

Curative potential:	Lymphomas (Hodgkin's and non-Hodgkin's disease)
	Germ cell tumors
	Acute leukemia
	Ovarian carcinoma
	Small cell carcinoma of the lung
	Pediatric sarcomas
Effective palliative potential:	
	Breast cancer*
	Prostate cancer*
	Gastric carcinoma
	Endometrial carcinoma*
	Medullary carcinoma of the thyroid
	Islet cell tumors of the pancreas
	Head and neck tumors
	Sarcomas

* Treatment solely with hormonal therapy can be very effective.

of the testes and prostate is indicated. Stools should be checked for occult blood. When additional information is learned, the exam should be repeated with the appropriate question in focus. If the issue is undifferentiated neoplasm, then a very thorough examination of the lymph nodes and the skin is needed. Discovering diffuse adenopathy in this setting would provide another biopsy site and might favor a diagnosis of lymphoma. In patients in which the anatomic site is being determined, possible primary sites such as the oral cavity, breast, pelvic organs, and prostate should be emphasized.

The Biopsy

It is mandatory that the biopsy be reviewed with the pathologist. The surgical pathologist's insight into the type of problem can be greatly extended by direct communication with the clinical oncologist. In such combined efforts, basic problems can be addressed, such as the adequacy of the biopsy tissue, the extent of differentiation, and the utility of special stains or other histological tests. Rarely, the actual diagnosis of cancer may prove to be erroneous after obtaining a correct clinical perspective; this is especially true for lesions which are sarcomatous-like or contain pleomorphic lymphocytic infiltration suggestive of lymphoma.

An important feature in determining the nature of a neoplasm is the architectural pattern, which is difficult to evaluate when only a few malignant cells are present, thus underscoring certain limitations of cytology. Larger specimens provide more tissue for microscopic examination and may reveal diagnostic elements that would be missed in a smaller biopsy. An example could be the discovery of teratomatous elements diagnostic of a germ cell tumor in a biopsy specimen, while the cytologic interpretation could simply be an undifferentiated carcinoma. After such a review it may be concluded that a repeat biopsy is needed. A detailed investigation can then be planned to maximize the diagnostic capabilities and to prepare for studies that may require fresh tissue for examination. There are a number of special studies that can be done on the biopsy of the tumor. They include special stains, immunohistochemical stains, biochemical assays, and electron microscopy.

Special stains usually refer to histochemical stains that are routinely provided in most histology laboratories. They include stains for mucin, fat, glycogen, and melanin. In the case of adenocarcinoma without a known anatomic primary, the demonstration of intracellular mucin makes such sites as kidney, prostate, and a number of endocrine organs less likely. Fresh tissue is needed for fat or glycogen. In the case of the latter, prompt placement of a portion of the specimen in alcohol increases the chance of demonstrating glycogen. This is a useful technique in tumors rich in glycogen such as Ewing's sarcoma and renal cell carcinoma.

The next major category of special studies that can be performed by a pathology laboratory is the testing with immunohistochemical stains using a number of immunoperoxidase reagents. This procedure can be applied to problems in which only formalin-fixed, paraffin-embedded tissue is available. Some of the reagents, however, do require fresh tissue. Review of the case with the surgical pathologist can help decide whether another biopsy for fresh tissue will be needed.

These immunoperoxidase reagents consist of polyclonal antibodies or more recently monoclonal antibodies derived from hybridoma technology.[8, 9] These reagents include antibodies that are directed at immunoglobulins, surface antigents, receptors for growth factors, cytoskelatal antigens, organelle antigens, and antigens which appear during selective stages of the cell cycle. Most tumor biologists and immunologists challenge the concept of the existence of tumor-specific antibodies and antigens. Nevertheless, organ-specific or selective antibodies to antigens shared by, for example, the normal prostate and prostate cancer, are highly useful. In addition, there are differentiation antigens such as oncofetal antigens, which may appear briefly during normal ontogeny and reappear in oncology. Despite this lack of absolute specifity, such antigens may also prove extremely helpful in diagnosis. The patient with an undifferentiated neoplasm is the ideal candidate for investigation with such a panel of reagents. Recently such an approach was utilized with success by Gatter et al. In 38 cases, using a battery of five immunoperoxidase antibodies, they were able to identify the patients who had lymphoma.[9] The identification of this group has obvious therapeutic implications. Furthermore, algorithms have been formed in order to develop an appropriate step-wise strategy in investigating such patients so that various epithelial malignancies including squamous, small cell, melanoma, and adenocarcinoma subtypes, various different lymphoma subtypes, and various different mesenchynal-derived malignancies are recognized. (see Fig. 22-1).[10]

Biochemical assays used to identify hormone receptors require fresh tissue, but immunoperoxidase reagents developed against estrogen receptors may obviate the need for these specimens. Identification of receptors for estrogen or other hormones can narrow down the likely type of malignancy.[11] The presence of estrogen receptors may indicate adenocarcinoma,[11] glucocorticoid receptors suggest leukemia, lymphoma, or possibly breast carcinoma, and androgen receptors may be positive in prostate carcinoma.[12] Ectopic ACTH, for example, has been demonstrated in a high proportion of cancers of lung origin, even though the presence of such hormones in blood is substantially less common and in the clinical syndrome still less so.[13] There is evidence for abnormal processing of polypeptide hormones in tumor tissues.[14] The proportion of pre-pro ACTH thus is substantially higher in ectopic sites (lung cancer) than in eutopic sites such as in this case, the anterior pituitary. It appears that while the transcription of ectopic hormones in patients with lung cancer would appear to be normal, translational and particularly post translational abnormalities occur which may serve as a basis for distinguishing certain forms of cancer.[15]

Examination of the tumor's genome may be a potential future use of molecular biology technology. Gene rearrangement for immunoglobulin synthesis provides the evidence for differentiation to the B cell before evidence of actual immunoglobulin formation.[16] In addition a number of oncogenes have been described which have been implicated in the pathogenesis of cancers.[17] The types of oncogenes formed in a specific cancer may be helpful in better identifying the lineage of the neoplastic cell.

A closely related area that also is rapidly advancing is cytogenetic technology. There are at least nine forms of human cancer wherein specific chromosome abnormalities have been identified.[18] The first example of this

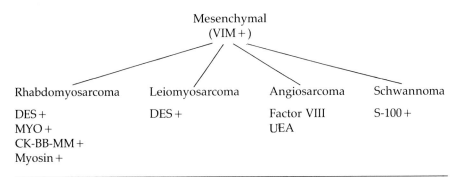

Mesenchymal
(VIM +)

Rhabdomyosarcoma   Leiomyosarcoma   Angiosarcoma   Schwannoma

DES +   DES +   Factor VIII   S-100 +
MYO +   UEA
CK-BB-MM +
Myosin +

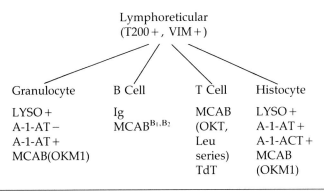

Lymphoreticular
(T200 +, VIM +)

Granulocyte   B Cell   T Cell   Histocyte

LYSO +   Ig   MCAB   LYSO +
A-1-AT −   MCAB[B1,B2]   (OKT,   A-1-AT +
A-1-AT +   Leu   A-1-ACT +
MCAB(OKM1)   series)   MCAB
                                    TdT   (OKM1)

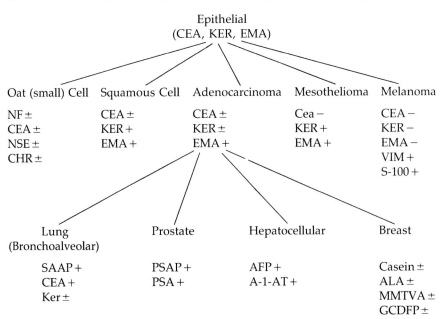

Epithelial
(CEA, KER, EMA)

Oat (small) Cell Squamous Cell Adenocarcinoma Mesothelioma Melanoma

NF ±   CEA ±   CEA ±   Cea −   CEA −
CEA ±   KER +   KER ±   KER +   KER −
NSE ±   EMA +   EMA +   EMA +   EMA −
CHR ±   VIM +
                                                               S-100 +

Lung   Prostate   Hepatocellular   Breast
(Bronchoalveolar)

SAAP +   PSAP +   AFP +   Casein ±
CEA +   PSA +   A-1-AT +   ALA ±
Ker ±   MMTVA ±
                                                              GCDFP ±

was the Ph1 chromosome for chronic myelogenous leukemia. More recently it has been found that 50–60 percent of patients with lymphoma of B cell origin have a specific cytogenetic abnormality involving chromosome 14. Direct air-dry cytogenetic analysis or analysis after short-term culture might allow for specific diagnosis in an undifferentiated neoplasm.

The distinction between hyperplasia might indeed be aided by cytogenetic studies since monoclonality can often be determined by chromosome studies. The sensitivity of banding technology can be increased markedly by the use of methotrexate-thymidine for arresting cells in late prophase and the use of premature chromosome condensation. For example, using the methotrexate-thymidine technique, essentially 100 percent of patients with acute myelogenous leukemia have been found to have chromosome markers, as compared to only 40–50 percent by standard banding techniques.[19] It is highly probable that cytogenetics will play an increasingly significant role in this clinical problem.

Another area of progress has been in tissue culture techniques, including the clonogenic assay which makes it possible to study human solid tumors and hematologic malignancies. In certain circumstances, neoplastic cells in short-term culture may undergo some degree of differentiation or may be induced by "differentiators," including compounds such as DMSO, butyric acid, azacytadine, and cisretinoic acid. The induction of any degree of differentiation, even in a minority of cells, should reveal haplotypic features which may allow for the identification of cell lineage.[20] It should be noted that if clonogenic assays prove useful in predicating treatment response, much of the emphasis on histologic identification may prove obsolete.

Returning to more conventional forms of analysis, electron microscopy

Figure 22-1. *Immunohistochemistry of undifferentiated malignant tumors.*[10] *AFP— alpha-fetoprotein; ALA—alpha-lactalbumin; A-1-ACT—alpha-1-antichymotrypsin; A-1- AT—alpha-1-antitrypsin; CEA—carcinoembryonic antigen; CHR—chromogranin; CK— creatine kinase; DES—desmin; EMA—epithelial membrane antigen; GCDFP—gross cystic disease fluid protein; Ig—immunoglobulin; KER—keratin; LYSO—lysozyme; MCAB— monoclonal antibodies; MMTVA—mouse mammary tumor viral antigen; MYO— myoglobulin; NF—neurofilament; NSE—neuron-specific enolase; PSA—prostate-specific antigen; PSAP—prostate-specific acid phosphatase; PTH—parathyroid hormone; SAAP— surfactant associated apoprotein; TdT—terminal transferase; TGB—thyroglobulin; T200— common leukocyte antigen (other common leukocyte antigens include PD7/26 and 2B11); UEA—ulex europeus agglutinin; and VIM—vimentin. [From personal communication with Drs. DeLellis and Yee, with permission.]*

(EM) can be very useful in patients who present with the problem of an undifferentiated neoplasm. EM can be used to identify evidence of epithelial lineage so that a lymphoma can be excluded. In addition, a number of malignancies have cytoplasmic structures which if recognized can pinpoint the type of cancer. Such cases are melanoma, small cell carcinoma, and endocrine malignancies. In patients with adenocarcinoma of unknown origin there have been studies suggesting that adenocarcinoma can be subdivided employing ultrastructural details.[21,22] Hickey and Seiler were able to separate colon from other adenocarcinomas solely on the basis of EM.[21]

Radiologic Studies

A radiologic search is usually considered in patients with cancer of unknown primary with the aim of determining an occult anatomic primary site. These investigations may subject the patient to many hours of inconvenience and discomfort when employed in a blind approach. In patients who have evidence pointing to a specific abnormality, such as occult blood in the stool or iron deficiency anemia, contrast studies of the gastrointestinal tract are indicated. Similarly, in a patient with flank pain or mass, or hematuria, image studies of the kidney are required. In the absence of such findings, however, ordering these tests by reflex is usually not revealing and can be misleading.[23] Computerized tomography (CT), with its increasing availability, appears to have a role in the search for the unknown primary. CT revealed an occult tumor in a third of cases in one series of patients with this problem.[24] Pancreas was the most common site identified in this study. The role of ultrasound, a less expensive method than CT, appears to be less effective in diagnosing primary sites.[25]

Mammography is usually done in women with adenocarcinoma of unknown primary. In screening programs, 33 percent of the breast carcinomas detected were diagnosed by mammography in women whose breasts were normal by physical examination.[26] In patients with metastatic disease it is less likely that the breasts will be found normal by physical examination. In one series of patients with cancer of unknown primary site, mammography was abnormal in 13 percent of the patients studied.[1] It appears justified and cost effective to obtain mammograms in women with adenocarcinoma of unknown origin, since an abnormal mammogram can sharpen the focus of the diagnostic and therapeutic choices and point toward a relatively responsive neoplasm.

Serum Tumor Markers

Although a number of biologic proteins may be associated with certain cancers, the lack of tumor specificity for many of these substances limit their usefulness in this clinical setting. Abnormalities of tumor markers thus need to be considered in the context of the overall clinical picture and other supporting clinical findings. In patients with an undifferentiated neoplasm, in which the differential diagnosis includes lymphoma and melanoma, an elevated CEA can mitigate against the possibility of melanoma.[27] On the other hand, studies evaluating peripheral blood lymphocytes for clonal excess may substantiate an equivocal morphologic diagnosis of lymphoma.[28-29] Again this area is undergoing rapid change with the production of a number of monoclonal antibodies directed against a specific tumor type. This permits the potential for measuring antibody activity in blood.

In patients with cancer of unknown primary, the combination of an elevated serum tumor marker and a specific radiological abnormality may provide support for identifying an organ as the probable primary site. In a patient with a poorly differentiated carcinoma, a high CEA and abnormal pancreas could support the suspicion of pancreatic carcinoma. More specific tumor markers such as galactosyl transferare II in conjunction with a positive CT scan, ultrasound, or ERCP apparently raises the probability of pancreatic carcinoma.[30] This type of approach may prove to be useful in the future as more clinical experience with these tumor markers is collected.

Treatment Options

Since the search for an unknown primary site of cancer can be fruitless, even at postmortem examination, in as many as 15–30 percent of cases,[1,3,31] there appears to be a limit to the success of investigative plans outlined above. Similar or lower success rates in identifying the specific type of an undifferentiated neoplasm might be expected in many centers. The clinician is therefore forced to make the most reasonable choices for therapy with the available information.

The pattern of metastases may be helpful but also deceptive in formulating a therapeutic strategy. Metastatic spread from tumors of unknown primary may not behave in the usual fashion, such as in the case of pancreatic carcinoma presenting with extensive bone metastases.[31] Consequently, there is no gold standard by which treatment plans can be made, but each individual patient has to be evaluated within the specific clinical context. If a precise diagnosis cannot be reached, therapy should include agents directed against responsive tumors that are possible in the given clinical setting.

Many patients present with lymph node involvement. Patients should be evaluated to see if the adenopathy is regional or generalized. In patients with regional adenopathy, clearly the drainage sites should be examined for a possible primary. The lymph node biopsy should closely be studied to determine cell lineage. The site of involvement can also be very helpful. For example, in patients who present with isolated cervical adenopathy which on biopsy reveals squamous carcinoma, a head and neck examination may be completely negative even if appropriate blind biopsies of the base of the tongue and nasopharynx are performed. Even in the absence of an identifiable primary, treatment for a presumed head and neck tumor should be considered in these patients, since substantial long-term survivorship has been reported with such an approach.[32–35]

In women presenting with isolated axillary adenopathy, investigation should exclude lymphoma and melanoma. Metastatic melanoma in as many as eight percent of cases can present with an unknown primary site.[36] If the patient has an undifferentiated carcinoma, studies should be directed at identifying an occult breast primary. Mammography should be done. Estrogen and progesterone receptor data is important in such patients, and even ultrastructural analysis may prove useful.[37] If necessary, a repeat biopsy should be obtained in order to do these studies. If evidence for breast carcinoma can be established then appropriate treatment can be instituted.

In patients with multiple sites of adenopathy without demonstrable disease outside the lymphatic system and with an undifferentiated neoplasm, aggressive histologic evaluation for a lymphoma should be pursued. Obtaining fresh tissue will permit greater utility of the immunoperoxidase reagents available as well as electron microscopy. If cell lineage remains unclear without evidence of either lymphomatous or epithelial differentiation, the treatment program used should probably include agents effective against lymphoma.

In young patients with multiple sites of disease including the midline structures of the chest and/or abdomen and biopsies revealing undifferentiated carcinoma, an extragonadal germ cell tumor should be suspected. Both serum and tumor should be evaluated for HCG and AFP. Aggressive treatment for this entity has been very encouraging.[38–41]

In women presenting with ascites and cytology revealing malignant cells, an ovarian primary should be considered even if a pelvic mass is undetectable. In this situation, evaluation of the tumor marker CA-125 may prove useful.[40] A laparotomy by a skilled gynecologic surgeon may be needed to answer this question. Debulking surgery followed by combination chemotherapy has recently yielded impressive survival results in advanced ovarian carcinoma.[41-45]

In patients presenting with isolated liver defects suspicious for cancer, a thorough evaluation of the biopsy should be carried out to avoid missing a treatable entity such as islet cell carcinoma. Immunohistochemical studies can prove very useful in this situation. Even if the diagnosis of adenocarcinoma is made, electron microscopy may separate the colon from other potential primary sites. This information could become more important if and when better treatment options become available for certain types of gastrointestinal adenocarcinomas.

Summary

The clinical problem of the patient with an undifferentiated neoplasm or a cancer of unknown primary has been reviewed. Although the focus differs in solving these two separate problems, our emphasis has been on the close examination of the biopsy with the surgical pathologist. Advances in the laboratory have provided the pathologist with an expanding number of tests. This area continues to develop rapidly and we have speculated on the potential use of other methods. After best utilization of the biopsy, the clinical data can be organized around diagnoses that can be potentially curable or effectively palliated. In this fashion, time will not be wasted and the patient's chance for the best outcome will be maximized.

References

1. Didolkar MS, Fanous N, Elias EG, et al: Metastatic carcinomas from primary tumors. Ann Surg 186:625–630, 1977
2. Holmes FF, Fouts TL: Metastatic cancer of unknown primary site, in Ariel IM (ed): Progress in Clinical Cancer, vol. 5. New York, Grune & Stratton, 1973, pp 427–435
3. Krementz ET, Cerise EJ, Foster DS: Metastases of undetermined source. Curr Probl Cancer 4:1–37, 1979
4. Moertel CG, Reitemeir RJ, Schutt AJ, et al: Treatment of the patient with adenocarcinoma of unknown origin. Cancer 30:1469–1479, 1972
5. Stewart JF, Tattersall MHN, Woods RL, et al: Unknown primary

adenocarcinoma: Incidence of overinvestigation and natural history Br Med J 1:1530–1533, 1979

6. Osteen RT, Kopf G, Wilson RE: In pursuit of unknown primary. Am J Surg 135:494–498, 1978

7. Frei E III: National cancer chemotherapy program. Science 217:600–606, 1982

8. DeLellis RA: Advances in Immunohistochemistry. New York, Masson Publishing USA, 1984, pp 1–30

9. Gatter KC, Alcock C, Heryet A, et al: Differential diagnosis of routinely processed anaplastic tumors using monoclonal antibodies. Am J Clin Pathol 82:33–43, 1984

10. DeLellis RA, Yee A: personal communication

11. Kiang DT, Kennedy BJ: Estrogen receptor assay in the different diagnosis of adenocarcinomas. JAMA 238:32–34, 1977

12. Lippman ME: In Levey GS (Ed), Glucocorticoid receptors, hormone-receptor interaction. New York, Marcel Dekker, 1976, pp 221–242

13. Menon M, Tannis CE, McLoughlin MG, et al: Measurement of androgen receptors in human prostate tissue utilizing sucrose density gradient centrifugation and a protamine precipitation assay. J Urol 117:309–312, 1977

14. Odell W, Wolfsen A, Yoshimoto Y, et al: Ectopic peptide synthesis: A universal concomitant of neoplasia. Trans Assn Am Phys 90:204–227, 1977

15. Odel WD, Wolfsen AB, Bachelot I, et al: Ectopic productions of lipoprotein by cancer. Am J Med 66:631–638, 1979

16. Korsmeyer SJ, Hieter PA, Ravetch, et al: Developmental hierarchy of immunoglobulin gene rearrangements in human leukemia pre-B-cells. Proc Natl Acad Sci USA 72:7096–7110, 1981

17. Krontiris T: Emerging genetics of human cancer New Engl J Med 309:404–409, 1983

18. Sandberg AA: Chromosomes of Human Cancer and Leukemia. New York, Elsevier/North Holland, 1980, pp 566–596

19. Yunis JJ, Bloomfield CD, Ensrud K: All patients with acute nonlymphocytic leukemia may have a chromosomal defect. N Engl J Med 305:135–139, 1981

20. Ruddon MW: Cancer Biology. New York, Oxford University Press, 1981, pp 94

21. Hickey WF, Seiler MW: Ultrastructural markers of colonic adenocarcinoma. Cancer 47:140–145, 1981

22. Dvorak AM, Monahan RA: Metastatic adenocarcinoma of unknown primary site. Arch Pathol Lab Med 106:21–24, 1982

23. Nystrom JS, Winer JM, Wolf RM, et al: Identifying the primary site in metastatic cancer of unknown origin. JAMA 241:381–383, 1979

24. Karsell PR, Sheedy PF II, O'Connell, MJ: Computed tomography in search of cancer of unknown origin. JAMA 248:340–343, 1982

25. McMillan JH, Levine E, Stephens RH: Computed tomography in the evaluation of metastatic adenocarcinoma from an unknown primary site. Radiology 143:143–146, 1982

26. Shapiro S: Evidence on screening for breast cancer from a randomized trial. Cancer 39:2772–2782, 1977

27. Koch M, McPherson TA: Carcino-embryonic antigen levels as an indicator of the primary site in metastatic disease of unknown origin. Cancer 48:1242–1244, 1981

28. Ault KA: Detection of small numbers of monoclonal B lymphocytes in the blood of patients with lymphoma. N Engl J Med 300:1401–1405, 1979

29. Smith B, Robert NJ, et al: Circulating monoclonal B lymphocytes in non-Hodgkin's lymphoma. N Engl J Med 311:1476–1481, 1984

30. Podolsky DK, McPhee MS, Alpert E et al: Galactosyltransferase isoenzyme II in the detection of pancreatic cancer: Comparison with radiologic, endoscopic and serologic tests. N Engl J Med 304:1313–1318, 1981

31. Nystrom JS, Weiner JM, Heffelfinger-Juttner J, et al: Metastatic and histologic presentations in unknown primary cancer. Sem Oncol 4:53–58, 1977

32. Jesse RH, Perez CA, Fletcher GH: Cervical lymph node metastasis: Unknown primary cancer. Cancer 31:854–859, 1973

33. Coker DD, Casterline PF, Chambers RG, et al: Metastases to lymph nodes of the head and neck from an unknown primary site. Am J Surg 134:517–522, 1977

34. Nordstrom DG, Tewfik HH, Latourette HB: Cervical lymph node metastases from an unknown primary. Int J Rad Onco Biol Phys 5:73–76, 1979

35. Leipzig B, Winter ML, Hokanson JA: Cervical nodal metastases of unknown origin. Laryngosope 91:593–598, 1981

36. Templer J, Perry M, Davis WE: Metastatic cervical adenocarcinoma from unknown primary tumor. Arch Otolarynyol 107:45–47, 1981

37. Lopez R, Holyoke E, Moore RH, et al: Malignant melanoma with unknown primary site. J Surg Onc 19:151–154, 1982

37. Iglehart JD, Ferguson BJ, Shingleton WW, et al: Ultrastructural analysis of breast carcinoma presenting as isolated axillary adenopathy. Am Surg 196:8–13, 1982

38. Muro AJ, Duncan W, Webb JN: Extragonadal presentation of germ cell tumors. Brit J Uro 55:547–554, 1983
39. Hainsworth JD, Einhorn LH, Williams SD, et al: Advanced extragonadal germ-cell tumors. Successful treatment with combination chemotherapy. Am Int Med 97:7–11, 1982
40. Richardson RL, Schoumacher RA, Fer MF, et al: Unrecognized extragonadal germ cell cancer syndrome. Ann Intern Med 94:181–186, 1981
41. Fox RM, Woods RL, Tattersall M: Undifferentiated carcinoma in young men: The atypical teratoma syndrome. Lancet 2:1316–1318, 1979
42. Bast RC, Klug TL, St. John E, et al: Radioimmunoassay using a monoclonal antibody to monitor the course of epithelial ovarian cancer. N Engl J Med 309:883–887, 1983
43. Griffiths CT, Parker LM, Fuller AF: Role of cytoreductive surgical treatment in the management of advanced cancer. Cancer Treat Rep 63:241–247, 1979
44. Young RC, Chabner BA, Hubbard SM, et al: Advanced ovarian adenocarcinoma: A prospective clinical trial of melphalan (L-PAM) versus combination chemotherapy. N Engl J Med 299:1261–1266, 1978
45. Greco FA, Julian CG, Richardson RL, et al: Advanced ovarian carcinoma: Brief intensive combination chemotherapy and second look operation. Obstet Gynecol 58:199–205, 1981

INDEX

Head and neck tumors
  cervical node metastases from, 104, 106
  hormone receptors in, 486, 494
Hemangiopericytoma, electron
      microscopy of, 236
Hepatic tumors. *See* Liver
Hepatomegaly, in metastatic
      adenocarcinoma, 123
Hexokinase as tumor marker, 90
Histaminase as tumor marker, 36, 89
Histiocytic lymphomas in childhood, 363
Histiocytoma, malignant fibrous, 248
  electron microscopy of, 236
  myxoid, 255
  pleomorphic, 254
  thymidine labeling index for, 523
  tumor markers in, 240
Histiocytosis X, electron microscopy of, 49
Histochemistry, 12–13, 544
HLA-DR antigen, in small round cell
      malignancies of childhood, 364
Hodgkin's disease, estrogen receptors in,
      494
Homovanillic acid excretion, in
      neuroblastoma, 347
Hormone receptors, 479–495
  analysis and interpretation of, 481–484
  assay methods for, 482
  in breast cancer, 479–480, 485, 488, 490
  in cystosarcoma phyllodes, 493
  in fibroadenoma, 493
  identification of, 545
  in lymphomas, 495
  nature of, 480–481
  problems with sampling of, 484
  therapy affecting, 484–485
Hormone tumor markers, 36, 83–85
  in lung cancer, 279–280
Hybridoma-produced monoclonal
      antibodies, 17
Hydatidiform mole, lactic dehydrogenase-
      Z in, 90
Hypercalcemia, in lung cancer, 278

Immunoblastic lymphomas, large cell, in
      childhood, 362–363
Immunocytochemistry, 6, 13–21
  in adenocarcinoma, 128
  avidin-biotin technique in, 15

commercial antisera in, 35
in endocrine tumors, 21–23
in genitourinary tumors, 23–26
immunofluorescence methods in, 13–14
lectins in, 18–19
in leukemias, 303
in lung cancer, 280
in lymphomas, 26–30
monoclonal antibodies in. *See*
      Monoclonal antibody studies
neuron-specific enolase in, 23, 36
in sarcomas, 238–246
selection of procedures in, 20–21
staphylococcal protein A in, 15
tumor markers in, 30–38
tissue preparation for, 422–425
unconjugated techniques in, 14–15
Immunofluorescence studies, 13–14
  double-labeling techniques in, 18
Immunoglobulins
  gene rearrangements in tumors,
      506–510, 545
  in lymphomas, 318
  as tumor markers, 37
Immunoperoxidase staining procedures,
      14–15, 20, 401, 423–425, 544–545
Incidence of undifferentiated tumors, 154
Inguinal lymph node metastases, 109–110,
      116, 117
  epidermoid or undifferentiated
      carcinoma in, 155, 169
  melanoma in, 178
Insulin production, by pancreatic tumors,
      23, 36
Insulinoma, neuron-specific enolase in, 91
Intermediate filaments, in tumor
      diagnosis, 31–33
Intestinal cancer
  in colon. *See* Colon cancer
  small cell carcinoma, 328–330

Kaposi's sarcoma
  progesterone receptors in, 492
  tumor markers in, 240–242
Karyotypes. *See* Chromosome analysis
Keratin
  in intermediate filaments, 31, 32
  as tumor marker, 37